THE TREATMENT

OF

DIABETES MELLITUS

WITH OBSERVATIONS BASED UPON
THREE THOUSAND CASES

BY

ELLIOTT P. JOSLIN, M.D. (HARVARD), M.A. (YALE)

CLINICAL PROFESSOR OF MEDICINE, HARVARD MEDICAL SCHOOL; CONSULTING PHYSICIAN
BOSTON CITY HOSPITAL; PHYSICIAN TO NEW ENGLAND DEACONESS HOSPITAL.

THIRD EDITION, ENLARGED, REVISED AND REWRITTEN

ILLUSTRATED

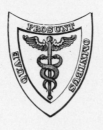

LEA & FEBIGER
PHILADELPHIA AND NEW YORK

PRINTED IN U. S. A.

TO

BANTING AND BEST

AND THE

TORONTO GROUP OF INSULIN WORKERS

PREFACE TO THE THIRD EDITION.

In the early months of the century Naunyn taught me with Case No. 8 that his methods enabled a diabetic of sixty years to live out the full expectation of life. In 1914 Allen's development of Guelpa's crude theories of undernutrition, together with insistence upon the patient's use of the Benedict test and of food scales, increased the average diabetic's outlook by two years. The courage of Newburgh and Marsh and of Petrén in giving a high-fat diet, empirically protected by low protein, and the scientific balancing by Shaffer and Woodyatt of the ketogenic antiketogenic food factors are adding another two years. Compared with the last decade the doctor now has twice as many diabetics to treat.

Today the men who have achieved progress in diabetes form a larger group than ever before in the history of the world. These contemporaries, and I omit the youngest, it has been my good fortune to know personally—the clinicians, Allen, Falta, Geyelin, Minkowski, Magnus Levy, Naunyn, Newburgh, von Noorden, Wilder, Williams and Woodyatt; the chemists, S. R. Benedict, Bloor, Folin, Shaffer and Van Slyke; the physiologists and metabolists, F. G. Benedict, Boothby, DuBois, Lusk and Macleod; the pathologist, Opie—and to have had for teachers, R. H. Chittenden and R. H. Fitz. All these are still alert with the exception of the last, and even he lives in his son. With such trained minds interested in diabetes the time was ripe for new discoveries. Yet, can the reader imagine the feelings of a doctor with a background of 1000 fatal cases, who has lived to see what the ages have longed for come true in the discovery of insulin by F. G. Banting with the help of his student friend, C. H. Best. I feel so sorry that Pavy is not here; he was such a fine Cyrano. And as for Bouchardat, Cantani, Külz, Lépine and all the other diabetic saints, how they would have enjoyed this year!

Insulin does not cure diabetes, but it is a priceless gift to the severe diabetic provided he be intelligent and faithful. Whereas formerly 10 per cent of all diabetics seen in a year died the same year, the mortality has now fallen to 6.7 per cent of my 293 patients treated with insulin. This drop is the more striking because this group excluded more than half of the patients seen, patients believed

(v)

too mild to need insulin.   Of the 48 children cared for in this period 46 remain alive, and the 2 deaths were accidental.

Who wants a vacation when he can watch mere ghosts of children start to grow, play and make a noise and see their mothers smile again, and read in the paper that his young colonel with the Victoria Cross after ten years of faithful dieting has nearly won the local golf championship.

Yet insulin is in its infancy.   New possibilities still continue to unfold.   One accomplishes in hours what formerly took days.   A widow with four children appears for the first time with one day free for treatment before vacation ends and work begins.   She comes to the hospital in the morning with 5 per cent sugar, is given insulin hourly with simultaneous urinary tests, is sugar-free at 3 P.M., on a full diet at 5 P.M., returns home at 7 P.M., fills her position the next day, and in a week reports still sugar-free. She is a type of other cases similarly treated.   The most recent of these administered her own treatment and Dr. Sisco made her do her own analyses that she might the better understand the process she was going through.   Such treatment is only safe when the family doctor coöperates and guarantees the intelligence of the patient.

The unit of insulin is changing as this book goes to press.   It is hoped that the new unit will shortly be accepted as the international unit.   Five of the new units equal seven of the old which have hitherto been employed in the United States.   It would be most unfortunate if patients transferred from the weaker to the stronger unit without allowance for its increased strength.   One should strive to lower rather than to raise the dose of insulin.

Next to the real pleasure of mixing the best dietetic ideas of clinicians like those mentioned with Banting's and Best's insulin, there has developed a keen though undramatic ambition to prevent diabetes in families or groups predisposed to the disease.   A patient confides that her fat husband lost 10 pounds in the ten days during which she was learning to get rid of and stay rid of her own 9 per cent sugar—simply because he was held up to the class as a promising candidate for conjugal diabetes.

A new and purer diabetes is described in this book.   It is a diabetes largely free from many of the complications which crowd and confuse the older monographs.   There are but 2 cases of alcoholism; only 1.6 per cent of the patients have had syphilis, but 6 per cent of the fatal cases have died of tuberculosis.   Notwithstanding these facts, the hospital treatment of diabetes today is largely devoted to the complications of diabetes rather than to the disease itself.   October 16, 1923, found 14 surgical diabetics on the service.

The greatest changes, among the thorough recasting of the book, may be worth a note. The insulin section is obviously new, and partly for that reason, partly for convenience, and partly because of its importance is placed first; the table of contents outlines its major parts, while its diffusion throughout the book may be traced by the index. New also are the sections on pathology, respiratory metabolism, levulose, duodenal ulcer, diabetes of twenty years' duration, the Newburgh and Marsh methods, and the modern conceptions of acidosis. Dr. E. M. Bailey's tables of diabetic and non-diabetic foods have no counterpart. They represent a gift from the Connecticut Agricultural Experimental Station in New Haven. The Harris and Benedict tables for predicting the metabolism are added and are so clear that he who runs may read. The technic of treatment with the diabetic creed and the Test and Maintenance diets are the outgrowth of the War which forced simplicity of management and the conviction that the hope for the diabetic lies in the general practitioner's adoption of the principles of diet. Last spring I was tempted to resume alkalis, but resisted the impulse, and have the satisfaction of recording Case No. 3382 on page 564, who recovered from coma without them. Surgery is entirely rewritten because diabetes is so often a surgical problem, more than one-fifth of all Boston diabetics dying of gangrene.

Gaps in our knowledge are plainly indicated even to the most casual reader with the hope they will be filled. Many represent enticing problems for patient, investigative medical students or general practitioners, whereas the errors and the frank beliefs, expressed occasionally with design, may stimulate others to confirm or confound.

Foreign nations have much to teach us. French books upon diabetes are rare. Hence I am glad to call attention to Labbé's book on *Diabetes Mellitus*, which has been translated by Cumston; it is rich in the discussion of symptoms and complications. Petrén's book is, unfortunately for most of us, in the Scandinavian language, but scattered through this text will be found abstracts of it, made possible through the assistance of Prof. Hilding Berglund.

So many have helped me with this book there is hardly space to mention their names. I am the debtor of all those cited in the text. The Carnegie Institution of Washington has allowed me to draw at will from my monograph on "Diabetic Metabolism with High and Low diets," just issued as Publication No. 323, and the same liberality has been granted by the *Journal of Metabolic Research*. The paragraphs or sentences in whole or in part taken from my Shattuck Lecture, which appeared in the *Boston Medical and Surgical Journal*, from two articles—one on "The Prevention of Diabetes" and the other on "The Causes of Death in Diabetes"—published in the *Journal of the American Medical Association*, and from material originally written for the Christian and Mackenzie *Loose Leaf Medicine*, I have endeavored to indicate in the text. Prof. Mallory helped me with the section upon the pathology of the pancreas and gave me the photographs, which do not do him justice because not reproduced in colors. Would that it were possible to thank individually all who have worked in the common cause in the clinic at the New England Deaconess Hospital, whether as assistants, secretaries, nurses, technicians, or last but not least patients. Many of their names appear here and there through the book.

The privilege of recording results with insulin is obviously the chief delight in writing this new edition. For this I am indebted to the courtesy of the Insulin Committee of Toronto and through their intervention to the Eli Lilly Company, well exemplified in the spirit of that insulin missionary, G. H. A. Clowes, who has ceaselessly wandered up and down the length and breadth of this land, untiring in his endeavor to be useful to all.

And as for my publishers, again I sincerely thank them for the courtesies shown from first to last, which only one, who has put together a book in betwixt compelling duties, can appreciate.

E. P. J.

Boston, November, 1923.

CONTENTS.

SECTION I.

Details to be Found in Index, p. 769.

INSULIN.

SECTION II.

THEORY, ETIOLOGY, INCIDENCE AND CURABILITY.

SECTION III.

PHYSIOLOGY AND PATHOLOGY.

SECTION IV.

THE EXAMINATION OF THE URINE, BLOOD AND RESPIRATION IN DIABETES.

SECTION V.

THE DIET IN HEALTH AND IN DIABETES.

SECTION VI.

TREATMENT.

SECTION VII.

THE MANAGEMENT OF THE DIABETIC IN OFFICE AND HOSPITAL.

SECTION VIII.

FOODS AND THEIR COMPOSITION.

SECTION IX.

HEIGHT WEIGHT SCALES, EQUIVALENTS AND TABLES FOR COMPUTING METABOLISM

TREATMENT OF DIABETES MELLITUS.

SECTION I.

INSULIN.

A. BANTING'S AND BEST'S DISCOVERY OF INSULIN AND THE EARLY WORK OF THE TORONTO SCHOOL.

F. G. BANTING, a young, orthopedic surgeon with zeal for research, undampened by four years' service at the front, discovered insulin, the hormone of the pancreas, which regulates carbohydrate metabolism. He received the assistance of his friend, C. H. Best, who, although a second-year medical school student, was trained in physiological research. Thus, just a generation elapsed since that other epoch-making discovery in diabetes by von Mering and Minkowski was announced, when they proved that fatal diabetes would follow complete removal of the same gland.

1. **Banting's Conception of a Method for the Extraction of the Pure Secretion of the Islands of Langerhans.**—Banting and Best write: "The hypothesis underlying this series of experiments was first formulated by one of us in November, 1920, while reading an article[1] dealing with the relation of the isles of Langerhans to diabetes. From the passage in this article, which gives a résumé of degenerative changes in the acini of the pancreas, following ligation of the ducts, the idea presented itself that since the acinous, but not the islet tissue, degenerates after this operation, advantage might be taken of this fact to prepare an active extract of islet tissue. The subsidiary hypothesis was that trypsinogen or its derivatives was antagonistic to the internal secretion of the gland. The failures of other investigators in this much-worked field were thus accounted for.

"The feasibility of the hypothesis having been recognized by Prof. J. J. R. Macleod, work was begun under his direction in May, 1921, in the Physiological Laboratory of the University of

2   (17)

Toronto.[2] Help was also generously rendered by Professsors Henderson, Fitzgerald, Graham, and Defries."

2. **The Preparation of the Original Extract and the Results Obtained.**—Using a chilled mortar, containing Ringer's solution, Banting macerated the half frozen gland of a dog whose pancreatic duct had been ligated weeks before and employed the filtrate in intravenous injections. On July 30, 1921, 4 cc of the extract of degenerated pancreas were injected intravenously into a partially depancreatized dog. Before the injection the blood sugar was 0.2 per cent; an hour later the blood sugar had fallen to 0.12 per cent; still an hour later 20 grams of glucose in 200 cc of water were given by stomach tube, and the animal excreted 0.2 gram of sugar in the following five hours in contrast to an excretion of 16 grams in the same interval after an intake of 25 grams of glucose, when no extract was administered. These results were confirmed, and it was demonstrated that the extract invariably exercised a reducing influence upon the percentage of sugar in the blood and the amount of sugar excreted in the urine, and that the extent and duration of the reduction varied directly with the amount of extract injected.

In other experiments Banting and Best proved that an extract of the whole gland would reduce the blood sugar, but much less actively than extract obtained from the gland atrophied by ligation of the pancreatic duct, that by boiling the extract was rendered inert, was destroyed by external pancreatic juice, and was ineffective if administered by rectum. When the pancreatic juice was exhausted by secretin and stimulation of the vagus below the diaphragm, an extract of the whole gland produced a definite effect, but it was accompanied by toxic symptoms, which were absent after injections of extracts from completely degenerated glands. An extract made with 0.1 per cent hydrochloric acid was also effectual in lowering the blood sugar. The therapeutic usefulness of the extract was demonstrated when it was shown that an extract prepared in neutral saline and kept in cold storage retained its potency for at least seven days.

3. **Fetal Calf Pancreas, a Source of Insulin.**—A new era was introduced in the investigation in November, 1921, by the utilization of the discovery that fetal calf pancreas of under five months' development did not contain digestive pancreatic juice, but did possess an internal secretion. Laguesse[3] had found in 1893, that the islands of Langerhans were comparatively more plentiful in the fetus and new-born than in the adult animal and suspected that they produced an internal secretion, though he made no mention of a possible relation between this hypothetical secretion and diabetes. Eighteen years later he reported[4] that in 2 rabbits three to four years after resection of the duct pancreatic tissue was lacking save for islands of Langerhans, and to these he ascribed

the prevention of diabetes. Ibrahim[5] had observed that proteolytic enzymes were absent from the pancreas of the fetus of under four months' development. Banting and Best, therefore, prepared a fetal calf extract by macerating the glands in Ringer's solution and filtering until a clear solution was obtained. This solution reduced the percentage of blood sugar in a 10 kilogram dog from 0.4 per cent to 0.15 per cent in three hours.[6] The percentage of blood sugar in another diabetic dog was reduced from 0.3 per cent to normal and the urine became sugar-free. In this way Banting and Best were able to obtain large quantities of the internal secretion of the gland and to avoid the destructive influence of the trypsinogen of the pancreative juice. When the extract was given subcutaneously, instead of intravenously, they found its action was slower and more prolonged, but not less effective.

4. **Beef Pancreas, A Source of Insulin.**—A Preparation for Clinical Use.—Two notable discoveries were then made in the preparation of the extract: (1) That antisepsis with 0.7 per cent tricresol did not sacrifice potency, whereas passing it through a Berkfeldt filter did, and (2) that the active principle was extractable with 95 per cent alcohol. This led to a successful attempt to secure the active principle from the whole gland. The method adopted was to mince the adult beef pancreas with an equal volume of 95 per cent alcohol acidified by the addition of 0.2 per cent hydrochloric acid. Fat was removed by washing twice with toluene and the alcohol removed by vacuum distillation at a low temperature, and the residue evaporated to one-fifth volume. The aqueous extract thus obtained was sterilized by filtering through a Berkfeldt filter. Sterile abscesses sometimes occurred owing to the presence of protein in the extract. Further purification for use in the first clinical cases at Toronto was made through the help of J. B. Collip.[7] To a small volume of 95 per cent ethyl alcohol freshly minced pancreas was added in equal amount. Eventually the mixture was strained and the filtrate treated with alcohol. The protein was thus largely removed and the active principle remained in solution. His method depends upon the fractional precipitation of the extract with alcohol. Later the lipoids were removed with ether and again the filtrate was distilled *in vacuo* to a pasty consistency. "Addition of 80 per cent alcohol and centrifugation then resulted in the formation of four layers, namely, a bottom layer of salt crystals, above it a saturated aqueous solution of salt, above this a flocculent layer of protein, and on top a clear layer of alcohol containing the entire active principle in solution. Extracts were prepared which were practically free from proteins, salts and alcohol-soluble substances. These could be made isotonic and injected subcutaneously without local reactions."[8]

The extract of the active principle obtained from the whole gland by this method was prepared in powder form, kept sterile, and in doses of 50 mg. dissolved in saline, gave a pronounced effect on the blood sugar.

By mouth, the extract lowered the blood sugar very slightly; *e. g.*, upon one occasion from 0.41 per cent to 0.28 per cent in four hours. Intravenous administration of the same extract made the blood sugar drop from 0.28 per cent to 0.11 per cent in three hours. Subcutaneous injection reduced the percentage of blood sugar in a diabetic dog from 0.35 per cent to 0.08 per cent in three hours and rendered the urine sugar-free.

5. **Standardization of Insulin.—The Unit.**—The standardization of insulin was essential for its practical application and it was found that the extracts could be tested with rabbits. In this investigation the previous investigators were joined by E. C. Noble. The average percentage of blood sugar in over 150 normal rabbits fed on oats was 0.133 per cent with a maximum of 0.186 per cent and a minimum of 0.095 per cent by the Shaffer-Hartman method.[9] Within an hour after an injection of insulin into a rabbit the blood sugar decreases and if sufficient insulin is employed, convulsions, coma, death ensue. The amount of insulin necessary to reduce the blood sugar of a 1 kilogram rabbit, starved about twenty hours, to 0.045 per cent or to produce convulsions within three hours is considered to be 1 unit of insulin. A new international unit has just been adopted by the Health Section of the League of Nations. It represents one-third the quantity of insulin required to lower the blood sugar of a 2-kilogram rabbit to the convulsive level, 0.045 per cent. A stable standard unit of reference is now being prepared by the Insulin Committee of Toronto. By November, 1923, all insulin will be sold on this basis. Five units of the new insulin will equal about 7 units of the old.

Characteristic symptoms, following the injection of insulin into rabbits, appear when the blood sugar reaches 0.045 per cent and hence this point was chosen for the standardization of the unit. A preliminary period of hyperexcitability ushers in the reaction to the injection of insulin. This gives place to a comatose condition in which the animal breathes rapidly, often periodically, and has sluggish conjunctival reflexes and widely dilated pupils. On the slightest stimulation violent clonic convulsions supervene, which last for one to two minutes, often recur without any apparent stimulation at intervals of about fifteen minutes, and frequently lead to death from respiratory failure. The maximum percentage of blood sugar in which these convulsions occurred in rabbits was 0.047 per cent, save in 1 of the 26 animals observed in which it was 0.067 per cent. The minimum percentage which was reached without development of convulsions was 0.037 per cent. Subcutaneous injections of glucose, 1 gram per kilogram body weight, restored the animal to normal condition within a few minutes.

Hypoglycemia appears a plausible mechanism underlying these symptoms, especially because of the observations of F. C. Mann[10] on dogs made hypoglycemic by the removal of the liver. He found that such dogs were promptly revived when they were given injections of glucose. No other sugar had the same effect as glucose, although temporary alleviation of the symptoms has sometimes been observed after injections of galactose and levulose. Injections of pentose or of salt solution had no effect. Rarely, recovery was possible without injections.

"Not only is the blood sugar lowered in rabbits that are normal but also in those rendered diabetic by any of the experimental methods usually employed to bring this about. These are puncture of the floor of the fourth ventricle (piqûre), asphyxia, poisoning by carbon monoxide gas, ether, or adrenalin. None of these causes hyperglycemia in rabbits after injecting them with sufficient amounts of pancreatic extract. There may occasionally be a slight increase in the percentage of blood sugar but never to anything like the extent usually observed without extract. The animals used for these experiments were always well fed with carbohydrates and the glycogen content of the liver determined. The importance of this result is that it shows us that even the purely experimental forms of diabetes have much in common with the clinical forms."[11]

6. **Glycogen and Fat.**—The sugar in the blood, the glycogen in the liver, and to a lesser extent the respiratory quotient, serve to register the extent of carbohydrate metabolism in the body. In the preceding sections it has been shown that the percentage of sugar in the blood invariably decreases after the administration of insulin. Insulin is also a potent factor in the storage of glycogen. With animals this can be proven by examination of the liver after death, but in man recourse must be had during life to indirect means, such as may be furnished by changes in the respiratory quotient.

Following total extirpation of the pancreas Minkowski found that the glycogen in the liver of dogs decreased from the normal, which is 1 to 10 per cent, to 0.5 per cent. This was not increased by the administration of carbohydrate, save when levulose was given, when the quantity of glycogen deposited in the liver varied from 0.72 to 8.14 per cent. Cruickshank[12] believed that even levulose would not form glycogen provided extirpation of the pancreas was actually complete. Banting and Best likewise fed depancreatized dogs for several days preceding death with large quantities of sucrose and found that the glycogen in the liver of two such animals

varied between 0.06 per cent and 1.32 per cent. When insulin
and sucrose were given by Banting and Best to three totally depancreatized dogs they observed that the quantities of glycogen in the
liver varied between 4 per cent and 13 per cent and as reported
later by Macleod to 20 per cent. It would appear, therefore,
from these striking differences in depancreatized animals fed with
sugar, with and without insulin, that the insulin stimulates the
glycogenetic function of the liver. With large doses of insulin
the glycogen of the liver is usually reduced, as is that of the muscles
(M'Cormack and O'Brien, and Dale and Dudley), and it is conceivable that the glycogen of the muscles is called upon first for
body needs, as suggested by Macleod in a lecture before the recent
Physiological Congress in Edinburgh.

In contrast to the lowered percentage of glycogen in the liver
of depancreatized animals is the increased percentage of glycogen
in the heart of the depancreatized dogs as compared with the normal
animal. The quantity of glycogen in the heart of 6 normal dogs
was found by Cruickshank[12] to average 0.5 per cent, but in 16
depancreatized dogs the average was 0.7 per cent. During starvation Macleod and Prendergast[13] found the glycogen in the ventricle
to be increased, amounting in 2 normal dogs to 1.03 per cent. In
the present investigations of the Toronto School the glycogen in
the heart muscle of depancreatized dogs fed sucrose was found to
vary between 0.79 and 0.98 per cent, but in the hearts of 4 other
depancreatized animals to whom insulin as well as sucrose was given
the values for glycogen were 0.725, 0.6, 0.57, 0.296 per cent. These
few observations, therefore, would indicate that insulin decreases
the glycogen in the heart of diabetic animals to within normal
limits, just as it raises the glycogen in the liver of depancreatized
animals likewise to normal limits.[14]

The metabolism of fat is so intimately connected with the metabolism of carbohydrate and the supposed antagonism between the
simultaneous deposition of fat and carbohydrate in the liver has
appeared to be so well grounded that the effect of insulin upon
the deposition of fat, particularly in the liver but also in the heart
and blood, is of especial interest. The normal quantity of fat
in the liver of normal laboratory animals is about 5 per cent. In
the Toronto experiments large quantities of sucrose were fed to 3
depancreatized dogs and the per cent of fat in the liver determined
as fatty acid varied between 10 and 14 per cent.

When 3 similarly depancreatized dogs were given insulin and
sugar, the percentages of fat were lessened, and varied between
2 per cent and 7 per cent. The total fatty acids in the heart
showed far less change between the treated and untreated animals,
but the total fatty acids in the blood of 3 depancreatized animals

decreased from 1.2 per cent to 0.27 per cent and 0.53 per cent. In 2 dogs, however, the fat in the liver was not found to be reduced following insulin. Even after large doses of insulin these dogs died, and in 1, 10.3 per cent and in the other 26.4 per cent of fatty acid were found in the liver.

The observations above recorded demonstrate that insulin given to sugar-fed diabetic animals causes the fat to become reduced in the liver at the same time as glycogen accumulates, and that, contrary to the supposed antagonism between glycogen and fat in the liver, a stage exists following the administration of insulin when both are present in considerable per cent. Since the extract acted but slightly when an animal was anesthetized, it appears reasonable to suspect that the glycogenetic function of the liver is in some way involved, as it is known that glycogen is not built up during anesthesia.

7. Insulin, the Consumption of Sugar, and the Respiratory Quotient.—In this connection may be mentioned experiments by Hepburn and Latchford[15] upon the rate of consumption of sugar by the isolated mammalian heart. When the rabbit's heart is excised and perfused with 0.2 per cent glucose the rate of disappearance of the sugar is 0.8 mg. per gram of heart per hour, but when insulin was added to the perfusing fluid, the average rate of disappearance of glucose was over 3 mg. per hour. It would thus appear that the action of the insulin was related to the tissues rather than to the blood alone. It has not yet been determined whether this more rapid disappearance of glucose with insulin was due to its increased combustion, or to its deposition as glycogen. It is therefore uncertain whether this experiment should be taken as an index of the action of insulin in general.

As yet, no experiments *in vitro* with insulin have been successful, and the Toronto School has been unable to demonstrate that the addition of insulin will hasten the disappearance of glucose from incubated extracts of muscle. No experiments appear to have been made to determine whether perfusing the liver with insulin immediately after death of the animal will prevent the customary disappearance of glycogen from that organ.

That the respiratory quotient of depancreatized animals would rise after the administration of insulin might easily be predicted from what has been recorded in the preceding paragraphs. In their depancreatized animals the previous writers with Hepburn found the respiratory quotients varied between 0.68 and 0.74, but when these same animals were treated with insulin and sucrose, the quotients rose to 0.85 and 0.94. In one animal after depancreatization the respiratory quotient was 0.63, and rose to 0.77 an hour and a half after the ingestion of 20 grams of sucrose. Seventy-four hours after the operation this same dog was given 25 grams of sucrose by mouth and 10 cc of insulin subcutaneously. In thirty-one minutes the quotient had risen to 0.86, and in an hour and a half to 0.9. The animal was again given 20 grams of sucrose and 8 cc of insulin and the respiratory quotient rose within fifty minutes to 0.91 and in one hour and thirty-seven minutes to 0.94. On the next morning the quotient had fallen to 0.68 but with 20 grams sucrose alone rose to 0.82 and 0.85. On the next day with a similar quantity of sucrose it rose from a basal level of 0.7 to 0.81 in one hour and after the injection of 10 cc of insulin to 0.9.

Since glycogen is stored in the liver of depancreatized dogs, following the administration of carbohydrate and insulin, and since the respiratory quotient under the same conditions will rise markedly, it is therefore evident that the beginning and end of carbohydrate metabolism is dependent upon insulin.

8. **Insulin and Acidosis.**—The effect of insulin upon the production and excretion of ketone bodies was also determined in 3 depancreatized dogs. Following the administration of insulin the excretion of acetone bodies was reduced to zero. In 1 of these dogs without insulin the acetone bodies in the urine amounted to 100 and 187 mg. daily for two days. Following a single injection of insulin the acetone bodies disappeared from the urine for the next three days. After this they gradually increased rising to 34, 55 and 114 mg. on three successive days to be removed a second time by another injection of insulin.

The length of life of a depancreatized dog is approximately fourteen days. Banting and Best were able to prolong the life of such animals for notable periods. One such dog lived nineteen days, a second twenty-one days, and a third was chloroformed at the end of seventy days. This animal at autopsy showed a complete depancreatization, save that in the submucous layer of the intestine there was found a nodule of pancreatic tissue about 2 mm. in diameter. On serial section this showed acinar tissue and no islands.

Insulin is a hormone which is capable of lowering the sugar in the blood and storing carbohydrate in the form of glycogen, allowing oxidation to take place as shown by a rise in the respiratory quotient. Secondary phenomena dependent upon carbohydrate combustion take their course in diabetic animals and man treated with insulin as is the case in health. Thus, fat is burned and ketone bodies banished from the urine. The hyperglycemia and glycosuria which can be produced by various well-known experimental procedures is prevented by insulin. The only exception to this statement is that when very large doses of adrenalin are given there appears to be an antagonism between insulin and adrenalin and it is possible adrenalin may serve as a means of standardization of insulin.* Cannon, McIver and Bliss[22] noted that as the blood sugar is reduced by the injection of 10 units of insulin in the cat there occurred an increased production of adrenalin—a new factor of safety for the maintenance of the physiological percentage of blood sugar.

9. **The First Therapeutic Tests of Insulin with Human Diabetics.**—The striking results attained with insulin in depancreatized dogs led to the test of its efficacy in patients with diabetes. Such an experiment was justifiable because of the knowledge acquired with animals. Despite all these carefully acquired data, Banting took no chances and injected the first dose of insulin into himself and only after that did he begin the treatment of a diabetic boy. It is not generally known that of the first 7 injections given a diabetic patient 6 resulted in abscesses. But these investigators were undaunted, overcame temporary difficulties, and had the satisfaction of seeing their efforts with human beings as successful as those with animals.

The use of the extract with human diabetics was begun with the coöperation of W. R. Campbell and A. A. Fletcher at the Toronto General Hospital in the clinic of Duncan Graham. The date of the injection of the first extract into a human case by Banting and Best was on January 10, 1922.[16]

By February 22, 1922, the Toronto investigators reported that: "The effects of these preparations have been observed in 7 cases of diabetes mellitus and it is now evident that certain definite results can be obtained by their administration. The effects observed in depancreatized animals have been paralleled in man. The fall in blood sugar occurs and in 2 cases, repeatedly examined, a rise in the respiratory quotient, indicating carbohydrate utilization, occurs more or less coincidently with the attainment of a normal blood-sugar level. Patients report a complete relief from the subjective symptoms of the disease. The sugar excretion shows marked decrease, or if dosage be adequate, disappears. Ketonuria is abolished. These results taken together have been such as to leave no doubt that in these extracts we have a therapeutic measure of unquestionable value in the treatment of certain phases of the disease in man. In agreement with observations of other investigators on laboratory animals, it has been found that without careful control severe toxic reactions may be encountered and this will undoubtedly be a factor in the evaluation of the ultimate therapeutic utility of the method."[11]

---

* If a subcutaneous injection of pituitary extract is given along with insulin, the fall in blood sugar usually produced by insulin is reduced, abolished or replaced by a rise. Burn: Jour. Phys., March 21, 1923, **57,** 38.

It can be said that when insulin is administered subcutaneously in adequate dosage it is capable within a remarkably short time of removing the cardinal symptoms of diabetes for a period of several hours. Treatment must be repeated at frequent intervals and so far time has not elapsed to show whether a cure of the disease can be brought about. Even should this not be the case, it is well to remember that in a somewhat analogous disease, myxedema, the first patient given thyroid by Murray in 1891 died in 1919, aged seventy-four years, from heart disease.[17] [18]

In certain of the bony fishes the islet tissue is collected into nodules separated from the zymogenous tissue and in the Lophius, angler fish, the principal islet may attain the size of the adrenal of the rabbit. Extracts made from the principle islets of both angler fish and sculpins by Macleod[19] lowered the blood sugar of a rabbit from 0.098 per cent to 0.046 per cent in one hour, and in another experiment to 0.01 per cent, but an extract from the zymogenous tissue had no effect. "The very definite nature of these results leaves little doubt that insulin is present only in the islet tissue and not in the zymogenous."

The name insulin was given, at the suggestion of Sir E. A. Schafer, to the pancreatic extract discovered by Banting and Best.

A substance, similar to insulin has been prepared from yeast by Winter and Smith[20] and from various vegetable sources by Collip[21] to which he has given the name "Glukokinin." Certain properties of insulin and of the extract of yeast prepared by Winter and Smith are very similar. Both contain organic phosphorus and carbohydrate. Seliwanoff's reaction is positive in each case after hydrolysis.

Best and Scott;[23] recently have prepared insulin from the submaxillary, thymus and thyroid glands and from liver, spleen and muscle tissue and in fact insulin was present in every tissue investigated. They also found it in the urine and believe it excreted in somewhat greater amounts by pregnant women than by normal men.

BIBLIOGRAPHY.

In the Journal of Metabolic Research for August, 1922, F. M. Allen has abstracted in considerable detail most of the following articles upon which the preceding summary is based.

1. Baron: Surg., Gynec. and Obst., 1920, **31**, 437.
2. Banting and Best: Jour. Lab. and Clin. Med., 1922, **7**, 251.
3. Laguesse: Compt. rend. Soc. Biol., 1893, **45**, 819.
4. Laguesse: Jour. de physiol. et de path. gen., 1911, **13**, 5.
5. Ibrahim: Bioch. Ztschr., 1909, **22**, 24.
6. Banting and Best: Communication to the Academy of Medicine (Toronto), February 7, 1922.
7. Collip: Trans. Royal Soc. of Canada, Third Series, 1922, **16**, Section 5.

8. Banting, Best, Collip and Macleod: Trans. Royal Soc. Canada, Third Series, 1922, **16**, Section 5.
9. Shaffer-Hartman: Jour. Biol. Chem., 1920, **1**, 349.
10. Mann: Proc. Am. Physiol. Soc., December, 1920.
11. Macleod: Canadian Med. Assn. Jour., 1922, **12**, 423.
12. Cruickshank: Jour. Physiol., 1913, **47**, 1.
13. Macleod and Prendergast: Trans. Royal Soc. Canada, 1921, Section V, 37.
14. Banting, Best, Collip, Macleod and Noble: Trans. Royal Soc. Canada, Third Series, 1922, **16**, Section 5.
15. Hepburn and Latchford: Am. Jour. Physiol., 1922, **62**, 177.
16. Banting, Best, Collip, Campbell and Fletcher: The Canadian Med. Assn. Jour., 1922, **12**, 141.
17. Macleod: British Med. Jour., 1922.
18. Banting, Campbell and Fletcher: British Med. Jour., January, 1923, p. 8.
19. Macleod: Jour. Metab. Research, 1922, **2**, 149.
20. Winter and Smith: British Med. Jour., 1923, **1**, 705; also Jour. Phys., 1923, March 21, **57**, 40.
21. Collip: Jour. Biol. Chem., 1923, **56**, 513.
22. Cannon, McIver and Bliss: Boston Med. and Surg. Jour., 1923, **189**, 141.
23. Best and Scott: Jour. Am. Med. Assn., 1923, **81**, 382.

B. PREVIOUS AND CONTEMPORANEOUS RESEARCHES IN PANCREAS THERAPY.

1. **Use of Entire Gland or "Principal Islet."**—Von Mering and Minkowski[1] in 1889, more than two centuries after the first attempt by Conrad Brunner in 1682, demonstrated that total pancreatectomy in dogs was followed by severe and fatal diabetes. Coming as it did almost in conjunction with the discovery by Murray[2] in 1891 that the hypodermic administration of an extract of the thyroid gland to a patient with myxedema would effect a cure, the hope was awakened that a similar type of treatment would be successful in diabetes. This was soon tried by a score of clinicians, but it was found by Sandmeyer[3] that, instead of the feeding of raw pancreas decreasing the glycosuria, the reverse took place, and his experience was universally confirmed. The explanation for the three to fourteen times increase in the glycosuria which Sandmeyer[3] found has generally been ascribed to the better absorption of the protein in the pancreas due to its content of trypsin and the other digestive ferments, and to the formation of carbohydrate from the protein of the gland itself. In 1903, Rennie[4] having noted a "principal islet" in teleosteal fishes to be quite distinct from the acinar tissue and, believing it to furnish an internal secretion whose function had some relation to the utilization of dextrose, he with Fraser[5] in 1907, fed this islet tissue, both in the boiled and raw state, to diabetic patients, but the results were not conclusive. Perhaps Rennie's experiments discouraged Allen,[6] because although he wrote in 1913, "Apparently no one has ever tried the interesting possibility of feeding the glands of new-born or fetal animals, in which the islets have a relatively high development and little

external secretion," he did not pursue the thought. Wegele's[7] one case of supposed pancreatic atrophy in a man aged fifty-two years, in whom glycosuria entirely disappeared on pancreas feeding is not convincing. Allen[6] in his summary of the literature cites the experiments of Pratt and Spooner[8] as the only positive results of the usefulness of pancreas feeding in dogs. They fed pancreas to a dog in which the pancreas had been separated entirely from the duodenum and had eventually atrophied. By feeding the animal during a period of six weeks with fresh pancreas, the tolerance of the dog steadily rose until it stood above normal, but it "*did not fall for more than a month*" after the feeding ceased!

Lepine[9] early explained that the diabetes resulting from pancreatectomy might be due to the withdrawal of an internal secretion of the pancreas which was necessary for the complete metabolism of sugar. Minkowski likewise conceived this possibility and endeavored to discover the internal secretion of the pancreas by feeding fresh pancreas and by subcutaneous injections of pancreas, but failed.[10]

2. **Use of Pancreatic Extracts.**—The difficulty which all investigators encountered who sought to secure an extract which would contain the internal secretion of the pancreas was seemingly insurmountable, because of the active proteolytic ferment, trypsinogen, in the gland. In 1907 and 1908, Zuelzer[11] studied the antagonism between adrenalin and the suspected anti-diabetic hormone of the pancreas. He reported a series of experiments in which he attempted to obtain at the height of digestion an extract of the pancreas with anti-diabetic power. Even at that date he recognized the importance of removing the protein from the extract and did this so thoroughly with alcohol that the pancreatic filtrate barely gave a biuret reaction. Zuelzer preserved the hormone in a 4 per cent solution of sodium chloride. He demonstrated by intravenous injections that there was an anti-diabetic substance in his extract of the pancreas by experiments on rabbits, and he even went so far as to designate as an unit that amount of the extract which would prevent the glycosuria caused by an injection of 1 mg. of adrenalin. Clinically, in 2 depancreatized dogs and in 8 human cases he showed by subcutaneous and intravenous injections the efficacy of his preparation in completely suppressing acidosis and glycosuria. One comatose patient revived and lived five days and in 1 surgical case the use of the extract very likely saved the life of the patient. Acidosis disappeared first and the glycosuria disappeared the next day and the effect of the extract ceased on the fourth day. The occurrence of fever and chills prevented the general application of this method of treatment.

Forschbach,[12] working with Zuelzer's pancreatic extract intravenously in 1909, confirmed Zuelzer's results in diabetic dogs and patients, but the toxic effects were severe and there was no genuine benefit therefrom. The question arose in his mind as to whether the glycosuria might not have decreased on account of the fever, but in the light of today's knowledge there is little doubt that both he and Zuelzer had a potent extract. In the next year, 1910, Crofton[13] pointed out independently that failure of such experiments might be explained on the ground that the hormone in the pancreas which controlled the metabolism of the sugar might be destroyed by the trypsin of the gland, and he consequently prepared an extract free from the external ferments. It was kept heated for three hours at 80° C. to precipitate all proteins and to destroy all ferments. He administered this orally and intramuscularly, but the results were not clear cut.

One cannot but feel that, if these early pioneers in pancreatic therapy had had simple blood sugar methods available, they might have succeeded in their quest, because then they would have recognized how near they were to their object.

3. **Utilization of Opie's and Ssobolew's Discovery of Islands of Langerhans, and the Cause of Diabetes.**—The demonstration by Opie[14] in 1901 and Ssobolew[15] in 1902 that the islands of Langerhans, first described by Paul Langerhans in his Inaugural Dissertation in Berlin in 1869, were the elements of the glands involved in pancreatic diabetes gave a new impetus to the search for a pancreatic ferment. Ssobolew was so far-seeing as to write: "Jetzt aber haben wir in der Unterbindung des Ausführungsganges ein Mittel, die Inseln auf anatomischem Wege zu isoliren und den Chemismus dieser Elemente gesondert, mit Ausschaltung der Verdauungs-Fermente, zu studiren. Diese anatomische Isolirung der Inseln gestattet aber auch in rationeller Weise eine Organo-Theraphie des Diabetes zu erproben." And he further adds and predicts: "Da es sehr schwierig ist, in grösserer Quantität Drüsen zu beschaffen, in denen nur die Inseln erhalten sind, so könnte man sie durch Drüsen von Neugeborenen Thieren, z. B. von Kälbern, ersetzen, bei denen die Inseln im Verhältniss zum Verdauungs-Apparat sehr gut entwickelt sind; dazu käme noch, dass die Bauch-Speicheldrüse der Neugeborenen wenig befähigt ist zur Verdauungs-arbeit und man also hoffen darf, dass ihre Verdauungssäfte die Wirkung der von den Inseln ausgearbeiteten Stoffe nicht beeinträchtigen wird. Auf alle Fälle darf man hoffen, dass es der nächsten Zukunft vorbehalten ist, die Frage zu lösen, ob es auf diesem Wege gelingt, die Leiden der Diabetiker zu lindern." It was mentioned above that Rennie and Fraser[5] fed the islet tissue of teleosteal fishes with this in mind, though to no avail. Laguesse[16] in 1893, also suspected the source of a pancreatic internal secretion in the

islands, though he made no mention of any relation to diabetes at that time, and he further pointed out the greater abundance of these in the fetal and new-born than in adult animals. Arnozant and Vaillard[17] noted in 1884 that ligation of the pancreatic duct in rabbits caused an atrophy of the gland without glycosuria, but Ssobolew[18] was the first to point out that the atrophy was confined to the acinous tissue, and hence no resulting glycosuria, but that when it did involve the islands after upward of one hundred and twenty days glycosuria developed. The significance of this latter observation and Ssobolew's suggestion that a method was thus available for studying the secretion of the islands was overlooked for a decade until Scott recognized its importance in his experiments, but it was Banting almost a decade later still who made the vision a reality. Ssobolew's work was confirmed by Kamimura[19] in 1917, who traced the degenerative changes in the parenchymatous tissue after ligation of the ducts in rabbits and proved that the animals did not develop glycosuria as long as the islands remained intact. In the previous year Sir E. A. Schafer[20] had crystallized the common belief of the source of the internal secretion of the pancreas by giving the name "insulin" to it.

The idea of ligating the external ducts of the pancreas in order to eliminate proteolytic enzymes by causing atrophy of the acinous tissue, though originally suggested by Ssobolew in 1902, was first utilized by E. L. Scott[21] in 1912, in his search for the internal secretion, "but after several attempts in the dog which proved futile so far as complete atrophy was concerned, this method was abandoned as impracticable." He further sought, like Zuelzer, to eliminate trypsinogen by using alcoholic extracts of the pancreas, evaporating the alcohol under vacuum and eventually dissolving his extract in 0.85 per cent sodium chloride for injection. He found, however, that the alcoholic extracts were less active in decreasing glycosuria than when the extracts were made with water slightly acidulated with acetic acid. In preparing his extracts the temperature was never allowed to go above 65° C. "Intravenous injections of the pancreas extract, prepared as above, into dogs rendered diabetic by complete pancreatectomy diminish temporarily the sugar excretion and lower the D:N ratio in the urine. . . .The injections are usually followed by a slight temporary rise of the body temperature, and this may be a factor in the lowered sugar output. The first three dogs showed no depression following the injection, and, *if one dared say it*, seemed even brighter for a time after the injection than before it."

Waterman[22] writing in 1920, claims to have shown in 1913,[23] that the disappearance of glycogen from the liver of a dog, kept for a long time under chloroform narcosis, was diminished greatly if blood taken from the pancreatic vein was infused into the blood stream or if an *alcoholic extract of pancreas* was so used. He also claims to have shown that the active substance was *thermo-stable*.

Credit is given by Waterman to De Meyer[24] for having detected the alcoholic solubility of the active substance of the pancreas in 1910.

In the following year, 1913, two other Americans, Murlin and Kramer,[25] began a series of researches upon the pancreas which have continued, save for an intermission due to the war, to the present day. They were the first to employ the respiratory quotient as a measure of the combustion of glucose resulting from the use of pancreatic extracts. Most of the extracts were made from dog's pancreas. A few of the extracts used were made from cow's pancreas with Ringer's solution and "kept acid with HCl until after boiling. In one instance after filtration and neutralization with Na$_2$CO$_3$, one-half of the total filtrate (500 cc) was injected subcutaneously in the evening and the other half the following morning." They give the following summary of their work.

"Intravenous infusion of pancreatic extract made from cow's pancreas by Knowlton and Starling's method raised the D:N ratio on the days immediately following, when the urine was collected in twenty-four-hour periods. When the urine was collected in short periods, a similar extract produced a slight fall in the hourly dextrose elimination and in the D:N ratio in the hours immediately following injection. A mixed extract made in the same manner from dog's pancreas and duodenal mucosa produced a greater fall and in one instance complete disappearance of the urinary sugar. The fall, however, was followed in three to ten hours by a compensating increase. A similar quantity of Ringer's solution made alkaline to about the same degree as the medium for the extract, produced an effect on the glycosuria almost identical. A 2 per cent Na$_2$CO$_3$ solution likewise caused a sharp decline in the excretion of sugar and a 2 per cent HCl solution by stomach tube, produced a sharp increase. The increase in the one case continued for about the same length of time as the decrease in the other and both are probably to be explained by the effects of the medium on glycogenesis and glycogenolysis. It is possible also that the pancreatic extract affected the renal permeability. Neither extract of pancreas alone nor the double extract of pancreas and duodenal mucosa produced, within the time of maximal effect on the glycosuria, any effect on the respiratory quotient which could be interpreted as an index of increased combustion of carbohydrate. . . .We conclude that neither the use of the Knowlton-Starling extract nor the transfusion of normal blood is yet a measure of any practical importance in restoring to the depancreatized dog the ability to burn sugar."

Murlin and Kramer's purpose in using an extract of duodenum as well as pancreas was that the secretin of the former might activate the anti-diabetic hormone of the latter, and this summary shows they believed this to be the case. In the text of their article they are more definite than in No. 3 of their summary and write "the effect of injection was immediate and resulted in complete disappearance of sugar at the end of two hours. . . . Sugar was completely absent for at least four hours and perhaps longer." With their next experiment (Ex. VI) there was a fall in sugar elimination almost as great as in the previous experiment. The blood was analyzed for sugar at 4.00 P.M., one hour before injection and at 8.15 P.M., nearly three hours after the injection ceased. The results show a rise from 0.128 to 0.148 per cent. Since they noted, when a solution of alkali alone was employed, the "dextrose elimination per hour and the D:N ratio reached the same level at the end of four hours as when the extracts were given," they were led to ascribe undue importance to the alkali, yet they saw that the alkaline Ringer's solution alone was not so immediate in its action and that the absolute fall in the sugar excretion was not so great. When they gave the dog 200 cc of a 2 per cent solution of HCl, the results were reversed. Again, contrary to No. 7 of their summary, in the text of their article they record *the respiratory quotient of a depancreatized dog rose after an injection of duodenum and pancreas from 0.69 to 0.73* and the protocol presents good evidence that this was not accidental. There is considerable evidence that Murlin and Kramer had a potent extract. They worked with boiled material, whereas the favorable results of Zuelzer, Forschbach, Kleiner, Paulesco, and Banting and Best were with unboiled extracts, but we know today from the work of Murlin in Rochester that boiling does not destroy insulin at a pH of 6.7 to 7.2 though the hormone is destroyed (Murlin) at pH 4.4 to 5.7. The thermo-stable quality of the active substance of the pancreas, Prof. Murlin writes me, was first described by Waterman in 1913, as mentioned above.

In a subsequent paper in 1916, Murlin and Kramer[26] studied in more detail the influence of alkali and acid upon glycosuria and hyperglycemia and conclude:

"Sodium bicarbonate and potassium bicarbonate administered by stomach tube may be without immediate effect on the glycosuria and the hyperglycemia of the depancreatized dog. . . . The normal anhydrous salt of sodium, Na_2CO_3, may, on the contrary, reduce the sugar in the urine materially when given by mouth, and when given by vein invariably does so, especially when added to Ringer's or Locke's solution to the amount of about 1 per cent."

According to a later report Kramer, Marker, and Murlin[27] stated that glucose thus retained is not held back as glycogen, and so the alkali does not act like an anti-diabetic hormone. . . . "Dilute HCl given by mouth or subcutaneously to the depancreatized dog has just the opposite effect of alkali—increasing the sugar in the urine without affecting materially the nitrogen elimination—and without causing any effect on the blood."

In a third paper in 1916, Murlin and Kramer[28] continued their study of the influence of alkali on the respiratory metabolism after total and partial pancreatectomy, and also used with it at this period the unboiled extract of pancreas. They gave the solution orally, save with dog 54 in which it was administered intravenously and "failed completely" to raise the quotient. The good results of other successful experimenters, such as Zuelzer, Forschbach, Kleiner, Paulesco, and Banting and Best, have been with the intravenous method or subcutaneous method. "Our conclusion after some three years' intermittent occupation with the problem is that in the totally depancreatized dog in good condition, *i. e.*, not moribund, the alkali alone is almost always without effect on the respiratory metabolism. An increase of a few points at most in the respiratory quotient may be obtained. With the partially operated animal, however, the result is striking and immediate. . . . We have obtained some evidence, also, that pancreatic material (whether merely as an extract or in virtue of the presence of living cells we are not yet prepared to say) is, when administered with alkali, of distinct benefit to the diabetic organism." In the depancreatized dog 51, the respiratory quotient rose from a basal level of 0.69 to 0.72 with 1 per cent $NaHCO_3$ in Ringer's solution given by mouth, but when pancreas, which had been allowed to macerate for two months under toluene in the ice box, was given in the same manner with glucose, the respiratory quotient rose to 0.87. "An increase of ten points in the quotient, with an accompanying dynamic action, in an animal known to be completely deprived of internal pancreatic function at a time when the deficiency was most serious, is the most hopeful sign we have encountered in our work that it may yet be possible artificially to restore this function not only to operated dogs but also to men suffering with diabetes mellitus." In another dog 53, they also found that the respiratory quotient rose from 0.67 and 0.69 to 0.83 on one day and to 0.77 and 0.79 on two others after the administration of pancreas and dextrose in Ringer's solution with 0.05 per cent NaOH. On the other hand, it must be pointed out that when glucose and alkali were given intravenously to dog 20, upon whom later the autopsy revealed no pancreatic tissue the respiratory quotient rose to 0.9. This dog had exhibited perfect Minkowski ratios but twelve days after operation did not show glycosuria, and had a blood sugar of 0.11 per cent before he was given the glucose. Perhaps he was not diabetic though this is not certain, because the severest human diabetics in inanition may show high respiratory quotients and die of hypoglycemia and it is quite possible that the dog presented this same peculiarity on this occasion. Further, their most decisive experimental animal, dog 51, on May 31, after 30 grams glucose by mouth, gave a quotient of 0.79 and it was following another dose of glucose, but with pancreas, that the quotient reached 0.87 some three hours later on the same day.

Kleiner[29] was successful in showing that the unfiltered aqueous extracts of fresh pancreas diluted with 0.9 per cent sodium chloride, when administered slowly and intravenously, usually resulted in a marked decrease in the blood sugar of dogs. His experiments were preceded by those of Kleiner and Meltzer, who found that large quantities of sugar introduced intravenously in normal animals[30] were promptly lost from the circulation; in diabetic animals[31] this occurred very slowly, as was shown by the fact that even an hour and a half after the infusion the blood sugar was still far above its original level. Five normal dogs showed 0.2 per cent sugar before the injection and 0.27 per cent sugar an hour and a half after the injection; 9 depancreatized dogs showed 0.38 per cent before the injection and 0.86 per cent at a similar time afterward. Kleiner's modification of Kleiner's and Meltzer's experiments was to add an emulsion of pancreas to the glucose solution to be injected, and he found that the diabetic animal handled the sugar in nearly a normal manner. They employed a simple water extraction with subsequent dilution with saline, and in order to imitate what presumably takes place in Nature, they introduced the pancreatic preparation by the intravenous route very slowly, since they expected the results to be observed during the injection and only a few hours thereafter. The first few experiments were briefly reported in 1915.[32] In their experiments the blood sugar fell in one depancreatized dog from 0.31 per cent to 0.13 per cent within two hours after the injection of the pancreatic emulsion; in another the percentage of blood sugar fell in two hours from 0.21 per cent to 0.08 per cent. Their experiments were controlled with emulsions of other organs. They proved that the reduction in glycemia was real and not due to dilution of the blood, and that it was not an accident, was proven by the fact that it occurred to a marked degree in 10 out of 16 experiments, and to some extent in 15 out of 16. The elimination of sugar was decreased in every experiment except one.

A search for the internal secretion of the pancreas was continued in another manner by A. H. Clark[33] with the isolated living mammalian heart. He demonstrated that glucose was more rapidly removed from the perfusing Locke's fluid when that had been perfused through the bloodvessels of the pancreas than when a fresh solution of Locke's fluid was employed. He observed that the solution was inactivated by boiling and unstable. Doubtless his thought of testing the pancreas in this way was instigated by Knowlton and Starling's experiments[34] on the heart, in which they deduced, though perhaps erroneously, that the heart of a depancreatized animal was less capable of utilizing sugar perfused in solution through it than the normal heart, and that the addition of a boiled extract of pancreas to the blood circulating through the heart of a diabetic animal restores to the latter the power of utilizing the glucose of the circulating blood.

It is thus seen that prior to the discovery of the utility of using pancreatic extracts in the treatment of diabetes by Banting and Best[35] many writers had earnestly sought and closely approached a solution of the problem. The latest of these was Paulesco[36] who, in 1921, showed the reducing effect of the entire pancreas of a dog, removed under sterile precautions and extracted with 0.7 per cent solution of sodium chloride, upon sugar, urea, and acetone, in both the blood and urine of depancreatized animals following its intravenous injection. He observed hypoglycemia and transitory disappearance of glycosuria and records that the effect of the extract began immediately, reached a maximum in two hours, and lasted for twelve hours. The effect of the extract varied with the amount of the pancreas employed to prepare it. Even in a non-diabetic he found if one injected the extract, there was a notable diminution in glycemia.

In 1921 Murlin with his co-laborers Clough, Stokes, Gibbs, and Stone[37] resumed the work which he had carried on with Kramer between 1913 and 1916, confirming and extending it. They showed that perfusates of the pancreas of the dog, cat, and pig made with Ringer's solution or Locke's solution either with 0.2 per cent sodium bicarbonate or glucose of 0.5 or 1 per cent would raise the respiratory quotient of a completely diabetic animal. At times these unboiled alkaline perfusates were given intraperitoneally and at others subcutaneously and intravenously. Extract given by stomach tube caused very little or no fall in blood or urinary sugar. Although in several instances they noted that there was a perceptible increase in the quotient in an animal previously incapable of oxidizing glucose, these were not strong enough to be of practical significance. Consequently, in June, 1922, Murlin and his associates[38] employed acid perfusates of the pancreas and with considerable success.

They were led to employ an acid solution because of Scott's experiments above cited[21] and Murlin's and Kramer's experiments with $\frac{N}{5}$ hydrochloric acid in 1913.[39] By perfusing the pancreas with 300 cc of a solution containing chiefly sodium chloride with potassium chloride, calcium chloride, and water for seventy-two minutes, they obtained a perfusate which in 7 doses kept a depancreatized dog alive for thirty days. They showed that the active internal secretion of the pancreas could be extracted by perfusion of the pancreas with acidulated Ringer's solution more readily than with the same fluid made slightly alkaline, and demonstrated that in this way enough of the internal secretion was obtained to cause a marked fall in blood sugar and D:N ratio. When such a perfusate was administered intravenously and glucose given by mouth, the respiratory quotient rose to 0.81 and 0.85 from the diabetic level.

In a final report on the aqueous extracts of the pancreas and their influence on carbohydrate metabolism of depancreatized animals[40] Murlin and his co-workers state: (1) That their experiments show that the acid extracts of the cats' pancreas raise the respiratory quotient; (2) that the acid extracts of the pancreas of the pig and ox are about equally effective in reducing the blood sugar and D:N ratio of depancreatized dogs whether given intravenously, subcutaneously, or intraperitoneally; (3) that the extracts of the pancreas obtained with acidulated water are quite as effective as those with acidulated alcohol. They emphasized (4) the extreme toxicity of pancreatic extracts if the trypsin is not completely destroyed and the acid not completely neutralized; and asserted (5) that boiling in a slightly acid medium does not destroy insulin; though (6) filtering through charcoal and Lloyd's reagent removes a large amount of it. They report (7) the presence of two substances in their extracts (*a*) a substance that lowers blood sugar and D:N ratio but increases the respiratory quotient, and (*b*) another substance which increases blood sugar of both normal and depancreatized dogs and may lead to an abrupt fall in the respiratory quotient. Since (8) the abrupt fall occurs quite regularly, but then rises again, they conclude it is not due to exhaustion of the insulin. Finally, (9) they record that the oral administration of their pancreatic extracts to depancreatized dogs gives results which are almost universally positive in raising the respiratory quotient.

R. L. Mackenzie Wallis[41] reports upon the oral administration of the pancreas of pigs kept without food for twenty-four hours before being killed. The divided pancreas was heated with alcohol at 60° C. for one hour and the alcohol later distilled in vacuo during thirty hours. The filtrate was eventually evaporated in an electric oven at 100° C. When the dried, unstable, deliquescent extract is incubated with fresh blood, to which sugar has been added, the sugar rapidly disappears. Three clinical cases are reported, but these are not convincing. Data for carbohydrate, protein and fat at the beginning and end of the periods are not given. The weights of the patients at beginning and end of treatment are omitted. Accurate urinary analyses fail. "A number of cases have shown no response at all, so pancreatic treatment has been discarded." In one case of diabetic coma the extract was given intravenously and the patient lived for four days.[42]

BIBLIOGRAPHY.

1. von Mering and Minkowski: Arch. f. exp. Path. u. Pharm., 1889–1890, **26**, 371.
2. Murray: Brit. Med. Jour., October 10, 1891, 796.
3. Sandmayer: Ztschr. f. Biol., 1894, **31**, 12.
4. Rennie: Jour. Anat. and Phys., 1903, **37**, 375.
5. Rennie and Fraser: Biochem. Jour., 1907, **2**, 7.
6. Allen: Glycosuria and Diabetes, W. M. Leonard, Boston, 1913, 814.
7. Wegele: Fortschritte d. Med., 1902, **20**, 313.
8. Pratt and Spooner: Arch. Int. Med., 1911, **7**, 665.
9. Lepine: Le Diabete Sucre, Paris, 1909, 54.
10. Minkowski: Arch. f. exp. Path. u. Pharm., 1893, **31**, 85, 175.
11. Zuelzer: Verh. d. Kong. f. inn. Med., 1907, **24**, 258; also, Ztschr. f. exp. Path. u. Ther., 1908, **5**, 307; Zuelzer, Dohrn and Marxer, Deutsch. med. Wchnschr., 1908, **34**, (2), 1380.
12. Forschbach: Deutsch. med. Wchnschr., 1909, **35**, (2), 2053.
13. Crofton: Dublin Med. Jour., 1910, **129**, 332.
14. Opie: John Hopkins Hosp. Bull., 1901, **12**, 263.
15. Ssobolew: Virchow's Arch. f. path. Anat., 1902, **168**, 91.
16. Laguesse: Compt. rend. Soc. Biol., 1893, **45**, 819.
17. Arnozant and Vaillard: Arch. de Physiol. Norm. et Path., Paris, 1884, **3**, 287.
18. Ssobolew: See 15 above.
19. Kamimura: Mitt. med. Fak. d. Univ. zu Tokyo, 1917, **17**, 95.
20. Schafer: The Endocrine Organs, Longmans, Green & Co., 1916, 125.
21. Scott: Am. Jour. Physiol., 1912, **29**, 306.
22. Waterman: Arch. Neerland. de Physiol. de l'Homme et des Animaux, 1920.
23. Waterman: Vzrsl. en meded. Kon. Acad. v. Wetensch., March 12 and July 31, 1913.
24. De Meyer: Arch. Internat. de Physiol., 1910, **9**.
25. Murlin and Kramer: Jour. Biol. Chem., 1913, **15**, 365.
26. Murlin and Kramer: Jour. Biol. Chem., 1916, **27**, 481.
27. Kramer, Marker and Murlin: Jour. Biol. Chem., 1916, **27**, 499.
28. Murlin and Kramer: Jour. Biol. Chem., 1916, **27**, 517.
29. Kleiner: Jour. Biol. Chem., 1919, **40**, 153.
30. Kleiner and Meltzer: Am. Jour. Physiol., 1914, **33**, xvii; also, Kleiner, Jour. Exp. Med., 1916, **23**, 507.
31. Kleiner and Meltzer: Proc. Soc. Exp. Biol. and Med., 1914, **12**, 58.
32. Kleiner and Meltzer: See 30, 31.
33. Clark: Jour. Exp. Med., 1916, **24**, 621; also, Jour. Exp. Med., 1917, **26**, 721.
34. Knowlton and Starling: Jour. Physiol., 1912, **45**, 146.
35. Banting and Best: Jour. Lab. and Clin. Med., 1922, **7**, 251.
36. Paulesco: Compt. rend. de Soc. de Biol., 1921, **85**, 555; also, Arch. Internat. de Phys., 1921, **17**, 85.
37. Clough, Stokes, Gibbs, Stone and Murlin: Proc. Soc. Exp. Biol. and Med., 1922, **20**, 66; also, Murlin, Clough, Stokes: Am. Jour. Phys., April, 1923.
38. Murlin, Clough, Gibbs and Stone: Am. Jour. Phys., April, 1923.
39. Murlin, Kramer and Sweet: Jour. Metab. Research, 1922, **2**, 19.

40. Murlin, Clough, Gibbs and Stokes: Proc. Soc. Exp. Biol. and Med., 1922, **20**, 67; also, Jour. Biol. Chem., May, 1923.

41. Mackenzie Wallis: Lancet, 1922, **203**, 1158.

42. Further investigations, in the main unsuccessful, are not cited here. They were summarized in an address given before the Rochester Medical Association, November 10, 1922 by Professor Murlin, to whom I am indebted for various references which had not come to my attention.

C. INSULIN IN THE TREATMENT OF DIABETES.

1. Introduction and Summary.—The use of insulin in the treatment of my series of diabetic cases was begun August 7, 1922, and since that date has been employed with 358 patients of whom 293 were treated in the first twelve months. Seven of the first 100 diabetics coming for treatment received it, but with succeeding hundreds the number treated with insulin has risen progressively so that in May it had changed to 64 in 100 and by September, 1923, to 77 in the last 100 hospital admissions. These statistics show my confidence in and dependence upon insulin.[1]

The types of patients treated with insulin have ranged in severity from the severest to the mildest; in age from one year to seventy-eight years; and in duration of the diabetes from four weeks to twenty-three years.

The policy adopted in the treatment of diabetes with insulin has been to utilize along with it all those measures which have proved of the greatest value in the treatment of diabetes without insulin. These are: Adherence to a diet which will keep the urine sugar-free, avoidance of over- or extreme undernutrition, and a method of life compatible with the strength such a diet affords.

Insulin does not cure diabetes.[2] Insulin does not allow a diabetic to eat anything he desires. It is a potent preparation alike for evil and for good. Thomas D., Case No. 1305, omitted insulin for five days, continued his relatively high diet, developed a mild infection, and entered the hospital to die seven and a half hours later of coma. A patient with a tolerance for 114 grams carbohydrate took 1 unit and the blood sugar fell to 0.03 per cent. Conversely, Miss M., our first case and the severest diabetic on our list, who had gone down to the street from her apartment but once in nine months, felt able after six weeks of treatment to walk

[1] All the insulin used in the treatment of the patients and in the investigations here recorded came originally through the instigation of the Insulin Committee of Toronto and upon their recommendation to the Eli Lilly Company. For the privilege of using insulin and its prompt and generous supply I am profoundly grateful. Whenever the word insulin is used in the text in connection with my patients, it means "iletin," the trade name of the insulin manufactured by the Eli Lilly Company.

[2] Certain sentences and paragraphs in what follows appeared in articles by the author in the Jour. Am. Med. Assn. (1923, **80**, 1581) and Jour. Metab. Research (1923, **2**, 651).

with ease 4 miles daily, has gained 31 pounds in nine and a half
months, and now does all the work save the washing for the household, and has reduced her insulin from 35 to 28 units. Mrs. M.,
Case No. 2980, with rapidly ascending gangrene, fever, 5 per cent
sugar, and marked acidosis, was first seen on a Sunday, brought
to the hospital the same evening, given insulin, and the thigh amputated at 10 o'clock the next morning by R. C. Cochrane. After
eight days the 30-unit daily dose of insulin was omitted; ten days
later she became sugar-free and remains so August, 1923, eight
months later, while upon an adequate diet.

Insulin is a remedy primarily for the wise and not for the foolish,
be they patients or doctors. Everyone knows it requires brains
to live long with diabetes, but to use insulin successfully requires
more brains. Two ignorant patients, who were helped by insulin
and needed it, went home without it, and their physicians, though
living nearby, did not take the trouble to come to the hospital
either to see the patients or learn about insulin. An alert little girl of
fifteen years, after two weeks of our best efforts with dietetic treatment seldom could keep sugar-free, yet she was wise and with
insulin has gained 32 pounds from the lowest level reached since
insulin treatment began—49 per cent of her body weight. Her
elderly, over-worked country doctor traveled nearly 200 miles to
see for himself this new form of treatment and to take her home.
We have had no coöperation in doctor and patient greater than this.

Insulin is no more dangerous than morphine, and it has these
advantages: Whereas an excess of morphine leads directly to sleep,
coma, and death, an overdose of insulin causes a warning train of
symptoms beginning with nervousness and extreme hunger as the
blood sugar drops below 0.07 per cent, progressing to sweating and
tremor, subconscious or evident, and ending with unconsciousness
as the blood sugar reaches 0.03 per cent. Death is possible. Again
unlike morphine poisoning recovery follows the simplest of measures,
the juice of an orange or 1 to 3 teaspoonfuls of sugar, and takes
place promptly within five or ten minutes.

Insulin has revolutionized diabetic treatment in more ways than
one: (1) It can give more food, strength, and weight, but (2) to
do this it demands not only a knowledge and respect for the diabetic
diet on the part of the doctor and patient, but adherence to the
same if the diabetic wishes to get his money's worth for the insulin
he injects.

For the wise, who may be rich or poor, young or old, and for the
innocent, who can be cared for, insulin is a benefit, but for the
ignorant, who likewise may be rich or poor and young or old, it
can be dangerous, and a gift of free insulin to such is like casting
away pearls.

Twenty deaths have occurred among the 293 patients, of whom all have been traced, who were treated with insulin during the first year of its use in my practice ending August 7, 1923. Two of these died from diabetic coma within eight hours after admission to the N. E. D. Hospital and 4 from coma elsewhere. The other patients have succumbed to diseases not directly attributable to diabetes, cirrhosis of the liver with pulmonary tuberculosis, pulmonary tuberculosis, meningitis, angina pectoris, coronary thrombosis, apoplexy, nephritis, cancer of pancreas, erysipelas, pneumonia and septicemia. It is, therefore, evident that with insulin we shall learn the remote rather than the acute results of diabetes. How profound a change this is will be pointed out on many occasions in this book.

The first cases of diabetes treated in August, 1922, were those who were the most severe. Thirty were selected for this reason. Later cases of milder degree were added to the list, including several representing surgical emergencies. Still later others were added to the list who were distinctly less severe in type, yet quite unable to maintain weight and do their daily tasks. A certain number of children with acute onset have been chosen for treatment, and the last four months the majority of the cases entering the hospital have received insulin in order to shorten the hospital stay. An incidental result of this has been the necessity to revise the system of Test and Maintenance Diets, because the insulin allowed the patients to progress from one diet day to another more rapidly. Among the group treated are many so-called (to use Woodyatt's term) "pedigreed" diabetics in that they have already found their way into medical literature. These are Cases No. 632, 866, 1305, 1542, 1794, 2174, 2560.

The first dose of insulin has usually been 1 unit and this has been increased by 1 unit, one, two or three times daily until the requisite number of calories could be taken by the patient to secure a gain in weight and strength. In February, 1922, a summary was made of 53 selected cases treated for an average period of sixty-three days, and at that time the average quantity of insulin taken daily by each patient was 11 units, and this was the same dose for 127 cases summarized in May, 1923. The average gain in weight of the early group of patients was 1 pound for every fifteen days of treatment. Frequently at the beginning of treatment patients lost weight because of the restriction of diet adopted along with the administration of insulin in order to render the urine sugar-free. Throughout treatment insulin has been added to the regular program of dietetic management and in no instance has this dietetic program been altered because of the insulin. With insulin the principles of the diabetic diet are utilized, not replaced.

The dose of insulin has been decreased in many cases and omitted in some, particularly as the total number of diabetics receiving insulin has grown. A few patients are taking more insulin than formerly. So far, fear that insulin would fail in the course of time to control the diabetes has been groundless, provided the patient would adhere to the diet. Thus, 14 cases treated for thirty days or less received 11 units per day, and the same number of units were taken daily by 13 cases treated between sixty-one and ninety days. In February there were 3 patients receiving 30 or more units daily, and when the total number of patients treated had increased from 83 to 219, the number of cases receiving over 30 units had not changed. Writing in August, 1923, after one year of the use of insulin, there are but 18 patients among 293 so treated who have received over 30 units daily, save for temporary emergencies. Patients with diabetes as severe as that represented in this group have not been encountered in the last six months. The Jewish race which includes so many mild diabetics is not represented in the list and in fact but 7 per cent of the patients taking insulin are Hebrews.

A few units of insulin will do much for mild cases of diabetes. Thirteen cases of children under fifteen years of age received less than 6 units daily, and these patients in the course of three months have added 8 per cent to their body weight, a gain equivalent to the normal rate of growth for children.

Additions to the diet have been made in the form of carbohydrate, protein, and fat. The carbohydrate taken daily by the early group of 53 patients at the beginning of treatment was 37 grams and two months later 45 grams. The greatest increase in carbohydrate recorded for any one patient was 132 grams and the least increase was 1 gram. The protein was also increased from an original quantity of 36 grams, which oddly enough represented exactly 1 gram per kilogram body weight for the 53 patients under discussion, to 55 grams. The greater proportionate increase in protein was due to the inclusion of many children in the table. These children require more protein per kilogram body weight than adults. The calories were added chiefly in the form of fat, and the average quantity rose from 62 grams at the beginning to 105 grams at the end. The ketogenic-antiketogenic ratio for the first diet was 1.1 and for the later diet 1.2, each being a ratio well below the limits of acidosis.

The average quantity of glucose made utilizable by the 11 units of insulin daily in this series of cases is easily determined from figures already presented. The total glucose for the first series of diets was 65 grams and for the second series of diets was 88 grams. In other words, 1 unit of insulin was responsible for the utilization of 2 grams of glucose in this particular series of cases.

The average percentage of blood sugar at the beginning and end of treatment is proof of the better utilization of the diet. Since the blood sugar values are taken more than twelve hours after the last dose of insulin, they are of especial significance. With the extra food allowed I expected that the morning blood sugars would be increased, but the contrary was the case. The average fasting blood sugar at the beginning was 0.24 per cent and at the end 0.19 per cent. It will be of value to compile similar data months later, because such data will indicate the course the disease is taking.

TABLE 1.—EFFECT OF INCREASE IN DIET AFTER LONG-CONTINUED UNDERNUTRITION—NO INSULIN. CASE NO. 866.

Date.	Diacetic acid.	Sugar in urine, gm.	Average daily diet.				Blood sugar.	
			C.	P.	F.	Cals.	Date.	Per cent.
October:								
14–24 inc. . .	0	0	31	74	75	1095	Oct. 22	0.13
25–31 inc. . .	0	0	36	84	79	1191	Oct. 30	0.14
31–Nov. 5 inc.	0	0	43	86	86	1290	Nov. 6	0.19

The increase in the well-being of the patients not only in weight and strength, but also in spirit, was remarkable soon after the beginning of treatment. Since many of these patients were of the severest type of undernourished diabetics and were given far more food than they had had for months or years, the question arose as to whether diet or insulin was responsible for the improvement. Consequently, Mr. P., Case No. 866, who had had diabetes for eight years, whose original weight was halved, whose metabolism was the lowest of any reported diabetic in the world, was asked to return to the Clinic and undergo an increase of diet exactly like that of our first case, Miss M., Case No. 1542. The results obtained with Mr. P., are summarized in Table 1. This table shows that on a diet of 1095 calories the fasting blood sugar was 0.13 per cent and the urine sugar-free. When this diet was increased by 100 calories or 10 per cent, the urine remained sugar-free as before, but the blood sugar rose to 0.14 per cent. Again the diet was increased by 100 calories, making a total increase of 20 per cent from the original diet. The urine still remained sugar-free, an index of the long years of faithful following of dietetic rules by this patient, but the blood sugar at the end of the period had risen to 0.19 per cent. Sugar soon appeared in the urine. With insulin this patient tolerated an increase in diet perfectly well and gained 10 pounds in weight, but I am very sorry to say that on March

10, 1923, he succumbed to erysipelas, though in no wise connected with his treatment with insulin. See page 97, Table 26, and page 98.

Menstruation returned in 1 case treated with insulin and reported by Allen. It has returned in 2 of my patients. In the Carnegie series of 46 female patients treated without insulin there was 1 such case.

The ages of the patients treated ranged from one year to seventy-eight years. Case No. 3019 is the youngest of the group coming for treatment at the age of one year and seven months. This child was sugar-free only twice during the two weeks he was at the hospital. Since he returned home he has done well. He is now sugar-free and his weight has risen from 23 pounds on February 5, 1923, to 25 pounds on April 29, 1923, and to 28 pounds on September 10, 1923. He receives 15 units of insulin today. Kenneth S., Case No. 2978, who developed diabetes at one and seven-tenth years and came for treatment twelve months later, was a most pitiable object, weighing 19 pounds. He resembled Major's[1] extraordinary patient whose pictures before and after treatment appear in his article. With 2 units he had a convulsion, though there is doubt whether this was due to a reaction. There was very slow improvement at first, but now, eight months later, in his own home his weight has risen to 34 pounds, 80 per cent, and he is sugar-free with 14 to 20 units. Both of these patients made their gains after leaving the hospital, confirming my belief in home treatment for diabetics. Mrs. H., Case No. 2972 coming for treatment at the age of sixty-eight years with 6 per cent sugar, ++ acidosis and weighing 69 pounds, has gained in the course of five months 20 pounds, thus adding one-third to her body weight. Mrs. P., Case No. 2040, at the age of seventy-eight years started treatment and is in better condition today than for two and a half years, when her disease began. Therefore, both extremes of life respond satisfactorily to treatment with insulin, though not rarely for the first few weeks both appear refractory. Thus, Olive O., Case No. 2815, originally reported as an unfavorable result[2] is now, September, 1923, usually sugar-free on a diet of carbohydrate 36, protein 40, fat 67, calories 907 and taking 14 units of insulin daily. Her weight dressed is 33½ pounds. At the other extreme of life Mr. S., Case No. 2626, at sixty-one years of age, having resisted all efforts to get sugar-free, has eventually been able to accomplish this with 10 units daily and a distinct increase in diet. Similarly, Mrs. L., Case No. 2908, aged seventy-two years, who for months showed glycosuria while recovering from several oper-

---

[1] Major: Jour. Am. Med. Assn., 1923, **80**, 1597.
[2] Joslin: Jour. Metab. Research, 1922, **2**, 661.

ations for gangrene, is now sugar-free, has gained weight, and is taking carbohydrate 110 grams and calories 2255.

2. **Dosage.**—Small doses of insulin from the start have characterized my method of treatment for several reasons. First, with one patient whose carbohydrate tolerance was 114 grams the injection of 1 unit lowered the blood sugar to 0.03 per cent. Allen has reported a similar result with half a unit (Allen, Case No. 1194).[1] The possibility that this might occur with other patients whose tolerance was far less, indicated the necessity for the use of small doses in the routine treatment of large numbers of cases remaining in the hospital for short periods or by physicians in general practice, and it is especially for the latter group that my system of diabetic treatment is planned. Consequently it has been the rule to give 1 unit of insulin for the first dose, 2 units for the second, 3 for the third, 4 for the fourth and 5 for the fifth, and thereafter 5 units three times a day and then increase or decrease the quantity as glycosuria and calories required. Usually the noon dose is omitted and the dose before breakfast made somewhat larger than the dose before the evening meal. A second reason for small dosage was the sad experience with a boy, Thomas D., my second case, who during the absence of his local physician and with other serious illness in his home gave up insulin for five days, failed to restrict his diet, developed a slight infection, and went into coma, from which he died seven and a half hours after entrance to the hospital. Unquestionably large doses of insulin will allow patients to take more food and thus gain weight very rapidly, but with large doses of insulin the patient is walking on longer insulin stilts and his equilibrium is therefore correspondingly endangered. With small doses progress is more gradual, but quite as sure and certainly safer. A third reason for using small doses was the fear, not entirely groundless, that as time went on the dosage of insulin might need to be increased; and fourth, that the patient would be unable to tolerate for months the larger injections. This last apprehension was warranted. It was real at the beginning, and time enough has not elapsed to show that it is wholly without basis. Thus, Carolyn, Case No. 2801, who is 1 of the 3 patients to have received more than 30 units daily for one hundred and thirty-nine days, developed, as a result of her early injections of a more dilute preparation, various hard, indurated masses at the sites of the injections. Excision of one of these showed the development of much scar tissue, and it is quite evident that insulin injected into this tissue would not readily be absorbed. In fact, it was because of the irregularity of the action of the insulin in her especial

---

[1] Allen: Jour. Metab. Research, 1922, **2**, 866.

case that the section of skin was removed. The child preferred the injections in the areas where the lumps had formed, because in such areas less pain developed. At present with insulin in the strength of 20 units to 1 cc it is probable that this complication can be avoided. This patient after indiscretions in diet and excitement went into coma, was brought out of it by Dr. Shedd, but nine weeks later succumbed to another attack, preceded by an infection.

A fifth reason against large doses of insulin was still more fundamental. The treatment of diabetes with insulin should follow the best lines of treatment of diabetes without insulin. In other words, overfeeding should be discountenanced, and overfeeding results when large doses of insulin are given.

The cost of insulin is the sixth reason which deters from large doses. Most patients with diabetes are in moderate circumstances. It is unfair to treat patients in the hospital with large doses of insulin without cost and then to send the same patients home expecting them to pay for that dosage of insulin indefinitely. We believe that the sale of insulin is a boon rather than a detriment to insulin therapy in general, but the expense should be kept low. When a patient pays for insulin, he is far more likely to use it wisely. Patients become very keen and learn at which meals following insulin the carbohydrate can be increased or decreased with surprising readiness, often adjusting the dose far more skillfully than can their physicians, who are seldom as familiar with all their conditions of life. Success with diabetic patients depends largely upon their willingness to make sacrifices for hospital board, treatment, and now insulin. The diabetic dependent upon charity seldom does well, just as it is hard for a rich diabetic to conform to rules, though he is far more apt to attempt it today than formerly.

How foolishly insulin is used was illustrated by one patient, a physician, Case No. 3346, who took 80 units daily on account of a trace of sugar in his urine. His blood sugar percentage both before and after meals was normal. It was instructive to learn that he did not have a reaction.

The amount of carbohydrate which a diabetic patient can take with the help of insulin is unknown. Geyelin writes: "We have as yet found no evidence that the degree of carbohydrate tolerance which any case of diabetes can achieve with insulin is limited by anything except the amount of insulin which can be given."[1] One should not misinterpret this statement of Geyelin. He by no means implies that one should give as much carbohydrate as possible.

Olmsted and Kahn[2] state that "in using insulin on more than 40 diabetic patients, we have never used less than 10 units a day."

[1] Geyelin: Jour. Metab. Research, 1922, **2**, 789.
[2] Olmsted and Kahn: Jour. Am. Med. Assn., 1923, **80**, 1903.

3. **Standardization of the Unit.**—One unit of insulin originally represented the quantity of insulin which was necessary to lower the blood sugar of a rabbit weighing 2 kilograms, fasting for twenty-four hours, to 0.045 per cent within four hours with the production of convulsions. This was found to be too large a unit for clinical purposes. The clinical unit at present employed may be defined as one-third the amount of insulin which is necessary to lower the percentage of blood sugar to the convulsive level, 0.045 per cent, within three to five hours in rabbits weighing 2 kilograms which have been starved twenty-four hours. It would be convenient to know the value of 1 unit of insulin in terms of glucose which it could metabolize. Various estimations have been made and agree in general that 1 unit renders utilizable to the body from 0.75 gram glucose to 2 grams glucose. With my patients 1 unit of insulin has allowed approximately 2 grams glucose material to be taken in addition to the previous diet. There are, however, wide variations. Fifty-three of my patients during sixty-three days of treatment were taking 65 grams of total glucose at the beginning of treatment and with an average daily dose of 11 units of insulin were receiving 88 grams of glucose at the end of the average period. See page 20.

Wilder and Boothby and their associates[1] have studied this method of assay of insulin very carefully. A standard preliminary diet was given their patients based upon the basal metabolism requirements with protein at 0.67 gram per kilogram body weight and carbohydrate and fat adjusted to preserve a safe ketogenic-antiketogenic ratio. On this closely calculated basis they found that 1 unit of insulin assays between 1.5 and 2 grams of glucose.

Russell and Bowen[2] also found 1 unit to be capable of utilizing about 2 grams of glucose. Woodyatt[3] found the equivalent of 1 unit of insulin in the form of glucose to vary between 1 and 1.5 grams.

An assay of the value of 1 unit of insulin in terms of glucose is quite theoretical. Our estimations of the foods entering into the diet are crude, and our estimations of the actual quantities of carbohydrate, protein, and fat burned by the body are still cruder. They vary greatly from day to day. Nearly all the patients taking insulin are gaining weight, and thus the values for the nitrogen determinations are of little consequence, because tissue protein is undoubtedly being built up. Allen[4] has shown that calories,

[1] Wilder, Boothby, Barborka, Kitchen and Adams: Jour. Metab. Research, 1922, **2**, 701.

[2] Russell, Bowen and Pucher: Bull. Buffalo Gen. Hosp., 1923, **1**, 41.

[3] Woodyatt: Jour. Metab. Research, 1922, **2**, 793.

[4] Allen: Jour. Metab. Research, 1923, **3**, 61.

quite independently of glucose, may increase greatly the insulin requirement. He goes so far as to write: "Just as it was formerly proved that reductions of total calories and body weight raised the tolerance, even when carried to an extreme degree in extremely severe cases, so now it has been demonstrable that every increase of the diet with any kind of food has required an increase of insulin dosage in these patients." Furthermore, cases are often changing in severity and one cannot be sure of constancy of the disease without prolonged observation. Finally, it depends upon the individual patient or the doctor how much glucose can be utilized by 1 unit of insulin, just as it does upon the chauffeur quite as much as upon the automobile as to how many miles may be secured from 1 gallon of gasoline. Skill counts. Just as various makes of automobiles vary in capacity to utilize gasoline, so do patients with their manifold varieties of diabetes vary in their ability to utilize glucose. Two instances alone will suffice. Olive H., Case No. 2962, entered the hospital on January 11, 1923, with 9 per cent sugar, with onset of the disease within four weeks. She became sugar-free on a Test Diet containing carbohydrate 34 grams, protein 15 grams, fat 30 grams, was transferred to Maintenance Diet 7; carbohydrate 74 grams, protein 52 grams, fat 88 grams, and progressed rapidly to $C_{12}PF_{12}$; carbohydrate 159 grams, protein 84 grams, fat 135 grams. During this time she received 5 to 9 units of insulin daily. She was discharged from the hospital, soon entered school, and one morning on coming home felt vague symptoms of weakness, and the next morning these were accentuated by an unusual hunger, and she recognized that she was having a reaction from insulin. The effect did not wholly disappear until after her second meal. At the time this patient was taking 156 grams of carbohydrate and but 4 units of insulin. It is almost inconceivable that this child who had been doing well for days should have so exhausted her carbohydrate stores that as little as 8 grams of carbohydrate were not available as such or derivable from protein to offset the 4 units which she was receiving. (See page 55 and Table 4.) The other case is that of Miss P., who usually takes 14 units of insulin three times a day and upon this dose is constantly sugar-free. By accident one day she received at morning and noon twice the quantity without the slightest sign of a reaction.

The effect of insulin upon one of the patients treated for some years with a high carbohydrate diet warrants report, because with this patient calories could be increased, but not carbohydrate, with the amount of insulin allowed. The case is that of an extraordinarily faithful boy, H. H., Case No. 1889, who developed diabetes in October, 1918, at the age of thirteen years and came under our observation on August 9, 1920. He was then able to take carbohydrate 121 grams, protein 66 grams, fat 61 grams, amounting to 43 calories per kilogram body weight, which was then 66 pounds. Between that date and re-entrance to the hospital on November 9, 1922, his weight had fallen to 61.5 pounds and his tolerance to carbohydrate 60 grams, protein 45 grams, fat 60 grams, 34 calories per kilogram body weight. Attempts to increase calories by addition of carbohydrate, protein, or fat always resulted in glycosuria. During sixty-four days of treatment with 13 units of insulin daily his weight rose to 73 pounds, his diet to carbohydrate 71 grams, protein 64 grams, fat 113 grams, or 46 calories per kilogram body weight. On January 18, 1923, he walked 10 miles, measured by a carefully adjusted pedometer, and perhaps was over-enthusiastic on returning to the hospital when he remarked that he was ready to walk 10 miles more. This boy developed several reactions while at the hospital, the most instructive of which followed one of his long walks, and it was therefore necessary to adjust his diet and insulin to the amount of exercise he was taking, although the carbohydrate in his diet was never below 61 grams when receiving insulin. With his increased diet he had one digestive upset during which 43 grams of sugar appeared in the urine in twenty-four hours, even though the insulin was 20 units. Since returning home his weight has increased to 81 pounds and his diet is now carbohydrate 60 grams, protein 55 grams, fat 110 grams, 53 calories per kilogram body weight, but he reports that he requires 24 units of insulin daily. His increased well-being is such that he is now occupying a salaried position in a bank. The increase in calories in six months has been 51 per cent, but there has been no increase in carbohydrate and the increase in total glucose amounts to but 11 grams, corresponding to only 0.5 gram for each unit of insulin, in contrast to 2 grams for my first series of cases. Calories, not glucose, have here demanded insulin.

Insulin has been given to 358 of my patients. The average daily dosage for 127 of these patients for an average period of one hundred and seven days has been 11 units daily. Twenty-nine diabetic patients in the hospital on August 22, 1923, were receiving an average of 18 units. It is significant that this group includes 5 of the 18 patients who have been given 30 or more units regularly at any time in the last year. These are Cases Nos. 1469, 1542, 2256, 2296, 2448, 2687, 2784, 2801, 3008, 3194, 2729, 2909, 1930, 3241, 1895, 1500, 2618 and 2702. With 31 children the average dosage has been 10 units during an average period of one hundred and twenty-two days, but with 13 children under the age of fifteen years, the average dosage has been 4 units for an average period of eighty-nine days. The largest quantity of insulin taken daily by a patient, excepting in coma has been 63 units, Case No. 2256. Case No. 2801 has taken 45 units and Miss M. (Case No. 1542) at times has received 35 units. The first cases treated erred in receiving too little, and it is possible that if I had given insulin more freely to Mr. P., Case No. 866, he would have gained more than 10 pounds in thirteen weeks and would have resisted erysipelas better.

The quantity of insulin required varies with the severity of the diabetes, with infections, with acidosis, food, exercise, and weight. Allen says that the minimum insulin requirement of children is lower than that of adults but the kilogram requirement of weight is considerably higher. Very likely this may be due to growth. The difference in dosage between that necessary for maintenance of weight and that demanded for growth is all-important.

The minimum insulin requirement compatible with sugar-freedom can be crudely estimated in depancreatized animals and in patients with maximally severe diabetes in a state of extreme inanition. This requirement may apparently be as low as 4 units per day in a young child, but is probably 12 units or more for an adult. Any diet sufficient for maintenance of life even on the lowest plane of nutrition probably requires a doubling of these figures. The need for insulin is related quantitatively to the body mass as well as to the quantity of food to be metabolized. (Allen.)

Dosage has not increased in our series after the patient has gained weight, and is maintaining it, as much as it has increased while the weight has been advancing. This statement is made as an impression, but is supported by some facts. Addition of diet, however, has caused an increase in the amount of insulin required even though the tolerance appeared to be improving. Miss M., Case No. 1542, when weighing 30 kilograms and receiving 1200 calories, required in the neighborhood of 30 units of insulin daily. With the same diet but with her weight at 40 kilograms or 30 calories per kilogram body weight she required 10 units. When the diet was then increased 5 per cent, it was necessary to increase the insulin as well. Now that her weight has risen to 46 kilograms and the calories to 1310 or 29 per kilogram, the insulin needed is much more. In this instance and in some others the quantity of insulin required appeared to depend chiefly upon the amount the diet was in excess of actual body requirements. For gain in weight more insulin was required than for maintenance of weight. It is the surplus diet and the gaining weight, therefore, which demand increasing units of insulin rather than the weight already added.

4. **Method of Administration.**—The routine method of administration of insulin has been cited above—the dose to be increased carefully from 1 unit before a meal to 5 units before each of the

4

three meals in a day and thereafter decreased or increased as required in order to enable the patient to receive sufficient calories. The dietetic management of the case goes on with insulin as without insulin, save that it can proceed more rapidly. For this reason repetition of the dietetic treatment of diabetes will not be given here, but reference is made to pp. 490 to 513, where it is summarized. In Table 2 will be shown empirically how this can be brought about.

TABLE 2.—ADJUSTMENT OF INSULIN AND CARBOHYDRATE TO DISPEL GLYCOSURIA.

	A.			B.			C.		
	Insulin.	Carbo-hydrate.	Sugar.	Insulin.	Carbo-hydrate.	Sugar.	Insulin.	Carbo-hydrate.	Sugar.
Insulin	5	..	..	8	..	..	10	..	..
Breakfast	..	10	..	..	10	..	..	12	..
Urine	..	..	+	..	..	0	..	..	0
Insulin	5	..	..	2	..	..	0	..	..
Dinner	..	10	..	..	10	..	..	8	..
Urine	..	..	0	..	..	0	..	..	0
Insulin	5	..	..	5	..	..	5	..	..
Supper	..	10	..	..	10	..	..	10	..
Urine	..	..	0	..	..	0	..	..	0

Section A of the table shows that the patient is receiving 5 units before each meal and that at each meal 10 grams of carbohydrate are in the diet. The urine which is voided after breakfast contains sugar, but the urine which is voided after the noon and night meals is free from sugar. Since multiple doses of insulin are to be avoided, and since it is wiser to give the insulin as many hours apart as possible in the day and thus imitate the action of the pancreas, the noon dose is the one first to be omitted. This would appear to be safe, because no sugar appears in the urine after the noon meal; consequently, section B, has been rearranged: The insulin before breakfast amounts to 8 units, the insulin at noon has been reduced to 2 units, and at night the insulin continues at 5 units; but the same quantity of 15 units is employed during the twenty-four hours. With this plan no change is made in the carbohydrate at the three meals, and it will be observed that the urine after breakfast has been sugar-free as well as after the other meals, but in order to get rid of the noon dosage of 2 units a new arrangement of insulin and diet is made in section C. Here it will be seen that the insulin has been changed to 10 units in the morning and, on account of the extra number of units and the giving up of insulin at noon, 2 grams of carbohydrate have been taken from the noon meal and added to the breakfast, but no change has been made in either insulin or carbohydrate at supper. The patient remains sugar-free throughout this period.

Various modifications of this schedule must be made to adjust the insulin to the carbohydrate in the diet. Woodyatt reports that in 90 per cent of his cases insulin is given but once a day, namely, before breakfast. Allen, on the other hand, in exceptional cases has given insulin four times in twenty-four hours. I have been unable to secure good results with a single dose and have seldom been compelled to resort to four doses, but there are very few of my patients who receive insulin more than twice a day. The severer cases only keep sugar-free throughout the twenty-four hours with 2 doses by adopting the expedient of less carbohydrate at noon than at the other meals, and by arranging for an *early* breakfast and a *late* supper. Often at the hospitals breakfasts are served at 8.00 A.M. and suppers at 5.00 P.M. The meals of diabetic patients must be further separated, and with severe cases I have found that breakfast and supper should be nearly twelve hours apart. With Case No. 2256, Miss A., if her nurse sleeps overtime and thus delays insulin until after 6.30 in the morning and postpones breakfast until after 7.00 A.M., with supper at about 7.00 P.M. the night before, glycosuria results.

Bliss[1] working with a depancreatized dog found that hypoglycemic collapse occurred if the insulin was given at one dose, even if all the food for the day was crowded into five hours.

Wilder, Boothby and their associates,[2] however, also favor the administration of insulin in a single early dose. They write: "Maximal results seem to be obtained from a given daily dose of insulin with a single injection of the entire amount about thirty minutes before the breakfast and with food distributed equally between breakfast at 8.00 A.M., dinner at noon, and supper at 5.30 P.M. . . Serial examinations of the blood sugar level after single and multiple injections of iletin also suggest that a single morning injection of a given amount will produce as low a blood-sugar curve for the twenty-four hours as can be accomplished by dividing the dosage." They present a typical experiment on an elaborate chart, which is not convincing to me of the advisability of this method. Barborka,[3] writing somewhat later, from the Mayo Clinic, states that "In cases of such severity as to require more than 30 units satisfactory results are accomplished by two distributed injections, . . ."

---

[1] Bliss: Jour. Metab. Research, 1922, **2**, 385.

[2] Wilder, Boothby, Barborka, Kitchen and Adams: Jour. Metab. Research, 1922, **2**, 708.

[3] Barborka: Med. Clin. North America, 1923, **7**, 25.

The dosage of insulin can be regulated very accurately by hourly quantitative tests of the urinary sugar with micro-analytical methods. This is shown in Fig. 1 placed at my disposal by Irwin H. Page of the Eli Lilly Laboratory. The same method is also applicable to the diagnosis of incipient diabetes and this is illustrated by Figs. 2 and 3 for a normal individual and a potential diabetic. Mr. Page will publish a micro-method which can be used by patients.

Fletcher and Campbell[1] and the Toronto group call attention to the development of acidosis in the later hours of the day if insulin is given but once in the twenty-four hours. It is my impres-

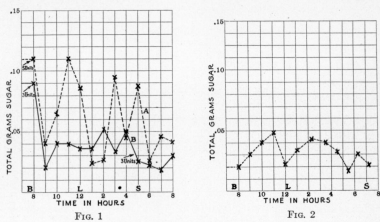

Fig. 1   Fig. 2

Fig. 1.—Regulation of insulin dosage by hourly urinary tests for sugar. (I. H. Page.)
  A. Diabetic with improper insulin regulation.
      Total, C = 80; P = 45; F = 185. Total glucose = 125°.
      The diet was equally divided throughout the meals.
  B. Same individual with proper insulin regulation. Diet was the same as
      before.
Fig. 2.—Hourly excretion sugar in a normal individual. (I. H. Page.)
  Normal individual; breakfast: C = 62; P = 23; F = 47. Lunch, C = 125;
  P = 16; F = 50. Supper, C = 58; P = 35; F = 53. Total, C = 245; P = 74;
  F = 150. Total glucose, 303.

sion that in giving insulin twice a day I am simply following the example of the Toronto workers as in many other respects.

With children who have devoted mothers it is often possible to omit an occasional evening dose, and with Billy B., Case No. 2560, this is often done for several days at a time. I question, however, the advisability of endeavoring to see with how few units a patient can get along. If the urine of the patient is kept sugar-free constantly throughout the twenty-four hours, such an attempt is quite justifiable; but otherwise not.

[1] Fletcher and Campbell: Jour. Metab. Research, 1922, **2**, 637.

A sugar-free urine is just as necessary in my opinion with diabetic patients treated with insulin as diabetic cases treated without insulin.   I believe that unless the urine is kept sugar-free during the additional length of life these patients will enjoy, complications due to hyperglycemia and glycosuria will ensue.   Hitherto there has been comparatively little opportunity to determine what the effects of hyperglycemia for long periods would be, but with the avoidance of death from coma the lives of these patients will be so much prolonged that the effects of hyperglycemia will be mani-

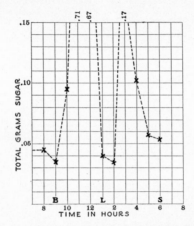

Fig. 3.—Hourly excretion sugar in a potential or suspected diabetic.   (I. H. Page.)
    Potential or suspected diabetic—Breakfast, C = 81; P = 13; F = 37.   Lunch, C = 70; P = 9; F = 22.   Supper, C = 68; P = 40; F = 81.   Total, C = 219; P = 62; F = 140.   Total glucose = 269.

fest.   Until proof accumulates that hyperglycemia is not accompanied by distressing complications such as cataract and arteriosclerosis, it appears wiser to maintain urine and blood as nearly normal as possible.

The status of the patient is known with difficulty if glycosuria is present.   The presence of more than a trace of sugar involves innumerable quantitative analyses.   The whole virtue in modern treatment has been the abolishment of quantitative analyses and elaborate methods.   To bring these all back into practice will retard the advance we have laboriously attained without insulin. One cannot have frequent quantitative analyses of sugar in the urine year in and out and so one loses control of the utilization of the diet.

Glycosuria is not only tolerated but encouraged by several clinicians highly skilled in the treatment of diabetes.   Even 20 grams of glucose in the urine are allowed with design. To this plan of treatment I am emphatically opposed. Diabetics for years have been taught to keep the urine sugar-free and it has been the general opinion among the best men treating diabetes hitherto that the danger attending diabetics with urines free from sugar is less than when the urine does contain sugar. If one faces about, allows or encourages the presence of sugar in the urine today, one breaks the patient's morale. If it is immaterial to success in the treatment of diabetes whether the urine is free or not free from sugar the patient will see no reason why he should not deliberately take food sufficient to allow the presence of sugar in the urine: Success in the treatment of diabetic children lies in keeping their urine sugar-free. If sugar appears, a penalty follows. Take away the necessity to keep the urine sugar-free and the control of that diabetic child is gone forever.

5. **Insulin in Diabetes of Varying Duration.**—The shorter the duration of diabetes, the more effectively insulin acts. The response of early discovered cases to insulin is as prompt as to diet. The duration of the disease in the first group of patients who were given insulin is shown in Table 3. This varied from four weeks (Olive H., Case No. 2962) to twenty-three years (Mrs. R., Case 2201). Measured by percentage gain in weight the cases of shortest duration advanced the most. If estimated by the number of days required to gain 1 pound in weight, the early cases again had the advantage. The average number of days required for a gain of 1 pound varied for the different years of duration between eight and nineteen days.

TABLE 3.—DURATION OF DIABETES AND GAIN IN WEIGHT IN AN EARLY SERIES OF PATIENTS TREATED WITH INSULIN.

Years.	Total number of cases.	Cases available for statistics.	Gain in weight.		Average number of days for gain of 1 lb.
			Lbs.	Per cent.	
Under 1 year	11	8	7	9	9
1– 2	14	12	6	8	10
2– 3	11	7	5	7	12
3– 4	9	6	8	11	11
4– 5	10	7	6	8	11
5– 6	7	4	4	5	19
6– 7	4	2	3	3	14
7– 8	3	2	2	1	13
8– 9	3	2	6	6	18
9–10	3	1	8	6	8
10–20	7	2	5	4	13
20–30	1	0			

An endeavor was made to determine the effect of insulin upon patients who had developed diabetes most recently. The case of shortest duration was Olive H., Case No. 2962. With this girl of twelve years, diabetes developed December 10, 1922, and she was brought for treatment on January 11, 1923, showing 9 per cent sugar in the urine. She was placed upon the routine test diets, became sugar-free in four days, beginning insulin on the third day, and eventually developed a tolerance for 155 grams carbohydrate and 41 calories per kilogram body weight. Olive's case is of especial interest because some weeks later while taking 4 units twice a day she developed a reaction, scarcely recognized the first forenoon, but definite the next, and since February 9, 1923 has not required insulin. Cases of short duration often make remarkable gains in tolerance, but seldom if ever has the gain in tolerance for carbohydrate and for calories as well been as great. From Table 4 it will be seen that insulin was used, beginning with 1 unit on the second day of treatment, and continued up to the last day in the hospital, January 31, 1923, the doses being increased to 4 units twice a day, thereafter 3 units twice a day until February 9, when it was discontinued and had not been resumed September 8 because the urine is sugar-free and the blood sugar 0.11 per cent.

TABLE 4.—DIABETES OF ONE MONTH'S DURATION. REMARKABLE GAIN IN TOLERANCE. INSULIN OMITTED. OLIVE H., CASE NO. 2962.

Date.	Diacetic acid.	Urinary sugar, per cent.	Diet in grams.				Naked weight (lbs.)	Blood sugar, per cent.	Insulin (units).
			C.	P.	F.	Cals.			
1923									
Jan. 11	..	9.0							
12–13	..	5.3	23	13	14	200[1]	90		{1
13–14	0	0.6	66	24	37	693	90	0.20	{2
14–15	0	0	35	15	30	466	89	....	{2 {3
18–19	0	0	73	51	70	1126	90	0.08	{3 {3
23–24	0	tr.	155	68	88	1684	90	....	{3 {3
25–26	0	tr.	155	68	88	1684	90	0.10[2]	{3 {3
29–30	0	0.1	155	66	88	1676	90	0.10[3]	{4 {4
Mar. 9	0	0.1	155	66	88	1676	92[4]	0.11	0
June 5	..	0	155	66	88	1676	95	0.07	0
Sept. 8	0	0	155	66	88	1676	99[4]	0.11	

[1] Supper only.
[2] Fasting one hour after insulin.
[3] Two hours after breakfast. Two and a half hours after insulin.
[4] Dressed weight.

Another early case was a little Finnish child, aged three years, Aune N., Case No. 2979. The symptoms of diabetes began October 4, 1922, and sugar was discovered December 3, 1922. The patient entered the hospital upon December 18, with 4.5 per cent of sugar and +++ acidosis. This did not immediately decrease, and five days later at midnight there were warning symptoms of coma. Insulin had not been started when she entered the hospital, but was then begun and three doses of 2, 4 and 4 units given during the remainder of the night and continued in similarly small quantities from then on. Thirty-six hours later the child had so far recovered that she sat up in bed, played at the window, and threw a kiss at the doctor on his leaving the room. Twelve units of insulin were then being given daily. The diet was steadily increased, and on January 15, 1923, the carbohydrate was 76 grams, protein 37 grams, and fat 46 grams, calories 866. Insulin was omitted occasionally before supper, and in consequence a trace of sugar appeared in the urine, promptly to disappear the next day when insulin was resumed. On March 31, the little girl returned for a morning visit, was sugar-free, and indeed had been constantly sugar-free, and was continuing her original diet, which had been arranged with design to be of extraordinary simplicity. It consisted of oatmeal 60 grams, orange 200 grams, eggs 3, 20 per cent cream, 120 cc, 5 per cent vegetables, 360 grams. August 25 she is reported sugar-free with 9 units.

An early case that surprised us by failing to respond well was that of a young girl, Case No. 2801, with an enlarged adolescent thyroid gland. Diabetes had developed acutely on June 27, 1922, been recognized on July 26, and on July 28, the patient came for treatment, showing 6 per cent of sugar and ++++ acidosis. The metabolism was +17 per cent when compared with the Girl Scout group and —20 per cent on the DuBois scale. Various methods of dieting were unsuccessful, but with insulin, begun on August 19, 1922, the patient has gained from a weight of 82 pounds to 95 pounds in the course of two hundred and fifty-four days. However, 35 units were required daily to enable this patient to utilize carbohydrate 49 grams, protein 63 grams, fat 144 grams, calories 1744. This patient is cited elsewhere as an example of the danger of the withdrawal of insulin and her death in coma reported on page 45.

Another early juvenile case, stubborn without insulin, hopeful with, was Alice S., Case No. 2802, aged fifteen years. She had resisted treatment by undernutrition during two weeks, and the outlook appeared very grave. Insulin was started, and at once improvement began. Upon admittance on August 11, 1922, which was five months after onset of diabetes, her weight was 67.5 pounds.

When insulin was begun the weight was 66.3 pounds. She left the hospital on November 2, 1922, weighing 69.3 pounds, and at present she shows a gain from the lowest weight after insulin was started of 32.5 pounds. This little girl now weighs more than she ever has in her life, regulates her own diet, and carries out her own treatment with the help of her mother.

Overweight as a result of insulin is plainly manifested by the appearance of Alice S., and she suggests a possible danger of insulin to which Allen has called attention. I had not seen her for five months when she and her doctor came to a clinic given by my patients at the Academy of Medicine in New York City. To my query she said she was taking but 1100 calories, but I am quite sure she must have been receiving more. She reports difficulty in keeping the urine sugar-free upon 24 units of insulin. A case of this sort should have the diet reduced until there is cessation of gain in weight, exercise should be promoted, and an endeavor made to increase the tolerance for carbohydrate along with diminution of the calories. This was done and on July 19, 1923, she was sugar-free on carbohydrate (28 grams), protein (51 grams) and fat (91 grams), while taking 24 units. Her fasting blood sugar was 0.33 per cent.

The keenest professional happiness of all has been to watch the resurrection of some of the frail but faithful cases who have been under care for many years. The oldest of these is Colonel P., Case No. 632. This patient developed diabetes in August, 1912, and has been reported in detail elsewhere.[1] Treatment along Naunyn's lines failed to render the patient sugar-free, but with undernutrition in 1916, this was accomplished and he lived successfully, carrying heavy responsibilities in a war office for several years, but in 1921 was forced to give up golf in which he was a champion in his Canadian city. On account of his remarkable dietetic record and excellent condition for a youthful diabetic of a decade's duration, he was not brought back for treatment until November 28, 1922, when experience had been attained with a considerable number of other cases doing less well. At that time he was living, as had been the case for many months and almost years, upon carbohydrate 15 grams, protein 69 grams, fat 103 grams. Various tests were first made with levulose and dextrose for comparison with similar tests conducted with this same subject in 1917. (See p. 541.) Following 8 units of insulin per day and levulose, the diet of this patient has been increased from carbohydrate 15 grams to carbohydrate 43 grams, and the total calories from 1263 to 1826. In the following nine months of treatment the weight has increased 14 pounds, 13 per cent from the lowest

---

[1] Joslin: Diabetic Manual, Second Edition; also Metabolism in Diabetes with High and Low Diets, Publication No. 323, Carnegie Institution of Washington, 1923.

record weight, and I have recommended that it not advance above 20 per cent below the standard weight for his age and height.

A similar case of improvement in diabetes of long standing is that of Mr. P., Case No. 866, described on p. 42.

Another patient in the Carnegie series with diabetes of fourteen years' duration, Mrs. M., Case No. 263, also returned for treatment. With 10 units of insulin daily glycosuria disappeared for the first time in many years and the diet was raised to carbohydrate 68 grams, protein 57 grams, fat 117 grams, calories 1553, or 28 calories per kilogram.

Still another case of eight years' duration and a similar length of time under my care is Case No. 812. Originally she came for treatment showing 6.4 per cent of sugar during her sixth month of pregnancy and later was successfully confined by Cesarean section at the hands of Dr. J. C. Hubbard. (See p. 649). She returned for treatment in April, 1923, and was able to take a diet of carbohydrate 107 grams, protein 62 grams, fat 119 grams and remain sugar-free with 8 units of insulin. The increase in general well-being far surpassed the increase in diet.

Cases of long standing in elderly people react to insulin slowly just as they react to dietetic treatment slowly and patience is necessary to await results. Particularly is this true with arteriosclerotic patients. With these cases the comparatively large doses of insulin may fail to render the urine sugar-free for weeks, but persistence in diet and treatment evolves success out of an apparently hopeless condition. Such an instance is that of Mr. S., Case No. 2626, who was reported in my article in the *Journal of Metabolic Research* as refractory, but he is now doing well taking 115 grams carbohydrate, sugar-free, with 10 units of insulin.

TABLE 5.—DEATH FROM ANGINA PECTORIS IN A DIABETIC, AGED SIXTY-SIX YEARS, WEIGHT 80.4 KILOGRAMS.

Date.	Urine, vol.	Diacetic acid.	Sugar, per cent.	Diet.					Blood sugar.	Insulin units.
				Gms.	C.	P.	F.	Cals.		
1922										
Nov. 16	s. s.	0	2.2	24					0.18	2
17	2400	0	0.5	12	65	28	26	606	0.18	2
18	1300	0	0.4	5	35	33	56	776	....	4
19	1900	0	0.3	6	35	33	56	776	....	4
20	2200	0	0.2	7	40	49	78	1058	....	6
21	1000	0	0.2	2	40	57	83	1135	....	6
22	....	..	...	..	44	65	99	1327	....	6

Mr. B., Case No. 705, aged sixty-six years who developed diabetes fourteen years ago, was first seen in February, 1914. He entered

the hospital November 16, 1922.   He received 28 units in the course
of six days, and died in the hospital of angina pectoris.   Death
occurred in the early morning hours of November 23, 1922, and
could not so far as we could see be attributed to insulin.   The
importance of the case merits the inclusion of the hospital chart.

Two surgical emergencies in diabetics of eleven years' and six
years' duration responded satisfactorily to treatment with insulin,
the first slowly because of the continued infection of a carbuncle
even after operation, but the second rapidly following the removal
of the infection by the amputation of the leg.   Mrs. D., Case
No. 1245, has had diabetes eleven years.   She developed a carbuncle
and later a second carbuncle which required an incision 10 inches
long.   With the help of 37 cc insulin and with the surgical assistance
of Dr. R. C. Cochrane her acidosis disappeared, she became sugar-
free and remained so.   Insulin was taken for twenty days only
and was not employed for the next eighteen weeks.   Although
she remained sugar-free and free from acidosis for much of the
time, the diet was so restricted that she has just resumed insulin.
The other patient was a Swiss, Case No. 3174, a man aged sixty-
four years with extreme arteriosclerosis and diabetes of twenty
years' duration.   Upon admittance to the hospital the sugar in
the urine was 5 per cent, acidosis +, and fever present.   Amputation of the leg was performed under spinal anesthesia by Dr. L. S.
McKittrick after three days.   He received 5 units of insulin three
times a day and eight days from entrance to the hospital was
sugar- and acid-free upon 1063 calories.

6. **Technic of Administration of Insulin.**—It is a mercy that at
present insulin becomes inert when given by mouth and that its
use is restricted to a syringe.   The medical profession cannot be
too grateful to the Insulin Committee of Toronto for limiting the
supply and the distribution for the first few months following its
discovery.   Consider for a moment what would happen if morphine
was the drug discovered and then was at once sold over the counter.
The useless pancreatic preparations of the past required no supervision; insulin does, because it is potent.

The time for the administration of insulin varies from one-
quarter of an hour to one and a half hours before meals, depending upon the rapidity of absorption of carbohydrate from the
stomach and insulin from the subcutaneous tissue as estimated
from observation of each individual patient.   As a rule, my patients
receive insulin from thirty to fifteen minutes before a meal.   With
this arrangement few reactions are obtained.   I do not believe in
deliberately producing reactions in patients.   This is contrary to
the advice and custom of many other clinicians, and time alone
will show which is the better practice.   If one gives little insulin

and in divided doses, there will be few reactions. The patients may not gain weight quite as rapidly, but it is my impression they will in the end gain as much as they should. The advantage of giving larger doses and producing hypoglycemia in patients is the development in the patients of a familiarity with its symptoms which will allow for prompt recognition and treatment. The actual injection of insulin is not an indifferent procedure. It is true that abscesses seldom develop, but "insulin burns" will develop if the insulin is injected into the superficial layer of the skin, and these should be avoided.

7. **Insulin in the Home.**—The million members of the Diabetic Club of America occasionally spend a few days in their various hospital clubhouses, but for the greater part of the time, like most club members, they live at home. If insulin is to be of permanent help in diabetes it must be usable by diabetics in their own dwellings. Constantly reference has been made to the improvement which patients have obtained after leaving the hospital. In most cases the improvement has been fully as great and in many instances greater than before they were discharged. Our attitude toward the treatment of diabetic patients in general has governed us in this regard and dosage with insulin has been kept low and calories in the diet have been kept low as well, in order that the home treatment of insulin might be safe. In the second month of treatment Thomas D., a little boy, died in coma, apparently as a result of having omitted insulin in his home. He felt so much better, had so much confidence in the good that he had received from insulin that he probably believed, as did his family, that the omission of it for a few days would be of little consequence. We have not forgotten the lesson which his case teaches. If insulin is to be used in the home, the patients must not only be educated in dietetic treatment but they must be educated in treatment with insulin. For this reason our efforts to teach patients the fundamentals of diabetes have been trebled and special exercises are given four days each week in the morning and afternoon on the diet and treatment with insulin. This has led to happy and unlooked for results. The increased attention given to education and to insulin has called forth greater coöperation on the part of the patients, and it is quite evident that the increased cost of treatment due to insulin has been offset by decreased cost of medical attendance and the shortening of hospital stay. Three-fourths of the exercises given for doctors, in connection with the John D. Rockefeller, Jr., gift for insulin, have been opened for patients.

One of the best examples of improvement of treatment in the home is Miss Pauline C., Case No. 2422, a school teacher who had become much discouraged with her diet and returned to the hospital for treatment with insulin on November 22, 1922. She then weighed 81 pounds and was 47 per cent under standard weight. During thirty days of hospital stay with dietetic treatment, supported by an average daily dose of 10 units of insulin, glycosuria and acidosis disappeared and she gained 5 pounds. On December 16, 1922, the carbohydrate of this patient was 54 grams, when levulose was added to it in 5-gram doses three times daily. This she tolerated and along with the levulose extra calories were given in the form of fat. Upon discharge from the hospital she continued to take levulose made by Mr. Bean in Prof. Folin's laboratory. Improvement continued at home and she returned a month later with a further gain of 2 pounds and without glycosuria. She answered the query ofttimes raised as to whether insulin is worth the cost, by resuming her work as a school teacher which had been abandoned for four and a half months. Her experience has been duplicated by two other teachers, by doctors, lawyers, salesmen, a policeman and even by day laborers.

Many other such cases of patients returning to work or working with far more efficiency than before the advent of insulin are available. There is no question but that accidents due to insulin in the future will occur and they must be expected, but the advantages gained by home treatment with the resumption of work more than offset prolonged periods of hospital stay. Each insulin diabetically trained patient sent home to his physician I consider the best sort of diabetic missionary. These patients are taught to coöperate with their doctors at home and to help in the details of treatment which doctors, seeing few cases, have little time to learn. If I felt the only good accomplished in the treatment of diabetes was in the treatment of my few cases under supervision the reward would seem slight, but if these patients help their physicians in the treatment of other cases then painstaking teaching is worth while. The law in Massachusetts also favors coöperation in treatment with insulin between the patients, the doctor and the hospital physician. The law declares that hypodermic syringes shall not be given, sold or kept in the possession of individuals in Massachusetts save physicians and nurses. In order to conform to the law therefore, syringes must be placed in the hands of the patient's physician and not in the hands of the patient. If the syringe is given to a patient the doctor should protect himself by a written guarantee that it is to be used by the patient alone, and only for insulin and is to be returned if the need for it ceases.

It is alluring to see patients gain weight, but it is our belief that it is safer to increase the diet so moderately and to give insulin in such conservative doses that dangers from its omission or from complications as a result of diet or the disease will be lessened.

The result of an excess of insulin and the changes which take place when the dosage and food are larger are very effectively described by Allen. "One very noticeable early effect of insulin treatment is a filling out of the face which may become noticeable within a day or two or even within a few hours after the first dose of insulin. This fullness of the face persists, and certainly in the early stage and possibly also in later stages of the treatment it is out of proportion to the general gain of weight. The skin is generally noticeably clear. The patients seem to tend readily to become obese, and it is questionable if there is not an undue proportion of fat deposited on the trunk in comparison with the limbs. The general appearance of patients who have thus been unduly fattened with insulin is more or less suggestive of the so-called dystrophia adiposo-genitalis. With proper insulin dosage and diet, adults undoubtedly recover normal musculature and strength, and children grow and develop well. Only one girl (No. 1065) has had a return of menstruation under insulin treatment. The continued absence of it in patients, such as No. 3, who have been nourished even to the point of obesity, is somewhat surprising. It will be a matter of interest to note the return of menstrual function in the cases in which it has been suppressed through many years of severe diabetes, and its delay may possibly be explained merely by organic changes during the interval. From every standpoint, however, physicians should be on their guard against the possible consequences of flooding the body with one of its most powerful hormones."[1]

Directions of various descriptions regarding insulin are given patients during their stay in the hospital, and these directions are copied below.

DIRECTIONS FOR PATIENTS TAKING INSULIN. 1. Insulin is prepared in solutions of different strengths. Know your dose in units (not in cubic centimeters) and how to measure the amount of solution to give that number of units.

2. An insulin reaction usually occurs one to two hours, but may occur as late as six hours, after an injection, and can be recognized by the sudden onset of severe hunger, weakness, sweating, trembling, or pallor. The first dose of a new preparation should always be half the last dose of an old.

3. A reaction should be treated by eating an orange, or by taking the carbohydrate portion of the next meal.

4. At present it is not prudent to use insulin without daily examinations of the urine.

5. If your usual exercise is not obtained, on that day reduce your diet.

---

[1] Allen: Loc. cit., p. 44.

6. Arrange for a supply of insulin for ten days in advance.

7. If your supply of insulin fails

    (*a*) Notify your doctor by telephone or telegraph, and

    (*b*) Omit one-third of your diet.

For the instruction of patients who receive insulin, the following directions have been prepared.

INSTRUCTIONS FOR GIVING INSULIN SUBCUTANEOUSLY.—A. STERILIZING.—Wash the hands thoroughly with soap and water. Wrap the cylinder and the piston of the syringe separately in a piece of cloth and cover them and the wired needle with cold water in a dish, heat to boiling, and let boil for three minutes. Pour off the water, being careful not to touch anything in the dish, and allow to cool by standing. Paint the top of the insulin bottle with medicated alcohol.

B. LOADING.—Draw out the piston so that the syringe contains a little more air than the amount of insulin needed.

Push the needle cautiously but firmly through the rubber cap until the point is just seen, invert the bottle; force the air from the syringe into the bottle and then withdraw as much insulin as is desired. By holding the syringe and needle-point upward air is easily expelled from the syringe before withdrawing it from the bottle.

C. INJECTING.—The desirable site for injecting insulin is one where the skin is loose. It is well to change the place with every dose. For example, the left thigh on Monday, the right thigh on Tuesday, the left arm on Wednesday, the right arm on Thursday, the left leg on Friday, the right leg on Saturday, and so forth.

Having decided on the site for injection, rub gently an area as large as a walnut with alcohol.

Pick up a fold of the skin between the thumb and forefinger of the left hand, and with the syringe held parallel to the skin, push the needle quickly and firmly into the fold nearly up to the butt. The tip of the needle should then feel loose in the soft tissue between the skin and the muscle.

Then change hands so that the butt of the needle and the end of the syringe are held in the thumb and first two fingers of the left, and the piston is held by the right hand.

Force the insulin gradually out of the syringe, while withdrawing the needle slowly, so that the insulin may not all be left in one spot.

If the insulin has been given too close to the upper layers of the skin a white blister-like elevation will appear.

Touch the spot lightly with clean cotton until the insulin has been absorbed.

D. CLEANING UP.—Rinse the syringe and needle with cold water immediately. Dry the syringe and needle with a cloth and blow air through the needle repeatedly with the syringe. Rub off any irregularities of the point on a fine stone such as a razor hone. A fine wire should always be kept in the needle

E. NEEDLES.—The needle found at the New England Deaconess Hospital most satisfactory for the administration of insulin has been one of 25-gauge and ⅞ inches long. A shorter needle, ⅝ inch, is advisable for beginners, because it requires less skill to use, and is less apt to break, but the longer penetrates to the deeper sub-cutaneous tissue. Some of the patients have used at home a gold needle with success, and this may prove to be especially adapted for continuous treatment. So far platinum needles have been only moderately satisfactory.

8. **Pain from Injection. Abscesses. Oral Administration. Omission of Insulin.**—The pain of an insulin injection is slight. Otherwise children would not so readily give it to themselves. Their little fingers are so delicate that often they can administer it with less discomfort than their elders, and this they soon recognize. With injections of insulin at the hospital no accident has occurred and but one abscess resulted. Indeed, of all of the patients who have received insulin in our series we have heard of but four instances of an abscess, either in or outside the hospital, and both of these promptly healed. One of these was in a girl, Case No. 3008, who clandestinely broke her diet, took up Christian Science and developed multiple abscesses and yet recovered. The other occurred in the hospital in a negro whose skin was most sensitive to insulin. "Insulin burns" due to the injection of insulin into the superficial layers of the skin were caused in a few instances. Presumably these were due to the tricresol used as a preservative rather than to the insulin. They were not of importance. Case No. 2448, however, had so much annoyance from the insulin which he was receiving in dilute form that he gave it up and brought himself near death's door despite our previous warnings. So soon as a stronger preparation, namely, 20 units in 1 cc was given him, his troubles disappeared. This patient was a severe case and had his diet been greater in quantity, due to larger doses on insulin, it is questionable whether recovery would have taken place. As it was, the change for the better was so great in forty-eight hours that in astonishment his uncle fainted on entering the room. On two other occasions he nearly went into coma by breaking diet or giving up insulin or both combined.

Other avenues for the administration of insulin have been sought to replace the subcutaneous method. In coma it is desirable to give the first dose of insulin intravenously, because it acts more promptly, but otherwise there is universal agreement that the subcutaneous injection is the one to be employed. Repeated trials have been made with preparations of insulin furnished by the Eli Lilly Company and two other investigators for administration by mouth. All of these tests have been unsuccessful, though at first hope was entertained that insulin so administered was yielding good results because the glycosuria was so low for one, two or three days after the subcutaneous method of injection had been omitted and the oral adopted. By the fifth day with all patients and in two days with one of the severest cases the futility of the oral method was manifest. In the last trial 450 units by mouth failed to replace 10 units insulin subcutaneously. Deprived of their insulin, the patients wilted. Already attention has been called with design on several occasions to the distressing result which transpired when the little boy, Thomas D., gave up insulin for five days. Invariably when insulin is left off the diet should be reduced at least one-third and the patient watched with closest care.

TABLE 6.—OMISSION OF INSULIN SUBCUTANEOUSLY AND ITS ADMINISTRATION BY MOUTH. MISS M., CASE NO. 1542.

Date.	Di-acetic acid.	Sugar in urine, gms.	Diet.					Glucose balance, gms.	Blood sugar, per cent.	Insulin.	
			C.	P.	F.	Cals.	Total glucose.			Subcutaneously, units.	By mouth, units.
October											
23	0	0	14	32	98	1066	43	+43	0.23	16	
24	0	0	14	32	98	1066	43	+43	....	16	
25	0	0	14	32	98	1066	43	+43	....	8	24
26	0	12	14	32	98	1066	43	+31	....	0	60
27	0	34	14	32	98	1066	43	+ 9	....	0	84
28	0	36	14	32	98	1066	43	+ 7	....	0	96
29	0	29	14	32	98	1066	43	+14	....	0	96
30	0	33	14	32	98	1066	43	+10	0.29	0	192
31	+	49	14	32	98	1066	43	+ 6	0.25	0	396
November											
1	0	11	14	32	98	1066	43	+32	0.26	16	
2	0	8	14	32	98	1066	43	+35	....	16	
3	0	5	14	32	98	1066	43	+38	....	20	
4	0	0	14	32	98	1066	43	+43	....	20	

Examples of the substitution of the oral for the subcutaneous method of administration of insulin follow:

Miss M., Case No. 1542, our first case, was free from glycosuria on a diet containing carbohydrate 14 grams, protein 32 grams, fat 98 grams. She was receiving 8 units of insulin twice daily. This was omitted and a special preparation, furnished us through the courtesy of the Eli Lilly Company, was substituted by mouth. The first day she received 24 units, the second day 60 units, the third day 84 units, the fourth day 96 units, and upon the last day 396 units. The results are shown in Table 6. During this period the diet remained unchanged. It will be seen that at once sugar appeared in the urine, that it did not increase materially for the first day, but eventually rose to 49 grams. Along with the sugar there was development of slight acidosis. At the end of the period insulin subcutaneously was resumed, and in four days the patient had regained her former tolerance. The change in the appearance of the patient during these few days was definite. The habitus of a severe diabetic returned—the dry skin, the drawn look, the bright flush in the face, and the decreased brightness of the eye.

Two months later a similar test of the oral administration of insulin was made with Miss Q., Case No. 2687, and as before, with the full approval of the patient. This test was conducted with a preparation which was thought especially desirable for such a purpose. The insulin was given in capsules. The results are to be found in Table 7. Though the patient was essentially free from glycosuria on a liberal diet, while taking 26 units of insulin daily, she promptly developed glycosuria, and, as in the case of Miss M., this increased irregularly and progressively during the period she was receiving the insulin by mouth. As with the former patient, along with the sugar in the urine acidosis developed. A similar experience was also noted by Russell and Bowen. With their Case 1, during the first three days of omission, there were only traces of glucose in the urine, but upon the sixth day the excretion had increased to 40 grams. Four days elapsed with 10 units daily before the urine again became sugar-free. I have also tried with a child, who was sugar-free on 2 units of insulin, the substitution of a pancreatic extract supposed to be equivalent to 60 units, but the result was a failure.

TABLE 7.—OMISSION OF INSULIN SUBCUTANEOUSLY AND ITS SUBSTITUTION BY MOUTH. MISS Q., CASE NO. 2687.

Date.	Di-acetic acid.	Sugar in urine, gms.	Diet.				Blood sugar.	Alveolar air, mm. Hg.	Insulin.	
			C.	P.	F.	Cals.			Subcuta-neously, units.	By mouth, units.
Dec.										
24–25	..	0	32	55	120	1428	......	..	26	
25–26	0	0	32	56	116	1396	......	..	26	
26–27	0	2	32	54	116	1388	......	..	26	
27–28	0	5	32	56	116	1396	0.20	..	0	68
28–29	0	12	32	55	116	1392	......	..	0	135
29–30	..	9	32	55	116	1392	0.19	..	0	270
30–31	..	30	32	55	116	1392	0.26—6 P.M.	..	0	540
31–Jan. 1	..	6	32	55	116	1392	0.26—9 A.M.	46	20	210
1– 2	..	0	32	55	116	1392	......	..	26	
2– 3	..	2	32	55	116	1392	......	..	26	
3– 4	..	10	32	54	116	1388	......	..	26	
4– 5	..	6	32	58	116	1404	......	..	26	
5– 6	..	4	32	58	116	1404	......	..	30	
6– 7	0	0	22	40	48	680	......	..	30	
15–16	0	0	31	57	115	1387	......	..	30	

Insulin has also been given intranasally, by rectum and by vagina. Telfer[1] is the only author who claims any degree of success by other than oral methods, and he employed inunctions.

Omission of Insulin.—The experience with the cases just cited, who have omitted insulin, is a definite warning of the danger of this omission by any patient whose diet has been increased with its help. Too much emphasis cannot be laid upon the danger of continuing the high diet when insulin is discarded. The foundations for the increased diet are certainly removed when insulin is omitted. All patients upon discharge from the hospital should be thoroughly instructed to reduce the diet if for any reason they do not obtain insulin or if for any reason they suspect the insulin has deteriorated in strength. They should be warned that the danger creeps on slowly and gains in intensity from day to day. With increased diets due to insulin they are walking on insulin stilts. The longer the stilts, the greater the danger of a fall when they are taken away. In this diabetic game one is treating patients for years and the closer one keeps to the ground, the better.

With gastro-intestinal upsets, especially when accompanied by vomiting and diarrhea, when less food is taken, insulin should be reduced, but here from a different danger, namely, hypoglycemia. Yet these upsets may be complicated by acidosis, so that it requires a clear head to detect what is going on. Bed, nursing, liquids, a little carbohydrate in the form of orange juice or a cracker or two (5 grams carbohydrate) and expectant treatment, will enable one usually to weather the squall.

The correct balancing of carbohydrate given, and insulin injected is a nice problem. Emergencies of this kind have not developed in my practice but I realize the possibility and the importance of the advice from other writers. Precautions have been taken to have glucose accessible for an emergency. Whereas it is advisable that the glucose solution should be fresh and sterilized, Allen states that this is not an absolute prerequisite and a filtered glucose solution can be substituted. The percentage of glucose commonly employed is 5 per cent and the quantity given 500 cc, but one can employ 20 per cent solution of glucose and give a correspondingly smaller quantity.

Insulin can, however, be discontinued fairly abruptly in at least three types of patients: Those recovering (1) from surgical emergencies; (2) from acute infections; and (3) from severe acidosis in mild diabetes. In severe acidosis, by common consent, it should be diminished very gradually. Rapid changes in insulin dosage may be made under close observation in the hospital, but only gradual changes should be attempted in the home.

[1] Telfer: British Med. Jour., 1923, **1**, 715.

Insulin can be omitted gradually in certain cases of recent onset, even in children, and with increasing frequency in elderly patients. Time enough has not elapsed to show whether it is for a temporary or a prolonged period. Case No. 2962 and Case No. 3078 represent the former type (see pages 55 and 74) and Case No. 3310 the latter.

The total number of omissions of insulin among those treated during the first year was 35. The number is so considerable, because insulin was used to shorten hospital stay and later was found unneccessary in order to maintain weight and strength and a carbohydrate intake of about 70 or more grams. There were 24 cases of this type. Some 6 cases later were able to omit it after recoveries from operations for prostatectomy, gangrene and cataract. The two little girls, often mentioned, are the most striking examples of gain in tolerance.

9. Protein Reactions.—Reactions due to the injection of insulin other than those caused by a lowering of the blood sugar were reported with the use of the first preparations employed. Such reactions have developed at most with but 4 of our patients. With Case No. 2802 urticarial wheals occurred with pruritus, and these were relieved by bathing with sodium bicarbonate and a whitewash. Severer reactions, however, have been noted by others, though with very rare exceptions. Wilder and Boothby[1] obtained these in but 3 of their patients, and likewise their experience was confined to the early days of the production of insulin. They described such a reaction as follows:

"The patient in Case 2, had been without insulin for five days, and received, December 2, 1922, at 8.10 A.M., 30 units of iletin 722845, followed by a light breakfast. At 8.15 A.M. he was nauseated, his face flushed, and he vomited. Severe pain developed in the epigastrium followed by diarrhea and profuse sweating. The pulse, at first full and bounding, became weak and slow, 50 each minute. At 8.50 A.M. he was drowsy, the epigastrium pain was less severe, but persisted as a dull ache. One hundred grams of orange juice were given by mouth. At 9.00 A.M. he was more alert and by 9.10 A.M. all the symptoms had disappeared and the pulse was strong, with a rate of 86 each minute. This reaction was believed to be due to hypoglycemia, particularly because the symptoms abated so promptly after the orange juice was given. We were disillusioned, however, as soon as the report of the blood sugar reached us. Blood drawn at 8.45 A.M. contained 270 mg. of sugar for each 100 cc. At 10.00 A.M. a moderate urticarial rash developed around the arm, and to some extent, on the face support-

---

[1] Wilder, Boothby, Barborka, Kitchen and Adams: Jour. Metab. Research, 1922, **2**, 701.

ing the evidence that the reaction was not due to hypoglycemia, but was a protein effect."

A severe protein reaction was also obtained in one patient treated by Williams.[1]

"Case 1524 for several months was given the extract prepared by the University of Toronto from the pancreas of beef animals. Later, when the preparation of the Lilly Company was substituted, which is made from pancreas of the pig, the patient experienced promptly most severe anaphylactic reactions which apparently could not be overcome. All attempts to use highly purified and practically protein-free extract have proved futile and have had to be abandoned. The following is a description of the phenomenon observed after an injection of the pork material September 23, 1922. Patient apparently normal, no pruritus, urticaria or edema evident. Five cubic centimeters insulin injected intramuscularly. Three minutes later patient stated that upper lip felt stiff and swollen, followed rapidly by dry mouth. In ten minutes lips became greatly swollen. Small wheals then appeared on all parts of the body. The reaction increased in violence for two hours, during which time the wheals became larger and coalesced. No nausea or vomiting occurred. Patient very weak and prostrated. Heart sounds rapid, regular, clear. Lungs normal. Adrenalin, 15 minims subcutaneously and atropine sulphate $\frac{1}{100}$-grain by mouth were given, affording slight relief. Twenty-four hours later patient had recovered from the reaction, but was very weak. The weakness and prostration persisted for four days. During this time much skin exfoliated from various parts of the body. It is interesting to note that this patient has been having beef extract since May 17, 1922, to February 1, 1923. . . .The patient has exhibited no evidence of sensitivity against beef material, which dispels the fear one time entertained that he might become sensitive to this and other proteins and make the administration of the extract a difficult problem."

It is not right to administer insulin to a patient without understanding the influence which it exerts in decreasing the sugar, fat, and ketone bodies in the blood and presumably in the body tissues generally and the indirect influences which are thereby exerted upon the metabolism of the patient. Therefore, these topics will be considered in some detail.

10. **The Effect of Insulin upon** (a) **Sugar of the Blood.**—The effect of insulin upon the fall in the blood sugar is most easily studied. Case No. 3129 entered the hospital on April 20, 1923, with 5 per cent sugar in the urine, $+ + + +$ acidosis, and a blood

[1] Williams: Jour. Metab. Research, 1922, **2**, 729.

sugar of 0.40 per cent two hours after food. Following a subcutaneus injection of insulin of 10 units at 11.30 o'clock and 10 units four hours later, the blood sugar fell in five hours to 0.08 per cent.

Fig. 4 placed at my disposal by R. Fitz shows graphically the descent of the blood sugar curve following a single injection of 15 units of insulin with the passing of the phenomenon and a beginning rise by the end of ten hours. Table 8, shows the lowering in blood sugar following the administration of 20 units of insulin to a series of diabetic and non-diabetic patients and Table 9 the fall of blood sugar in 2 patients who were given varying amounts of insulin, as observed by Fletcher and Campbell.

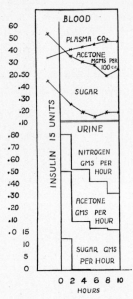

Fig. 4.—Effect on blood and urine of a single dose of insulin. (Fitz.)

The extent to which the blood sugar drops in different individuals with the same dose of insulin varies greatly. The percentage fall is less in non-diabetics than in diabetics, and the actual fall is, as is to be supposed, of far less degree. The limits of variation are so wide with the same number of units that it is not safe to predict what change a single unit will produce. In general, the greater the number of units, the greater the fall in percentage of blood sugar, but the fall is not proportionate to the amount of insulin used. Thus, with 10 units the decrease in blood sugar was 0.057 per cent, with 20 units 0.082 per cent, but with 30 units it was only 0.1 per cent. With another case 10 units lowered the blood sugar 0.037 per cent, 20 units 0.083 per cent, 30 units 0.081 per cent, but upon another day 0.118 per cent, and 50 units lowered the blood sugar even less; *i. e.*, 0.088 per cent.

It is well to bear these varying possibilities in mind in the administration of insulin, because they awaken caution and further hint at the futility of large doses of insulin.

The lowest percentage of blood sugar after insulin may be reached at variable periods, from one-half hour to as late as twelve hours, and the blood sugar likewise returns to normal at a variable rate.[1] The tendency of the blood sugar to fall during fasting and the variations which the blood sugar will naturally undergo when the body is or is not supplied with a moderate quantity of glycogen

---

[1] Fletcher and Campbell: Loc. cit., p. 638.

undoubtedly exert an influence upon the action of insulin. The higher the blood sugar, the greater its fall, as a rule, following injections of insulin in normals as well as in diabetics.

TABLE 8.—FALL IN BLOOD SUGAR FOLLOWING THE ADMINISTRATION OF TWENTY UNITS OF INSULIN IN DIABETIC AND NON-DIABETIC PATIENTS. A. A. FLETCHER AND W. R. CAMPBELL.[1]

Case No.	8 A.M.	9 A.M.	10 A.M.	11 A.M.	12 Noon	1 P.M.	2 P.M.	3 P.M.	Lowest blood sugar.	Initial blood sugar minus lowest B.S.	Blood sugar fall in per cent of initial B.S.
1*	.089	.090	.083	.120	.080	....	....	....	.080	.009	10.1
2*	.094	.079	.070	.064	.075	....	....	....	.064	.030	31.9
3*	.10	.083	.068	.064	.063	....	....	....	.063	.037	37.0
4*	.113	.071	.091	.077	.107	....	....	....	.071	.042	37.1
5	.118	....	....	.071	.071	....	....	....	.071	.037	31.3
6*	.12	.093	.096	.088	.099	....	....	....	.088	.032	26.6
7	.133	.099	.089	.077	.082	....	....	....	.077	.056	42.1
8	.148	.133	.125	.102	.100	....	....	....	.100	.048	31.0
9	.154	.163	.153	.089	.088	....	....	....	.088	.066	42.8
10	.160	.147	.133	.107	.077	....	....	....	.077	.083	51.8
11	.161	.172	.137	.090	.068	....	....	....	.068	.093	57.7
12	.163	.143	.122	.094	.090	....	....	....	.090	.073	44.7
13	.182	.174	.141	.10	.10	....	....	....	.10	.082	45.0
14	.20	.192	.182	.120	.097	....	....	....	.097	.103	51.5
15	.20	.178	.138	.097	.086	....	....	....	.086	.114	57.0
16	.208	.186	.175	.128	.110	....	....	....	.110	.098	47.8
17	.208	....	....	.182	.160	....	....	....	.160	.048	23.0
18	.280	....	....	.21	.170	....	....	....	.170	.110	39.2
19	.330	....	....	.182	.158	.174	.154	....	.154	.176	53.3
20	.360	....	....	.270	.217	.199	.20	.207	.199	.157	44.0

TABLE 9.—FALL IN BLOOD SUGAR FOLLOWING THE ADMINISTRATION OF VARYING AMOUNTS OF INSULIN IN PATIENTS H AND D. A. A. FLETCHER AND W. R. CAMPBELL.[1]

Case.	Amount of insulin.	8 A.M.	9 A.M.	10 A.M.	11 A.M.	12 Noon	1 P.M.	2 P.M.	3 P.M.	Lowest blood sugar.	Initial B.S. minus lowest B.S.
H.	10 units	.170	.196	.166	.137	.113	....	....	....	..113	.057
	20 units	.182	.174	.141	.110	.10	....	....	....	.10	.082
	30 units	.185	.152	.085	.091	....	....	....	....	.085	.100
	Later 20 units	.118	....	....	.071	.071	....	....	....	.071	.047
D.	10 units	.172	.189	.147	.138	.135	....	....	....	.135	.037
	20 units	.160	.147	.133	.107	.077	....	....	....	.077	.083
	30 units	.182	.164	.178	.120	.101	....	....	....	.101	.081
	30 units	.20	.142	.132	.106	.082	....	....	....	.082	.118
	50 units	.152	....	....	.077	.074	.068	.072	.064	.064	.088

[1] Fletcher and Campbell: Jour. Metab. Research, 1922, **2**, 640.

* Non-diabetic patient.

[2] Fletcher and Campbell: Loc. cit., p. 643.

The maximum period of influence exerted by insulin upon the percentage of blood sugar is eight hours. The highest blood sugars, therefore, should be found before breakfast, because this is usually fourteen hours removed from the last injection of insulin. It was, therefore, a gratifying surprise to learn that in my series of 53 diabetics who were treated for sixty-three days with insulin the average morning blood sugar had fallen from 0.24 per cent before insulin to 0.19 per cent at the end of the period despite the higher diets instituted.

The lowering of the blood sugar is explained by Forrest, Smith and Winter[1] on the basis that the alpha and beta glucose is transformed into gamma glucose.

(1) *Hypoglycemia.*—Hypoglycemia is the result of an overdose of insulin. This state may occur in diabetics, however, quite apart from insulin administration, and on p. 174 various instances are cited. In diabetics the fall in blood sugar below normal is usually accompanied by a definite train of symptoms. These may appear when the blood sugar falls to 0.08 per cent, though they are frequently not manifest until the blood sugar is 0.07 per cent. Hunger and tremor are the outstanding symptoms, but nervousness and weakness are also present, as well as pallor, flushing of the face, dilated pupils and increased pulse-rate.

At 0.07 per cent to 0.05 per cent of sugar in the blood sweating, anxiety, vertigo and faintness appear with emotional instability, hypotonia and diplopia may be manifest. These symptoms are all accentuated with further lowering of the sugar in the blood. Aphasia and delirium may occur and even convulsions, which, as in rabbits under similar conditions, may alternate with coma. The subject may go into a collapse with low blood-pressure and low temperature, though but 1, or at the most 2, of my cases have been unconscious or even on the verge of unconsciousness. With others bradycardia has appeared and during unconsciousness a loss of control of the sphincters.[2]

Symptoms do not invariably develop when the blood sugar falls to 0.05 per cent, and in a single instance in one of my cases symptoms of a reaction were absent when the blood sugar was as low as 0.03 per cent. With this patient, Case No. 2909, the percentage of sugar in the blood was carefully checked and the observation must be regarded as reliable. Fletcher and Campbell report their lowest blood sugar as 0.025 per cent. This was found in their patient during the course of an influenzal bronchial pneumonia, but with glucose the patient recovered from the hypoglycemia. However, with a blood sugar at 0.035 per cent, according to the experience

[1] Forrest, Smith and Winter: Jour. of Phys., 1923, **27**, 113.
[2] Fletcher and Campbell: Loc. cit., p. 645.

of Fletcher and Campbell, the patient is usually unconscious. A reaction is also more severe and more prolonged with undernourished patients, just as Macleod found it with dogs deficient in glycogen. The experience of Fletcher and Campbell, and our experience at the hospital coincides with this. Woodyatt[1] writes that another patient "received in extreme inanition, ... but free of glycosuria, was given a large increase of diet and a calculated dose of insulin. This case developed hypoglycemic convulsions and the blood sugar was then at a level too low to read. Sugar administration restored hyperglycemia and gross glycosuria, but the patient died without regaining consciousness."

Clinically, it is important to remember (1) that the patients who are most undernourished are the ones who receive the most insulin; (2) that any diabetic has a far smaller glycogen factor of safety than a normal; (3) that in coma and fever larger doses of insulin may be required temporarily and that the need soon passes; (4) that insulin should be counterbalanced by a meal at least within an hour; (5) that oftentimes patients improve in tolerance for carbohydrate and a formerly suitable dose of insulin becomes an overdose; (6) that exercise taken in unusual amount may act like an additional dose of insulin and hasten a reaction.

(2) *Hypoglycemic Reactions.*—The cause of hypoglycemic reactions cannot wholly be explained by the low percentage of blood sugar. Blood sugar percentages as low as 0.06 are not so very rarely observed in the course of any series of blood tests. Indeed, children show these low percentages of blood sugar quite frequently. The accumulation of some toxic substance in the blood appears responsible for the effects, such an accumulation being rendered possible by variations of sugar in solution. "It may possibly be that through the lowering of blood sugar certain oxidative processes become depressed to such a degree that the brain cells are affected in much the same manner as in asphyxia."

A description of a reaction in the language of one of my patients, Miss Q., Case No. 2687, follows: She had received her insulin at 7.00 A.M. and her breakfast at about 7.30 A.M. "About 10.30 A.M., while in the kitchen helping the nurse to get out lunches, I began to feel rather warm about the neck and forehead. I opened the door to get a little fresh air, as I thought the heat from the stove made me feel warm. I then began to feel a little nervous and shivery about the legs and body, and when one of the girls spoke to me I sort of looked blank and my voice seemed trembly. Right then I knew I was having a reaction and immediately tested my urine. I found I was sugar-free, so reported to Miss Kenseth.

---

[1] Woodyatt: Jour. Metab. Research, 1922, **2**, 793.

I lay on my bed, and Dr. Gray took my blood. After that I rested five to ten minutes and that peculiar feeling left, so I did not eat the 100 grams of grapefruit which the nurse brought in."

Hypoglycemic reactions have been purposely produced in some clinics with the object of acquainting patients with their character. When one uses small quantities of insulin and changes the dose but an unit at a time, such reactions are neither common nor severe and it has seemed unnecessary to subject patients to a toxic dose of insulin any more than to a toxic dose of any other drug. At the New England Deaconess Hospital hypoglycemic reactions have never been induced with design.

False hypoglycemic reactions are not uncommon. Fear that they might be simulated in order to obtain additional carbohydrate as the antidote led us to suspect one little boy, who in pre-insulin days had so frequently broken his diet. He became so accustomed to blood-sugar tests upon the occasion of a reaction that in answer to the query put to the Diabetic Class—"What do you do if you have a reaction?"—invariably he would reply—"Have a blood sugar test." He never deceived us, for his blood sugar tests were always low. Several patients, two young men and a professor, were quite sure they were having reactions when their blood sugar percentages were 0.29, 0.22 and 0.24. Case Nos. 1978, 2784 and 1078. The appearance of two of the young men so closely resembled patients who were having a true reaction as to mislead a nurse and an assistant of great experience. In such a dilemma the presence of sugar in the urine may solve the situation, but should glycosuria be absent a blood test alone would be conclusive. Six months after two young girls, Case Nos. 2962 and 3078, had given up insulin, because of gain in tolerance they felt on several occasions that they were experiencing a reaction. This occurred near the time of catamenia.

Treatment for an hypoglycemic reaction consists in the prompt administration of any carbohydrate out of which glucose can be quickly formed.[1] Orange juice acts very well and is especially suitable, because while peeling the orange the patient has time to reflect and decide as to whether he is actually having a reaction due to an overdose of insulin and thus not take the carbohydrate unnecessarily and therefore harmfully. An orange is less temptation to a child than two or three pieces of sugar or even of candy. Honey or corn syrup can be given if the patient does not swallow easily. Any solution of sugar of this type could be administered by stomach tube, by intranasal catheter or by rectum. If the condition of the patient is critical, the glucose may be given in a

---

[1] Noble and Macleod: Am. Jour. Phys., 1923, **64**, 547.

solution of 5 to 20 per cent strength, the total amount given not exceeding 25 grams. Raffinose and rhamnose are types of sugar which are ineffective in insulin hypoglycemia.[1]

Protein, also, may serve as an antidote to insulin, but according to Sherrill[2] "protein ranks below preformed carbohydrate in respect to glycosuric effect and insulin requirement when the substitution is made on a basis of either equal caloric value or theoretical glucose content. Though hypoglycemia may be prevented by sufficiently large quantities of protein, this influence is surprisingly feeble and by no means in proportion to the theoretical value."

Epinephrin has been employed as an antidote to insulin. Indeed, it was with the hope of standardizing epinephrin with extract of the pancreas which led Zuelzer to seek for an active pancreatic extract. It will act even more quickly than carbohydrate in overcoming an hypoglycemic reaction. The dose is 1 cc, 15 minims, of a 1:1000 solution. Though epinephrin is a valuable antidote with diabetics whose carbohydrate store is not utterly exhausted, it is probably useless in greatly undernourished cases, unless accompanied by the ingestion of carbohydrate.

In none of my 350 or more cases treated with insulin has it been necessary to use either glucose solution intravenously or to give epinephrin.

(*b*) **Blood Fat.**—The changes which the fat in the blood undergoes after insulin have been studied less than the alterations in the sugar. In the discussion of the experiments upon animals by the Toronto workers attention has already been drawn to the decrease of storage of fat in the liver. One might, therefore, expect a similar decrease in the accumulation of fat in the blood.

TABLE 10.—DECREASE OF BLOOD FAT WITH DIET AND INSULIN. CASE NO. 2448.

Date.	Diacetic acid.	Sugar in urine.		Diet.				Blood fat, Bloor, per cent.	Insulin, units.
		Per cent.	Gms.	C.	P.	F.	Cals.		
1922									
Oct. 18	..	6.5	169	110	18	0	512	2.28	8
Oct. 20	..	2.4	82	64	29	19	543	1.74	12
Oct. 23	sl.–	0.3	5	3	2	0	20	1.56	16
Oct. 26	0	0	0	17	27	52	644	1.50	16
Oct. 30	0	0	0	55	51	68	1036	1.57	16
Nov. 6	0	0	0	67	66	106	· 1486	0.94	16

NOTE: The diet, urinalyses, and insulin dosage are given for the twenty-four hours preceding the date of the fat determination.

[1] Campbell and Fletcher: Jour. Am. Med. Assn., 1923, **80**, 1641.
[2] Sherrill: Jour. Metab. Research, 1923, **3**, 59.

My own data upon the changes in the fat of the blood of diabetics treated with insulin are not numerous. Mr. C., Case No. 2448, showed a fall in percentage of total fat in the blood from 2.28 per cent on October 17, 1922, to 0.94 per cent on November 6. The urinary findings, the diet, and dosage of insulin during this period are given in Table 10.

The change in blood fat in Miss M., Case No. 1542, our patient longest under treatment with insulin, is also definite. On August 2, 1922, the fat in the blood was 3.18 per cent and on October 2, 1922, it was 0.67 per cent.

TABLE 11.—DECREASE OF BLOOD FAT WITH DIET AND INSULIN. CASE NO. 1542.

Date.	Diacetic acid.	Sugar.		Diet.				Blood fat, Bloor, per cent.	Blood sugar, per cent.	Insulin.
		Per cent	Gms.	C.	P.	F.	Cals.			
1922										
Aug. 2	+	1.4	59	13	26	82	894	3.18	0.35	0
Aug. 7	+	0.8	22	13	26	82	894	1.72	0.33	0
Aug. 9	+	1.4	46	24	29	83	959	2.82	0.30	0.6 c.c.
Aug. 11	+	1.1	47	24	29	83	959	2.20	0.30	2.0 c.c.
Aug. 14	+	1.0	40	24	29	83	959	3.00	0.32	0
Aug. 18	Sl. +	0.5	20	24	29	89	1061	1.46	0.25	4.0 c.c.
Aug. 28	0	0.6	35	33	37	96	1144	1.80	0.24	0
Sept. 5	0	0.2	11	33	45	99	1203	1.70	0.24	4.0 c.c.
Oct. 2	0	0.6	30	33	45	101	1221	0.76	0.31	6 units.
Oct. 11	0	0.4	18	22	30	68	820	0.89	0.26	12 units.
Oct. 23	0	0	0	14	32	98	1066	0.88	0.23	16 units.
Nov. 6	0	tr.	0	16	33	98	1078	0.67	0.14	20 units.
Dec. 2	0	0.5	..	25	36	81	973	....	0.24	20 units.
1923.										
Jan. 18	0	0.3	10	25	47	104	1224	....	0.22	20 units.
Mar. 26	0	0	0	26	43	105	1221	....	....	25 units.
Apr. 30	0	0	0	30	50	110	1310	....	....	11 units.
May 23	0	0.1	2.5	30	50	110	1310	....	0.26	15 units.
May 25	..	...	..	30	50	110	1310	1.00	0.19	15 units.

A really strikingly rapid fall in the percentage of fat in the blood took place with a patient who presented lipemia retinalis.[1] Here the blood fat amounted to 6.3 per cent on the day after admission, fell to 2.95 per cent in four days, and in six days to 2.2 per cent. During this interval the amount of insulin given was 63 units.

Still more rapid was the decrease of lipemia in one of the cases reported by Bock, Field and Adair.[2] In this patient's blood on January 29, at 7.30 P.M., the total fat was 10.5 per cent; at 11.30 P.M., 6.27 per cent, and on January 31, 11.30 A.M., 4.37 per cent.

(c) **Ketone Bodies.**—*Acidosis.*—A decrease in acidosis registered by a fall in the ketone bodies can be anticipated from the changes which have been shown to take place in the sugar and fat of the blood. If the sugar is burned and the fat is burned, the ketone bodies must decrease, and this in fact takes place. This fall in

[1] Gray and Root: Jour. Am. Med. Assn., 1923, **80**, 995.
[2] Bock, Field and Adair: Jour., Metab. Research, to be published.

ketone bodies is strikingly shown in a chart which Reginald Fitz constructed from studies upon the blood chemistry of one of his cases of diabetic coma and by his courtesy is inserted herewith. Fig. 5 also exhibits the accompanying changes in blood sugar and blood CO_2.

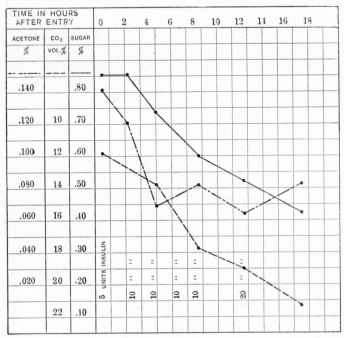

Fig. 5.—The effect of insulin on the blood chemistry of a case of diabetic coma. (Reginald Fitz.)

During sixteen hours there was a precipitous descent of ketone bodies from 140 to 60 mg., and the percentage of blood sugar from 0.6 to 0.14 per cent along with the administration of 65 units of insulin. In passing it should be noticed that the rise in carbon dioxide in the blood was not commensurate with the fall in ketone bodies. For Bock's and Fitz' explanation of this phenomenon see p. 86. This discrepancy between acetone bodies and CO_2 was also observed by Banting, Campbell, and Fletcher, and by others. The curves also demonstrate that the percentage of sugar in the blood falls more rapidly than the decrease in percentage of ketones and that ketones both disappear later from the urine and return earlier than glycosuria as observed first in Toronto.

Banting, Campbell and Fletcher[1] also have published an excellent

[1] Banting, Campbell and Fletcher: Jour. Metab. Research, 1922, **2**, 547.

table showing the two-hourly output of sugar and ketones in the urine for a twelve-hour period following injection of insulin Table 12.

TABLE 12.—VARIATIONS IN SUGAR AND KETONES IN URINE AND BLOOD AFTER INSULIN. BANTING, CAMPBELL AND FLETCHER.

Time.	Volume, c. cm.	Sugar.		Ketones.	
		Per cent.	Grams.	Mg. per liter.	Mg. per 2 hrs.
7– 9	40	0.75	0.3	1737	70
9–11	250	0	0	262	66
11– 1	520	0	0	0	0
1– 3	460	0	0	0	0
3– 5	470	0	0	213	100
4– 7	240	0.43	1.16	491	115

TABLE 13.—INFLUENCE OF INSULIN UPON CARBOHYDRATE AND NITROGENOUS METABOLISM OF A DIABETIC. REGINALD FITZ.

Time, hours.	Nitrogen excretion per hour, grams.	Urine.			Blood.			Insulin, units.
		Sugar excretion per hour, grams.	Total acetone excretion per hour, grams.	Sugar, per cent.	Acetone mg. per 100 c.c.	CO_2 vol., per cent.		
Entry.	Urine excreted at entry before insulin was injected had 5 per cent sugar and a + + ferric chloride reaction. The acetone was 0.26 per cent.			0.47	55.0	35.2		15
0.2	0.82	13.00	0.52					
2	...	.....	...	0.27	36.9	42.6		
4	...	.....	...	0.20	31.8	44.5		
2.5	0.53	Trace	0.10					
6	...	.....	...	0.17	29.0	46.5		
5.8	0.43	None	0.04					
8	...	.....	...	0.20	20.0	48.4		
8.10	0.33	None	0.03					
10	...	.....	...	0.20	26.4	48.4		

The influence of insulin upon the carbohydrate and nitrogenous metabolism of a diabetic patient and incidentally upon the acidosis is beautifully exhibited in Table 13 furnished me by R. Fitz. His moderately severe diabetic was given a ten-hour "Insulin Fast Day" and analyses of the blood and urine made at two-hourly intervals. The urine excreted at entrance to the hospital before insulin was given contained 5 per cent sugar, the ferric chloride reaction ++, and the acetone as total acetone bodies was 0.26

per cent. The blood sugar was 0.47 per cent, blood acetone 55 mg. per 100 cc, and the carbon dioxide in volumes per cent 35.2. Fifteen units of insulin were then given.   Within six hours the blood sugar was 0.17 per cent and the glycosuria had disappeared.   During ten hours the nitrogen excretion fell from 0.82 gram per hour to 0.33 gram per hour and the total acetone excretion from 0.52 gram per hour to 0.03 gram per hour.   It is true that fasting alone would lower the hyperglycemia, nitrogen excretion, and acidosis, but no one could expect such marked reductions in so short a period as ten hours.

The influence of insulin upon carbohydrate metabolism has been sufficiently discussed elsewhere, but it is appropriate here to mention its effect upon protein metabolism.   That this is reduced the table of Fitz would indicate, but the subject is by no means simple.   In this special instance we have: (1) The influence of fasting, which in itself would lower protein metabolism, not only on account of the temporary absence of food, but because of the permanent effect of fasting; (2) the sparing action of the combustion of carbohydrate which saves calories otherwise required from protein and fat; (3) the saving of calories indirectly, because of better utilizability of fat.   In observations of longer duration in which nitrogenous metabolism has been observed to change from a minus to a plus basis all these factors come into play, and also another factor which in long continued observations is of greater importance, namely, the extra amount of food which the patient is given and, because of its utilization, is able to retain and use for the formation of new tissue.   The change in nitrogen metabolism is therefore an indirect, rather than a direct, result of insulin.

The influence of insulin upon acidosis can easily be predicted from its effect upon the metabolism of carbohydrate.   When carbohydrate burns freely, acidosis disappears.   Even a fasting diabetic with little store of carbohydrate in the body is shown by insulin to have enough carbohydrate available for combustion, when properly burned, to allow the complete combustion of fat.   Insulin shows that the diabetic has more depots of carbohydrate at his disposal than have been credited to him.   That insulin plus carbohydrate should dispel acidosis could be anticipated, but that insulin plus carbohydrate already existing in the body should so quickly dispel acidosis is another of the marvelous properties of this extract. From where does the carbohydrate come which is burned?   To a considerable extent from the blood, as shown by the falling blood sugar, though perhaps not more than (4000 cc blood x 0.0047) 12 grams in this way, though an additional quantity may come from sugar in solution in the tissues, for we must not forget the body is about 60 per cent water, and hence presumably the balance from the oxidation of carbohydrate derived from the protein metabolized—(0.82 gram nitrogen per hour x 2) + (0.53 gram x 3) + (0.43 gram x 2) x 3.65 = 13 grams. This experiment with insulin shows at one stroke how little total glucose is required to lessen acidosis, providing it is completely oxidized.

Coma and its Treatment with Insulin in Various Clinics.—Insulin has improved the results of treatment in acidosis and coma to a remarkable degree. "From January 1, 1912, to January 1, 1923 of a total of 844 cases of diabetes mellitus admitted to the Massachusetts General Hospital 68 died in coma, and no case recovered from this state except one. . . ." write Bock, Field and Adair[1] —and then proceed to report 5 cases of diabetic coma cured.

TABLE 14.—RECOVERY FROM IMPENDING COMA WITHOUT ALKALI OR INSULIN.

Case No.	Date.	$FeCl_3$.	NH_3 gm. (24 amt.)	Plasma CO_2 combining power, vols. per cent.	Alveolar CO_2 mm. Hg. tension.	Notes.
755	Apr. 15, 1917	+	1.6	....	18	
786	June 11, 1916	++	3.9	....	18	
938	Nov. 2, 1917	++++	1.3	....	18	
942	July 13, 1916	++	3.7	....	17	
1011	Sept. 25, 1917	++++	4.3	....	15, 15, 16	
	Sept. 26, 1917	++	....	....	18	
1012	Sept. 13, 1917	+++	....	....	14, 15	Deep respiration.
	Sept. 14, 1917	++	2.5	30	16	
1120	Sept. 7, 1916	+	....	....	18	Deep breathing.
1196	Dec. 10, 1916	+++	3.3	....	18	Nausea, vomiting, air hunger.
1200	May 29, 1917	+++	2.3	....	18, 18	Nausea.
1410	Oct. 21, 1917	++++	....	....	16, 16	
	Oct. 22, 1917	++	....	....	16, 17, 16	Air hunger, vomiting.
1566	June 30, 1919	+++	....	18	12	
	July 1, 1919	++++	3.4	....	15	
	July 2, 1919	++	3.2	33	21	
1673	Sept. 7, 1920	++	3.1	26	18	
	Sept. 24, 1920	+	3.05	....	18	
	Sept. 30, 1920	+	5.5	....	14	Weak and drowsy.
	Oct. 4, 1920	+	....	27	..	
	Oct. 5, 1920	+	7.2	....	..	
	Oct. 9, 1920	+	....	....	16	
2074	Nov. 16, 1921	+++	....	23	18	Air hunger.
2218	June 13, 1922	++++	....	....	18	Air hunger.
2366	Sept. 29, 1921	++++	3.0	15.9	14, 11	Soft eyeballs, vomiting. Kussmaul respiration, stuporous but could be roused.
	Sept. 30, 1921	+++	4.4	....	22, 22, 22	
	Oct. 1, 1921	++	....	....	26, 28	
	Oct. 3, 1921	+	3.8	33	32, 30	

[1] Bock, Field and Adair: Jour., Metab. Research, to be published.

Cases of severe acidosis may recover without insulin but rarely a case on the border line of actual coma has come back to life. Examples of this kind are presented in Table 14. In this table 15 cases of recovery are reported from acidosis when the CO_2 percentage in the alveolar air was between 11 and 21 or the CO_2 volume combining power of the blood plasma between 15.9 and 33 volumes. Since such results are obtained without insulin, reference here will be made to but 4 of our own cases treated with insulin which are of equal severity. Cases of coma treated with insulin which have resulted fatally teach less than the successfully treated cases, because of early errors in the use of insulin. "In a multitude of counsellors there is wisdom" and I shall therefore draw freely from the experience of other clinics which has been more extensive than my own in actual coma. Before insulin is considered a failure in diabetic coma one should await the report of the autopsy.

Wilder and Boothby[1] record 2 cases of acidosis similar in severity to those described in the series in Table 14 treated prior to the use of insulin. They write, "Two patients (Case 9, A411219 and Case 10, A409679) both with plasma carbon dioxide combining power of 18 volumes per cent, 1 with a blood fat of 9 per cent, were restored to symptomless and safe serological conditions within thirty-six hours. One patient received a total of 50 iletin units in 3 doses, and the other, 60 units. Each had 600 grams of orange juice. No alkalis or other drugs were employed. We have not found it necessary to accompany the doses of insulin in these cases with other than small doses of carbohydrate, and we do not believe it advisable to resort to larger doses of sugar intravenously or otherwise. The tissues of these acidotic patients are saturated with sugar and considerable quantities of insulin should be tolerated without danger of hypoglycemia. Adding sugar should merely delay results." To these sentiments I heartily subscribe and until discouraged by untoward results shall continue to administer in coma and precoma moderate doses of insulin, moderate doses of carbohydrate and no alkalis. Particularly would it appear undesirable to give much carbohydrate. Allen has shown in dogs and men that hyperglycemia is harmful; Petrén lays great stress upon the dangers of marked hyperglycemia and Blum, Schmid and Schwab at the Fifteenth French Congress of Medicine have anew pointed out its toxic action.

Thus far I have had an opportunity to use insulin in few cases of this type.[2] Perhaps our experience at the New England Deaconess Hospital is unusual; at any rate it must be said that of 477 cases coming for treatment for diabetes on my service since insulin was

---

[1] Wilder, Boothby, Barborka, Kitchen and Adams: Jour. Metabolic Research, 1922, **2**, 714.

[2] See page 564 for report of a recent case; also Joslin: Med. Clin. North America, 1923, Boston Number; Rort, idem, and Shedd, idem.

begun August 7, 1922, up to August 7, 1923, there have been but 2 cases of actual coma of purely diabetic origin and 2 deaths. The other cases of acidosis promptly recovered with insulin varying . in amount from 14 units to 50 units the first twelve hours and not over 30 units any twelve hours subsequently. One of the patients who died was the little boy Thomas D., the first severely acidotic case to be treated. His death occurred October 20, 1922, seven and a half hours after entrance. Whether with the knowledge of the experience of other clinics he could now be saved is a possibility. At that time insulin was so new that we gave him only 8 units on admission, three hours later 16 units more, and in the following two hours which preceded his death the remaining 16 units. During this interval the blood sugar rose from 0.41 per cent to 0.54 per cent. At entrance the plasma CO_2 was 7 volumes per cent. The other case had been in coma one entire day before admission, was brought about 100 miles in an automobile and died within seven hours. My other cases deserve mention simply in the form of a table because they so readily recovered.

TABLE 15.—RECOVERY FROM ACIDOSIS WITH INSULIN.

Case No.	Date.	$FeCl_3$.	Plasma CO_2 combining power vols., per cent.	Alveolar CO_2 mm. Hg. tension.	Insulin units in 12-hour periods,		
					1	2	3
2687	Nov. 27, 1922	+++	31	17	14	12	8
2448	Apr. 24, 1923	++++	21	17	50	30	0
3129	Apr. 20, 1923	++++	29.9	22	25	10	20
3137	May 13, 1923	++++	20	14, 15	40	20	30

The above groups of cases from the Mayo Clinic and the Deaconess Hospital are encouraging, but the occurrence of coma in other clinics has allowed more striking results to be obtained.

W. H. Olmsted at Washington University, St. Louis, has had a remarkable series of 10 patients in precomatose or comatose condition. Six of these had blood alkalies below 15 volumes per cent. Many of these patients were actually in coma according to his definition. "When I speak of coma I mean a patient showing the following signs and symptoms: (1) Mental condition in which the patient will not respond to questions, or is not oriented as to time or place; (2) typical air hunger; deep forced inspiratory motions; (3) blood alkali below 20 volumes per cent; (4) diacetic acid in the urine in large amounts."[1] Bock, Field and Adair define coma somewhat differently. "A diabetic patient who, without other

---

[1] W. H. Olmsted: Personal communication, April 13, 1923.

cause is oblivious to his environment, who is not roused at all or with great difficulty, and who is incapable of any complicated response, is in coma. In this clinical state the tension of alveolar CO_2 is usually below 15 mm. of mercury and hyperpnea is invariably present."[1] To the latter definition of coma I can subscribe except for the last four words. One of my patients, Case No. 1070, described in detail on page 660, was in diabetic coma *without* hyperpnea. This appeared so extraordinary to Dr. F. G. Benedict at the Carnegie Laboratory and to my assistants, that we asked Dr. Francis Peabody's technician, Miss Barker, to confirm our analyses of blood and alveolar air, and this she did. The analyses for the CO_2 in the alveolar air as made in the laboratory at the New England Deaconess Hospital and in the laboratory at the Peter Bent Brigham Hospital were respectively as follows: CO_2 in alveolar air 12 mm. 15 mm.; CO_2 in volume percentage in blood 23.2, 27.5. To the first definition of coma the fourth criterion of Olmsted has been made perhaps irrelevant since it was written by the work of Bock and his confréres soon to be presented. However, Olmsted writes; "Of these symptoms, it seems to me, the two last are by far the most important. I believe that the symptoms of air hunger and coma depend on the response of the patient to a certain amount of diacetic acid in the blood. It has been my observation that older patients with arteriosclerosis will show signs of coma more quickly than a younger patient. An old person may show coma with a blood alkali of 25 or 30 volumes per cent, whereas a younger person will not show evidence of coma before the blood alkali is below 20 volumes per cent, and it is for these reasons that I think the laboratory data is the true basis for coma. I have never seen a blood alkali below 20 volumes per cent where the patient was not comatose."[2]

For the privilege of inserting this series of studies upon coma from Washington University I am most grateful to Dr. Olmsted. In Fig. 6 will be shown the remarkable rise in the few hours of the volume per cent, of the CO_2 in the blood of 9 patients. Nothing equal to this series has been known hitherto in the treatment of diabetic coma. In Table 16, which I have compiled from data also furnished by Olmsted, are given other facts relating to his cases which will be discussed subsequently to the presentation of an even still more extraordinary group of patients showing recovery from coma studied by Bock, Field and Adair.[1]

The important discovery in the 5 cases of diabetic coma treated at the Massachusetts General Hospital centers around Case 4 in

[1] Bock, Field, Adair: Jour., Metab. Research, 1923.
[2] W. H. Olmsted: Personal communication, April 13, 1923.

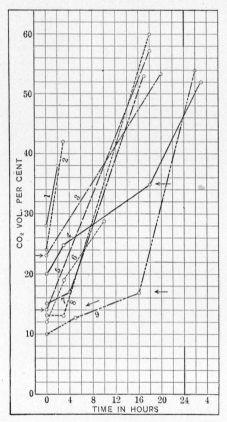

Fig. 6.—Recovery from coma, or severe acidosis in nine cases of diabetes.
(W. H. Olmsted.)

TABLE 16.—AMOUNT OF INSULIN AND ALKALI NECESSARY TO BRING BLOOD ALKALI
TO NORMAL. W. H. OLMSTED.

Case No.	Age.	Blood sugar, per cent.	CO_2		Insulin units.	Alkali, grams.	Result.		
							Immediate	Remote.—Dead.	
			Vol. per cent.	Alv. air.				After days.	Cause.
I	18	0.407	14.0		90	36	Recovery	35	Unable to get insulin.
II	14	1.40	27.7		27	0	Death	..	Uremia.
III	76	0.39	20.2		65	24	Recovery	16	Bronchopneu.
IV	39	.....	23.0		25	20	Recovery		
V	40	0.58	12.6		70	0	Recovery	6	Gangrene.
VI	39	0.75	14.5		150	0	Recovery		
VII	50	0.39	13.6		27	56	Recovery	42	Septicemia.
VIII	73	0.31	10.0		118	40	Recovery		
IX	73	0.36	24.0		17	8	Recovery	17	Gangrene(?)
X	23	0.36	13.6		130	32	Death	..	Pul. T. B.

Date.	Hour.	Insulin, units.	C. G.	P. G.	F. G.	NaHCO G.	Diacetic acid.	N. G.	Sugar G.	Blood sugar, per cent.	Arterial.	Venous.	Alkali reserve, vol. per cent.	CO₂ alveolar mm.	pH.
							Case 1								
Jan. 4	19	50[1]	54	0	0	6	+++	27.0	270.	0.41	7.5	8.5		8.7	7.17
5	1		144			6	+++			0.28		17.6	23.2	26.5	7.25
	7	75					Lost			0.31	26.9	30.3	53.9	30.7	7.38
6	15		81	0	0		0	26.5	30.0	0.23	41.1	42.7		35.2	7.38
7	12	30	40	40	0		0	17.2	40.0	0.26		44.2			
8	11	30	20	20	0		0	13.7	18.0	0.17	47.8	49.9	59.2	35.2	
		10													
							Case 2								
15	9	90[2]	200	0	0	19		9.9	154.0	0.45	11.2	19.1[3]		12.5	7.20
16	9	45	99	0	0			18.0	63.8	0.29	39.5	45.1		29.4	7.38
17	10	20	58	20	0			20.0	73.5		35.3	38.5		26.0	7.39
18	9	15	40	20	0			10.9	28.5	0.20	51.0	53.4		37.8	7.38
19		10	10	20	0		0	12.8	44.0	0.22					
							Case 3								
9	11	80[4]	110	0	0	9	++	3.8	30.0	0.33	7.1	9.4	15.9	8.3	7.17
23										0.21		24.0			
10	8	75	75	50	0		0		15.0	0.30	34.7	35.8	25.0	25.0	7.39
	16									0.29		41.8			
11	15	30	25	50	0		Trace	5.8	0	0.15					7.57
							Case 4								
29	19	60[5]	105	0	0		+++			0.45	6.2	9.9	13.8	9.7	7.03
30	6	210	93.5	0	0	24	+++	3.4	8.8	0.42	11.8	17.1	22.6	10.5	7.29
	15									0.30	19.3			15.7	7.34
31	11	95	72	0	0	12	0	2.3	Trace	0.11	34.6	36.2	42.8	21.4	7.46
Feb. 1	8	35	64	40	0	4	0	3.1	0	0.18	34.0			33.5	7.41
2	8	35	40	40	50	21	0	2.8	0	0.41	21.0			16.9	7.36
3	16										35.0				7.44
4	9	15	40	40	50	27	0	2.7	0	0.36	26.5			19.7	7.38
5	10	15	40	40	50	22	0	5.3	5.2	0.29	50.5	52.8			7.49
		15	40	40	50			6.5							
							Case 5								
Jan. 16	17	34[6]	63	7	3	32	+++		60.0	0.34		11.1	18.1		
	20									0.37		8.5	14.6		
17	24	68	123	6	3	44	+		52.0	0.39		9.4	16.9		
	8									0.25		24.3	35.0		
18	16	44	60	30	0		Trace		23.5	0.21		43.8	55.8		
19		18	40	30			0		43.8	0.24		50.1	61.9		
										0.12		56.8	68.0		

[1] 7.30 P.M. to 12.00 M.   [2] 9.30 A.M. to 12.00 M.   [3] Variation between arterial and venous values due to tourniquet.   [4] 11.30 A.M. to 12.00 M.   [5] 7.30 P.M. to 12.00 M.   [6] 5.00 P.M. to 12.00 M.

Table 17. With this patient Bock, Field and Adair observed that after 60 units of insulin, "and notwithstanding the fact that considerable quantities of ketones must have disappeared, very little change with respect to CO_2 in the blood was found. A possible explanation of this phenomenon was that some other acid than the ketone group was responsible for the persistence of acidosis, and it was therefore decided to give alkali to take up the extra acid. After alkali therapy was begun the response was slow, as inspection of Table 17 will show, but it was satisfactory and we believe that the use of alkali in this patient was life saving. As noted above, on two occasions there was a return of acidosis following the omission of soda although the absence of ketones by the ferric chloride test was continuous and complete. On the occasion of the first relapse into acidosis on the fifth day and for several subsequent days, the titration of the urinary acidity, after the technic of Van Slyke and Palmer,[1] gave the following results, the figures as given being for grams per liter."

TABLE 18.— URINARY ACIDITY IN DIABETIC COMA. BOCK, FIELD, AND ADAIR.

Date.	Total organic acid, 0.1 N.	Total[2] acetone, 0.1 N.
February 2	2610	43
3	960	0
4	380	109
5	190	35
6	200	10

[1] Van Slyke and Palmer: Jour. Biol. Chem., 1920, **41**, 567.
[2] "These analyses were made for us at the Peter Bent Brigham Hospital by Drs. R. Fitz and P. Starr."

These really exquisite series of investigations which at once saved the lives of 5 human beings and advanced scientific knowledge were made possible in part by a clause in a will, originally written by President Eliot. At the time of its writing, President Eliot pointed out to me that it was unwise to make a gift for one special disease, because one never could tell when the need for that special disease would pass.

The clause was as follows.—"To the President and Fellows of Harvard College and their successors I give $50,000, the same to constitute a fund to be known as the Proctor Fund for the Study of Chronic Diseases: The income of said fund to be devoted to the care in a hospital or hospitals of persons afflicted with chronic diseases, and to investigations into the nature and treatment of the same: The special disposition of the income of said fund to be under the control of the Heads of the Departments of Theory and Practice, Clinical Medicine and Pathology in the Harvard Medical School."

Subsequently, another sum of $50,000 was added to the fund by a relative of the donor. The fund has been well expended. The Committee has systematically selected a disease for investigation for a period of years, presented to the larger hospitals in Boston a plan of campaign for the study of this disease, received their cordial coöperation and in return for financial help the hospitals have on their part placed at the disposal of the investigators free beds. This originally modest fund has done much to amalgamate scientific with philanthropic work, as well as the activities of the Harvard Medical School with those of the Boston City Hospital, the Massachusetts General Hospital, and the Peter Bent Brigham Hospital.

Bock, Field and Adair continue the discussion of their cases as follows: ". . . The nature of the organic acid remains unknown but of its existence there can be no doubt. A review of the cases of diabetes dying in coma at the Massachusetts General Hospital from January 1, 1912 to January 1, 1923, has disclosed the fact that 15 of a total of 68 died with either a very slight ferric chloride test for diacetic acid in the urine or none at all. A number of them had a high output of ammonia. It seems not unlikely that certain of these cases may belong to the same group as does the case under discussion here. The cases reported by Rosenbloom,[1] McCaskey,[2] and Starr and Fitz[3] are possibly in the same category. Apart from its merit as a therapeutic agent, the value of insulin must be emphasized in this connection. It enabled us to recognize at once the existence of a type of acidosis that must be considered in every case of severe diabetic acidosis."

"The Administration of Insulin.—The amount and rate of administration of insulin in these cases have varied greatly. In Case 5, our first case, we proceeded with more caution than in the subsequent cases, giving the patient 8 units every two hours during the first twenty-four. Case 1, was given 10 units intramuscularly and 20 units intravenously at once followed by 10 units an hour for 2 doses, then 10 units every two hours. Case 2, was given 10 units an hour for five hours, then every two hours. Case 3, received an initial dose of 15 units, then 10 units every hour for six hours, then every two hours. Case 4, received 15 units each for four hours, then 10 units every hour. The total amount of insulin given in each case is recorded in the tables.

"During the period of eight or ten hours after treatment with insulin has been started and when most of the ketones are being eliminated or destroyed, we have administered from 50 to 100 units of insulin. For two or three days following this period it seems essential in our experience to give from 30 to 50 units daily since the patient recovering from coma has very little if any sugar metabolism for a period approximating this time. And 20 to 30 units daily may well be continued for a week or ten days after recovery from coma in order to prevent as far as possible the tissue destruction that goes on apace in most cases. We overstepped the amount of insulin necessary in Case 4 by about 150 units, failing to realize at the time that the action of insulin might be negligible when acids other than ketones are present.

"The clinical experience and experiments of Banting and his

[1] Rosenbloom: New York Med. Jour., 1915, **102**, 204.
[2] McCaskey: Jour. Am. Med. Assn., 1916, **66**, 350.
[3] Starr and Fitz: Personal communication.

associates[1] appear to demonstrate that insulin promotes the combustion of glucose. It therefore follows that carbohydrate should always be available in the body when insulin is being employed. We have found that in states of coma it is necessary to give about 1 gram of carbohydrate for each unit of insulin injected. After the coma has cleared up as much as 4 grams of carbohydrate may be burned with 1 unit of insulin or else other features of an improved metabolism account for the increase. A safe guide to follow would be to have a small amount of sugar appearing in the urine during the time when insulin is being pushed."

"*The Use of Alkali in Diabetic Coma.*—The objection to the administration of alkali is directed chiefly against the promiscuous use of it, while the argument for its use is based on the fact that normally bicarbonate of soda is one of the most important elements in the blood and necessity demands a replacement when there has been a serious loss of it.

"Our experience in the treatment of 5 successive cases of coma leads us to advocate the restricted use of bicarbonate of soda in diabetic acidosis on grounds that we believe are rational, safe and essential for the patient's welfare. Four of 5 cases received alkali, 3 in very small amounts and 1 a total of 76 grams. Each of these 4 might have done as well without alkali as with it so far as our evidence goes. In the remaining case, on the other hand, the failure to respond to insulin therapy and the presence of large amounts of unidentified organic acid were strong indications for the use of soda. Until it is possible to differentiate clinically the latter type of cases from the others, it seems advisable to use alkali in the early hours and days of treatment in every case of coma. If frequent examinations of the blood for CO_2 are possible, alkali need not be given unless it is found after four or five hours of insulin therapy that the CO_2 of the blood has not increased. This delay, however, may be attended with risks. If the patient is not in hospital, alkali should be given until the danger from acidosis is passed.

"The manner of administration and dosage of alkali are important considerations. We have employed in general a regime advocated by Stillman[2] in which 3 grams of bicarbonate of soda dissolved in a tumbler of water are given by mouth every hour. If it may not be given by mouth, we give 5 grams dissolved in 6 ounces of water by rectal injection every two or three hours. The alkali is given until the acidosis has essentially cleared up. It is not necessary to continue giving alkali until the reaction of the urine is alkaline,

[1] Banting, Best, Collip, Campbell and Fletcher: Canadian Med. Assn. Jour., March, 1922.
[2] Stillman: Arch. Int. Med., 1919, **39**, 261.

but it must not be continued if the urine is no longer acid in reaction.[1]
We feel that the intravenous use of bicarbonate of soda, except in
small amounts, is contraindicated on grounds mentioned by Allen,
Stillman and Fitz:[2] 'It is probably bad policy to try to force a low
blood alkalinity suddenly up to or above normal by large alkali
dosage, especially intravenously. Progress is favorable if the
level of the plasma bicarbonate tends distinctly though gradually
upward.' With the use of insulin large doses of alkali appear to
be unnecessary. The object to be accomplished can be met with
an amount of soda approximating 25 to 40 grams a day and this
need not be continued for more than two or three days in most
cases."

To the management of cases of diabetic coma there is little to
add to the suggestions of Wilder, Olmsted, Bock and Fitz and
their co-workers. As for the cases in the Mayo Clinic and the
New England Deaconess Hospital when the CO_2 in the blood was
above 20 volumes per cent or the CO_2 in the alveolar air above 15
the amount of insulin required to relieve the situation was comparatively small, varying from 17 units upwards. So soon, however,
as the percentage of CO_2 in the blood or alveolar air fell below this
level, greater and greater quantities of insulin were employed.
Thus, with patients whose CO_2 in the blood was 15 volumes per
cent, or below, Olmsted gave his patients respectively 90, 70, 150,
27, 118, 130 units of insulin in twenty-four hours. Bock and his
co-workers on the other hand with equally severe cases employed
respectively 50 units in the first four and a half hours with
Case 1, 90 units in the first fourteen and a half hours with Case
2, 80 units in the first twelve and a half hours with Case 3, 60
units in the first four and a half hours with Case 4, and 34 units
in the first seven hours with Case 5. These data therefore allow
a general rule for the administration of insulin to be formulated
somewhat as follows: With patients whose alveolar air shows CO_2
above 15 mm. pressure and CO_2 in the blood above 20 volumes per
cent, 10 units of insulin may be injected intravenously every hour
for four doses unless rapid improvement occurs and thereafter 10
or 5 units may be injected every two hours for another four doses
to be followed by about 30 units per day. Improvement in such
cases is apt to be so rapid that over-dosage from a sugar-free urine
or hypoglycemia must be carefully sought. When the alveolar
air is below 15 mm. mercury and the percentage of CO_2 in the
blood below 20 volumes per cent the first intravenous dose of
insulin should be 20 units and 20 units more in the next hour.

[1] Stillman: Loc. cit., p. 88.
[2] Allen, Stillman and Fitz: Total Dietary Regulation in the Treatment of Diabetes, New York, 1919, p. 113.

From then onward doses greater than 10 units an hour are allow-able only when laboratory data are available for immediate and accurate control of the condition of the acidosis and of the percent-age of the blood sugar. Yet one must not be too dogmatic because Dr. G. H. Shedd, of New Hampshire, brought one of my patients out of complete coma with 240 units of insulin. Cases almost in coma recover without insulin. A few units of insulin should insure not only greater safety for this comparatively large group of acidosis cases, but should rescue those who present a somewhat greater intensity of acidosis. Indeed, the number of patients requiring heroic doses of insulin, because of the severity of their acidosis, must be extremely small.

The administration of alkalis in these cases must be determined by each practitioner. It is obvious that if alkalis are required, the dosage is small in comparison with that formerly advised. In no instance was more than 56 grams of sodium bicarbonate given in twenty-four hours by Olmsted or Bock.

Any treatment of diabetic coma will result disastrously unless the closest attention is directed to the general condition of the patient. Methods which resulted in successful treatment of severe cases of diabetes without insulin all apply here but to avoid repeti-tion reference is made to p. 551.

Pneumonia complicated a case of coma at the Peter Bent Brigham Hospital and a case of severe acidosis at the New England Deaconess Hospital. A tabular record of the former case was kindly furnished me by Reginald Fitz and is shown in Table 19.

TABLE 19.—THE EFFECT OF INSULIN ON THE BLOOD CHEMISTRY OF A CASE OF DIABETIC COMA COMPLICATED BY PNEUMONIA.[1]

| Hours after admission. | Blood. | | | Insulin, units subcuta-neously. Per cent. |
	Sugar per 100 cc. Gm.	Acetone bodies as acetone per 100 cc. Gm.	Plasma carbon dioxide. Volume.	
0	0.84	0.139	11.9	5
$1\frac{1}{2}$	0.84	0.120	....	10
$3\frac{1}{2}$	...	....	....	10
$5\frac{1}{2}$	0.73	0.073	13.9	10
$7\frac{1}{2}$	0.60	0.081	17.8	10
$11\frac{1}{2}$	0.52	0.063	18.7	20
$16\frac{1}{2}$	0.41	0.081	21.4	20

The story of the case at the New England Deaconess Hospital is as follows: Mr. C., Case No. 2446, carried coal upstairs and was feeling fairly well on the morning of December 8. He had a chill

[1] Fitz, Murphy, Grant: The Effect of Insulin on the Metabolism of Diabetes. From the Medical Clinic of the Peter Bent Brigham Hospital, 1923.

at 2 P.M., of the same day and entered the hospital at 8.30 P.M. on December 9. He was drowsy, but not unconscious. Respiration was typically Kussmaul in type and no doubt the depth and noisy character of his breathing helped obscure signs of the true condition of his lungs. He was energetically treated with subcutaneous injections of salt solution, given 80 grams of carbohydrate by mouth and rectum and all the details of treatment for coma carried out. Upon entrance to the hospital the urine contained 2.8 per cent of sugar and the acidosis was $+++$. During fourteen hours in the hospital he received 100 units insulin. The blood sugar *increased* from 0.41 per cent to 0.57 per cent and the CO_2 in the blood rose also from 14 volumes per cent to 22 volumes per cent. During the night the clinical picture changed. Grunting respiration and cough appeared and respiration became shallow. The appearance of diabetic coma changed. He died suddenly at 10.50 A.M., December 10. At autopsy lobar pneumonia of the right upper lobe in the stage of gray hepatization was found. Table 20.

TABLE 20.—RELIEF OF ACIDOSIS BUT NOT OF HYPERGLYCEMIA DURING LOBAR PNEUMONIA. CASE NO. 2446.

	Urine.		Blood.		Insulin, units.
Date and time.	Diacetic acid.	Sugar, per cent.	Plasma CO_2, vol. per cent.	Sugar, per cent.	
December 9–9 P.M.	$+++$	2.8	20.7	0.41	
December 9–9.30 P.M.	$+$	2.8	31.9	0.57	100
to					
December 10–10 A.M.					

These 2 cases are useful because each showed improvement in the severe acidosis and did not die of it, but of pneumonia. They are also useful for comparison because in the case of Fitz the blood sugar fell steadily from 0.84 per cent to 0.41 per cent, whereas with my patient it rose from 0.41 per cent to 0.57 per cent. The dosage of insulin given in the 2 cases was approximately the same, but my patient received carbohydrate and that of Fitz received none.

The quantity of carbohydrate given to patients in severe acidosis or coma along with the insulin has been small in most of the successful cases and there is general agreement in this regard between clinicians at the Mayo Clinic, New England Deaconess Hospital, Washingtom University, Massachusetts General Hospital and the Physiatric Institute. The general consensus of opinion favors the use of about 50 grams of carbohydrate in the form of 500 cc of orange juice. Someone has written: "The rising blood sugars act as a stimulus to pancreatic activities for a time. High blood sugars appear rapidly to fatigue the insular tissues." If this

Table 21.—Disappearance of Acidosis with Insulin. Case No. 2687.

Date.	Diacetic acid.	Sugar in urine.		Alveolar air, mm. Hg.	Blood total acetone, mgm. 100 cc.	Blood CO₂, volume per cent.	Blood sugar, per cent.	Diet in grams.				Insulin, units.
		Per cent.	Gms.					C.	P.	F.	Cals.	
Nov.												
27–10 P.M.	+++	2.5	..	17	....	30	0.45					
27–28 (12 hr.)	++	2.6	31	..	....	..	0.39–8 A.M.	50	6	0	224	14
28–29	+	1.8	28	27	30.6	..	0.34–5 P.M.	52	29	24	540	12
Dec.												
4– 5	++	1.3	22	..	....	..	0.30	24	51	97	1173	18
8– 9	++	0.4	5	36	....	..	....	25	50	98	1181	22
11–12	0	...	..	..	....	..	0.24	27	51	103	1239	24
15–16	0	...	..	36	....	..	....	32	55	108	1320	30

In July, 1923, this patient was reported to have broken her diet. In August she temporarily gave up scales and was brought back to the hospital in her city in coma. With 25 units of insulin every two hours for 4 doses she regained consciousness. Will this patient repeat the experience of Case No. 2801, pages 44 and 45? Case No. 2448 has several times returned to the hospital on the verge of coma, when he has broken diet and discarded insulin. Moral: Diabetic patients must not overeat either taking or not taking insulin. For the case of coma most recently treated at the New England Deaconess Hospital, see Case No. 3382, page 564.

is true and it would seem probable, there is all the more reason for not giving large quantities of glucose along with insulin in the treatment of coma. In the early cases in Toronto rather more carbohydrate was employed and Allen also recommends larger doses under certain circumstances. In certain of the early cases of coma treated at Toronto as well as in certain of the cases of coma treated by Allen, larger and even heroic doses of insulin were employed, but the results do not appear to be superior to those at Washington University or at the Massachusetts General Hospital. Allen raises the question as to whether in addition to the harm of hypoglycemia which may result from large doses of insulin there may also be a toxic effect of the insulin itself when 200, 300 or more units are used. As yet this is unproven.

Following recovery from coma there is also general agreement that the patient should be protected with 10 units or more of insulin administered three times a day for several days, even though the acidosis and hyperglycemia have greatly decreased. Failure to observe this rule has led to a recurrence of symptoms.

(*d*) **Metabolism.**—With such striking changes as have been reported for the sugar, fat, and ketones in the blood one might expect equally striking changes in the metabolism of these patients, particularly with reference to the respiratory quotient. The effect of insulin upon the metabolism of diabetic patients can be studied in several ways: (1) The immediate effect, and (2), the effect during the course of a period of weeks. Obviously the former method furnishes more direct data, because the changes in body tissue and body weight which take place in patients over a period of time also influence the metabolism and conceal the picture.

The immediate effect of insulin on the basal metabolism was negligible with Case No. 2448 and Case No. 2801. To the latter 15 units of insulin were given and three observations of the metabolism made in the following fifty-six minutes. Breakfast was then taken by the patient and the metabolism at once rose, reaching a maximum of 14 per cent at the end of two hours, and again at noon the patient received 15 units of insulin and after a meal the metabolism rose steadily in the subsequent eighty-eight minutes to a maximum of 21 per cent. Similar results were obtained with several other individuals to whom insulin was given. The effect of the ingestion of levulose upon the metabolism of a patient, both with and without insulin, was also determined, and the details of these tests are shown in Tables 22 and 23. On the day without insulin, following the ingestion of 75 grams of levulose the basal metabolism rose to a maximum of 14 per cent and the respiratory quotient rose from 0.77 to a maximum of 0.98 thirty-four minutes after levulose. (See Table 24.) A similar observation was repeated thirteen days later, save that 12 units of insulin were given the patient prior to his taking levulose. (See Table 25.) Following the insulin and levulose, the metabolism rose to a maximum of 19 per cent and continued higher for a longer period than in the experiment without insulin. The respiratory

TABLE 22.—IMMEDIATE EFFECT OF SIX UNITS OF INSULIN ON BASAL METABOLISM AND RESPIRATORY QUOTIENT, OCTOBER 20, 1922. CASE NO. 2448, AGE NINETEEN YEARS, HEIGHT 172 CMS., WEIGHT 43.5 KGS.

Time, hours and minutes.	Oxygen consumed per minute, cc.	Carbon dioxide eliminated per minute, cc.	R. Q.	Calories per 24 hours.	Blood sugar, per cent.
Average basal	198	150	0.76	1355	0.28
		6 units of Insulin.			
12′ p. insulin	208	143	0.69	1406	
23′ "	209	147	0.70	1410	
1° 0′ "	198	143	0.72	1339	
1°10′ "	197	139	0.71	1329	1°19′ 0.24
1°50′ "	203	151	0.75	1384	
2° 0′ "	196	139	0.71	1321	
2°36′ "	190	131	0.69	1285	
2°46 "	198	145	0.73	1345	3° 0.22
Average	200	142	0.71	1352	

TABLE 23.—EFFECT OF INSULIN UPON THE METABOLISM AND RESPIRATORY QUOTIENT OF CASE NO. 2801 WITHOUT AND. WITH FOOD, JANUARY 2, 1923. AGE, SIXTEEN YEARS; HEIGHT, 161 CM.; WEIGHT, 38.1 KG.

Time. Hrs. and min.	Oxygen consumed per minute, cc.	Carbon dioxide eliminated per minute, cc.	R. Q.	Calories per 24 hours.	Per cent increase.	Blood sugar, per cent.
Average basal	179	130	0.73	1215	....	0.40
	15 units of inulin at 9.26 A.M.					
36′ p. insulin	177	123	0.70	1149 ⎫		
46′ "	179	130	0.72	1212 ⎬	−2	
56′ "	176	131	0.74	1198 ⎭		
		C P F	Cals.			
Breakfast	8	13 34	390 at 10.55 A.M.			
35′ p. breakfast	194	143	0.74	1318	+9	
43′ "	192	146	0.76	1314	+8	
52′ "	95	146	0.75	1331	+10	
1° 2′ "	197	152	0.77	1349	+11	1°12′
						0.30
1° 52′ "	197	144	0.73	1336	+10	
2° 2′ "	202	156	0.77	1387	+14	
	15 units of insulin at 1.19 P.M.					
	C P	F Cals.				
Dinner	18 31	44 592	at 1.54 P.M.			
1° 8′ p. dinner	207	146	0.71	1397	+15	
1° 18′ "	213	153	0.72	1440	+19	
1° 28′ "	217	158	0.73	1471	+21	

quotient, on the other hand, did not rise quite as high after insulin as it did in the experiment without it, but it continued higher from about one hour after the insulin than in the other test. Whereas insulin and levulose together failed to raise the respiratory quotient to as high a level as levulose alone, the increase of metabolism when insulin and levulose were given together was greater. Davies[1]

TABLE 24.—EFFECT OF LEVULOSE ON BASAL METABOLISM, NOVEMBER 7, 1922. CASE NO. 2729, AGE, TWENTY-TWO YEARS; HEIGHT, 181 CM.,; WEIGHT, 48.2 KG.

Time. Hrs. and mins.		Oxygen consumed per minute, cc.	Carbon dioxide eliminated per minute, cc.	R. Q.	Calories per 24 hours.	Per cent increase,	Blood sugar, per cent.
Average basal		139	107	0.77	954	..	0.22
			74.5 gms.	levulose.			
16' p. levulose		147	117	0.80	1014	+6	..
25'	"	149	133	0.89	1054	+11	..
							1°17'
34'	"	150	147	0.98	1083	+14	0.31
1° 18'	"	151	134	0.89	1069	+12	..
1° 27'	"	149	135	0.91	1057	+11	..
2° 16'	" 2	142	113	0.80	982	+3	2°0.35
							3°12'
3° 41'	" 2	139	114	0.82	966	+1	0.34
							5°50'
5° 35'	" 2	142	111	0.78	975	+2	0.28

TABLE 25.—EFFECT OF LEVULOSE AND INSULIN UPON THE METABOLISM AND RESPIRATORY QUOTIENT OF A DIABETIC PATIENT. (NOVEMBER 20, 1922.)

CASE NO. 2729. AGE, TWENTY-TWO YEARS; HEIGHT, 181 CM; WEIGHT, 47.1 KG.

Time. Hrs. and mins.		Oxygen consumed per minute, cc.	Carbon dioxide eliminated. per minute, cc.	R. Q.	Calories per 24 hours.	Per cent increase	Blood sugar, per cent.
Average basal		143	113	0.79	986	..	0.21
	12 units	insulin and	73.5 gms.	levulose	at 8.16 A.M.		
21' p. ins. and lev.		149	130	0.87	1046	+6	
30'	" "	165	147	0.89	1168	+19	
39'	" "	157	144	0.92	1118	+13	
48'	" "	156	143	0.91	1112	+13	
57'	" "	157	136	0.87	1106	+12	1° 0.25
1° 31'	" " 2	151	145	0.96	1081	+10	2° 0.27
2° 41'	" " 2	149	131	0.88	1049	+6	
4° 2'	" " 2	145	126	0.87	1020	+3	4° 0.24
5° 50'	" " 2	150	116	0.78	1031	+5	6° 0.20

[1] Davies, Lambie, Lyon, Meakins and Robson: British Med. Jour., 1923, **1**, 847.
[2] Average of two nine-minute periods.

and his co-workers give another explanation for the failure of the respiratory quotient to rise after insulin as high as the fall in blood sugar would lead one to expect. They suggest that the liberation of the alkali consequent upon the removal of the acetone bodies might result in a compensatory retention of carbon dioxide.

The basal respiratory quotients and basal metabolic rates were found by Wilder and Boothby[1] to be unaffected by the insulin. Following the administration of 20 units of insulin to 1 case the respiratory quotient rose from 0.75 to 0.85 in two hours with a gradual fall to 0.79 at the end of four hours. This was accompanied by a decrease in the percentage of blood sugar from 0.282 to 0.082 in the same period. Epinephrin 0.5 mg. was then injected subcutaneously. Subjective improvement followed, and this was accompanied by both an increase in the metabolic rate and in the respiratory quotient. In the subsequent period forty minutes later there was a fall in the respiratory quotient and basal metabolic rate, although the blood sugar was still further increased. The experiment, the writers point out, confirms the value of epinephrin as an emergency measure, but shows that it must be immediately followed by carbohydrate to counteract the increased metabolism due to the epinephrin. Insulin does not affect the metabolism as do thyroxin and epinephrin.

Observations with dextrose and levulose with and without insulin were also made in the Mayo Clinic. With dextrose thin, rather severe diabetics showed no increase in respiratory quotients and a depression in the first half-hour was noted as with normals. With levulose no such depression occurred and a definite though slight elevation was manifest. The metabolism was increased slightly more with the levulose. The blood sugar was elevated about equally by both sugars. In the insulin experiments with these sugars there was the initial depression in respiratory quotient after dextrose, followed, however, by a definite rise in one case, but insignificant in the other. Levulose and insulin, on the other hand, led to an immediate and profound rise in quotient. The metabolism curve rose somewhat more with the levulose and insulin. The blood sugar was less elevated by levulose and subsequently fell to a lower level.

The more remote effects of insulin are shown by the changes which the basal metabolism of patients undergoes in the course of weeks or months of treatment. Of 11 patients so studied during an interval of eighteen to one hundred and eleven days all but 3 presented a material increase in basal metabolism. The greatest increase in basal metabolism was that of Case No. 2801, who showed a gain of 262 calories in eighty-eight days, or 24 per cent, with a gain of weight in the same period of 4 per cent.

[1] Wilder and Boothby: Jour. Metab. Research, 1922, **2**, 720.

TABLE 26.—CASE NO. 866, BONNIE P. AGE AT ONSET IN APRIL, 1914, THIRTY-ONE YEARS. LOW BASAL METABOLISM.

Date	Weight, net kg.	Urine		Blood sugar, per cent.	Diet in grams.				Basal metabolism before and after treatment with insulin.[1]				
		Diac. acid.	Sugar, per cent.		C.	P.	F.	Cals.	Oxygen consumed per minute, cc.	Carbon dioxide eliminated per minute, cc.	R. 2.	Computed calories per 24 hours, cals.	± Variation from standard H. and B., per cent.
1915 May 22	54.1	0	4.0	....	....	....	....	....					
June	52.7	0	0	....	33	91	158	1918					
1918 Jan. 29	50.9	0	0	0.24	40	105	144	1876					
1922 Oct. 13	....	0	0	0.12	31	74	75	1095	124	99	0.79	854	−33
Oct. 14	39.9	0	0	....	31	74	75	1095	108	87	0.81	749	−43
Oct. 16	42.1	0	0	0.13	31	74	75	1095	124	100	0.80	857	−35
Oct. 23	42.9	0	0	....	31	74	75	1095	122	97	0.78	840	−36
Oct. 25	41.6	0	0	0.14	37	80	81	1197	124	102	0.83	864	−34
Oct. 30	41.8	0	0	0.19	32	104	65	1059	125	105	0.84	873	−33
Nov. 6	41.5	0	0	0.23	51	93	94	1422	130	106	0.81	901	−31
Nov. 10	41.8	0	0.1	....	51	73	105	1441	135	111	0.82	938	−29
Nov. 24	42.5	0	0	0.27	51	73	105	1441	139	111	0.80	961	−27
Dec. 12	42.6	0	0	0.22	52	74	109	1485	148	116	0.79	1021	−22
Dec. 15	42.8	0	0.2	....	52	74	121	1593					
1923 Jan. 23	43.0	0	0	0.17	52	74	121	1593	141	114	0.81	977	−26
Feb. 5	45.9	0	0										
Mar. 10	Erysipelas and Death												

Treatment with insulin began November 11, 1922. (See page 42.)

The patient with the lowest metabolism in the series of the patients taking insulin and of the entire series of patients studied at the New England Deaconess Hospital and Nutrition Laboratory and, in fact, in the literature upon diabetes, was Mr. P., Case No. 866. His diabetes was of eight and a half years' duration. His weight had fallen to 50 per cent below normal standard. On October 14 and 16 his basal metabolism was 854 and 749 calories, respectively; in other words, -33 to -43 per cent by the Harris and Benedict standard. These values were well supported by values for the ensuing three weeks. Ten weeks later the metabolism showed a material gain, but he still was 26 per cent below the normal level. In March, 1923, this most faithful patient contracted erysipelas and died. Upon an average of 12 units insulin daily he had gained 10 pounds in weight.

Russell and Bowen[1] record a rise in metabolism in Case 5 of their series from -38 per cent to -27 per cent with a gain in weight of 11 pounds.

In Table 27 the basal metabolism of Case No. 2801 is shown for 7 observations between October 7 and January 15. The favorable rise at the beginning of treatment is brought out and the uniformity of the results early in the course of treatment and at the end. In this patient there was a fairly steady gain in metabolism upon successive days and the respiratory quotient rose as well. The basal metabolism of the patient on October 7 was -20 per cent and finally came to as near normal as -5 per cent on January 15.

TABLE 27.—BASAL METABOLISM DURING TREATMENT[2] WITH INSULIN. CASE NO. 2801, AGE, FIFTEEN YEARS; HEIGHT 161 CM.

Date.	Weight (net), kg.	Oxygen consumed per minute, cc.	Carbon dioxide eliminated per minute, cc.	R. Q.	Computed calories per 24 hours.	± Per cent variation from standard (DuBois),
1922.						
Oct. 7 . .	39.3	167	118	0.71	1128	-20
Oct. 10 . .	38.9	158	112	0.71	1067	-24
Oct. 19 . .	38.0	161	116	0.72	1090	-21
Oct. 24 . .	38.6	158	116	0.74	1079	-22
Dec. 29 . .	38.4	186	140	0.75	1269	$- 8$
1923.						
Jan. 2 . .	38.1	179	130	0.73	1215	-11
Jan. 15 . .	39.5	196	147	0.75	1338	$- 5$

11. The Behavior of Insulin in Infections During the Course of Diabetes.—Infections whether general or local are always looked

---

[1] Russell, Bowen and Pucher: Bull. of Buffalo Gen. Hosp., 1923, 1, 41.
[2] Treatment with insulin begun in August, 1922. See also pages 44, 56, 94.

upon with dread in diabetes. Tolerance for carbohydrate and weeks of hospital treatment are lost in consequence. An infection lowers tolerance and acidosis is therefore favored, which the increased metabolism, due to fever, accentuates. Surgical aid cannot be sought too early to remove the source of the infection. To insulin and the increased diet which it has allowed must be attributed the more favorable course which such infections take today and also perhaps the greater freedom from infections. Children have easily withstood measles, whooping-cough and scarlet fever, as well as infections of the upper air passages. The tendency to a return of glycosuria is always evident, but I have seldom tried to control it entirely, because in the first place it has been but slight and as the event has proved with the subsidence of the infection the glycosuria has disappeared and the former tolerance been regained. Banting, Campbell and Fletcher report that during infections they have been able to keep the urine sugar-free.

Serious infections occurred with several patients, and in these insulin was of no avail. A young man, Case No. 2046, who had had diabetes for two years, entered the hospital with septicemia, proved by blood culture. The result of the blood culture was not known for the first few days, and he was given insulin. Neither good nor harmful effect was noted with the 77 units which he received during the eight days until it was discontinued. His death from septicemia was unrelated in any way to insulin. Case 866 succumbed to erysipelas; he did not develop coma. Whereas 12 units of insulin kept him sugar-free before he acquired the erysipelas, during the erysipelas many more units of insulin daily were without effect. Case No. 523 died of cerebrospinal meningitis, streptococcus viridans, thirty-six hours after its onset, six weeks subsequent to an operation for abscess near to but not involving the mastoid. The wound was healed and the man attending to his business when the flare-up occurred. He entered unconscious. At first the case was difficult to diagnose, but a lumbar puncture explained the situation. He had been given 20 units of insulin before coming to the hospital and I will confess that we gave 10 units more before the true diagnosis was made. The blood sugar was 0.26 per cent, and glycosuria persisted to the end.

The instance of tuberculosis in the diabetic patient, Case No. 2148, who also had cirrhosis of the liver, has been cited. Insulin was of service at first, but, when the tuberculosis became active was no longer needed, because the tolerance for carbohydrate had risen rapidly up to 76 grams. Insulin allowed another patient with hopelessly advanced phthisis to eat a little more liberally.

Patients with local infections have recovered more quickly with insulin than under the customary, unaided, dietetic and surgical treatment. The case of Mrs. D., Case No. 1245, has already been cited.　Case No. 2192 showed distinctly better improvement following his operation for mastoid when insulin was begun.　Case No. 2980, Mrs. M., we consider our best case of recovery following amputation from rapidly ascending gangrene accompanied by fever.　The management of infections is discussed at length in the section upon Surgery.

12. CAUSES OF DEATH OF DIABETIC PATIENTS TREATED WITH INSULIN.

During the year August 7, 1922, to August 7, 1923, there were 20 deaths among the 293 patients treated with insulin.　The details are presented in Table 28.　Two of the deaths from coma occurred in the New England Deaconess Hospital and have been described above.　Coma was responsible for nearly one-third of the total deaths.　To show how far the present treatment of diabetes was from the ideal, the deficit in years of life expectancy has been inserted in the table.　The average duration of the disease in these 20 fatal cases was six and eight-tenths years, as compared with six years for 597 fatal cases since June, 1914, and prior to insulin medication.

TABLE 28.—CAUSES OF DEATH OF DIABETIC PATIENTS TREATED WITH INSULIN, AUGUST 7, 1922 TO AUGUST 7, 1923.

Case No.	Diabetes.		Deficit in life expectancy calculated from age at onset years.	Cause of death.
	Age at onset, years.	Total duration, years.		
523	54	9	9	Septicemia.
705	52	14	5	Angina pectoris.
866	31	9	26	Erysipelas.
1305	11	5	43	Coma.
2046	37	2	28	Septicemia.
2148	40	13	15	Pulmonary tuberculosis.
2192	28	3	34	Coma.
2304	47	4	19	Uremia.
2446	36	1	30	Pneumonia.
2585	37	2	28	Coma and pulmonary tuberculosis.
2725	16	4	41	Coma.
2960	55	8	9	Cerebral hemorrhage and hypoglycemia.
3034	39	2	27	Coma.
3058	45	13	12	Pulmonary tuberculosis.
3079	61	0.3	13	Septicemia.
3109	55	0.3	17	Carcinoma of pancreas.
3176	41	17	10	Pulmonary tuberculosis.
3240	16	0.5	44	Coma.
3242	27	25	12	Septicemia.
3148	49	1.4	20	Coronary thrombosis.
Average . . .		6.8	22	

The percentage of deaths from coma to the total deaths in patients treated with insulin was 32 per cent.

The four cases of septicemia were proved by positive blood cultures.

SECTION II.

THEORY, INCIDENCE, ETIOLOGY AND CURABILITY.

A. DEFINITION OF DIABETES MELLITUS AND GLYCOSURIA.

1. DEFINITIONS of diabetes are unsatisfactory, but it is safe to say that diabetes is a disease in which the secretion of the islands of Langerhans is deficient and, as a result, the normal utilization of carbohydrate is impaired and glucose is excreted in the urine. Glucose is all important according to Woodyatt, irrespective of its source in carbohydrate, protein, fat or whether exogenous or endogenous, provided only it is metabolized; and upon the glucose in the diet and in the urine he builds the disease diabetes. Allen's structure is on a broader foundation. In addition to carbohydrate he includes all the protein, fat and total calories, believing all are involved in the injury the body undergoes from deficiency in the secretion of the islands of Langerhans.

My rule in the treatment of diabetes is to consider any patient who has sugar in the urine demonstrable by any of the common tests, to have diabetes mellitus and treat him as such, until the contrary is proved. This method of procedure is safer for the patient than to make use of the term glycosuria, which begets indifference (see p. 471).

Sugar, meaning thereby glucose (dextrose, $C_6H_{12}O_6$), is a normal constituent of the urine, occurring in varying quantities. Folin[1] was able by means of his technic to demonstrate the presence of sugar in nearly one hundred tests made on the urines of normal persons, and he adds: "The amount of sugar present in normal human urine is therefore probably much greater than is indicated by the negative findings recorded on the basis of the clinical qualitative tests for sugar in current use." Myers[2] concludes that normal urine appears to contain between 0.08 and 0.2 per cent sugar.

[1] Folin: Jour. Biol. Chem., 1915, **22**, 327.
[2] Myers: Proc. Soc. Exp. Biol. and Med., 1916, **13**, 178.

Benedict and Osterberg[1] by their special method of analysis find about 0.07 per cent sugar normally in the urine, of which about half is fermentable and they believe this is increased by food, so that by the urine one can predict a rise in blood sugar. Folin and Berglund[2] doubt this and by a series of carefully conducted experiments demonstrated that normal individuals have a glucose threshold for the blood and that sugar never appears in excess in the urine, no matter what the amount given unless this blood sugar threshold is exceeded. Their results are differently interpreted by Benedict and Osterberg[3] who still adhere to their original contention. Given health and time these four investigators will find the truth. At present, therefore, alimentary glycosuria is theoretically in abeyance, so that in practice I still adhere to my rule and disregard alimentary glycosuria. This was a troublesome point for Naunyn[4] and he suggested the administration of 100 grams of dextrose two hours after a breakfast of a large cup of coffee and milk and 80 to 100 grams of bread. If sugar is then demonstrable in the urine in a quantitatively estimable amount, diabetes mellitus exists.

The drug glycosurias and those of traumatic and emotional origin are almost invariably of a temporary nature, so that doubt concerning the diagnosis of diabetes mellitus vanishes when sugar is constantly found in the urine. To this there is one exception, renal glycosuria, for a discussion of which and of glycosuria in pregnancy, which is somewhat related to it, see pages 649 and 663.

B. NAUNYN'S CONCEPTION OF DIABETES MELLITUS.

Naunyn[5] thoroughly believed in the unity of diabetes, notwithstanding the manifold, and even doubtful, causes which appeared to lead up to it. It must be a great satisfaction to this Nestor of the disease to find his theory proved correct by Banting and Best. He sees in heredity the common bond which unites the different forms, or as he says, "to speak more exactly, the heredity of the diabetic tendency." Variety in the etiology of diabetes becomes understandable if one sees in the disease the development of an individual tendency. Almost any illness or injury, no matter how slight it may be, may serve as a cause. Furthermore, the experience that an individual, who at one time has been diabetic or even has had a suspicious glycosuria which has passed for years as cured and has even dropped out of memory, perhaps for decades, may

[1] Benedict and Osterberg: Jour. Biol. Chem., 1918, **34**, 261.
[2] Folin and Berglund: Jour. Biol. Chem., 1922, **51**, 259.
[3] Benedict and Osterberg: Jour. Biol. Chem., 1923, **55**, 769.
[4] Naunyn: Der Diabetes Mellitus, Wien, 1906, p. 37.
[5] Loc. cit. p. 159.

again become diabetic under favoring influences, is in conformity with this view.

This diabetic tendency is generally congenital—indeed, in many cases hereditary, and this heredity is demonstrable in 20 per cent of the cases. The cases in which heredity is demonstrated differ in nowise from those in which heredity is not demonstrated.

According to the manner in which the development of the diabetes stands to the diabetic disposition, Naunyn distinguishes three forms of the disease:

1. The diabetes of young people, chiefly between thirty and forty years of age: Naunyn's "true[1] diabetes." In this group the congenital weakness of the sugar metabolism, of itself or often in conjunction with some accompanying circumstance (illness, accident, exertion, excesses), may lead to an insufficiency of the metabolism of sugar even without the addition of the disease of a diabetic organ. In this type one must conceive of an especially severe tendency to the disease and this accounts partly for the especial severity of its form, but only in part, for this severity depends in high degree upon the great demand which youth makes on metabolism.

2. The diabetes, usually mild, of elderly people. In this type, the tendency is less severe. The disease comes late to development, and for this it requires a lowering of the vitality which comes with age. The age of a man depends on the condition of his arteries. So here, too, arteriosclerosis comes into play, and with the arteriosclerosis come to the front all those conditions which favor the development of diabetes—overnutrition, luxurious living, and, especially, excesses in alcohol. Syphilis, which is so important according to many authors in the cases of arteriosclerosis, strange enough to say, appears to play no great rôle here.

3. The Organic Diabetes.—The rôle which the tendency plays in the different cases of this group varies. In general, the tendency is present, although it need not be. To the organic type of diabetes belong those cases in which the disease of the diabetic organs appears as the cause of the diabetes. Thus, diseases of the liver, of the nervous system, whether organic, functional, or traumatic, diseases of the thyroid gland and of the pancreas are here found, and the pancreas, according to experiment and autopsy, holds the first place. In these organic diseases arteriosclerosis is important, and in this way arteriosclerosis may be the cause of diabetes.

C. TENDENCIES TO LOSS AND GAIN IN TOLERANCE.

Hitherto, most writers have been unanimous in the belief that the tendency of the diabetic glycosuria, particularly if untreated,

[1] Pure.

is to increase. There are numerous exceptions to the rule if the diabetes has been treated, but I know of none where the disease has been allowed to take its course without medical intervention. Since A. A. Hornor and I paid especial attention to the group of diabetics of fifteen and twenty or more years' duration, a good many cases have come to light in which the disease has shown little if any progress. All of these patients, however, have been treated to a certain extent and though the treatment may have been very slight, strictly speaking, it has been enough to take them out of the class of untreated cases. If treatment has been thorough the question changes, but even then I must acknowledge, with my methods of treatment without insulin, I have been unable to guarantee to the patient that the severity of his disease would remain unaltered. Even with my most conscientiously treated cases the diabetes has become more severe. In the future I believe it will continue to do so, although in a much smaller number of instances. This cheerful forecast is based upon the favorable course in the past of many mild cases and the ease with which cases rather more severe in character are now controlled.

Case No. 8 shows this tendency of the glycosuria to increase. The case dates back many years and, of course, strictly modern methods were not followed, yet the patient was carefully treated. The description of the case is as follows:

A woman showed the first symptom of diabetes in the spring of 1899, at the age of sixty years, and 5 per cent of sugar was found in June. She had gradually lost 20 pounds during the preceding fifteen years and weighed 165 pounds when the diagnosis was made. Under rigid diet the urine promptly became sugar-free; the tolerance rose to 130 grams and, save for very transitory intervals, remained so for nine years, until 1908. During 1908, and until the autumn of 1909, it returned, but except at one analysis was less than 1 per cent. In October, 1909, the sugar amounted to 4.6 per cent, and a carbuncle appeared. With prompt surgical care, vaccines, the restriction of carbohydrates, and the temporary utilization of the oatmeal diet, the sugar disappeared, and the carbuncle healed promptly. But the urine did not remain permanently sugar-free, although only about 30 grams of sugar were excreted daily. In the spring of 1911, the sugar again rose at the time of an attack of lobar pneumonia, but as recovery took place and a restricted diet was instituted, the sugar disappeared. Evidently the patient could be freed from sugar, but upon a diet containing only about 30 grams of carbohydrate. This seemed too narrow (compare treatment in 1912 and now) for the patient after thirteen years of dieting, so that it was practically impossible to keep the urine free from sugar continually. Residence in a hospital for a few days in September, 1912, in order to have several teeth removed, lowered the sugar to 0.8 per cent.

Except for the brief periods of illness due to the carbuncle and pneumonia, the patient remained well during all these years, and was unusually strong and vigorous for a woman of seventy-three years. She finally succumbed to a lingering illness subsequent to a hemiplegia, and death finally occurred due to a terminal pneumonia in 1913.

Yet I confess that doubt arises as to the progressive character of the disease when one sees cases of diabetes untreated for years, who were able to become sugar-free with restricted diet, and apparently able to acquire a considerable tolerance for carbohydrates. If the disease was actually progressive, then such a patient should ultimately, barring death from accidental causes, lose all tolerance for carbohydrate, but a case of this type has not yet come to my observation. I confess that these long-standing, neglected cases are, apparently, easily amenable to modern treatment, but the question arises as to whether they can be kept in a sugar-free condition and maintain weight consistent with life without insulin. Cases Nos. 436 (see p. 129) and 632 (see p. 57) are examples of very slow progression of diabetes. Case No. 2201 has had diabetes for twenty-three years, and has a carbohydrate tolerance for 100 grams for weeks at a time, though when she first came under my observation in 1921 she was excreting 7 per cent sugar. However, her blood sugar is elevated and even with insulin it is difficult to reduce it to 0.15 per cent. Despite her high tolerance for carbohydrate, she takes insulin hoping to prevent further disease of the retina.

Further evidence of value would be afforded by a study of very mild cases of diabetes discovered by routine or insurance. If such cases, often very little treated, remained stationary for years, it would be evidence against a progressive tendency. This special group is not available for study, but it can be said that cases of diabetes discovered by insurance live an unusual length of time. Then, too, my group of 65 cases of diabetes of twenty or more years duration also offer some information. Forty of these patients are now living and in most of them the disease appears to be stationary.

A low percentage of blood sugar in cases of long duration is also evidence against a progressive tendency. Thus, in the 65 cases of twenty or more years' duration, of the 44 analyses of blood sugar which have been made, 22 were 0.2 per cent or below, 8 were between 0.21 and 0.25 per cent, and 14 between 0.26 and 0.49 per cent.

Sherrill's[1] observations at Allen's clinic, from a study of 5 cases of

---

[1] Sherrill: Jour. Metab. Research, 1922, **1**, 667.

diabetes under strict control for considerable periods, "are opposed to the belief in a mysterious, spontaneous progressiveness of typical diabetic cases. They support the view that functional deterioration in diabetes can be traced to definite causes, particularly infections and dietary excesses, that downward progress clinically depends upon the different susceptibilities of different patients to these injurious influences, and that by the strict avoidance of such influences downward progress can be largely or wholly prevented."

Newburgh and Marsh[1] express themselves quite as categorically: "it is true that we have not as yet observed loss of tolerance in patients who have adhered to the diet" (a maintenance diet that will control glycosuria and acidosis) "as long as three years." Yet on an earlier page these authors give a table of cases treated by themselves and the writer which admits of different interpretation.

TABLE 29.—DIABETIC PATIENTS TREATED FROM APRIL 1, 1919 TO DECEMBER 31, 1921, ON JANUARY 1, 1922.[2]

	Newburgh and Marsh.		Joslin.	
	Number.	Per cent.	Number.	Per cent.
Cases, total	124	100	536	100
Cases, traced	117	94	508	95
Deaths in hospital	10	8	11	2
Deaths in and outside hospital	26	21	118	23

In my opinion cases of diabetes carefully treated do infinitely better than those cases which are neglected. In each group exceptional examples of the disease can be found in which there is little tendency to progression, but careful investigation usually shows that an advancing tendency exists.

One must not forget that wide fluctuations in severity occur in one and the same diabetic largely owing to treatment or its neglect. A case untreated today may simulate severity, and if carefully treated for the subsequent three years may appear no worse, but was the original estimation of severity correct? Case No. 983 appeared severe in 1916, but a few weeks sufficed to prove the disease mild which her condition in 1923 substantiated, but it is quite another matter to demonstrate that it remains as mild as when first seen. My cases ought to furnish more evidence upon this interesting question of loss of tolerance in the course of years, and I shall seek it.

The tendency of the diabetic patient to gain in tolerance for carbohydrates when the urine becomes sugar-free is the fundamental principle upon which all treatment has been and is rightly based, and that by which the value of all therapeutic measures is deter-

[1] Newburgh and Marsh: Arch. Int. Med., 1923, **31,** 455.
[2] Newburgh and Marsh: Loc. cit.

mined. This proposition is a reverse of the preceding, and it would appear to hold, so far as evidence is available, both experimentally and clinically, yet here again the evidence should be far more carefully weighed than heretofore. The employment of the test and maintainance diets gives many striking opportunities to observe gains in tolerance. (See p. 55.) Among the older cases, Case No. 194 is an excellent illustration of this gain in carbohydrate tolerance in a child and its later loss when the treatment was interrupted.

TABLE 30.—VARIATIONS IN CARBOHYDRATE TOLERANCE. CASE 194.

Date.	Volume, c.c.	Diacetic acid.	β-oxybutyric acid, gm.	Nitrogen, gm.	Ammonia, total gm.	Sugar in urine. Reduction, gm.	Sugar in urine. Rotation, gm.	Carbohydrate in diet, gm.	Carbohydrate balance, gm.	NaHCO₃, gm.	Naked weight of patient, kilos
1908											
April 18–19	1800	+	..	..	..	..	50	90	+40	8	
19–20	2610	−	..	..	1.9	..	78	90	+10	8	49.2
20–21	1710	++	..	..	..	..	44	64	+20	8	49.2
21–22	1890	++	..	..	..	..	60	60	..	8	49.2
22–23	1600	+	..	20.1	1.9	..	42	60	+20	8	49.4
23–24	1650	+	..	..	..	..	20	40	+20	8	49.5
24–25	1650	+	..	..	..	..	17	20	+5	8	49.6
25–26	1590	+	..	..	..	..	16	15	−	8	50.2
26–27	2970	+	..	..	1.5	0	12	10	−	8	50.4
27–28	1650	0	..	..	..	0	−	12	+10	8	50.0
May 1– 2	1830	0	..	13.0	..	0	−	16	+15	0	50.2
Nov. 11–12	1500	0	..	..	..	0	..	50 ±	+50	0	53.6
1909											
Feb. 1– 2	1520	0	..	..	..	0	..	90 ±	+90	0	
May 10–11	....	0	..	..	..	0	..	90 ±	+90	0	55.9
July 27–28	....	..	..	..	..	0	..	90 ±	+90	0	55.9
Sept. 18–19	2820	−	..	13.6	0.5	17	11	15	−	20	53.0
22–23	3280	+++	13.0	11.2	0.6	42	24	15	−25	20	52.9
23–24	2577	+++	14.3	8.0	0.5	50	43	165	+115	20	52.3
24–25	2410	+++	14.1	10.0	..	19	−	15	−5	20	52.6
1910											
Oct. 25–26	2300	+++	..	15.9	2.4	80	64	−	−	−	53.6
Nov. 29–30	2000	+++	..	..	..	+	64	−	−	−	52.6
Dec. 10	Death in coma.										

Female, born August 16, 1893, single, no occupation, onset of diabetes at age of fourteen years in February, 1908; sugar in the urine March, 1908; came under observation April 18, 1908; died in coma December 10, 1910. There was no history of diabetes in the family. Father died of pneumonia, mother and brother well. The past history included scarlet fever, dysentery at three years of age, measles, mumps, whooping-cough, chicken-pox, enuresis nocturna which ceased at the age of four years. (I have repeatedly observed this symptom in the early history of diabetic children).

Always a voracious appetite, sometimes eating six potatoes at a meal; ate much candy. During the year preceding the onset of the disease the patient developed rapidly both in height and weight. In February, 1908, she showed weariness. Early in March polydipsia, polyuria and polyphagia were present, and sugar was demonstrated in the urine. In the previous year the urine was normal.

During the whole period of illness the patient remained in good condition and attended school with comfort. *The diet was rigidly adhered to and not relaxed except when the diagnosis was at one time doubted by the local physician. Catamenia was established for the first time in March,* 1909. The patient died in coma on December 10, 1910. The harmfulness of doubting a diagnosis is well illustrated by this patient's career. She was an ideal case for faithful treatment and even without insulin with present day treatment this patient should have lived at least four years longer. Remembering her tragic end I am always very slow to tell a patient he does not have diabetes if any doctor has ever found sugar present in the urine or thought it present. I tell such patients to have their urine examined each month for a year and thereafter at least every six months for life, even though I find no proof of diabetes.

Case No. 564 (see p. 456) shows a remarkable gain in tolerance from a minus carbohydrate balance of 70 grams to a positive balance of 50 grams, lasting for years. Case No. 203 (see p. 161) also illustrates a gain in tolerance, for now, March, 1923, this boy is able to take a free diet without the appearance of sugar. Case No. 653 showed 5.8 per cent and 174 grams sugar on a free diet in September, 1913, but now, three and a half years later, at the age of fifty-six years, eats between 200 and 300 grams carbohydrate and is free from sugar. This patient, like several others, takes comparatively little fat. The remarkable case of Geyelin and DuBois,[1] who progressed from a minus carbohydrate balance of 75 grams to a positive balance of 160 grams, is another striking illustration of gain in tolerance. Case No. 30 showed sugar for eighteen years, and yet now, 1923, on a very liberal diet, is sugar-free. Case No. 321 had a tolerance for 90 grams carbohydrate in 1910, at the age of fifty-six years, but now takes carbohydrate 181 grams, protein 57 grams and fat 102 grams, without a trace of sugar. Case No. 632 (see p. 57) had difficulty in becoming sugar-free in July, 1913, at the age of thirty-one years, upon carbohydrate 15 grams, but in 1917 maintained an active life, played golf better than ever, and reached a position of eminence in his country in his military vocation, yet he kept sugar-free upon a diet of carbohydrate 29 grams, protein 85 grams, and fat 150 grams. This tolerance again fell by 1922 and

[1] Geyelin and DuBois: Loc. cit., p. 209.

he was forced to give up exercise. His diet was carbohydrate 15 grams, protein 69 grams, fat 103 grams. With 8 units of insulin daily it was raised to carbohydrate 43 grams, protein 76 grams, fat 150 grams and in the six months ending in May, 1923, he has gained 14¼ pounds and been able to take up golf and work. I recall no other patient who has lived accurately by the scales for six years on so low a carbohydrate diet.

The best writers are all most emphatic in their approval of the endeavor to promote tolerance for sugar by rendering the patient sugar-free. Naunyn says, "From my experience I consider it highly probable that among the early, strictly treated cases which passed in the beginning as severe, but later took a favorable course, there is many a one for which one must thank this early strict treatment; moreover, on the other hand, there can be no doubt that the cases which run ultimately a severe course have undergone little, if any, energetic care." And again he urges not to be "content to maintain the patient for a time in just an endurable condition, but rather to strive to improve the diseased function, or at least to check further inroads on the same." So universal are the two principles that there is an increase in severity the longer the disease lasts and that the progress of the disease is checked by making the patient sugar-free, that it makes any glycosuria, no matter how inconsiderable, worthy of energetic treatment.

D. INCIDENCE.

1. **Increase in the Incidence of Diabetes Mellitus.**—If diabetes should continue to increase in the next thirty years at the same rate at which statistics show it to have increased between 1880 and 1910, it would rival tuberculosis as a cause of death, and should this rate progress for another generation it would be responsible for almost the entire mortality of the world. In 1880, the death-rate from diabetes was 2.8 per 100,000 in the registration area of the United States, and thirty years later, in 1910, it was 14.9 per 100,000. This astounding rate of increase then ceased. In the decade which has elapsed since 1910, the death-rate on the same basis has advanced to but 16.1 per 100,000. In the intervening years it rose above this figure, notably in 1915, when it reached its acme of 17.5 per cent. Thereafter it steadily fell until it reached in 1919, the same death-rate as in 1910. In the two years since 1919, it has again begun to rise.

Such a rapid rate of increase as took place between 1880 and 1910, is evidence of itself that a fallacy exists somewhere in the statistics. Convincing proof that this is the case is furnished by a comparison of the statistics for the registration area of the United

States during the years 1910, 1911, 1912 and 1913, because during these years the death-rate for diabetes was nearly stationary. Such a sudden halt in the progressive frequency of the disease could not have been brought about without some obviously remarkable improvement in treatment, preventive or otherwise. This we know did not take place in 1910. This striking interruption in the advancing incidence of the disease is also indicated by the statistics of New York and Boston. Thus, in Boston during 1912 and 1913, the death-rate from diabetes was less than during 1910 and 1911. But since 1913, a remarkable advance is registered throughout the country, and in New York and Boston as well. This rapid rise in mortality in 1914, 1915 and 1916, I believe attributable to the increased attention devoted to this disease by the medical profession and by the newspapers following the announcement of a new method of treatment by F. M. Allen.

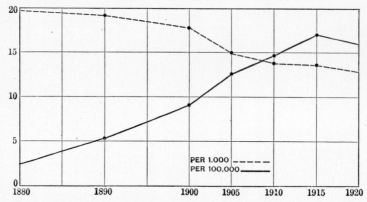

FIG. 7.—The falling total death-rate per 1000 and the rising diabetic death-rate per 100,000 between the years 1880 and 1920 in the registration area of the United States.

In Fig. 7 and Table 31, are displayed the falling rate of deaths from all causes per 1000 and the rising rate of deaths from diabetes per 100,000 during the last forty years in the registration area of the United States.

The decrease in the diabetic death-rate, beginning with 1915, may be explained first, by the general tendency to eat less food during the war, and second, by the less accurate observation of the civilian population due possibly to the withdrawal of physicians from general practice and their entrance into the army. It is, therefore, not surprising that in 1920, the rate began to rise because these two factors had ceased to be operative. It is a safe prediction that it will continue to rise, irrespective of the actual cases of diabetes in the country, because of a third factor, namely, the discovery of insulin, which has focused attention upon this disease. Indeed, an increase in the diabetic death-rate will probably continue until examinations of the urines of each individual in the community are made, not only with each illness, but also once or twice yearly. Only in that way will the actual number of latent cases of diabetes be disclosed.

TABLE 31.—TOTAL AND DIABETIC MORTALITY IN THE REGISTRATION AREA OF THE UNITED STATES.

Census year.	Population in registration area, per cent.	Deaths from all causes.		Deaths from diabetes.		Diabetic deaths to total deaths, per cent.
		Number.	Rate per 1000 population.	Number.	Rate per 100,000 population.	
1880 . .	17.0	169,453	19.8	237	2.8	0.14
1890 . .	31.4	386,212	19.6	1,089	5.5	0.28
1900 . .	37.9	512,669	17.8	2,693	9.3	0.53
Calendar year:						
1900 . .	. .	539,939	17.6	2,996	9.7	0.55
1901 . .	. .	518,207	16.5	3,212	10.3	
1902 . .	. .	508,640	15.9	3,312	10.4	
1903 . .	. .	524,415	16.0	3,681	11.3	
1904 . .	. .	551,354	16.5	4,259	12.9	
1905 . .	. .	545,533	16.0	4,397	13.0	0.81
1906 . .	. .	658,105	15.7	5,331	13.0	
1907 . .	. .	687,034	16.0	5,801	13.9	
1908 . .	. .	691,574	14.8	6,274	13.9	
1909 . .	. .	732,538	14.4	7,024	14.4	
1910 . .	58.3	805,412	15.0	8,040	14.9	0.91
1911 . .	. .	839,284	14.2	8,805	14.9	
1912 . .	. .	838,251	13.9	9,045	15.0	
1913 . .	. .	890,848	14.1	9,660.	15.3 .	
1914 . .	. .	898,059	13.6	10,666	16.2	
1915 . .	. .	909,155	13.6	11,775	17.5	1.31
1916 .	. .	1,001,921	14.0	12,199	17.1	
1917 . .	. .	1,068,932	14.3	12,750	17.0	
1918 . . .	. .	1,471,367	18.1	12,927	15.9	
1919 . .	. .	1,096,436	12.9	12,683	14.9	
1920 . .	82.2	1,142,558	13.1	14,062	16.1	1.22
1921 . .	. .	1,032,009	11.6	14,933	16.8	1.40

Save for the diseases of the arteries, diabetes has increased more rapidly as a cause of death in the registration area of the United States in the first decade of this century than cancer, cerebral hemorrhage and apoplexy, organic diseases of the heart cirrhosis of the liver, or Bright's disease.[1]

The percentage of diabetic mortality to the total mortality has risen even more rapidly than the actual increase in diabetic deaths.

[1] Dublin: Popular Science Monthly, 1915, **86**, 313.

This is partly accounted for by the fall in deaths from all causes throughout the United States. Whereas in thirty years the death-rate from diabetes increased five-fold its share in the total mortality, during forty-one years diabetes has increased ten-fold. There is justification for the added attention devoted to the study of diabetes in the last few years. Future practitioners are destined to have far more cases of diabetes to treat than their fathers.

All age groups are about equally represented in the statistical increase in diabetes. This is shown by a study of Table 32, in which the relative proportion of the population of the United States in the registration area at different groups is given for the years 1890 and 1920, along with the corresponding percentage of deaths from diabetes. In this table the decreasing percentages of population under twenty years of age in 1920, compared with 1890 is manifest. This is due in part to the marked prolongation of life (see Table 42) and, doubtless, in part to a falling birth-rate. The feature of the table which caused its insertion into the text is, however, the right-hand column. This shows that the diabetic mortality per 100,000 in 1920 per decade, as compared with 1890, has about doubled. Closer inspection of the table shows that this approximate doubling of mortality holds for each age period. It is true that for the period forty-five and over the mortality has nearly trebled, rising from 20.6 to 57.3, but this can be accounted for by the decrease in mortality for unknown age groups from 13.75 in 1890 to 3.36 in 1920.

TABLE 32.—RELATIVE PROPORTION OF THE POPULATION OF THE UNITED STATES IN THE REGISTRATION AREA AT DIFFERENT AGE GROUPS IN 1890 AND IN 1920 WITH CORRESPONDING PERCENTAGE MORTALITY FROM DIABETES.

1890.

Age group, years.	Population.	Per cent of total.	Percentage mortality per 100,000.	
			Total.	Diabetic.
Under 5	2,392,447	12.2	5591.70	0.96
5– 9	2,373,440	12.0	589.86	0.85
10–14	2,204,293	11.2	318.60	2.22
15–19	2,055,305	10.5	562.40	1.90
20–44	7,244,021	36.9	1196.00	3.63
45 and over . . .	3,339,050	17.1	3927.50	20.60
Unknown	50,884	0.003	4180.00	13.75
Total	19,659,440	99.9		

1920.

Age group, years.	Population.	Per cent of total.	Total.	Diabetic.
Under 5	9,239,058	10.75	2688.80	2.03
5– 9	9,014,012	10.37	300.10	2.83
10–14	8,409,709	9.68	234.20	4.32
15–19	7,527,480	8.65	411.20	4.65
20–44	33,876,531	38.98	718.70	6.46
45 and over . . .	18,711,942	21.52	3005.30	57.30
Unknown . . .	119,047	0.001	1349.00	3.36
Total	86,897,779	99.95		

New York City's total mortality per 1000 population has been halved in the last forty years, but the diabetic death-rate per 100,000 population has increased six-fold, and the percentage of diabetic to total deaths has increased ten-fold. The data are given in Table 33.

TABLE 33.—TOTAL AND DIABETIC MORTALITY IN NEW YORK CITY.

Year.			Deaths from all causes.		Deaths from diabetes.		Diabetic deaths to total deaths, per cent.
			Number.	Rate per 1000 population.	Number.	Rate per 100,000 population.	
1880	.	. .	937	26.4[1]	44	3.6[1]	0.14
1890	.	. .	203	24.9[1]	130	8.0[1]	0.32
1900	.	. .	70,872	20.6	357	10.4	0.50
1910	.	. .	76,742	16.0	768	16.0	1.00
1915	.	. .	76,193	14.6	1109	20.2	1.45
1916	.	. .	77,801	14.7	1118	20.0	1.44
1917	.	. .	78,575	14.6	1153	21.0	1.47
1918	.	. .	96,989	17.9	1011	18.0	1.04
1919	.	. .	74,131	13.4	955	17.0	1.29
1920	.	. .	73,393	12.9	1075	19.0	1.46
1921	.	. .	64,257	11.2	1120	19.0	1.74
1922	.	. .	69,690	12.3	1448	25.0	2.08

TABLE 34.—TOTAL AND DIABETIC MORTALITY IN BOSTON.

Year.			Deaths from all causes.		Deaths from diabetes.		Diabetic deaths to total deaths, per cent.
			Number.	Rate per 1000 population.	Number	Rate per 100,000 population.	
1880	.	. .	8,531	23.5	[2]	[2]	[2]
1890	.	. .	10,181	22.7	31	6.9	0.3
1900	.	. .	11,678	20.8	77	13.7	0.7
1910	.	. .	11,574	17.2	135	20.1	1.2
1915	.	. .	12,018	16.1	195	26.1	1.6
1916	.	. .	12,760	16.8	192	25.2	1.5
1917	.	. .	12,728	16.5	148	19.2	1.2
1918	.	. .	17,447	22.2	133	16.9	0.8
1919	.	. .	11,689	15.6	171	23.0	1.5
1920	.	. .	11,601	15.4	175	23.0	1.5
1921	.	. .	10,220	13.5	149	19.7	1.5
1922	.	. .	11,420	15.0	222	29.1	1.9

Boston shows a higher mortality from diabetes than that of any city which has come to my attention, but New York has the highest percentage mortality to total mortality. In 1922, the diabetic death-rate in Boston reached the peak of 29.1 per 100,000. In New York in 1922, the deaths from diabetes were 2.08 per cent of all the deaths. The decrease in percentage of diabetic death-rate appeared here during the war as well as the decrease in percentage of diabetic deaths to total deaths. It will be of great interest, statistically, to note whether the mortality in other sections of the

[1] Old City of New York included present Boroughs of Manhattan and the Bronx.
[2] 1880 data not available.

8

country continues to approach the level reached here. To a certain extent the city with the highest mortality is an index to which the mortality in other communities may be expected to rise. In Malta the rate is 38.4 per 100,000, according to Hoffman,[1] whose article upon the statistics of diabetes should be consulted.

TABLE 35.—TOTAL AND DIABETIC MORTALITY IN BERLIN.

Year.	Deaths from all causes.		Deaths from diabetes.		Diabetic deaths to total deaths, per cent.
	Number.	Rate per 1000 population.	Number.	Rate per 100,000 population.	
1871–1875	..	..	..	1.7	
1876–1880	..	..	..	3.0	
1881–1885	..	..	..	3.6	
1886–1890	..		..	5.1	
1891	33,394	21.0	91	5.7	0.27
1892	32,696	20.3			
1893	36,038	22.1	120	7.4	0.33
1894	30,961	18.8	149	9.1	0.48
1895	33,627	20.2	131	7.9	0.39
1896	30,578	18.0	152	8.9	0.50
1897	30,622	17.7	152	8.8	0.50
1898	30,574	17.2			
1899	34,011	18.7	167	9.2	0.49
1900	35,411	19.0	193	10.3	0.55
1901	34,096	18.1	261	13.8	0.77
1902	30,741	16.2	281	14.8	0.91
1903	31,882	16.6	310	16.1	0.97
1904	33,425	17.0	395	20.1	1.18
1905	34,451	17.1	324	16.1	0.94
1906	32,648	15.9	414	20.1	1.28
1907	32,353	15.6	374	18.1	1.16
1908	32,408	15.7	367	17.8	1.13
1909	31,844	15.5	406	19.8	1.28
1910	30,152	14.6	391	19.0	1.30
1911	32,307	15.6	441	21.3	1.37
1912	29,981	14.4	459	22.0	1.53
1913	28,067	13.5	409	19.6	1.46
1914	29,664	14.6	468	23.1	1.63
1915	28,572	15.2	385	20.5	1.35
1916	27,147	15.1	332	18.5	1.22
1917	34,138	19.6	246	14.1	0.72
1918	35,764	20.7	204	12.0	0.57
1919	31,307	18.5	185	10.9	0.59
1920	30,982	18.6	178	10.9	0.57

Certain foreign cities present statistics which will serve for comparison with those in this country. Berlin formerly had a higher diabetic death-rate than any of our American cities, but in the later years of the war the death-rate from diabetes was cut in halves. One must not forget that the civilian population received less medical attention there as well as here, and this may partially account for the fall in death-rate, but few will gainsay that the

---

[1] Hoffman: Boston Med. and Surg. Jour., 1922, **187**, 135.

outstanding cause for the precipitous decrease in diabetic mortality was due to undernutrition. Confirmation of this conclusion will

TABLE 36.—TOTAL AND DIABETIC MORTALITY IN PARIS.

		Deaths from all causes.		Deaths from diabetes.		Diabetic deaths to total deaths, per cent.
Year.		Number.	Rate per 1000 population.	Number.	Rate per 100,000 population.	
1880	. . .	55,706	25.4	..	6.3	
1890	. . .	54,566	22.8	..	13.5	
1900	. . .	51,725	19.6	413	17.0	0.82
1910	. . .	45,814	16.2	468	18.4	1.02
1911	. . .	48,942	16.9	451	16.9	0.92
1912	. . .	47,059	16.3	483	17.7	1.05
1913	. . .	44,624	15.4	424	16.0	0.95
1914	. . .	45,972	15.9	406	14.3	0.89
1915	. . .	43,068	14.9	382	13.2	0.89
1916	. . .	43,450	15.0	387	13.4	0.89
1917	. . .	44,597	15.4	392	13.5	0.88
1918	. . .	49,658	17.4	279	9.6	0.56
1919	. . .	44,936	15.5	297	10.3	0.66

TABLE 37.—DIABETIC MORTALITY IN DIFFERENT COUNTRIES AND CITIES ON DIFFERENT DATES COMPARED (RATE PER 100,000).

Countries.	1880.	1900.	1910.	1915.	1916.	1917.	1918.	1919.	1920.	1921.	1922.
United States[1]	2.8	9.7	14.9	17.5	17.1	17.0	15.9	14.9	16.1	16.8	
England[2] . .	4.1	8.6	11.0	13.0	13.0	11.2	10.6	10.5	10.0	10.8	
Germany . .											
France . . .											
Italy . .	1.4	3.3	4.7	5.3	5.0	5.2					
Japan[3] . . .	..	..	2.2	3.0[4]	3.1	3.2	3.6	2.9	3.1		

Cities.	1880.	1900.	1910.	1915.	1916.	1917.	1918.	1919.	1920.	1921.	1922.
New York[1] .	3.6	11.4	18.6	24.1	22.8	24.3	22.3	21.2	23.4	24.1	25.0
Boston[1] . .	..	15.2	20.8	27.1	26.6	21.3	19.6	23.5	24.2	19.8	29.0
London[5] . .				11.9	11.4	10.0	8.1	8.7	8.0	9.3	
Berlin . .	..	10.3	19.0	20.5	18.5	14.1	12.0	10.9	10.9		
Paris . . .	6.3	17.0	18.4	13.2	13.4	13.5	9.6	10.3			
Rome . . .											
Tokyo . . .	..	..	2.9	3.2	2.6	2.7	2.4	2.5	2.2		

[1] Registration area exclusive of Hawaii: 1900, from Mortality Statistics, U. S., 1900 to 1904; 1910, from Mortality Statistics, U. S., 1910; 1915 to 1921, from Mortality Statistics, U. S., 1921.

[2] 1900, from report Registrar-general, England and Wales, 1911; 1910, from report Registrar-general, England and Wales, 1920; 1915 to 1921, from report Registrar-general, England and Wales, 1921.

[3] Based on civilian deaths and civilian population.

[4] 1915 to 1918, from Statistique Causes de Dérès, Japan, for each year; 1919, from Résumé Statistique de Mouvement de la population, Japan, 1919; rates worked from population and deaths in each report.

[5] 1915 to 1921, from reports Registrar-general, England and Wales, for each year. Rates worked from population and deaths in each report. Figures are for London administrative county, which is Greater London, exclusive of "Outer Ring." In 1921 report *only* are deaths from diabetes shown for Greater London; Greater London, population 7,535,582, deaths from diabetes, 746, rate per 100,000, 9.9; London Administrative County, population 4,524,000, deaths from diabetes, 422, rate per 100,000, 9.3.

be furnished by the mortality statistics for the next few years, during which they should rise. Today the demonstration of the importance of undernutrition in the treatment of diabetes appears to be beyond doubt.

Paris shows almost as striking a variation in the statistical mortality from diabetes as Berlin, because from 1912, when the diabetic mortality in Paris reached its acme, 17.7 per 100,000 population, it fell in 1918 to 9.6

The diabetic mortality in different countries and different cities on different dates is compared in Table 37. All data in the table, save those in heavy type, were placed at my disposal by the Department of Commerce, Bureau of the Census, Washington, through the courtesy of William H. Davis, M.D., Chief Statistician for Vital Statistics. There are various regrettable gaps in the table which it is hoped some one can fill. The general tendency is about the same. England shares with Berlin and Paris in presenting a falling diabetic mortality for the years subsequent to 1915 to 1920 with an almost insignificant rise in 1921; but why is the diabetic death-rate so low in England?

TABLE 38.—TOTAL AND DIABETIC MORTALITY IN ENGLAND AND WALES.

	Deaths from all causes.		Deaths from diabetes.		
Year.	Number.	Rate per 1000 population.	Number.	Rate per 100,000 population.	Diebetic deaths to total deaths, per cent.
1850 . . .	368,995	20.8	422	2.4	0.11
1860 . . .	422,721	21.2	536	2.7	0.13
1870 . . .	515,329	21.6	735	3.3	0.14
1880 . . .	528,624	19.5	1059	4.1	0.20
1890 . . .	562,248	19.3	1863	6.5	0.33
1900 . . .	587,830	18.2	2767	8.6	0.47
1901 . . .	551,585	16.9	2964	9.1	0.54
1902 . . .	535,538	16.2	2769	8.4	0.52
1903 . . .	514,628	15.4	2844	8.5	0.55
1904 . . .	549,784	16.2	3133	9.3	0.57
1905 . . .	520,031	15.2	3174	9.3	0.61
1906 . . .	531,281	15.3	3342	9.7	0.63
1907 . . .	524,221	14.9	3360	9.7	0.64
1908 . . .	520,456	14.5	3610	10.3	0.69
1909 . . .	518,003	14.3	3698	10.4	0.71
1910 . . .	483,247	13.2	3937	11.0	0.81
1911 . . .	527,810	14.2	3853	10.6	0.72
1912 . . .	486,939	13.0	4051	11.1	0.83
1913 . . .	504,975	13.5	4311	11.8	0.85
1914 . . .	516,742	13.7	4507	12.2	0.87
1915 . . .	562,253	14.8	4658	13.2	0.82
1916 . . .	508,217	13.4	4544	13.2	0.90
1917 . . .	498,922	13.5	3816	11.3	0.77
1918 . . .	611,861	17.1	3568	10.6	0.58
1919 . . .	504,203	13.3	3857	10.5	0.77
1920 . . .	466,130	12.1	3749	10.0	0.80
1921 . . .	458,629	11.5	4092	10.8	0.90

The detailed diabetic mortality in England and Wales is given in Table 38. It is a striking fact that the percentage of diabetic deaths to total deaths in England and Wales for 1921, was only one-half that in Boston. What is the explanation?

The low total and percentage diabetic mortality in Italy, as well as the constancy in the mortality, is noticeable in comparison with the mortality in other countries. This low mortality is only exceeded by that in Japan. The same upward tendency, however, in the prevalence of diabetes is noted in Japan. This is shown in Japan and Tokyo by statistics furnished by Muryama and Sakaguchi with death rates calculated by H. Gray and by Iwai's[1] reports of admissions to the Red Cross Hospital and the Hospital of the Imperial University of Tokyo, as exhibited in Table 40.

TABLE 39.—TOTAL AND DIABETIC MORTALITY IN ITALY.

	Deaths from all causes.		Deaths from diabetes.		Diabetic deaths to total deaths, per cent.
Year.	Number.	Rate per 1000 population.	Number.	Rate per 100,000 population.	
1890	795,911	27.3	637	2.1	0.08
1891	795,327	27.3	680	2.2	0.09
1892	802,779	26.8	792	2.6	0.10
1893	776,713	26.3	704	2.3	0.09
1894	776,372	25.1	700	2.3	0.09
1895	783,813	25.4	771	2.5	0.10
1896	758,129	24.1	833	2.6	0.11
1897	695,602	21.9	882	2.8	0.13
1898	732,265	22.9	894	2.8	0.12
1899	703,393	21.9	1026	3.2	0.15
1900	768,917	23.8	1082	3.3	0.14
1901	715,036	22.0	1071	3.3	0.15
1902	727,181	22.2	1154	3.5	0.16
1903	736,311	22.2	1139	3.5	0.16
1904	698,604	21.2	1242	3.8	0.18
1905	730,340	22.0	1322	4.0	0.18
1906	696,875	20.9	1394	4.2	0.20
1907	700,333	20.9	1535	4.6	0.22
1908	770,054	22.8	1503	4.4	0.20
1909	738,459	21.7	1551	4.6	0.21
1910	682,459	19.9	1608	4.7	0.24
1911	742,811	21.4	1714	4.9	0.23
1912	635,788	18.2	1658	4.7	0.26
1913	663,966	18.8	1818	5.1	0.27
1914	643,355	17.9	1838	5.1	0.29
1915	741,143	20.4	1942	5.3	0.26
1916	721,847	19.7	1827	5.0	0.25
1917	682,311	19.2	1835	5.2	0.29

For the total number of diabetics in the United States no accurate figures are available. Since approximately 1 death out of each 50 in New York and Boston is due to diabetes, one might be tempted

[1] Iwai: Le Diabete Sucre chez les Japonais, Tokyo, translated by Le Goff, Paris, Masson et Companie, Editeurs, 1916.

to assume that 2 per cent of the population have or will have the disease. On this basis the number of diabetics for the United States would be nearly 2,000,000! Granted the average length of a diabetic's life to be ten years, the number of fatal cases would be 200,000 instead of the actual number reported for the registration area, which was approximately 15,000 for 1921. Support for using the New York and Boston figures for an estimate of the total diabetics in the country is furnished by the statistics of Barringer,[1]

TABLE 40.—TOTAL AND DIABETIC MORTALITY IN JAPAN, TOKYO AND TWO HOSPITALS IN TOKYO.

JAPAN.

Year.	Deaths from all causes. Number.	Rate per 1000 population.	Deaths from diabetes. Number.	Rate per 100,000 population.	Diabetic deaths to total deaths, per cent.
1909	1,091,264	21.7	1057	2.1	0.10
1910	1,064,234	17.7	1089	1.8	0.10
1911	1,043,906	20.0	1212	2.3	0.12
1912	1,037,016	19.8	1331	2.5	0.13
1913	1,027,252	19.3	1373	2.6	0.13
1914	1,101,815	20.3	1467	2.7	0.13
1915	1,090,000	19.9	1609	2.9	0.15
1916	1,187,832	21.4	1737	3.1	0.15
1917	1,199,669	21.3	1801	3.2	0.15
1918	1,493,162	26.3	1995	3.5	0.13
1919	1,281,965	22.8	1625	2.9	0.13
1920	1,422,096	25.4	1725	3.1	0.12

TOKYO.

Year.	Number.	Rate per 1000 population.	Number.	Rate per 100,000 population.	Per cent.
1909	36,407	22.3	44	2.7	0.12
1910	35,870	19.8	53	2.9	0.15
1911	36,789	19.3	41	2.2	0.11
1912	35,283	17.6	37	1.8	0.11
1913	36,593	18.1	43	2.1	0.12
1914	36,765	17.5	50	2.4	0.14
1915	39,270	17.5	73	3.2	0.19
1916	39,397	17.2	59	2.6	0.15
1917	42,596	18.1	64	2.7	0.15
1918	46,815	20.3	55	2.4	0.12
1919	49,198	20.9	60	2.5	0.12
1920	50,516	21.1	52	2.2	0.10

RED CROSS HOSPITAL.

Year.	Admissions.	Cases of diabetes.	Per cent of admissions for diabetes.
1891–1893	1,134	7	0.61
1897–1900	1,367	13	0.95
1901–1903	1,449	17	1.17
1906–1908	1,006	16	1.59

HOSPITAL OF IMPERIAL UNIVERSITY, TOKYO.

1900–1902	24,424	59	0.24
1903–1906	39,016	135	0.34
1907–1910	47,289	207	0.43

[1] Barringer: Arch. Int. Med., 1909, **3**, 295.

TABLE 41.—DIABETES MELLITUS. ADMISSIONS, DEATHS, DISCHARGES FOR DISABILITY, AND DAYS LOST FOR THE PERIOD OF THE WAR. APRIL 1, 1917 TO DECEMBER 31, 1919, INCLUSIVE.

Disease.	Admissions.					Deaths.					Discharges for disability.					Days lost.				
	Total Army officers and enlisted men, including native troops.	Total officers.	Total enlisted men, including native troops.	Total American troops.	Total native troops.	Total Army officers and enlisted men, including native troops.	Total officers.	Total enlisted men, including native troops.	Total American troops.	Total native troops.	Total Army officers and enlisted men, including native troops.	Total officers.	Total enlisted men, including native troops.	Total American troops.	Total native troops.	Total Army officers and enlisted men, including native troops.	Total officers.	Total enlisted men, including native troops.	Total American troops.	Total native troops.
Absolute numbers	718	83	635	632	3	104	6	98	97	1	330	14	316	315	1	39,062	5453	33,609	33,520	89
Ratios per 1000	0.17	0.40	0.16	0.16	0.08	0.03	0.03	0.02	0.02	0.03	0.08	0.07	0.08	0.08	0.03	0.03	0.07	0.02	0.02	0.01

based upon the frequency with which sugar was found in the urines of 72,000[1] adults examined for life insurance in New York City. His method of investigation showed that nearly 2 per cent[2] of this large group of the adult population in a city had diabetes. It would be unjustifiable to apply his statistics to the entire population, because diabetes is comparatively rare in the early part of life, but increases in frequency as age advances, and Barringer's data relate to adults. The incidence of diabetes might be far below 1 in 85 in the first and second decades of life and then increase to 1 in 40 of the population from the sixth decade onward. Today our information rests upon hypothetical grounds, but within a few years far more satisfactory information will be available. For the present it is probably safe to state that the number of individuals in the country who either have diabetes or will develop it is about 1,000,000.

Through the courtesy of Major W. B. Borden of the Surgeon-General's Office, I am enabled to give the records for diabetes in the Army during the World War (Table No. 41).

In explanation of this table, attention is called to the fact that "admissions" should be interpreted to mean cases admitted to such report with a primary diagnosis of diabetes mellitus, and does not include any cases which may have been discovered as an associate or as complications of the primary disease.

"Deaths" should be interpreted to mean the deaths occurring among those cases primarily admitted for diabetes mellitus, regardless of whether or not they may have had any associate disease or complication which could have been a contributing cause or actual cause of deaths, that is, all deaths were charged against the primary admission."

The Army percentage mortality of 0.03 per 1000 is less than half that for civilian life for the age group twenty to forty-four years. (See Table 32.)   This low army rate may be attributed to: (1) The initial exclusion from the army of recruits with diabetes by routine examination on enlistment. Omission of routine urines from the general physical in certain training camps under the stress of preparation in time of war, probably accounts for the fact that even as many as 718 cases were found in soldiers; (2) the freedom from overfeeding and sedentary living.

For diabetes in the negro, see page 606, and for a discussion of the increase of diabetes in the Philippines, see an article by Concepcion.[2] In the latter country the incidence is increasing, due apparently to a greater accuracy of vital statistics, but it is still less than that in other countries, including Japan.

---

[1] Actually 71, 729.   [2] 1.895 per cent.
[3] Concepcion: Phil. Island Med. Assoc. Jour., 1922, **2**, 57.

2. **The Explanation of the Statistical Increase in Diabetes.**—
(*a*) **Greater Accuracy of Vital Statistics.**—The increased accuracy
of vital statistics in recent years undoubtedly explains to a great
extent the apparent increase in diabetes. It is evident from the
study of the incidence of diabetes in different localities that the
rate is not always today the highest where one would expect the
statistics to be most trustworthy. The war introduced an entirely
new factor, and the results of this gigantic etiological and therapeutic
experiment in diabetes will be of great significance. Time enough
has not elapsed to furnish the control after-period, which, when
food becomes abundant again, should show an incidence comparable
to that of former days.

(*b*) **More Frequent Urinary Examinations.**—The chief cause for
the improvement in the vital statistics upon diabetes lies in the
increased frequency of routine urinary examinations. Urinary
examinations are comparatively recent. This is shown by the
records of a case of diabetes at the Massachusetts General Hospital
for the year 1866, where the words "urine tasted sweet" may be
seen in the handwriting of a house pupil, later a professor in the
Harvard Medical School, and now still vigorous.

(*c*) **General Increase in Duration of Life.**—The general increase
in the duration of life throughout the world is an important cause
for the apparent increase in the frequency of diabetes. This is
of more importance in studying the incidence of diabetes than it
would be with the infectious diseases. The infectious diseases are
common to the early years of life, and consequently prolongation
of life would affect their incidence comparatively little; but with
diabetes quite the opposite is the case. Just as in cancer so it is
with diabetes, the longer a person lives the more liable he is to the
disease. The general mass of the population is marching toward
the age of the greatest incidence of diabetes. This is very well
shown in Table 42, which presents the approximate age at death
from all causes in the registration area of the United States in
1860 and for following decades. This average has risen to forty-
two years. But a better figure to consider is the present average
expectation of life, which is a very different matter than the average
age at death. This expectation of life in the United States is now
estimated to be fifty-five years. In 1885, the average expectancy
of life for a new-born baby in Massachusetts was forty-two and
seven-tenths years; in 1920 it was fifty-five and one-tenth years.

TABLE 42.—AVERAGE AGE AT DEATH FROM ALL CAUSES IN THE UNITED STATES.

Year.	Age, yrs.	Year.	Age, yrs.
1860	22.7	1900	35.2
1870	25.2	1910	38.7
1880	26.9	1915	42.2
1890	31.1	1920	41.9[1]

[1] Unofficial.

(d) **Life Insurance Statistics.**—The increased frequency of urinary examinations is due to some extent to the increasing percentage of the population which is insured. In Table 43, the growth of the per cent of population to policies in force in the United States for successive periods is indicated. Further proof of the important part which insurance examinations occupy in the discovery of diabetes is shown by an analysis of my own diabetic statistics. Whereas between the years 1893 and 1916, 6 per cent of patients coming to me for treatment of diabetes reported the disease had

TABLE 43.—LIFE INSURANCE POLICIES IN FORCE IN THE UNITED STATES. RISING PERCENTAGE ACCORDING TO POPULATION.

Year.	Number of policies.	Population.	Per cent of population to policies in force.
1880	608,681	50,155,783	1
1890	1,276,167	62,947,714	2
1900	3,071,253	75,994,575	4
1910	6,040,617	91,972,266	7
1920	13,199,605	105,710,620	12

TABLE 44.—INCREASED FREQUENCY OF DISCOVERY OF DIABETES BY LIFE INSURANCE.

Period.	Number of cases in series.	Sex.		Discovered by life insurance.		
		Male.	Female.	Total per cent.	Males, per cent.	Females, per cent.
1893–1916 . . .	1000	594	406	6	10	0
1916–1920 . . .	1000	578	422	9	15	1
1920–1923 . . .	1000	524	476	13	22	2

been discovered by routine life insurance examinations, by 1923 the percentage had risen to 13. Indeed, the percentage in males, which was formerly 10 per cent, had changed by the latter date to 22.

(e) **Frequency by Decades at which Onset Occurs Now and Formerly.**—The increase in the incidence of diabetes has already been shown to be quite uniform for the different decades. Up to von Noorden's time the distribution of frequency of diabetes in the experience of men especially concerned in its treatment was approximately the same for different age groups and is shown in Table 45. These early writers lived at a time when urinary examinations were really not a part of the general routine of medical examinations. Von Noorden's statistics represent a later era, and it is noticeable that he had at least 50 per cent more cases in the first decade of life than earlier writers. My own statistics, being still more recent, make this still clearer, for they include three times as many as von Noorden's[1] 1.43 per cent. Of 608 cases of diabetes reported by

---

[1] von Noorden's: Die Zuckerkrankheit, Berlin, 1912, p. 59.

Iwai[1] in Japan not a single case was encountered in the first decade of life. The point may be raised that on account of my interest in diabetes and the general feeling of the hopelessness of the disease in children a proportionately larger number of young than of older diabetics may have come to me. This is undoubtedly true, but this argument applies to the other writers cited with even more force.

TABLE 45.—FREQUENCY OF ONSET OF DIABETES BY DECADES.

Decade.	1.	2.	3.	4.	5.	6.	7.	8.
Frerichs[2]	1.0	7.0	10.0	18.0	25.0	26.0	11.0	1.0
Seegen[3]	0.5	3.0	16.0	16.0	24.0	30.0	10.0	0.5
Grube[4]		1.7	2.8	11.2	23.1	39.5	18.1	3.4
Schmitz[5]	0.8	4.1	9.3	17.3	22.3	32.6	10.0	3.3
Pavy[6]	0.5	4.1	7.1	16.4	24.9	30.7	13.4	2.6
Kulz[7]	1.0	3.0	4.6	17.2	36.0	26.8	9.2	0.1
Von Noorden:[8]								
Mild	..	0.4	2.4	10.0	21.0	17.7	4.0	0.4
Severe and moderately severe	1.4	2.4	6.0	9.6	12.6	11.0	2.1	
Muryama, Yamaguchi[9] .	0.2	0.9	5.8	18.6	33.6	28.6	9.3	1.2
Joslin[10]	5.7	8.3	12.2	15.9	25.1	22.3	8.7	1.6

This increase in the percentage of cases in the first decade as compared with a generation ago speaks emphatically in favor of the better diagnostic methods of today rather than of actual increase in the frequency of the disease, and this statement is confirmed by a study of diabetes for different age groups in the United States shown in Table 32.

(*f*) **The Importance of Recognition of the Extent of Diabetes in the Community and its Influence upon Treatment.**—The recognition of the large number of diabetic individuals living in the United States is important. It determines the character of the treatment. The number of cases is so great that it at once becomes evident that their care must rest in the hands of the general practitioner. It is ridiculous to expect that the treatment of diabetics should

[1] Iwai: Loc. cit., p. 117.
[2] Ueber den Diabetes, Berlin, 1884.
[3] Der Diabetes Melitus, Berlin, 1870, 1st ed.; 1893, 3d ed.
[4] Diatetische Behandlung der Zuckerkrankheit, Bonn, 1898.
[5] Berl. klin. Wchnschr., 1873, **18**, 18; also Berlin, 1891, p. 373.
[6] On Diabetes, London, 1869; Differentiation in Diabetes, London, 1900.
[7] Klinische Erfahrungen über Diabetes Melitus, Herausg. von Rumpf, Jena, 1899.
[8] Die Zuckerkrankheit, Berlin, 1917, 7th ed., p. 74.
[9] Personal Communication. Age unknown 1.7 per cent.
[10] Compiled to July, 1922, 2611 cases.

be under the supervision of a specialist; neither can they all undergo hospital treatment. It is plain that a program of education not only for the diabetic patients themselves but the population as a whole must be instituted along similar lines to that which has been adopted in the treatment of tuberculosis. But first of all this program must begin with the doctor. The campaign against tuberculosis has given the community fresh air. A campaign for the prevention and treatment of diabetes should give the community a knowledge of diet, the danger of obesity, and the importance of physical exercise. The gain to the community from the dissemination of such knowledge will almost offset the harm caused by diabetes. In this campaign I would especially emphasize the importance of the education of the general practitioner in diabetics. To treat the 1,000,000 or more diabetic patients in the United States there were in 1921, 159,250 physicians. Formerly a physician would rarely see over 5 to 10 diabetics a year, but with the increased frequency of the disease in the future he is destined to see still more, partly because of the new cases which will be discovered, but also because of the increased duration of life of the existing cases. The Registrar's Office in the City of Boston shows that between 1895 and 1913 the average duration of life in the fatal cases of diabetes amounted to two and three-tenths years. For 1915 it was four and three-tenths years, but for 1920 it was five and three-tenths years. Consider what this change in duration from three years to five years means when applied to the million diabetic patients in the United States. It creates an addition of two million years of the disease diabetes which the general practitioner must treat. Furthermore, these additional two years of illness for each patient with diabetes require far more treatment, and more resourceful treatment than the earlier three years. The type of diabetes one sees today is very different from what it was before the war. This increase in the duration of life of diabetics was in pre-insulin days. How much greater the increase in duration of life is destined to be through insulin no one can predict.

3. **Sex Incidence.**—More men than women are treated for diabetes according to the authors, but more women than men die of the disease according to mortality statistics.

In illustration of the above the following table from von Noorden[1] is cited, to which are added my own statistics, and also a table showing the deaths from diabetes according to sex in the registration area of the United States during the years 1913–1921 inclusive. (See Table 46.)

---

[1] Von Noorden: Loc. cit., p. 122.

TABLE 46.—SEX IN DIABETES.

Sex in diabetes.			Diabetic deaths in registration area of United States.		
Name.[1]	No. of cases.	Males, per cent.	Year.	No. of cases.	Males, per cent.
Grube	177	77	1913	9,660	47
Külz	692	76	1914	10,666	46
Griesinger	225	76	1915	11,775	45
Seegen	938	75	1920	14,062	45
Von Noorden . . .	1960	73	1921	14,933	45
Frerichs	400	70			
Williamson	100	62			
Schmitz	2109	57			
Joslin	2800	57			

The apparent clinical preponderance of diabetes in men may be ascribed: (1) To the greater consideration which they receive; (2) to the large percentage discovered by life insurance examinations, amounting to 22 per cent of my male cases; (3) to the hesitancy of women to speak about their urinary troubles and their neglect to regard such seriously; (4) to the type of practice of those who have reported large series of cases. It is suggestive that in Japan 80 per cent of the cases of diabetes reported by Iwai[2] and 85 per cent of 900 cases treated at the Kyonndo Hospital of Tokyo between 1915 and 1922 (Muryama and Yamaguchi) were males, and that 70 per cent of the German cases reported are males, save the series of Schmitz, but in the United States only 57 per cent, according to my series, and 45 per cent for the registration area.

Morrison's[3] figures for the city of Boston between the years 1895–1913, like the national statistics, show 45 per cent of 1775 deaths from diabetes to have been males.

The fact that more men than women receive special medical treatment for diabetes and that more women than men die of the disease is evidence in favor of the usefulness of our present therapeutic procedures. In Table 47 the duration of the disease is given for males and females separately. These tables show clearly the longer duration of diabetes in males.

4. **Heredity Incidence.**—The influence of heredity in diabetes has always interested me, and I have taken great pains to secure data from my patients upon this point. Naunyn said that the more carefully he inquired into the family history, the more commonly he found heredity to be present, and I am quite sure that this rule holds. It is easy to exaggerate the importance of heredity, for diabetic patients naturally would be more liable to know of the presence of diabetes in the members of their families than would

---

[1] Arranged chronologically.
[2] Iwai: Loc. cit., p. 177.
[3] Morrison: Boston Med. and Surg. Jour., 1916, **175**, 54.

TABLE 47.—FATAL CASES OF DIABETES ARRANGED ACCORDING TO ONSET AND DURATION OF DISEASE.   DECEMBER 1, 1916.

Males.

Cases arranged by decade of onset	Un. 1 yr.	1 yr.	2 yrs.	3 yrs.	4 yrs.	5 yrs.	6 yrs.	7 yrs.	8 yrs.	9 yrs.	10 yrs.	11 yrs.	12 yrs.	13 yrs.	14 yrs.	15 yrs.	16 yrs.	17 yrs.	18 yrs.	19 yrs.	20 yrs.	21 yrs.	22 yrs.	23 yrs.	24 yrs.	25 yrs.	26 yrs.	27 yrs.	28 yrs.	29 yrs.	30 yrs.	31 yrs.	32 yrs.	33 yrs.	34 yrs.	35 yrs.	Total
0–10	6	6	1	1	1		1																															16
11–20	10	10	5	5	1	2		1																													34
21–30	1	5	11	3	3	2		1	1																											1	28
31–40	7	6	5	4	4	1	2		1	1	1	1	1													1											35
41–50	4	7	6	7	7	5	2	2	2	4	2	4	1	1	1	2	1	1	1	1	1																62
51–60		5	11	6	4	6	6	6	5	5	5	4	2	1	3	4					1																74
61–70	2	6	1	4	1	6	4	1	4			1	1				1																				32
71–80	2	2	3			1	1																														9
Total	32	47	43	30	21	23	16	11	13	10	8	10	5	2	4	6	2	1	1	1	2					1										1	290
Per ct.	11.0	16.2	14.8	10.3	7.2	7.9	5.5	3.4	4.5	3.4	2.8	3.4	1.7	.7	1.4	2.1	.7	.3	.3	.3	.7					.3										.3	

patients who did not have diabetes. This introduces a considerable error into the statistics of the heredity of diabetes. Among 100 non-diabetic patients, Heiburg found 7 who had relatives with the disease, and upon inquiry from 100 diabetic patients he learned that 18 had relatives similarly affected. Among 500 consecutive histories of my own non-diabetic patients 25 had relatives with the disease. Having seen the increase in diabetes in the community to be, at least in great part, apparent rather than real, I hesitate to attach too much importance to heredity. Undoubtedly, heredity will appear more prominently in the case reports of diabetes as time goes on, but this may reflect only the greater accuracy in vital statistics.

Evidence was not forthcoming that diabetes was transmitted as a Mendelian characteristic according to Buchanan.[1] He studied 34 families resulting from the marriage of 1 diabetic and 1 non-diabetic individual through the second and third generations.

Statistics upon heredity in diabetes are susceptible to criticism because of what is included under the term "hereditary." Often by this term familial as well as hereditary cases are included. So far as my own statistics are concerned "heredity" signifies the presence of the disease in a parent, and occasionally information about a grandparent was obtained, as well as uncle, aunt or child. The term "familial," on the other hand, embraces brothers, sisters, and cousins and it is quite evident from the literature that brothers, sisters and cousins are usually included in compiling statistics on heredity. Conjugal diabetes, of course, does not belong to either group. In securing statistics upon heredity, a record should always be made upon the history blank as to whether the information appears reliable, and is suitable for tabulation.

In 6 cases at least of my series, Cases Nos. 105, 473, 503, 954, 1285 and 1421, the diabetes developed in the child or children before it occurred in the parent

The age of onset and the duration of the disease in these 6 cases to death or the present time is shown in Table 48.

TABLE 48.—DIABETES IN THE CHILD AND PARENT COMPARED.

	Child.				Parents.		
Case No.	Age at onset.	Duration, years.	Condition.	Case No.	Age at onset.	Duration, years.	Condition.
105	15	2.8	Dead	339	47	5.7	Dead
	14	1.4	Dead	473	48	0.2	Dead
503	30	5.1	Alive	711	54	3.8	Alive
	2	1.0	Dead ⎫	954	49	1.0	Alive
	12	0.2	Dead ⎭				
1285	27	1.5	Untraced		55		
	23	2.5	Dead	1421	74	1.0	Dead

[1] Buchanan: Am, Jour. Med. Sci., 1923, **155**, 675.

A history of diabetes in grandparent, parent, uncle, aunt or child was obtained in 417 cases of my series of 2800 cases—in other words, 15 per cent. Of this number, 211 were males and 206 females On the other hand, the group of cases showing a familial tendency included 189 cases, or 7 per cent of my series. Of this group 96 were males, and 93 females. If we combine the two groups, we have 606 cases showing an hereditary or familial tendency, or 21 per cent of all the cases. Older writers record data which are similar. For comparison, Table 49, taken in part from von Noorden, is inserted:

(*a*) **Earlier Statistics.**—

TABLE 49.—HEREDITY IN DIABETES.

Author.	Date of compilation.	No. of cases.		Heredity, per cent.
Grube	..			8.0
Frerichs	..	400		9.8
Seegen	..	..		14.0
Schmitz	..	..		20.0
Külz	..	692		21.6
Williamson	..	500		22.0
Bouchard	..	..		25.0
Naunyn	1906	398		17.0
von Noorden . . .	1917		{ Hereditary, 18.5 { Familial, 6.9 }	25.4
Joslin	1923	2800	{ Hereditary, 15.0 { Familial, 7.0 }	21.0

A recent writer, Hoogslag,[1] reports that in 43 per cent of 207 cases, diabetes was known in the family.

(*b*) **Notable Diabetic Families Showing Heredity.**—The most interesting diabetic family history that I have encountered was furnished by a nurse, who stated that her mother and her mother's 11 brothers and sisters all died of diabetes save 1, who, like the rest, has the disease but is still alive. Two of her aunts each had a child with diabetes. To my repeated inquiries about the accuracy of the information, she writes: "I am positive that diabetes was proven by examination of the urine in the case of 5 of the first generation; the others are on record as having died of diabetes. All the patients were stout." (See Table 50.)

The family showing the most marked diabetic heredity with which I have personally come in contact was that of a Jewish patient, Case No. 759, who developed diabetes at the age of fifty-five years.

A brother died of diabetes and tuberculosis at sixty-eight years; a sister of diabetic coma at fifty-five years; a sister of acute indigestion at fifty-eight years, having had diabetes for many years; a sister of Bright's disease at fifty-six years, having had diabetes for ten years; a sister, who is living, has had acute indigestion and

[1] Hoogslag: Cit. Jour. Am. Med. Assoc., 1922, **2**, 1934.

also has diabetes; finally a brother died of influenza at sixty-two years, having had diabetes eight years. The father succumbed to paralysis at sixty-two years, and the mother to heart disease at sixty-five years. A niece, Case No. 436, also has had diabetes for fourteen years, during eleven of which she has been under my observation. She became pregnant in 1915, and the carbohydrate balance, which amounted to 15 grams for a year or more before pregnancy began, rose to about 65 grams. She had a normal delivery in April, 1916, nursed her baby for several months, and both mother and child are in excellent condition and were kind enough to go on to a Clinic at the Academy of Medicine in New York in May, 1923. The tolerance for carbohydrate fell after delivery and again when nursing was given up. No sudden change in tolerance, however, was observed.

TABLE 50.—A FAMILY WITH A DOZEN FAT DIABETIC BROTHERS AND SISTERS.

Preceding generation.	Date of birth.	Date of death.	Duration of life, years.	Cause of death.
Andrew	Oct. 18, 1803	1853	50	Lockjaw
Hannah his wife .	Aug. 9, 1805	1848	43	Childbirth
First generation:				
Emily	Feb., 1827	1881	54	Diabetes
Daniel	Aug., 1828	1843	15	"
Hannah	Mar., 1830	1905	75	"
George	Aug., 1831	1890	59	"
Elizabeth . . .	Jan., 1833	1883	50	"
Andrew	May, 1834	1874	40	"
Jane	Feb., 1836	1896	60	"
Addie	Dec., 1837	1904	67	"
Rachel	Oct., 1841	1873	32	"
William	Dec., 1843	1895	52	"
John	July, 1845	1878	33	"
Catherine . . .	Mar., 1848	Living	52 to date, December, 1915.	
Second generation:				
Jennie, daughter of Elizabeth			18	
Jane, daughter of Emily			42	

Landis[1] has reported a diabetic family in which the disease was transmitted to the 5 blonde but not to the 4 brunette children of a diabetic mother.

(c) **The Favorable Influence of Heredity.**—The influence of heredity upon the disease is not uniform. It may be serious, or it may be favorable. Naunyn has pointed out that the onset of the disease in successive generations is apt to take place at a successively earlier age, and consequently the diabetes is more apt to be severe. Von Noorden has emphasized the importance of the character of the diabetes in the progenitor as indicative of the character of the disease in the offspring. My cases of hereditary diabetes have usually been mild, so that I always look upon heredity as a favorable omen. Several cases in young people have been

[1] Landis: Trans. Assoc. Amer. Phys., 1921, **36**, 293.

9

unusually favorable.   Of a total of 34 living hereditary and familial cases who developed the disease under the age of twenty years, the duration of life is already three and two-tenths years.   Of a total of 31 fatal cases also with onset under twenty years of age the average duration of life was three and four-tenths years.

All cases which have come to my attention of youthful patients with diabetes living for very long periods of time have been hereditary.   The case of Schmitz quoted by Naunyn[1] was hereditary, and deserves regard because of its encouraging features.   This was a four-year-old child, whose mother and older sister were diabetics.   The urine was frequently examined for sugar, and always found sugar-free, the last examination being November 22, 1871.   November 26, 1871, a febrile attack, and evening urine of November 27, contained 5.8 per cent of sugar.   Patient put upon a strict diet.   December 3, 3.5 per cent; December 8, 2 per cent, and on December 13, was sugar-free.   The strict diet was continued for some time, and then gradually some bread and milk were allowed.   Sugar was constantly absent from the urine, and the child felt well.   The diet was made more liberal from year to year, and finally included the diet which most children much enjoy, fruit, chocolate, and puddings.   Everything went well, and at eighteen the strong, well-developed girl was married, and in 1892, presented the appearance of blooming health, and was the mother of two healthy children, sugar having never reappeared.

Naunyn's own famous cases Nos. 124, 173 and 32 were all hereditary cases and he refers on pages 96 and 97 of his book to other cases of long duration in which I find that heredity was manifest.

Teschemacher[2] has reported several cases of apparently cured diabetes.   The most remarkable feature is the simultaneous occurrence of diabetes in all four members of a family, father, mother, and two young children.   It is doubtless a coincidence rather than an evidence of the infectiousness of diabetes.   The father slowly became worse; the mother and both children apparently recovered completely; at any rate they remained sugar-free on a mixed diet for two years.

Riesman[3] has emphasized the mild character of some cases of diabetes in children.   Of the 4 cases which he reports one again finds the presence of a familial or hereditary history in 3.   Cases I and II were brother and sister; Case III showed neither familial nor diabetic heredity, but the mother of Case IV had had diabetes for nine years.

The duration of life of the fatal cases of hereditary diabetes is shown in Table 51 and in Table 52 are collected the data of those with a familial history.

[1] Naunyn: Loc. cit., p. 102, see p. 384.
[2] Teschemacher: Deutsch. med. Wchnschr., 1910, **36**, 401.
[3] Riesman: Am. Jour. Med. Sci., 1916, **161**, 40.

TABLE 51.—DURATION OF LIFE OF 96 FATAL CASES OF HEREDITARY DIABETES, 1894 TO SEPTEMBER 1, 1922.

Decades.	Under 1 yr.	1 yr.	2 yrs.	3 yrs.	4 yrs.	5 yrs.	6 yrs.	7 yrs.	8 yrs.	9 yrs.	10 yrs.	11 yrs.	12 yrs.	13 yrs.	14 yrs.	15 yrs.	16 yrs.	17 yrs.	18 yrs.	19 yrs.	20 yrs.	21 yrs.	24 yrs.	35 yrs.	Total.
0–10	3	1	1	..	..	1	1	..	..	..	..	..	..	..	..	..	..	..	..	..	..	..	..	..	7
11–20	1	1	3	..	1	1	..	..	..	1	..	..	1	..	..	..	..	..	..	..	..	1	..	..	10
21–30	2	..	2	1	4	..	..	..	..	..	..	..	..	..	..	..	..	..	..	..	..	..	..	..	9
31–40	2	2	..	2	1	1	..	..	..	..	..	..	1	..	..	..	..	1	1	..	..	..	..	1	12
41–50	3	2	2	1	2	..	1	1	3	4	4	3	..	..	1	1	..	1	..	1	1	..	..	..	31
51–60	1	2	1	..	..	2	2	..	2	1	..	..	..	..	..	..	..	2	..	..	..	1	..	..	14
61–70	1	..	2	..	..	3	2	..	..	..	..	..	..	..	..	1	..	..	..	..	..	..	..	..	9
71–80	1	..	1	..	..	..	2	..	..	..	..	..	..	..	..	..	..	..	..	..	..	..	..	..	4
Total	14	8	12	4	8	8	8	1	5	6	4	3	2	..	1	2	..	4	1	1	1	2	..	1	96
Per cent	14.5	8.3	12.5	4.2	8.3	8.3	8.3	1.0	5.2	6.3	4.2	3.1	2.1	..	1.0	2.1	..	4.2	1.0	1.0	1.0	2.1	..	1.0	

Average duration of 96 fatal cases of hereditary diabetes, 6.4 years.

TABLE 52.—DURATION OF LIFE OF 94 FATAL CASES OF FAMILIAL DIABETES, 1894 TO SEPTEMBER 1, 1922.

Decades.	Under 1 yr.	1 yr.	2 yrs.	3 yrs.	4 yrs.	5 yrs.	6 yrs.	7 yrs.	8 yrs.	9 yrs.	10 yrs.	11 yrs.	12 yrs.	13 yrs.	14 yrs.	15 yrs.	16 yrs.	17 yrs.	18 yrs.	19 yrs.	20 yrs.	21 yrs.	24 yrs.	35 yrs.	Total.
0–10	2	2			1																				5
11–20	1	4	2		2		2	1	1																13
21–30		2	2		2															1					7
31–40		2	3		1		1	1	1				1			1									11
41–50		2		3	3	1	1	1	2		1		3		1		1	1					1		21
51–60	1	1	3	4		2	2	1	2			1			1										18
61–70	1	2	1	2		4	1	2		1	1		1			1									17
71–80				1					1																2
Total	5	15	11	10	9	7	7	6	7	1	2	1	5		2	2	1	1		1			1		94
Per cent.	5.3	15.9	11.7	10.6	9.6	7.4	7.4	6.4	7.4	1.1	2.1	1.1	5.3	..	2.1	2.1	1.1	1.1	..	1.1	..	..	1.1	..	

Average duration of 94 fatal cases of familial diabetes, 5.5 years.

The average duration of life of 96 fatal cases of hereditary diabetes seen between 1894 and September, 1922, was six and four-tenths years, in contrast to the average duration of life of all fatal cases at that time, which was five and six-tenths years. The average duration of life of 94 fatal cases of familial diabetes seen between 1894 and September, 1922, was five and five-tenths years, in contrast to the average duration of life of all fatal cases at that time, which was five and six-tenths years.

5. **Conjugal Incidence.**—Twenty-four instances (27 cases) of conjugal diabetes occurred in my 3000 cases. Oppler and C. Külz found 10 such instances in 900 cases of E. Külz; Senator, among 770 cases, found 9 diabetic couples. Naunyn observed 8 instances in 775 cases. All agree that similarity of living rather than contagion accounts for this condition, and I subscribe to this opinion. It is exposure to good food rather than to one another.

Twenty-seven of the 48 individuals concerned were seen by me, and only 1 of these was thin; information is lacking about the weights of 15, 7 of the patients weighed 165 to 190 pounds, and 14 from 190 pounds to 251 pounds. These facts, together with the duration of the disease, are recorded in the following table:

TABLE 53.—CONJUGAL CASES OF DIABETES.

Case No.	Sex.	Age at onset, years.	Height, feet and inches.	Weight, pounds.	Weight above standard, per cent.	Duration, years.	Weight of consort, pounds.
2 . . .	F.	54	..	171	..	9.0	165
10 . . .	M.	38	..	147	..	12.0	248
111 . . .	F.	46	..	248	..	9.0	147
234 . . .	M.	77	..	165	..	2.0	171
403 . . .	F.	55	..	192	..	6.1	
730 . . .	F.	57	5'5"	205	+40.5	13.5	
778 . . .	M.	54	5'8¾"	204	+23.7	10.0	
830 . . .	M.	45	..	196	..	20.0	Obese
832 . . .	F.	54	5'3½"	251	+76.4	11.7	200
905 . . .	M.	55	..	205	..	4.3	
1007 . . .	F.	39	5'4"	139	+ 4.9	22.3	
1024 . . .	F.	69	..	163	..	10.0	
1072 . . .	M.	63	..	175	..	11.0	
1232 . . .	F.	30	5'5"	113	−10.9	6.0	
1520 . . .	F.	61	4'11"	135	+ 9.0	4.7	
1558 . . .	M.	56	6'	190	+ 4.7	2.7	
1645 . . .	F.	58	..	220	..	4.6	
1903 . . .	F.	59	5'5"	208	+42.5	6.0	Obese
2139 . . .	F.	51	5'5"	184	+27.6	8.0	
2294 . . .	F.	48	5'3¾"	199	+42.2	7.5	
2574 . . .	F.	58	5'2"	173	+29.8	2.0	
2657 . . .	M.	49	5'7¼"	185	+21.2	2.5	
2694 . . .	F.	55	..	208	..	14.8	170
2701 . , .	F.	57	5'	142	+12.6	0.5	200
2775 . . .	M.	53	5'7"	243	+56.2	5.4	200
2864 . . .	M.	46	5'4½"	170	+21.6	2.3	299
2865 . . .	F.	34	5'½"	229	+88.2	4.3	170

The information given above offers no support to the infectious theory, and makes it appear quite plain that obesity, probably associated with lack of exercise, led to the development of the diabetes. None of the cases suggested to me at the time the presence of syphilis.

6. **Racial Incidence.**—The evidence of heredity should be greatest among Jewish patients. Unfortunately comparatively few of these patients are accurately informed about the causes of death of their antecedents. However, the statistics are as follows: Among 417 cases showing an hereditary tendency 64, or 15 per cent, were Hebrews. One hundred and eighty-nine of my cases showed a familial tendency, and 29 of these, or 15 per cent, were Hebrews. Combining the two groups, we find an hereditary or familial tendency among 93 Hebrews, which represents 26 per cent of the total number of Jewish patients. Thus, so far as my statistics go, the incidence of diabetes in the Jewish race distinctly favors the etiological importance of heredity, because as said above many of these patients were not in a position to know of the causes of death of their relatives. Evidence against this explanation is furnished by a study of my cases of diabetes with onset under twenty years. Thus, 12.3 per cent of 2800 cases developed diabetes under the age of twenty years, but only 9.2 per cent of 355 cases of Jewish extraction. The Hebrew race ought to exercise more and eat less.

The frequency with which diabetes occurs in the Jewish race is proverbial. Wallach[1] found that the death-rate from diabetes among the Jews in Frankfort, as compared with the deaths from all other causes, was six times greater among the Jews than among the other inhabitants. Thus of 1487 diabetic patients treated by von Noorden in eleven years, 31.5 per cent were Hebrews.

TABLE 54.—PERCENTAGE OF JEWISH CASES FOUND IN SUCCEEDING GROUPS OF 100 PATIENTS.

Groups of 100 patients.	Percentage of Jewish cases.	Groups of 100 patients.	Percentage of Jewish cases.	Groups of 100 patients.	Percentage of Jewish cases.
1st	5	11th	8	21st	18
2d	3	12th	10	22d	24
3d	4	13th	12	23d	15
4th	4	14th	11	24th	15
5th	6	15th	13	25th	14
6th	6	16th	12	26th	15
7th	17	17th	15	27th	15
8th	11	18th	17	28th	17
9th	13	19th	18	29th	24
10th	16	20th	21	30th	14

Morrison[2] found 1775 deaths from diabetes in Boston between 1895–1913. Among Jews the ratio of deaths from diabetes to

[1] Wallach: Deutsch. med. Wchnschr., 1893, **19**, 779.
[2] Morrison: Loc. cit., p. 125.

Table 55.—Duration of Life of 57 Fatal Cases of Diabetes in Jewish Race. September 1, 1922.

Decades.	Under 1 yr.	1 yr.	2 yrs.	3 yrs.	4 yrs.	5 yrs.	6 yrs.	7 yrs.	8 yrs.	9 yrs.	10 yrs.	11 yrs.	12 yrs.	13 yrs.	14 yrs.	15 yrs.	16 yrs.	17 yrs.	20 yrs.	22 yrs.	Total.
0–10	2	1	1																		4
11–20		1	2		4																7
21–30	3	3	3	1					2	1											13
31–40		1	2	1			1						1		1		1		1	1	8
41–50			3	1	2		1		1							1		2			12
51–60		1	4				2					2									10
61–70	1																				1
71–80						1		1													2
Total	6	7	15	3	6	1	4	1	3	1		2	1		1	1	1	2	1	1	57
Per cent	10.5	12.3	26.3	5.3	10.5	1.7	7.0	1.7	5.3	1.7		3.5	1.7		1.7	1.7	1.7	3.5	1.7	1.7	

Average duration of life of 57 fatal cases of diabetes in Semitics, 5.2 years.

the total number of deaths was 0.018, in contrast to 0.007 among non-Jews. In other words, diabetes is nearly twice and a half as common in this vicinity among Jews.

The number of Jewish patients in my series is 355. Of this number there were 171 males and 184 females, an interesting contrast to the preponderance of males among the total group of patients which has been above recorded. The number of Jewish patients seen in each successive 100 cases is given in Table 54.

It shows little more than the increase in the Jewish population in the community during the period of observation.

What is, however, of much more interest than the percentage of Jewish patients to the total number is the course which the disease has taken among these individuals. This is shown in Table 55.

The statistics for the Jewish patients have also been arranged in a table showing onset by decades, and as in former instances, the duration of life of the fatal cases up to September 1, 1922, is given. It is surprising to me that the course of the disease among my Jewish patients was less favorable than the general average. The reason for this is not clear, but I believe it to be due to the fact that they understood the diet less well, and so have paid the penalty of poor coöperation. Their diabetes does not appear severe and the absence of a single member of the race among my 12 patients taking over 30 units insulin daily would tend to confirm this opinion. There does not seem to be a prejudice among Hebrews against insulin, although they constitute but 7 per cent of the 358 insulin cases under my care.

The causes of death of the 58 fatal Jewish cases were as follows:

TABLE 56.—CAUSES OF DEATH OF THE 57 FATAL JEWISH CASES.

Coma	22
Tuberculosis	4
Cardio-renal and vascular	10
Tonsillitis	1
Cancer of kidney	1
Cancer of gall-bladder	1
Sarcoma of liver	1
Suicide	1
Gangrene	1
Angina pectoris	2
Diabetes	2
Empyema	1
Unknown	11
	—
	58

E. ETIOLOGY.

Diabetes centers around the islands of Langerhans, but why should they become diseased or cease to functionate? This is clear in experimental hemochromatosis, where Mallory has produced the destruction of the islands by injections of copper, but bronze diabetes is rare. This does not explain the hyaline degeneration and atrophy of the islands which is the far more common condition. An antecedent pancreatitis would appear to be the most logical explanation, but the existence of such can seldom be proved. In lieu of the true cause attention can be directed with profit to the predisposing causes and among these obesity is preëminent.

1. **Obesity.**[1]—(*a*) **Relation to Diabetes.**—The association of obesity and diabetes has long been noted. Contrariwise, in the presence of a wasting disease, diabetes is practically unknown. A few years ago an analysis of 1063 of my own cases showed that in more than 40 per cent of the number marked obesity preceded the outbreak of the disease, and the prediction was made that if more exact data were available the percentage would be fully twice as great. Writers generally have observed this connection, and von Noorden not only emphasized the necessity of examining the urines of fat persons for sugar, but also suggested that examinations of the blood sugar of fat persons would disclose their approach to the disease when the urine was sugar-free. In other words, a prediabetic stage in fat persons has been recognized and recently demonstrated by Paullin,[2] Beeler and Fitz.[3] But the closeness of the dependence of diabetes on obesity demands still more elucidation.

"While compiling the data for age, height and weight of a series of 118 diabetics whose respiratory metabolism had been studied at the Nutrition Laboratory of the Carnegie Institution, it was found that persons above the age of fifty rarely acquired diabetes if their weight remained a little below normal. These statistics, although striking, were too few for generalities. Therefore, data from 1000 successive cases of diabetes in which the age, weight and height were known were compiled and are here reported.

"Such extensive and inclusive data have not been published heretofore. Even if one searches the best of the monographs on diabetes it will be found that the case records, while giving the weight frequently fail to give the height. This unfortunate practice is not limited to diabetes. Indeed, it is only too true that during life patients are weighed, and at death they are measured, but in neither life nor death are both height and weight taken. This may explain why the data in this series of 1000 cases throw additional light on obesity as a predisposing cause of diabetes, and at the same time suggest how the disease may be prevented.

---

[1] This paragraph and others on the succeeding 9 pages are taken or rewritten from an article published by the author: Jour. Am. Med. Asso., 1921, **76**, 79.

[2] Paullin: So. Med. Jour., 1922, **15**, 249.

[3] Beeler and Fitz: Arch. Int. Med., 1921, **28**, 804.

"The table shows that among 1000 diabetic persons there was no instance in which diabetes occurred when the maximum weight was 31 or more per cent below the normal zone, whereas there were 273 persons who developed the disease among those who were 30 or more per cent above it.

TABLE 57.—VARIATION FROM NORMAL OF MAXIMUM WEIGHTS, AT OR PRIOR TO ONSET, OF 1000 CASES OF DIABETES, CALCULATED FOR HEIGHT, AGE AND SEX.

Age, years.	Number of cases.	Below standard weight, per cent.			Normal average zone, per cent. +5 −5	Above standard weight, per cent.								Percentage of each decade below normal zone.
		30-21.	10-11.	10-6.		6-10.	11-20.	21-30.	31-40.	41-50.	51-60.	61-70.	71+.	
1-10 . .	16	0	3	2	5	3	2	..	..	1	..	..	..	31
11-20 . .	59	2	11	8	24	6	4	2	1	..	1	..	..	36
21-30 . .	131	..	15	13	41	15	29	9	4	..	3	..	2	21
31-40 . .	178	1	9	12	28	22	34	25	15	14	10	6	2	12
41-50 . .	291	2	8	7	31	19	59	59	40	30	18	10	8	6
51-60 . .	233	..	4	7	16	28	39	48	45	14	13	5	4	5
61-70 . .	84	..	..	2	8	10	17	23	14	7	1	1	1	2
71-80 . .	18	..	..	1	6	3	2	3	2	1	..	..	..	6
1-80 . .	1000	5	50	52	159	106	186	169	121	67	46	22	17	

"If one examines the next pair of groups nearer the normal zone, namely, those between 21 to 30 per cent below and above normal, it will be seen that these contain 5 cases below the normal in contrast to 169 above normal. Consolidating this pair of groups with those mentioned in the preceding paragraph, one might add that of 1000 persons with diabetes there were only 5 who showed a maximum weight 21 or more per cent below normal, while there were as many as 394 whose maximum weight was 21 or more per cent above normal. Therefore, in this series, when the persons were 21 or more per cent overweight, diabetes occurred 79 times as frequently as when in the corresponding degree of underweight." In the 6 to 20 per cent group underweight there are 102 cases, but in the corresponding group overweight there are 292 cases, or 3 times as many. Hence, persons in the community at large who are from 6 to 20 per cent above weight are from 6 to 12 times as liable to diabetes as their counterparts in the same group below weight.

"The table as a whole shows that of the 1000 diabetics considered, the maximum weights of only 10 per cent were below the standard weight zone, while 15 per cent came in that zone and 75 per cent above it."

To the relation between obesity and diabetes, Mr. Mead of the Lincoln National Life Insurance Company has recently made a valuable contribution. He finds that the frequency of constitutional diseases in general increases as age advances and particularly as obesity advances, but that diabetes is to this extent an exception to the rule; its incidence increases with age only in the fat, while in the thin it remains constant throughout life. This shows that diabetic patients, young and old, are akin, and the earlier clinicians were right in sharply differentiating the fat and the thin patient with diabetes. The effect of body weight on the death-rate in general is graphically shown in a diagram issued by the Postal Life Insurance Company. The diagram applies to those individuals between forty-five and forty-nine years of age. Until thirty-five years of age the mortality is low for the overweights. The most favorable weight for longevity in middle life is 10 to 20 pounds below the average weight and even 30 pounds below the average is safer than the average weight itself.

DIAGRAM I. — EFFECT OF BODY WEIGHT ON GENERAL DEATH-RATE.[1]

(Persons between 5 ft. 7 in. and 5 ft. 10 in. in height, and between forty-five and forty-nine years of age).

50 lbs. under-weight	100%	Mortality
40 " " "	94%	"
30 " " "	93%	"
20 " " "	92%	"
10 " " "	92%	"
5 " " "	93%	"
Average Weight	94%	"
5 lbs. over-weight	95%	"
10 " " "	99%	"
20 " " "	109%	"
30 " " "	122%	"
40 " " "	137%	"
50 " " "	153%	"

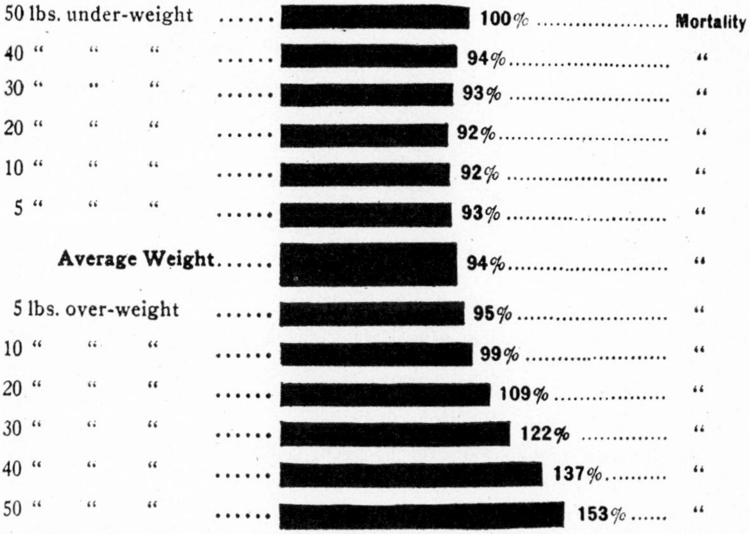

The black bars indicate, by their lengths, the proportionate mortality at different body weights, the number of pounds "underweight" and "overweight," recorded at the left, being the departures from the *average* weight for the specified heights and ages.

The figures recorded at the right of the bars are the specific

[1] Supplement to Health Bulletin No. 28, Postal Life Insurance Company.

mortality percentages for the corresponding underweights or overweights, the percentage for the average weight at this height and
age being 94.

*Note the greatly increased death-rate among the overweights, and that
the greater the excess weight the higher the death-rate. Only a little less
striking is the absence of increased death-rate among the underweights
except in the small class 50 pounds subnormal, whereas the increase
of mortality begins to be manifest as soon as the person becomes 5 per
cent too fat.*

"(*b*) **Diabetes.—A Penalty of Obesity.**—Diabetes, therefore, is
largely a penalty of obesity, and the greater the obesity, the more
likely is Nature to enforce it. The sooner this is realized by physicians and the laity, the sooner will the advancing frequency of
diabetes be checked. The penalty of taking too much alcohol is
well known, and a drunkard is looked on with pity or contempt.
Rarely persons who become fat deserve pity because of a real tendency to put on weight despite moderate eating, but usually most
should be placed in somewhat the same category as the alcoholic.
In the next generation one may be almost ashamed to have diabetes.
Jewish patients, sometimes hypersensitive to physical ills, but
often rightly anxious to take things in time, are already beginning
to realize this fact. I was told by the relative of one Hebrew
patient who died under distressing circumstances following laxity
in diet that the man's one desire was to avoid a death from diabetes,
because this had been so common in his ancestry.

"(*c*) **The Substandard Weight Patients.**—Patients in Table 57
who developed diabetes, though underweight, furnish a group for
very particular study. They should represent a purer, simpler
type of the disease. As this fact is now realized, subsequent cases
falling into this class will be better analyzed and the number
possibly reduced in size. On investigation of this series I have
already found that 29 of the 107 were really doubtful diabetics
according to the more accurate standards of today. They include
that dangerous group, "renal" diabetics, "insurance" diabetics
who are sometimes accepted as risks, and other extremely mild
cases. There may be further reductions because a considerable
number probably weighed more than is recorded, for the tendency
of the statistical error, as has been already said, is in the under-
statement rather than the overstatement of weight. An hereditary
and familial element was present in 24, and among these there were
8 examples of more than 1 case in the family. Several cases showed
stigmas of degeneracy, and it is my impression that greater familiarity on my part with such signs would increase the number that
should be classed in this way. Conversely, there were several extraordinarily severe cases, and yet in some of these very cases in which

the disease appeared severe, the patients withstood it for an un-usually long period. Indeed, it would seem justifiable to formulate this diabetic law: *It is rare for diabetes to develop in an individual above the age of twenty years who is habitually underweight, and when it does so develop the case will usually be found to be either extremely severe, extremely mild, or associated with a marked hereditary taint or degenerative stigmas.* The tendency to diabetes appears to be con-genital. It is most intense in childhood; but, escaping that period, the individual is less and less likely to acquire the disease if he remains underweight, whereas in the obese the tendency finds a fertile soil. In the fat the predisposition may be no greater, but the external cause is more provocative."

(*d*) **Obesity Predominant in Other Factors Often Mentioned in the Etiology of Diabetes.**—The preponderating influence of obesity in the development of diabetes explains various peculiarities in diabetic case histories and furnishes a new point of view from which to regard them.

1. *Conjugal Diabetes.*—Of 27 persons concerned in my series there was but 1 who was thin. Husband and wife were alike fat, and the implication is strong that they contracted the disease from exposure to good food rather than to one another.

2. *Frequency of Diabetes in the Jewish Race.*[1]—One has only to visit the Jewish quarter of a large city to be impressed with the frequency of obesity. Over-feeding begins in childhood and lasts to old age. Very likely with the increasing affluence of the Jewish race in this country, permitting indulgence in their well-known fondness for style, obesity will tend to diminish and along with it diabetes. The fashion plate makers are far ahead of insurance company presidents in their propaganda for a normal weight. All one needs to do is to glance at the morning paper to see ladies and gentlemen portrayed for our benefit whose sylphlike figures are models of weight and height—nay, more, they are invariably a trifle below the standard weight and so might bear the legend: "Immune to diabetes." Already obesity is seen less among the well-to-do than formerly. This applies not alone to the Jewish race, but to all races.

3. *Frequency of Diabetes Among the Richer Classes of Society.*— "On the broad street of a certain peaceful New England village there once stood three houses side by side, as commodious and attractive as any in the town. Into these three houses moved in succession 4 women and 3 men—heads of families—and of this number all but 1 subsequently succumbed to diabetes. The remaining member of the group died of cancer of the stomach at the age of seventy-seven years. A search for the cause of these

---

[1] See also page 134.

deaths, untimely in the majority of instances, led to the accumulation of the data on which this study of obesity was based.

"Although 6 of 7 persons dwelling in these adjoining houses died from a single cause, no one spoke of an epidemic. Contrast the activities of the local and state boards of health if these deaths had occurred from scarlet fever, typhoid fever or tuberculosis. Consider the measures that would have been adopted to discover the source of the outbreak and to prevent a recurrence. Because the disease was diabetes and because the deaths occurred over a considerable interval of time, the fatalities passed unnoticed. Even the insurance companies failed to grasp their significance, and yet probably no group of individuals in the community carried *pro rata* a higher amount of insurance than did these 6 diabetics." At the time these individuals lived, ideas of exercise for pleasure and the benefit of the body had not penetrated this rural region. Consequently, in this as in many other New England villages, though fortunately to a less extent now, the well-to-do were unusually fat. In fact, even today it is a common observation to note that country families tend more to obesity than their city cousins of similar means.

4. *Heredity.*—This may simply mean unusual exposure to an obetic environment. One should not forget that obesity is usually an acquired characteristic, and acquired characteristics are little subject to transmission from parent to child. The handicap of a diabetic heredity may be to a considerable extent counteracted by avoidance of overweight. What a comfort and stimulus to diabetic parents and gain to their children!

5. *Mental Workers in Contradistinction to Physical Workers.*— The former are more likely to be fat. But the probability of more frequent urinary examinations among the more intelligent and city dwellers might explain the apparent increase in frequency. Worms said that diabetes was so frequent among the mentally active in Paris that 1 in 10 had the disease.

6. *A Sequel to Infectious Diseases.*—Convalescents have big appetites, and unfortunately are almost fanatically overfed during a period of forced inactivity and at the very time when the pancreas must necessarily, like the rest of the body, be in a vulnerable state.

7. *Diabetes and Gout.*—Is it usual to see gout in the thin?

8. *Rarity of Syphilis in Diabetes.*—Statistics of the Peter Bent Brigham Hospital, those of von Noorden, and my own all agree in this regard—that syphilis is less common in diabetics than in the general population. Although data on the weights of syphilitic patients are not known to me, it is possible, first, that those who acquire the disease are more often thin than fat, and secondly, that they more often lose than gain weight after the disease has fully

developed. Who weighs and measures syphilitics? However, the shorter duration of life of patients with tuberculosis, cancer and syphilis in part explains the decreased frequency of diabetes in their presence.

9. *Age.*—The second decade of Table 57 proves an exception to those which follow in that there were more patients who developed diabetes below the standard weight than above it. This is almost the case in the first decade as well. In fact, obesity appears to play no part at this age, and so far as present evidence is available it must be acknowledged that these decades constitute an argument against the importance of obesity as a predisposing factor in the development of diabetes. Life insurance tables for prediction of longevity also give preference to persons in the first, second, third, and even a part of the fourth decade who are slightly above normal weight. Until more data concerning diabetic children are acquired, it is necessary to be cautious about conclusions, either pro or con, regarding obesity and diabetes at this age. In explanation of the many cases of diabetes in children who were not obese is Naunyn's conception of the virulence of the diabetic tendency in childhood which leads it to break forth without an external stimulus. Of the correctness of this interpretation, however, I am not quite convinced. It is possible that even here obesity is more of a predisposing agency than would appear. It might well be that a future compilation of children's cases would avoid errors of heights and weights unnoticed in this series, which began many years ago, when the cross-questioning of parents was less searching. The maximum weight of a child is even less frequently known than that of an adult. It should also be stated that in order to secure 1000 cases with definite data it has been necessary to exclude from the entire group of diabetics more cases from the first decade than from the others. Likewise in the second decade there is an added source of error because here more rapid accessions of weight occur and the peaks of these accessions often escape record. The subsequent histories of children once overweight should be compared with those of normal weight or below weight, and the incidence of diabetes in each group determined. Finally, the total number of cases in these decades is relatively small, making conclusions less justifiable. In the future, the proportion of cases of diabetes in children compared with diabetes in later years will probably continue to increase. Thus, if one examines the distribution by decades of onset of the disease prior to von Noorden's time, it will be found that six writers with an extensive diabetic practice recorded an average of only 0.7 per cent of all their cases as occurring in the first decade. Von Noorden's clientele showed 1.9 per cent, while, in my more recent series ending in 1922, this had risen to 5.4. Like-

wise, in the second decade fall 7.3 per cent of my cases, nearly twice the figure of most former observers. The relative disproportion of diabetes by age is, therefore, rapidly disappearing. At present the most common decades of onset are the fifth and sixth, in which the outstanding peculiarity, according to my table, is that there are more cases markedly overweight than in the other decades.

Kisch[1] directed attention to the frequency of the development of diabetes in the later lives of fat children, and I never see a fat child without thinking of this possibility, for a fat child, like a fat man, is prone to diabetes. Particularly serious must it be for a child or adult of slight stature to put on weight which would be excessive even for a man of large frame. Case No. 1142 first consulted me at the age of forty-one years, and I can just remember his little spindling legs and delicate frame as a boy before he entered the primary school; many years later he entered a grocery store, "worked like the dickens and ate the same way," until at the age of forty he was 60 pounds above the average weight, and sugar was found at a life insurance examination.

One of the most striking instances is that of a little child, Case No. 1139, a healthy baby until his second year, when he entered upon a series of rhinopharyngeal and bronchial attacks, including a mild bronchopneumonia. During eleven of the feverish illnesses exercise was curtailed and he was kept abed to safeguard his heart. A cow was bought that he might have fresh, rich milk, and to the 50 ounces of this milk which he daily consumed were added 3 tablespoonfuls of a malt preparation, amounting in nutritive value to 120 or more calories. At the end of his first year he was of normal weight, but at eighteen months his weight was above that of a child of two years. When two years old his weight had increased to that of a child of three years and a half, and when two years and a half old, his weight was above that of a child of four years. Is it surprising that when mumps developed in 1915, glycosuria appeared to the extent of 3.1 per cent. It vanished with a change in diet, to return three months later, during the presence of another mild febrile disorder, and again in six months after the removal of adenoids, but since this occasion the urine has remained sugar-free to date, 1923.

A poor musculature usually accompanies obesity. One-half of the carbohydrate in the body is stored in the muscles and a large part of the sugar of the body is burned in them. Therefore it does not appear strange that fat people develop diabetes. It would almost seem as if the muscles became so loaded with fat that they were unable to burn carbohydrate. At one time fat and glycogen in the liver were thought to be antagonistic to one another. Under

---

[1] Kisch: Jour. Am. Med. Assn., 1915, **64**, 1038.

the influence of insulin, the Toronto investigators found they could exist together.

10. *Dietary Excesses.*—Dietary excesses figure quite prominently in my records as precursors of diabetes. Allen's dogs artificially predisposed to diabetes by removal of a considerable portion of the pancreas became diabetic when overfed. It is, however, the excess of food rather than of carbohydrate which does the harm. Indeed, a high percentage of carbohydrate in the diet does not appear to predispose to diabetes. Thus, the Japanese live upon a diet consisting largely of rice and barley, yet so far as statistics show, the disease is not only less frequent but milder in that country than in this. In 1913, Germany consumed half as much sugar as was eaten in the United States, and yet diabetes was quite as prevalent there as here. The increase in the quantity of sugar consumed per capita in the United States during the last century is very great, as shown by Table 58, and when one compares this table with the rising incidence of diabetes shown in Tables 31 to 34, it would seem as if the two must stand in relation. Fortunately, the dietary habits and the statistics upon diabetes of Japan would seem to save us from this error, but I am not quite convinced, and shall be glad to study the more accurate figures for the incidence of diabetes in countries where carbohydrate food is predominant, which will come with time. It will also be of interest to learn the incidence of diabetes of workers in candy factories. Even yet this has not been thoroughly investigated.[1]

TABLE 58.—THE CONSUMPTION OF SUGAR IN THE UNITED STATES.

Years.	Population average for decade.	Pounds per capita, yearly average.	Diabetic death-rate per 100,000.
1800–1810	6,146,343	11	First and
1810–1820	8,280,041	8	last years
1820–1830	11,038,448	9	of de-
1830–1840	14,720,126	12	cades.
1840–1850	19,824,542	2	
1850–1860	26,905,025	26	
1860–1870	34,645,094	23	
1870–1880	43,777,206	33	
1880–1890	55,912,152	44	2.8– 5.5
1890–1900	68,818,801	56	5.5– 9.3
1900–1910	83,275,548	65	9.7–14.9
1910–1920	98,796,383	82	14.9–16.1
1921	107,064,455	84	16.8

The marked increase in the consumption of sugar, largely sucrose, shown in Table 58 might appear of great significance in seeking for a cause of the greater frequency of diabetes today were it not

[1] Von Noorden: Die Zuckerkrankheit, Berlin, 1917, 7th ed., p. 331.

10

for the fact that, whereas the consumption of sugar per capita between 1900–1921 has increased 17 per cent, the mortality from diabetes has nearly doubled.   Nevertheless, such a marked alteration in the diet of a nation is noteworthy and deserves attention."

2. **Multiple Etiology.**—The majority of diabetic patients present multiple causes for their diabetes.   This is well exemplified by the history of a gentleman, aged forty-nine years, Case No. 954, who consulted me on December 12, 1915.   One of his children died in 1901 at the age of two years, and another in 1913 at the age of twelve years, both of diabetes.   As a child he had measles, scarlet fever, and whooping-cough, and at twenty-four years was ill for eighteen months with inflammatory rheumatism, and the pericardium was tapped twice.

At the age of thirty-three years his weight was 200 pounds, and for his height—5 feet 11 inches—was 17 per cent above normal. Prior to this time he indulged in considerable alcohol three evenings a week, and his use of tobacco was more than moderate.   He was fond of sweets and occasionally ate half a pound of candy in an evening.   During the last two years he took little exercise, and recently led a strenuous life on account of his active business. An attack of gall stones, which was accompanied by an infection of the biliary tract, led to an operation on November 15, 1915. Prior to the operation the urine was examined and found normal. The anesthetic was ether.   Convalescence from the operation was satisfactory, but while at the hospital his friends, knowing his fondness for sweets, sent him much candy, which he ate.   On December 11, 1915, he observed polyuria, and later he recalled that when nervous and working hard this symptom had occurred off and on for a day's duration during several years.   On December 11, 1915, sugar was demonstrated in the urine, and upon the following day, when he came for treatment, the specific gravity was 1045 and the percentage of sugar was 7.2.   The weight of the patient was approximately 185 pounds shortly after the operation, and on December 13 was 177 pounds naked.   The patient began fasting by omitting his supper on December 12, and the twenty-four-hour quantity of urine ending December 14 contained only a trace of sugar, and even this was absent the following day.   Improvement was uninterrupted.

The important etiological factors of diabetes were all present in this case.   There was a tendency to diabetes, as illustrated by the death of his two children with the disease; obesity and dietary excesses existed; a strenuous life; nervous excitement connected with the operation; the presence of an infection; the trauma of the operation, and presumable local interference with the normal action of the pancreas and liver.

It was interesting that the disease did not break out earlier in the case of this patient, when one realizes that obesity had existed several years before. It plainly suggested that obesity alone was not a sufficiently strong factor to lead to the disease. Even when to this were added dietary excesses and the strenuous life, the disease still remained latent and only a multiplicity of influences, such as were brought about by the operation, were sufficient to make it declare itself.

3. **Heredity.**—The influence of heredity is elsewhere discussed. (See p. 125.)

4. **Nervous Element.**—A strenuous life has been considered by most writers as of importance in the etiology of diabetes, and it has so impressed me. Von Noorden records that 8 per cent of all his mild diabetic patients were physicians, and this can easily be connected with the strenuous life which medical work entails. The frequency of diabetes, among physicians, however, is undoubtedly in part due to the opportunity they have for detecting the disease. In my own series of male patients ending 1916, above the age of twenty, 10 per cent were physicians. Of these 15 had died by 1917, and the average duration of the diabetes was seven years; 47 were alive, and the average duration of the diabetes up to December 1, 1916, was likewise seven years.

The nervous element in diabetes has gained additional importance since the publication of the work of Cannon, Shohl and Wright[1] and the investigations of Folin, Denis and Smillie[2] upon the appearance of sugar in the urines of 192 insane patients. Of these, 22 showed sugar with the standard tests. The latter investigators also examined the urines of students after important examinations. "Of 34 second-year medical students examined before and after an examination, 1 had sugar both before and after the examination. Of the remaining 33, 6, or 18 per cent, had small but unmistakable traces of sugar in the urine passed immediately after the examination. A similar study was made on second-year women students at Simmons College. Since these students were younger, and presumably much more excitable than our medical students, it was thought that even more striking results might be obtained. This expectation did not prove to be well founded. Out of 36 taking the examination and showing no sugar in the urine on the day before, 6, or 17 per cent, eliminated sugar with the urine passed immediately after the examination." Even emotion caused by securing samples of blood for analysis may lead to a rise in blood sugar percentage. Case No. 10 developed severe diabetes when on an unusual business trip involving much responsibility. The appearance of

[1] Cannon, Shohl and Wright: Am. Jour. Phys., 1911, **29**, 280.
[2] Folin, Denis and Smillie: Jour. Biol. Chem., 1914, **17**, 519.

polyuria and polydipsia was acute, but he lived twelve years. In comparatively few instances in this series was the presence of an organic nervous disease demonstrated. Allen's conception of the functional nature of diabetes shows how the disease may be brought about through the nervous system by its action upon the pancreas. Thus the Claude Bernard puncture produced diabetes in one of Allen's dogs, predisposed to the same by the removal of a portion of the pancreas, and yet proved to be non-diabetic before the puncture. In this dog characteristic changes were found in the islands of Langerhans at autopsy.

Soldiers returning from the front did not show sugar in the urine. About 40,000 passed through the hospital center in Mesves, France, where I was consultant; yet, though the urines were systematically examined, but 2 cases of diabetes were discovered, or at least came to my attention. It would be instructive to note the incidence of diabetes in the same soldiers at a period some months later when added weight was the rule.

Children who have stood exceptionally high in their classes at school have figured largely among those children who have come under my observation with the disease. Because of the frequency of this association I have cautioned my medical friends whose children were exceptionally brilliant. Statistics are not of great service in this regard, but my associates H. Gray and H. F. Root confirm my observation. In August, 1923, a boy of seventeen years comes with diabetes who has just been admitted to Harvard without examination and already has two scholarships at his disposal!

5. **Infections.**—An infection lowers a diabetic's tolerance for carbohydrate and visibly increases the severity of the disease. In only a few instances have I been able to associate infectious diseases with diabetes. In fact, in but 15 per cent of 400 cases in my series. Geyelin[1] has seen 8 cases of diabetes originating in patients within five weeks of the beginning of the infection and all of these patients were known to be sugar-free before the infection commenced. Coleman, who with DuBois has had much experience with high diets in typhoid fever, tells me that in none of their cases did diabetes develop. When one considers the frequency of infectious diseases in a community and the rarity with which diabetes develops after the same, one is not inclined to assign great importance to infections. On the other hand, the marked lowering in tolerance for carbohydrates in the diabetic patients when an infection appears is an emphatic demonstration that this subject should be thoroughly investigated, and I certainly remain open-

---

[1] Geyelin: Annual Meeting of Connecticut State Medical Society, New Haven, Conn., 1923.

minded upon it. The loss of tolerance during an infection was recently discussed by Peters.[1] He reported several cases with striking decrease in tolerance during acute illness and later a recovery of tolerance even up to 275 grams carbohydrate. With another patient tolerance successively failed following a series of infections, but this could be related to breaking diet. With adherence to diet the loss of tolerance did not disappear.

The association of acidosis with an infection was also emphasized by Peters in a considerable series of cases of diabetic coma treated at the New Haven Hospital. There was but one admission of a patient with whom a recent infection did not play a factor. According to Peters an infection in a diabetic means—go to bed.

The importance which diseases of the teeth and gums play in the etiology of diabetes is often raised. The evidence in my data is pro and con. It is a routine practice at the hospital to have the teeth of all patients promptly cared for. I have observed in certain cases that diabetes has appeared shortly after many teeth have been extracted and have attributed this in part to the increased proportion of carbohydrate in the diet.

6. **Arteriosclerosis.**—The frequency of arteriosclerosis with diabetes is perhaps best explained by the increasing incidence of the disease as age advances quite as much as any effect the arteriosclerosis may have upon the blood supply of the islands of Langerhans.

7. **Syphilis.**—See pp. 142, 607. Syphilis is a rarity in a diabetic clinic.

8. **Trauma.**—If trauma were a factor in the causation of diabetes the war would have shown it. Above, see p. 148, attention is drawn to the infrequency of diabetes in soldiers returning from the front. My experience was not unusual. Von Noorden writes: "...... neurogenen Diabetes gibt es überhaupt nicht; die Kriegserfahrungen haben ihn vollends zu Grabe getragen."[2]

A definite history of trauma immediately preceding the disease was present in Cases Nos. 7 and 982 of my series. In Case No. 7 the patient observed the first symptoms of diabetes directly after being injured by a cow. He was seen by me once on October 25, 1898, four weeks later, and died in coma five months after the onset. No record of a previous urinary examination exists. Case No. 982 was seriously hurt in his back in a foot-ball game, in the fall of 1913, and became unconscious. A broken neck was suspected. In the following January he again had a serious fall in the woods and again injured his back, so that he was incapacitated for three weeks.

---

[1] Peters: Annual Meeting of Connecticut State Medical Society, New Haven, Conn., 1923.

[2] This statement occurs in an instructive address by von Noorden before the Berlin Medical Society, December 13, 1922, and was published by Julius Springer, Berlin, 1923.

At the expiration of this time he observed that his mouth was dry, and in February, sugar was found in the urine. This case too, ran a rather severe course and the patient died six years after onset in coma.

Case No. 954 (See p. 46) developed the diabetes after the trauma of an operation but there were many other etiological factors present, and furthermore such an event must be extremely rare. An operation represents trauma, yet after operation even with ether for an anesthetic, diabetes is almost unknown.

Case No. 1188 probably represents best of all the indirect harm which may result from trauma, though his case resembles most cases of the supposed influence of trauma upon diabetes by lack of evidence showing its absence before the accident. This patient was an ice-cream manufacturer in 1915, at the age of thirty-one, and weighed 242 pounds. He was in the habit of eating, in addition to his regular meals, two quarts of his own ice-cream. During the subsequent year, his weight fell to about 212 pounds, when on October 27, he was accidentally shot with a rifle, and his leg badly shattered, requiring frequent painful dressings. The urine was first examined on November 27, 1916, and sugar found. The quantity amounted to 3780 cc, and the percentage of sugar was large. Under treatment he gradually became sugar-free and acquired a tolerance for about 80 grams carbohydrate. He is (1923) alive and in good condition.

The fracture of an extremity is often accompanied by glycosuria. Among 61 cases at the Surgical Clinic at Kiel, 24 showed alimentary glycosuria, and in 3 unsuspected diabetes was discovered. Hyperglycemia was present in 31 out of 36 of the cases examined.[1] It would not seem strange if many of the cases of diabetes following trauma might be due to the enforced idleness and rest combined with forced feeding at the hands of friends.

Demonstrated septicemia, resulting from trauma, even though diabetic coma supervenes, should be reported as the primary cause of death.

9. **Hypophysis.**—The intimate relation of the hypophysis to glycosuria and diabetes has been emphasized by Cushing, and is described in detail by him.[2] I have recognized but one instance, Case No. 1155.

10. **Liver.**—The connection between diseases of the liver and diabetes has been frequently pointed out. Such an association is only demonstrable in my cases with gall stones. Out of 887 deaths there have been only 3 who have died in which cirrhosis of the liver appeared to figure as a cause of death, and but 8 of cancer

---

[1] Konjetzuy and Weiland: Jour. Am. Med. Assn., 1915, **65**, 2264.
[2] Cushing: The Pituitary Body and its Disorders, Philadelphia, 1912.

of the liver. The 73 cases (Table 182, p. 478) in which gall stones have been a factor probably should be credited etiologically to the pancreas.

11. **Gout.**—Gout is frequently mentioned as a precursor or companion of diabetes. So seldom has this occurred in my experience that I cannot attach much importance to it. Dr. J. H. Pratt, of Boston, who has seen an unusually large number of cases of gout, assures me that in but one instance was sugar found in the urine of his patients.

F. IMPROVEMENT IN TREATMENT STATISTICALLY PROVED.

For the successful treatment of a chronic disease it is essential that the physician be convinced that his methods of treatment are improving. In diabetes mellitus there has been no doubt about this improvement. Various factors have contributed indirectly to bring about this result and of these an earlier diagnosis, a more general knowledge of the diet, a clearer understanding of the disease, including the prevention of coma, and the far better treatment of surgical complications are the more important.

Success in the treatment of diabetes, as well as of tuberculosis, depends upon an early diagnosis. Naunyn especially urges the importance and good results of early treatment. All will agree, we are in a much more favorable position to make early diagnoses now than were the physicians of a former generation. Yearly urinary examinations and life insurance examinations help much. When a routine urinary examination is neglected, the damage done to the patient is considerable, but to the physician's reputation is extreme. The physician is *never* forgiven. The time is probably not far distant, if not already here, when the question will be asked of the diabetic: "How long did the disease exist before it was discovered?" and "Who was your physician?" We are familiar with the same questions in tuberculosis.

Already attention has been drawn to the increasing frequency of life insurance examination, and the growing percentage of my own cases who discovered diabetes in this way.

An accurate knowledge of the diet is responsible for a large share of the improvement in treatment. For this we are indebted— first to the publication by the United States Government of Bulletin No. 28,[1] and especially to the vigorous campaign conducted under the auspicies of the Connecticut Agricultural Experiment Station in bringing to common knowledge the carbohydrate content of

---

[1] Chemical Composition of American Food Materials, Bulletin No. 28, U. S. Department of Agriculture. This can be obtained by sending 10 cents in coin to Superintendent of Documents, Washington, D. C.

so-called diabetic foods. Twenty-five years ago a knowledge of the carbohydrate content of the food of an individual was almost negligible. One is free in making this statement because even today relatively few physicians can reckon up the carbohydrate in the diet of their patients. For this lack of instruction in diet medical teaching is largely responsible.

It is no longer considered almost miraculous for a patient to void urine with 11 per cent of sugar upon one day and a few days later to become sugar-free. It is recognized that a blood sugar of 0.4 per cent falls slowly and that with renal complications may not reach normal, and that under these circumstances sugar may persist for days or even weeks in the urine. Successes with bizarre methods of treatment, such as an exclusive buttermilk diet, are now explained by the accompanying undernutrition which they entailed.

The merits of a new method of treatment are more quickly determined today than a generation ago, and this contributes to better treatment. The number of new remedies exploited upon the profession and upon the laity has been growing less, though there are some indications that a new crop of remedies is about to mature. Physicians realize better than formerly that the value of any remedy in the disease must depend upon its power to increase tolerance for carbohydrate, and so far insulin has been the only remedy capable of bringing this about. The prevention of coma is plainly taught.

TABLE 59.—DURATION OF LIFE OF DIABETICS WHO DIED AT THE MASSACHUSETTS GENERAL HOSPITAL BETWEEN 1824–1917.

Duration, years.	1824–1898.		1898–1913.		1913–1917.	
	No. of cases.	Per cent.	No. of cases.	Per cent.	No. of cases.	Per cent.
0– 1	27	67.5	28	40.6	10	47.6
1– 2	7	17.5	13	18.8	1	4.8
2– 3	3	7.5	6	8.7	2	9.5
3– 4	1	2.5	6	8.7		
4– 5	..	..	2	2.9	3	14.3
5– 6	1	2.5	5	7.2	2	9.5
6– 7	1	2.5	1	1.4	1	4.8
7– 8	..	..	2	2.8		
9–10	..	..	1	1.4		
10–11	..	..	1	1.4	1	4.8
15–16	..	..	1	1.4	1	4.8
16–17	..	..	2	2.9		
20–21	..	..	1	1.4		
Unknown because of lack of past history	7	..	10	..	6	
Total deaths	47		79		27	
Percentage of diabetics treated	27		28		11	

Direct improvement is shown by statistics. The duration of life of diabetic patients for three epochs at the Massachusetts General Hospital are of especial value for comparative purposes and are shown in Table 59. The first period includes all cases from the beginning of the records of the hospital in 1824 to 1898 and the second from 1898–1913, a period which is sufficiently remote to exclude the results of modern treatment. The third period (1913–1916) represents the transition to the period of treatment by undernutrition as introduced by Allen. For the data of the first period I am responsible, having searched the records for a paper which was published conjointly with R. H. Fitz.[1] The statistics for the years 1898–1913 and 1913–1916 were collected, under my direction, by my secretary, Miss Helen Leonard, and the duration of each case verified by my former assistant, Dr. F. Gorham Brigham. For the privilege of inserting these data, I am indebted to the Superintendent and Staff of the Massachusetts General Hospital.

Of the total number of 172 diabetic patients treated during the first seventy-four years, 47 or *27 per cent* died within the hospital walls. Of the total number of 280 diabetic patients treated during the second period 1898–1913, 79 or *28 per cent* died. Whereas the percentage of patients who died in the hospital during the two periods was the same, it is evident that the duration of life of the patients was distinctly greater in the second period. The most striking feature, however, is the fall in mortality during the first year, namely from 67.5 per cent to 40.6 per cent. The statistics lend weight to the inference that the treatment of the disease as a whole in the community had improved, but that the intensive treatment of such cases as came to the hospital remained stationary. During the third period 243 cases of diabetes were treated at the hospital and the number of deaths was 27, or *11 per cent.*

The duration of life of the fatal cases of diabetes occurring in Boston for the period 1895–1913 and for 1915 are given in Table 60. Between 1895–1913, in Boston, the average duration of the disease was three and three-tenths years, for 1915, it was four and three-tenths years, but in 1920, it was five and three-tenths years.

Heiberg[2] has published a table which gives the duration of life of fatal cases of diabetes in Denmark. This table does not give comparative figures for different years but shows the duration for different age groups. Thus between the ages of fifteen and thirty years 25 per cent of the cases were dead at the end of six months

---

[1] Fitz and Joslin: Diabetes Mellitus at the Massachusetts General Hospital, 1824–1898, Jour. Am. Med. Assn., 1898, **70**, 139.

[2] Heiberg: Ztschr. f. klin. Med., 1921, **92**, 76.

and 100 per cent dead in fifteen years.   From this table comparison
can be made with subsequent tables of my own and a favorable
difference in mortality noted.

TABLE 60.—DURATION OF LIFE OF 1057 FATAL CASES OF DIABETES IN BOSTON
DURING 1895–1913 AND IN 1915.

Duration, years.	1895–1913.[1]		1915.	
	No. of cases.	Per cent.	No. of cases.	Per cent.
0– 1	309	32.7	32	27.3
1– 2	207	21.9	16	13.6
2– 3	102	10.8	18	15.3
3– 4	56	5.9	5	4.2
4– 5	71	7.5	8	6.8
5– 6	26	2.6	14	11.9
6– 7	24	2.5	2	1.7
7– 8	30	3.2	3	2.5
8– 9	8	0.8	3	2.5
9–10	59	6.3	1	0.8
10–11	4	0.4	4	3.4
11–12	8	0.8	1	0.8
12–13	4	0.4	3	2.5
14–15	17	1.8	2	1.7
15–16	4	0.4	2	1.7
17–18	3	0.3	1	0.8
20–30	8	0.8	2	1.6
	940		117	
Duration long, but uncertain .	207	..	20	
Unknown	567	..	54	
Diabetic gangrene	50	..	4	
Total	1764		195	

TABLE 61.—THE DURATION OF LIFE IN FATAL CASES OF DIABETES.   (HEIBERG.[2])

Sex.	Age.	25 per cent, years.	50 per cent, years.	75 per cent, years.	100 per cent, years.
Males . .	15–30	$\frac{1}{2}$	$1\frac{1}{4}$	$2\frac{1}{2}$	15
	31–50	$1\frac{1}{2}$	3	$4\frac{1}{2}$	20
	51 and over	$1\frac{3}{4}$	$4\frac{1}{4}$	9	20
Females . .	15–30	$\frac{3}{4}$	$1\frac{1}{2}$	$2\frac{1}{2}$	10
	31–50	1	2	$3\frac{3}{4}$	15
	51 and over	$1\frac{1}{2}$	$3\frac{1}{2}$	$7\frac{1}{4}$	20

Von Noorden[3] writing in 1917, says that diabetes in children
under ten years of age seldom lasts more than for one and a half
or two years; in the second decade it seldom exceeds two to four
years; in the third decade four to six years, occasionally even ten
years, but seldom longer.   People who acquire the disease after
the thirtieth year have a considerably greater length of life, and

[1] Morrison: Boston Med. and Surg. Jour., 1916, **175**, 54.
[2] Heiberg, K. A.: Ztschr. f. klin. Med., 1921, **92**, 76.
[3] Von Noorden: Die Zuckerkrankheit, Berlin, 1917, 7th ed., p. 342.

with favorable conditions the disease may last from ten to fifteen years or even longer. The first half of the fifth decade, however, is a more critical period, but when this corner is passed the tendency of the disease is to remain mild, provided doctor and patient are free from blame themselves. Such patients may live fifteen, twenty or even thirty years. Still, a length of life of more than twenty years belongs to the exception.

TABLE 62.—DURATION OF LIFE IN FATAL CASES OF DIABETES ARRANGED IN DECADES BEFORE AND AFTER JUNE, 1914.

Decades of onset, years.	Before June, 1914.		After June, 1914.	
	No. of cases.	Duration, years.	No. of cases.	Duration, years.
0– 9	25	1.2	47	2.7
10–19	39	2.9	69	3.3
20–39	80	3.9	162	5.3
40–59	137	6.9	216	8.1
60–89	50	4.5	103	6.1
0–89	331	4.8	597	6.0

The prolongation of life in my own series of cases is manifest just as in the Boston series. Prior to June, 1914, the average duration of life of my fatal cases was four and eight-tenths years and since 1914 has been six years. With advancing age periods the average duration of life has increased from the first to the seventh decade, when as might be expected the duration has again fallen off. Table 62.

The effect of insulin will not appear clearly in my own statistics until the completion of the second year of its use on August 7, 1924, and not fully for about a decade, because the average diabetic today following treatment with moderate care should live eight years without insulin. However, see Table 28, p. 100.

TABLE 63.—PERCENTAGE OF FATAL CASES AND AVERAGE DURATION OF SAME WHO OUTLIVED AN AVERAGE PERIOD OF SIX YEARS. ARRANGED BY DECADES FOR THE PERIODS BEFORE AND AFTER JUNE, 1914.

Decades of onset, years.	June, 1914.					Average, duration. years
	Before.—Cases.		Average duration, years.	After.—Cases.		
	No. of cases with duration over six years.	Percentage to total deaths in decades.		No. of cases with duration over six years.	Percentage to total deaths in decades.	
0– 9	0	0	0	3	6	7[1]
10–19	3	8	10	7	10	8
20–29	3	9	20	15	18	12
30–39	11	24	9	30	38	13
40–49	24	21	13	58	53	11
50–59	37	47	11	72	57	11

[1] Case No. 887 is omitted, as the duration of life was thirty-three years.

The number of diabetic individuals who have lived in excess of the space of years attained by my entire group of fatal cases is considerable. Thus in the seventh decade there were actually 18 who reached or exceeded the average normal expectation of life for this period. In Table 63 are shown 79 cases (23 per cent) out of the total number before 1914 who lived above the average period of six years, which was that for the cases after 1914, and 186 cases (31 per cent) out of the total number since 1914, who did the same. If one examines the table by individual decades it will be found without exception that the percentage surviving the six-year average was greater in the later than in the earlier series. Data for the seventh decade and over are omitted, because the expectancy of life for the general population is thirteen years or less after sixty years of age. See p. 678 for a series of diabetics who outlived their expectation of life. Regretfully it must be acknowledged that even in recent years some cases have died within a few weeks of onset. These are the deaths which must be eliminated if the average duration is to be strikingly increased, and fortunately this is an easy task.

The change in treatment in diabetes is registered by the decreasing number of patients who succumb during the year following the onset of the disease. Until 1898, at the Massachusetts General Hospital, 68 per cent of the patients who died showed a duration of less than one year, and even in the subsequent fifteen years this proportion was as high as 41 per cent. Returning to my own series of 331 fatal cases before June, 1914, 18 per cent succumbed during the first year; but of 569 fatal cases since June, 1914, the percentage has fallen to 12.

TABLE 64.—DECREASE IN DEATHS DURING FIRST YEAR OF THE DISEASE.

		Total deaths.	Deaths, first year, per cent.
Massachusetts General Hospital, 1824–1898	. .	69	68
1898–1914	. .	21	41
Author's series . . . . { 1898–1914	. .	331	18
1914–1922	. .	569	12

Data will be presented in different forms upon my own series of cases which will show improvement in various ways. It is appropriate to record these results, because they will serve as a basis for comparison with future series of cases treated with insulin. In December, 1916, only 1 of the 17 cases first seen prior to 1900 was alive while 14 per cent of those seen between 1901–1905 were living, and 31 per cent of those seen between 1906–1910. Of the 551 cases who first came under my observation during the previous five years there were 60 per cent alive, and 90 per cent of those seen during the twelve months ending December 1, 1916. *There-fore, in the year 1916 about 10 per cent of all cases coming for treat-ment died during the year. For comparison I can report 282 cases of diabetes, selected largely on account of their severity, who were treated with insulin for the year ending August 7, 1923. Of these patients, all but 1 have been traced and 7 per cent are dead.* One hundred and fifty-five other cases of diabetes were treated during the same period, but for one reason or another were not given insulin. They have not been traced because often they were mild and so not comparable. Insulin-treated diabetics should be the best, henceforth, for statistical purposes, because they will be more carefully selected, though it is true they may be more severe than the average diabetic.

TABLE 65.—VITAL STATISTICS OF DIABETIC PATIENTS ARRANGED ACCORDING TO PERIODS WHEN FIRST OBSERVED, IRRESPECTIVE OF PREVIOUS DURATION. DATA COMPILED IN 1916.

Period first observed.	Total cases traced.	Alive in 1916.	
		No.	Per cent.
1893–1900	17	1	6
1901–1905 . . . . : .	86	12	14
1906–1910	263	82	31
1911–1915	551	329	60
1915–1916	239	216	**90**
Total	1156	640	55

TABLE 66.—THE INCREASING DURATION OF LIFE IN DIABETES, BASED UPON FATAL CASES AT DIFFERENT PERIODS.

Duration, years.	Dec., 1893–1915.		Dec., 1893–1916.		Jan., 1893–1918.	
	No. of cases.	Per cent.	No. of cases.	Per cent.	No. of cases.	Per cent.
0– 1	69	16.9	74	14.8	85	14.4
1– 2	72	17.6	85	17.0	96	16.2
2– 3	64	15.7	80	16.0	90	15.2
3– 4	35	8.6	41	8.2	52	8.8
4– 5	23	5.6	27	5.4	36	6.1
5– 6	23	5.6	33	6.6	39	6.6
6– 7	17	4.2	27	5.4	31	5.2
7– 8	13	3.2	19	3.8	23	3.9
8– 9	18	4.4	20	4.0	27	4.6
9–10	14	3.4	19	3.8	22	3.7
10–11	10	2.4	10	2.0	14	2.4
11–12	12	2.9	15	3.0	18	3.0
12–13	9	2.2	11	2.2	15	2.5
13–14	4	1.0	5	1.0	6	1.0
14–15	6	1.5	6	1.2	6	1.0
15–16	4	1.0	7	1.4	8	1.4
16–17	2	0.5	3	0.6	4	0.7
17–18	3	0.7	4	0.8	4	0.7
18–19	1	0.2	1	0.2	2	0.3
19–20	2	0.5	5	1.0	5	0.8
20–21 and over .	7	1.7	8	1.6	9	1.6
Total . . .	408		500		592	

TABLE 67.—FATAL CASES OF DIABETES ARRANGED ACCORDING TO ONSET AND DURATION OF DISEASE. JANUARY 1, 1918.

Cases arranged by decade of onset.	Under 1 yr.	1 yr.	2 yrs.	3 yrs.	4 yrs.	5 yrs.	6 yrs.	7 yrs.	8 yrs.	9 yrs.	10 yrs.	11 yrs.	12 yrs.	13 yrs.	14 yrs.	15 yrs.	16 yrs.	17 yrs.	18 yrs.	19 yrs.	20 yrs.	21 yrs.	22 yrs.	23 yrs.	24 yrs.	25 yrs.	26 yrs.	27 yrs.	28 yrs.	29 yrs.	30 yrs.	35 yrs.	Total.
0–10	22	14	4	1	1	·	2	·	1	·	·	·	·	·	·	·	·	·	·	·	·	·	·	·	·	·	·	·	·	·	·	·	46
11–20	13	21	16	9	3	4	·	1	1	1	1	·	1	·	1	1	·	·	·	·	·	1	·	·	·	·	·	·	·	1	·	·	70
21–30	13	12	17	6	7	5	1	1	2	2	1	2	·	1	1	2	2	1	1	2	·	·	·	·	·	·	·	·	·	·	·	1	64
31–40	10	10	14	7	8	3	3	2	5	5	4	6	3	4	3	5	1	2	1	3	1	1	1	·	·	1	·	·	·	·	·	·	71
41–50	7	15	12	13	8	6	3	7	3	10	6	8	6	5	6	·	1	·	1	·	1	1	·	·	·	·	·	·	·	·	·	·	107
51–60	9	12	14	13	5	9	11	3	12	3	2	2	4	·	2	·	1	1	1	·	1	1	·	·	·	·	·	·	·	·	·	·	136
61–70	8	10	8	5	3	12	6	7	3	1	·	·	6	·	·	·	·	·	·	·	·	·	·	·	·	·	·	·	·	·	·	·	79
71–80	3	2	5	1	1	1	1	2	1	·	·	·	·	·	·	·	·	·	·	·	·	·	·	·	·	·	·	·	·	·	·	·	19
Total	85	96	90	52	36	39	31	23	27	22	14	18	15	6	6	8	4	4	2	5	2	3	1	·	··	1	·	·	·	1	·	1	592
Per cent	14.4	16.2	15.2	8.8	6.1	6.6	5.2	3.9	4.6	3.7	2.4	3.0	2.5	1.0	1.0	1.4	0.7	0.7	0.3	0.8	0.3	0.5	0.2	·	··	0.2	·	·	·	0.2	·	0.2	

LIVING CASES OF DIABETES ARRANGED ACCORDING TO ONSET AND DURATION OF DISEASE. JANUARY 1, 1918.

Cases arranged by decade of onset.	Under 1 yr.	1 yr.	2 yrs.	3 yrs.	4 yrs.	5 yrs.	6 yrs.	7 yrs.	8 yrs.	9 yrs.	10 yrs.	11 yrs.	12 yrs.	13 yrs.	14 yrs.	15 yrs.	16 yrs.	17 yrs.	18 yrs.	19 yrs.	20 yrs.	21 yrs.	22 yrs.	23 yrs.	24 yrs.	25 yrs.	26 yrs.	27 yrs.	28 yrs.	29 yrs.	30 yrs.	35 yrs.	Total.
0–10	2	9	5	2	·	1	1	1	·	·	·	1	·	·	·	·	·	·	·	·	·	·	·	·	·	·	·	·	·	·	·	·	22
11–20	3	9	7	8	3	1	2	1	1	·	·	·	·	·	1	·	·	1	·	1	·	·	·	·	·	·	·	·	·	·	·	·	38
21–30	11	10	12	10	4	1	6	·	2	5	2	2	4	2	·	·	2	1	2	·	2	·	1	1	·	·	1	1	·	·	·	·	81
31–40	12	15	14	15	7	6	13	15	7	3	3	3	9	4	6	1	4	3	3	3	2	3	1	·	·	·	·	1	1	·	·	1	114
41–50	15	16	19	22	13	17	16	13	15	13	19	10	11	3	6	3	1	1	·	2	1	1	1	1	·	·	1	1	1	·	·	·	224
51–60	6	23	17	23	18	11	13	13	7	4	3	7	1	4	6	·	1	1	·	2	1	·	·	·	·	·	·	·	·	·	·	·	188
61–70	5	·	6	7	8	1	3	2	5	1	·	2	·	·	·	1	·	·	·	·	·	·	·	·	·	·	·	·	·	·	·	·	63
71–80	2	4	1	1	3	1	·	2	2	1	·	·	1	·	·	·	·	·	·	·	·	·	·	·	·	·	·	·	·	·	·	·	18
81–90	·	·	1	·	·	·	·	·	·	·	·	·	·	·	·	·	·	·	·	·	·	·	·	·	·	·	·	·	·	·	·	·	1
Total	55	86	73	88	56	56	54	39	39	37	36	25	27	13	14	5	7	7	5	8	7	4	3	1	·	·	1	1	1	·	·	1	749
Per cent	7.3	11.5	9.7	11.7	7.5	7.5	7.2	5.2	5.2	4.9	4.8	3.3	3.6	1.8	1.9	0.7	1.0	1.0	0.7	1.1	1.0	0.5	0.4	0.1	·	·	0.1	0.1	0.1	·	·	0.1	

The duration of life of my own fatal cases arranged in successive periods is shown in Table 66. The decrease in mortality during the first year of the disease of my own cases for successive periods is definite. Although this change in mortality from 16.9 per cent in the first year of the disease to 14.4 per cent does not seem much, it is really greater than appears because the new cases added each year were handicapped by the averages of the original 408 fatal cases. Since 1914 the mortality has fallen to 12 per cent.

A clearer idea of the duration of life in diabetes will be obtained if both the age of the patient and the onset of the disease are considered. The statistics have, therefore, been rearranged with this in view and in Table 67, the duration of life of both fatal and living patients with onset in the different decades is recorded. The data are compiled to 1918. The number of cases treated in the last few years has been so large that it is questionable whether ever again as complete reports of cases can be secured.

Inspection of the table shows that nearly one-half of the cases dying under one year came from the first three decades of life. The mortality for the other decades is unquestionably far higher than it ought to be. It is plain that the year which followed the discovery of the disease was the diabetic's danger zone.

TABLE 68.—THE DURATION OF LIFE OF 749 LIVING CASES OF DIABETES.

Duration, years.	Dec., 1893–1915.		Dec., 1893–1916.		Jan., 1893–1918.	
	No. of cases.	Per cent.	No. of cases.	Per cent.	No. of cases.	Per cent.
0– 1	29	5.9	58	9.1	55	7.3
1– 2	66	13.5	56	8.8	86	11.5
2– 3	61	12.4	61	9.5	73	9.6
3– 4	47	9.6	66	10.3	88	11.7
4– 5	46	9.4	72	11.3	56	7.5
5– 6	43	8.8	60	9.4	56	7.5
6– 7	43	8.8	42	6.6	54	7.2
7– 8	27	5.5	34	5.3	39	5.2
8– 9	24	4.9	36	5.6	39	5.2
9–10	15	3.1	27	4.2	37	4.9
10–11	26	5.3	31	4.8	36	4.8
11–12	10	2.0	23	3.6	25	3.3
12–13	12	2.4	17	2.7	27	3.6
13–14	8	1.6	10	1.6	13	1.9
14–15	4	0.8	8	1.3	14	1.9
15–16	7	1.4	8	1.3	5	0.7
16–17	2	0.4	4	0.6	7	1.0
17–18	4	0.8	5	0.8	7	1.0
18–19	7	1.4	8	1.3	5	0.7
19–20	4	0.8	5	0.8	8	1.1
20–21 and over	5	1.0	9	1.6	19	2.5
	490		640		749	

1455 cases seen prior to Jan. 1, 1918. Statistically treated, 1341. Of remaining 114, 90 untraced and in 24 duration uncertain (May 14, 1918). Statistics compiled by Helen Leonard.

The duration of life for the living cases both up to December 1, 1915, and to January 1, 1918, is shown in Table 68. The large accession of new cases raised the percentage with a duration under one year, but the general tendency of the table is to show an increasing number of cases who have had the disease over a longer period than was indicated in the statistics of two years before. Thus, up to December, 1915, the percentage living over ten years was 12.6 and the later series shows 17.5 per cent.

G. THE CURABILITY OF DIABETES.

The course of diabetes occasionally ceases during the lifetime of an individual, but this happens very seldom. Both Naunyn and von Noorden believe that a diabetic patient may recover. I am unwilling to state that any of my patients have been cured. The term "arrested" instead of "cured" has found general acceptance in the literature of tuberculosis, and it is equally appropriate in diabetes. It is better for the present to take the conservative standpoint and be very slow to report cured or even arrested cases. One is constantly being told of patients who have been "cured," of which proof does not exist. It should be remembered that a sugar-free urine and a normal blood sugar do not constitute a cure; both should be normal for years.

The duration of the disease was fifteen or more years, in 1917 with 62 cases, or 6 per cent of the then total number, and now in 1923 there are 65 patients, or 2.2 per cent of the total, who have lived over twenty years.   Yet few if any of these long living diabetics are cured, though perhaps 41 per cent, according to A. A. Hornor who has studied the protocols for me, may be considered as arrested. Even if the disease has subsided so far as glycosuria and hyperglycemia are concerned, its complications remain in most instances. These cases, just as the groups of underweight diabetics, gall-stone diabetics, and the growing group with gastric or duodenal ulcer, deserve closer investigation.

Recovery is possible in three types of cases as described by Allen:

1. **Acute Diabetes Arising from Curable Causes.**—It is quite possible that diabetes which has followed trauma might subside, either with or without operation.   Recognizing the hyperglycemia which occurs in the course of infectious diseases, it is easy to understand that in a few cases glycosuria may develop, last several days, and after recovery from the infectious disease may disappear. Schmitz's remarkable case, already described on p. 130, might come under this heading and I hope Case No. 203, p. 161, will prove to be of this type. See also Case No. 1139, p. 144, who resembles very closely the patient of Schmitz.   I consider Case

No. 1139 about the best case of this type which I have seen. Undoubtedly more cases of this nature will appear as time goes on because of the frequency of urinary examinations during the infectious diseases of childhood. In fact so many of these are appearing in my records that it is beginning to complicate reports on the results of treatment.

Local infections in the neighborhood of the pancreatic gland, for instance those accompanying pancreatitis and gall stones, might give rise to a temporary diabetes. Thus Case No. 18, first seen by me in 1900, was treated for diabetes for years by my friend, Dr. Pfaff, and lived conscientiously upon a diet. After an interval of fifteen years, I saw her again and found the urine free from sugar, and it remained so until her death in 1922, save when her gall stones were removed in 1919.

Syphilis might be expected to furnish cases of diabetes with recovery, but no clear-cut case of this kind has developed in my series. (See p. 611.)

2. **Exceptional Cases in Childhood.**—A considerable number of cases of mild or temporary diabetes in children is beginning to appear in the literature, just as in my records. It is not easy to decide whether diabetes originally existed. (See Riesman, already cited, p. 130.) Case No. 203 of my series is instructive. This little boy first showed sugar at the age of seven, in 1908, although symptoms were present the preceding year. His mother has diabetes and is Case No. 155 having come for consultation in 1907. He was promptly put upon a careful diet by his mother and physician, Dr. Warren White, of Roxbury, Massachusetts, and has remained sugar-free during the subsequent fifteen years. He was very faithful to his diet and remains in good condition. By advice he is purposely keeping a trifle underweight, eating a normal diet save for less sugar. When his mother had had diabetes sixteen years, she "would not touch sugar any more than she would poison." Due to her faithfulness she is still living happily in 1923.

Von Noorden reports a striking case of a boy, aged seven years, who on a strict diet, constantly excreted 20 to 30 grams of sugar and considerable quantities of acetone bodies. He became sugar-free only with the help of oatmeal and vegetable days. He remained on this restricted diet for some years and at the age of twelve years was again seen by von Noorden, when he was in perfect health, eating an ordinary diet without a trace of glycosuria.

3. **Diabetes Associated with Organic Diseases.**—This group is subdivided by Allen into (1) those cases with nervous disorders, such as the cases described by Naunyn in association with tabes; (2) cancer involving the pancreas which may be followed by the disappearance of sugar. No instance of this kind has occurred

11

in my practice, though it is readily understood through the development of undernutrition in the patient; (3) neither has cirrhosis of the liver been observed to replace diabetes, such as Claude Bernard and Lepine describe; (4) on the other hand, with the development of severe nephritis, diabetes has ceased in a few cases, notably Case No. 354. In Cases Nos. 457 and 872 it developed; (5) the fifth group mentioned by Allen is tuberculosis. Naunyn and many other writers have observed the subsidence and disappearance of the disease following tuberculous infection. In Case No. 344 of my series, (see p. 574) the severest degree of diabetes, as shown by the urinary analyses of December 25–26, 1911, changed its character entirely, as proved by the urinary reports of March 17–18, 1912. During the interval pulmonary tuberculosis broke out and advanced rapidly. Weight decreased from 147 pounds to the neighborhood of 80 pounds, and the patient died without acidosis. Many diabetics are cachectic at the time of death, but this condition has by no means modified the disease. On the other hand, when cachexia, due to other cause than diabetes, occurs in a diabetic, it may be responsible for improvement in the diabetes.

SECTION III.

PHYSIOLOGY AND PATHOLOGY.

A. BLOOD SUGAR.

1. **The Blood Sugar in Health and Diabetes.**—The blood sugar of normal individuals fasting, *i. e.*, before breakfast, is most frequently 0.1 per cent. The average percentage found for 431 observations compiled from many sources by Gray[1] was 0.09 per cent, the minimum being 0.04 per cent and the maximum value, 0.16 per cent. With closer scrutiny of what constitutes a normal individual it is probable that the normal range would be more narrowly restricted.

In diabetes the percentage of sugar in the blood is increased. Adequate data for the fasting blood sugar in diabetics are not available, because nearly all patients have undergone more or less treatment when they come for examination. With 722 diabetics examined in my office or at the hospital, the average percentage of sugar in the blood fasting was 0.21 per cent, and with 619 diabetics at varying times of the day, not fasting, the average was 0.19 per cent.[2] Under treatment the blood sugar may fall to normal. In diabetics reduced by inanition the blood sugar may fall to below normal,[3] reaching as low a value as 0.017 per cent (Herman[4]) shortly before death. In a few cases values are obtained above 0.40 per cent. As a rule, such cases are on the verge of coma, complicated with nephritis or, as in Case No. 1015, p. 173, associated with suppression of urine. Olmstead reports a value of 1.40 per cent in coma. (See p. 84.) This is the highest value I have seen either in my own cases or in the literature. Petrén considers the case severe when the percentage of sugar in the blood is above 0.24 per cent.

The distribution of the fasting blood sugar between the blood plasma and corpuscles is so nearly equal that "no serious error is

[1] Gray: Arch. Int. Med., 1923, **31**, 241.
[2] Gray: Med. Clin. of North America. To be published.
[3] Joslin: Med. Clin. of North America, May, 1921, **4**, 1723.
[4] Personal communication. See p. 83.

involved in the use of whole blood for the analysis."[1] The plasma gives slightly higher figures. Thus far all of our analyses have been with the whole blood. Blood sugar values as reported by European observers are quite generally lower than the values obtained by methods employed in the United States.

2. **Sugar Absorption and Glycogen Formation.**[2]—In order to understand the variations in the sugar content of the blood it will be of advantage to refer to certain observations of Folin and Berglund. The mechanism of the prevention of the accumulation of sugar in the blood is not entirely due to glycogen formation in the liver, according to them, but more likely dependent primarily upon absorption of sugars by the tissues. These contain in the first instance glucose and presumably in as high a concentration as the blood and probably more. "The glycogen formation need not begin until the tissues have begun to possess a much higher concentration than that present in fasting. Much absorbed sugar can thus be distributed without any large increases of the sugar in the blood. But the kidneys receive their quota of sugar, just as do the other tissues, and this increase of sugar does not involve the slightest degree of strain. The strain comes only when the holding capacity for free sugar is reached and when the glycogen formation must come into play to keep the sugar concentration within normal limits. The speed of glycogen formation is of a much lower order than is the earlier process of merely absorbing the sugar from the blood. At this stage, therefore, the sugar backs up in the blood and the holding capacity of some tissues including the kidneys is exceeded. As a result of the strain thus produced the kidneys are finally compelled to make use of a more efficient process than the glycogen formation for reducing the sugar concentration in the kidney cells, and the elimination of sugar suddenly begins. That a real local strain has preceded the escape of the sugar is indicated by the fact that the sugar excretion once begun does not stop as soon as the blood sugar has fallen below the threshold, but, in fact, continues until the level of the blood sugar has gone away down, even to subfasting values (hypoglycemia").[3]

"Normally there is neither fructose nor galactose in the tissues, and within this enormous empty reservoir the galactose disappears as readily as does fructose and more readily than glucose. With respect to absorption and distribution galactose and fructose are alike. As far as excretion is concerned, the difference between the two is not even of a quantitative character. One is, the other is not

---

[1] Folin and Berglund: Jour. Biol. Chem., 1922, **61**, 241.
[2] This subject has been exhaustively considered by Geelmuyden in two recent numbers of Ergebnisse d. Phys., 1923, **21**, 273; ibid., 1923, **21**, Abt. II, 1.
[3] Folin and Berglund, loc. cit.

excreted. Such a qualitative difference in the matter of excretion cannot very well depend on quantitative differences in the speed with which the two sugars are transformed into glycogen. The sugar excretion observed after very small doses of galactose clearly points to the absence of a renal threshold for galactose. In the absence of such a threshold galactose will continue to be excreted as long as there is any galactose in the tissues, for a little of it will constantly leak back into the blood. The excretion would be like that of absorbed dextrin except for the fact that even galactose is gradually converted into glycogen thus diminishing and finally exhausting the supply of galactose." In later experiments these investigators suggested that the extent to which galactose is retained and utilized by the human organism depends upon the quantity of available glucose.

3. **The Glucose Threshold.**—The glucose threshold, or renal threshold, that is the percentage level of sugar in the blood above which sugar appears in the urine, has been carefully studied. The normal glucose threshold level lies between 0.16 and 0.18 per cent sugar for whole blood and somewhat higher, about 0.19 per cent for the plasma. These figures correspond to the highest normal level for the glucose threshold, because lower levels are frequently obtained and these lower levels eventually verge into renal glycosuria.[1] It also makes a difference in such determinations as to whether the threshold is determined on the basis of a rising or a descending curve of sugar concentration in the blood. The two may be quite different. Thus, Goto and Kuno[2] observed in one experiment that the sugar elimination began at 0.15 per cent of sugar in the plasma but continued until the sugar in the plasma dropped to 0.06 per cent. Also the level of the blood sugar is not the same in venous and arterial blood, according to Henriques and Ege,[3] though the blood sugar in venous and capillary blood are said to be the same. The threshold is characteristic for the individual according to John[4] and may be low or high and in untreated diabetics changes.

A levulose threshold, similar to the glucose threshold, appears probable from the researches of Folin and Berglund, but for galactose or lactose they find no such threshold exists.

"The tissues of the diabetic person should contain much higher concentrations of glucose than tissues of normal persons, and this is the immediate reason why the blood sugar rises so high after the intake of glucose in any form. The high concentration of glucose in

[1] Folin and Berglund: Jour. Biol. Chem., 1922, **51**, 213.
[2] Goto and Kuno: Arch. Int. Med., 1921, **27**, 224.
[3] Henriques and Ege: Biochem. Ztschr., 1921, **119**, 121.
[4] John: Jour. Metab. Research, 1922, **1**, 1.

the tissues would probably have little or no effect on their absorption of fructose. From the giving of fructose we should, therefore, get a much higher concentration of total sugar (glucose plus fructose) in the tissues without any material increase in the sugar of the blood."[1]

The concept comprised in the term "glucose threshold" is not only approximately true, but absolutely correct, however uncertain the exact figures given for the threshold may be. This appears proved, because even as much as 200 grams of glucose failed to yield a trace of sugar in the urines of normal individuals studied by Folin and Berglund, and also was without effect on the sugar excretion comprised in the term glycuresis. "Hyperglycemia definitely below the threshold does not normally produce the slightest leakage of glucose through the kidneys and normally not a trace of absorbed and circulating glucose is lost." To this conclusion Benedict and Osterberg[2] do not agree, basing their opinion largely on a different interpretation of the experiments of the writers quoted.

4. **Alimentary Glycosuria.**—From the preceding paragraph it is evident that the views of the leaders in the chemistry of the blood sugar are at variance upon this topic. If it exists at all it is of so slight a degree as not to lead to confusion with actual diabetes. "The term alimentary glycosuria has been used to express the fact that some apparently normal persons eliminate moderate quantities of sugar after the ingestion of cane-sugar, glucose, or even after starch." The term alimentary glycosuria is a misnomer, according to Folin and Berglund. "The sugar is excreted either because the level of the blood sugar has risen above the normal threshold or because the threshold itself is below the normal, as in renal glycosuria. There can be no doubt as to the existence of some mechanism by which the excretion of glucose is normally absolutely prevented."[3] The fact however remains that Holst[4] found glycosuria developed after carbohydrate meals in 31 of 159 individuals. He used the Benedict test.

5. **Food Tolerance Tests.**—After a meal the percentage of sugar in the blood of normal individuals rises promptly, but should not exceed 0.16 per cent. Since it frequently occurs that diabetic patients under treatment have normal blood sugar fasting values, various test meals have been proposed with smaller or larger quantities of glucose either selected arbitrarily or dependent upon the weight of the patient, and with other foods.

---

[1] Folin and Berglund: Loc. cit., p. 164.
[2] Benedict and Osterberg: Jour. Biol. Chem., 1923.
[3] Folin and Berglund: Loc. cit., p. 164.
[4] Holst: Ztschr. f. Klin. Med., 1922, **95**, 394.

The administration of 100 grams of glucose to normal individuals raises the percentage of sugar in the blood, and Jacobsen[1] has shown that this takes place within five minutes. The rise is greatest when the glucose is given fasting in the morning, being somewhat less after breakfast. The increase reaches on the average 0.14 per cent in half an hour, in one hour 0.12 per cent (300 curves), in two hours, 0.11 per cent, but in three hours the percentage drops to slightly below normal or 0.09 per cent. A peak value of over 0.16 per cent is usually considered abnormal. When the quantity of glucose given is between 150 and 200 grams, the values for the four periods are 0.16, 0.15, 0.12, and 0.10 per cent, and when the quantity is between 20 and 25 grams, 0.10, 0.12, 0.11 and 0.09 per cent. With normal individuals maximal and minimal values are obtained differing considerably from the averages above recorded, but it is probable, as with the normal fasting values, that a more careful selection of normals will eliminate the gross extremes. In the latter months of pregnancy the percentage of blood sugar may rise to as high levels or even above the threshold, but is not accompanied even then by glycosuria. See page 656.

TABLE 69.—AVERAGE BLOOD-SUGAR CURVES IN NORMAL PERSONS (COMPILED BY GRAY).[2]

Form of test.	Amount, gm.	Before.	Blood sugar.			
			½ hour.	1 hour.	2 hours.	3 hours.
Glucose . . .	150–200	..	0.16	0.15	0.12	0.10
	70–100	..	0.14	0.12	0.11	0.09
	50	..	0.14	0.14	0.10	0.10
	20–25	..	0.10	0.12	0.11	0.09
Sucrose . . .	50–100	..	0.15	0.14	0.12	0.12
Levulose . . .	100	..	· 0.14	0.13	0.12	0.11
Starch . . .	70–100	..	0.15	0.14	0.12	0.11
	50	..	0.14	0.12	0.19	
Fat	10–75	..	0.10	0.10	0.10	0.10
Mixed meal . .	..	..	0.13	0.12	0.11	0.11

EXPERIMENTS OF FOLIN AND BERGLUND.[3]

Glucose . . .	200	0.105	0.152	..	0.121	0.136
"	200	0.090	..	0.118	..	0.094[4]
Levulose . . .	200	0.100	0.102	0.101	..	0.098[5]
Maltose . . .	200	0.090	0.080	0.078	0.069	
Galactose . .	100	0.093	0.089	0.087		
" . .	100	0.094	0.079	0.082		
Glucose . . .	100	0.094	0.079	0.082		
Lactose . . .	200	0.094	0.101	..	0.088[6]	
Dextrin . . .	200	0.101	..	0.101	0.087	0.083
Starch, potato .	175	0.093	..	0.083	0.070	0.068
Olive oil . . .	200	0.096	..	0.070	..	0.088
Egg white . .	1000	0.108	..	0.102	0.101	0.098
Gelatin . . .	135	0.097	..	0.093	0.084	0.092

[1] Jacobsen: Bichem. Ztschr., 1913, **56**, 471.
[2] Gray: Arch. Int. Med., 1923, **31**, 241.
[3] Folin and Berglund: Jour. Biol. Chem., 1922, **51**, 213.
[4] Four hours.   [5] See Table XI.   [6] One hour, forty minutes.

The effect of various quantities and forms of carbohydrate and some other foods upon the blood sugar is shown in Table 69, which is compiled from two sources, first data accumulated by Gray from the literature and second the experiments of Folin and Berglund. The blood-sugar values obtained by Folin and Berglund in their experiments with maltose, glucose, dextrin and starch are somewhat lower than the levels attained by other investigators. They ascribe this partially to their subjects being medical students, and with these the influence of emotion would be less. Furthermore, in these experiments the blood was drawn from the veins rather than by puncturing the fingers, which causes distinctly more pain. In support of this theory they call attention to the reports of a group of investigators[1] who have obtained substantially the same degree of hyperglycemia from any kind of food, except fat, as they obtained from sugar or any other carbohydrates. These authors took the blood from the roots of the finger nails. Peculiar, high results from certain other laboratories using micro-methods are possibly open to suspicion for the same reason.

They mention one subject: "A medical student, S-g., never had any sugar in his urine (qualitative tests) either before or after the day of the experiment. When the preliminary sample of blood was taken, he grew pale and very faint. When the second sample was taken, he fainted completely. The plasma of this blood contained 210 mg. of sugar, whereas the first contained only 105 mg. In the course of the next hour the sugar content sank to 111 mg., and neither at this time nor later did the taking of the blood disturb him."[2]

A demand for refinement of the glucose tolerance test by washing out the stomach at a definite time after ingestion, and allowance for the recovered glucose, has been put forward by Beeler, Bryan, Cathcart, and Fitz.[3] Ohler[4] has not found material improvement from a study of 25 patients by both the usual and the advised technic, despite the fact that there was considerable variation in the amount of glucose absorbed from the stomach during the first hour.

Repetition of tolerance curves at approximately annual intervals has been carried out by Ohler[5] in 20 patients, with results which, together with the after-history, emphasize the fact that tolerance improves with proper attention to dietary restrictions and fails with neglect. Furthermore, in this series the relationship between decrease in tolerance and increase in weight has been striking.

---

[1] Cammide, Forsyth and Howard: British Med. Jour., 1921, p. 586.
[2] Folin and Berglund: Loc. cit.
[3] Beeler, Bryan, Cathcart and Fitz: Jour. Metab. Research, 1922, 1, 549.
[4] Personal communication.
[5] Ohler: Med. Clin. of North America, 1922, 5, 1465.

A recent study of blood-sugar curves in 25 Jewish and 25 non-Jewish patients with no apparent glycogenic disturbance indicates that race is not a factor, even though the Jew is also endowed with a nervous or emotional temperament.[1]

To the observers cited by Gray, who have obtained satisfactory curves with smaller amounts of glucose than 100 grams or 1.5 grams per kilogram body weight may be added W. R. Ohler, whose experience in Peabody's Clinic at the Boston City Hospital has made him feel that smaller amounts give information just as valuable, and that a determination two hours after a mixed meal will often give all the information required.

The hypoglycemia in normals observed to follow hyperglycemia in a sugar tolerance test is a regular and normal occurrence but is difficult to explain. It is of much practical importance. Food tests should be arranged so that the maximal and minimal values will occur within a two-hour period following ingestion of the test meal. Folin and Berglund say that "The fall of the blood sugar comes when there is reason to believe that all tissues are well supplied with available food material. It is an index of the fact that the need for sugar transportation from some tissues to others has temporarily fallen very low or ceased altogether." The latter alternative would seem to be indicated in those cases with the most extreme states of diabetic inanition. The most satisfactory test meal would appear to be 50 grams of glucose. This is a conservatively small quantity of food and after such a meal the average peak value is 0.14 per cent in half an hour and the blood sugar has returned to normal in two hours. A mixed meal is disadvantageous in that the blood sugar takes a longer and variable time to return to normal. Although levulose finds a place in the table, it should not be employed on account of the recent work of Folin and Berglund discussed elsewhere (see p. 297). Sucrose is unsatisfactory because it is a compound of two kinds of sugar. Fat is useless as it produced no glycemic reaction. Protein may or may not raise the blood sugar and is therefore unreliable as a food test.

Test meals given to diabetic patients raise the percentage of blood sugar higher and for a longer period than with normals. Following 100 grams of glucose, the blood sugar of 40 diabetic patients with a normal, fasting blood sugar rose to 0.18 per cent in half an hour, 0.20 per cent in one hour, 0.15 per cent in two hours, and 0.10 per cent in three hours. With 54 diabetic patients whose fasting blood sugar was 0.12 per cent or more the values were distinctly higher. These values are compared with normal values in Table 70. When the fasting blood sugar of the diabetics was 0.11

---

[1] Morrison, H., and Ohler, W. R.: Boston Med. and Surg. Jour., 1922, **188**, 852.

per cent or less, fasting, as in 6 individuals and these were given 50 grams of glucose, the increase in percentage of blood sugar was not abnormal until the second and third hours. Therefore, 50 grams of glucose cannot be accepted as a routine test unless blood values for at least two hours are obtained.

Fig. 70.—Glucose Tolerance Tests[1] in Diabetics and Normals Compared.

Diabetics, total number.	Glucose given, gm.	Blood sugar (fasting), per cent.	Diabetic blood-sugar curves.				
			Fasting.	½ hour.	1 hour.	2 hours.	3 hours.
40 . . .	100	Normal	0.09	0.18	0.20	0.15	0.10
54 . . .	100	0.12 or more	0.17	0.25	0.27	0.25	0.21
6 . . .	50	0.11 or less	0.08	0.12	0.12	0.14	0.13
Normals							
300 . . .	100	. . . .	0.09	0.14	0.12	0.11	0.09

In normals the blood sugar rises less after the mid-day meal than after breakfast if the interval between is three hours. This difference is not constant in normals and still less so in diabetics. In the latter the greater the severity, the greater the advantage in separating the meals instead of approximating them.[2] Maclean[3] found that the blood-sugar curve following the administration of 50 grams of glucose to fasting diabetics might be high and prolonged. After feeding the patients for a time, though starting at the same blood-sugar level, the same amount of glucose produced a reaction which was not as high or lasted as long and to this extent indicated improvement of the patient. Sakaguchi[4] explains the above phenomena on the basis that at breakfast-time glycogen formation by the liver is at a low ebb. The indication, therefore, would be not only to make the carbohydrate at breakfast less than at the other meals, but to precede breakfast with a small amount of carbohydrate. Gray's[5] experience with divided meals in my clinic is a practical confirmation of these observations.

Diabetes can be diagnosed in the vast majority of cases without the use of a glucose tolerance test. I always use such a test with reluctance, and for two reasons: (1) I fear that my patients will not understand why it is justifiable for me to give them sugar when I say it is harmful for them to take it; (2) although I have never

---

[1] Gray: Arch. Int. Med., 1923, **31**, 241.

[2] Sakaguchi and Sato: Mitt. d. med. Fakultät d. Kais. Universität zu Tokyo, 1920, **23**, 373;

[3] Maclean: Modern Methods in the Diagnosis and Treatment of Glycosuria and Diabetes. Constable and Co., London, 1922.

[4] Sakaguchi: Ibid., 1918, **20**, 439.

[5] Gray: Boston Med. and Surg. Jour., 1922, **186**, 763.

seen a diabetic patient whom I considered injured by a glucose tolerance test, I cannot forget Allen's statement: "In the early stage, glucose is more powerful than starch in producing diabetes, and animals which are progressing toward complete recovery on starch diet can be sent into hopeless diabetes by admixture of glucose."[1]

6. **The Blood Sugar in Other Diseases.**—Other diseases or states than diabetes are accompanied by abnormal blood-sugar percentages. Of these hypertension, nephritis, pregnancy, hyper- and hypothyroidism, diseases of the liver and of the pituitary body are the most common. Gray[2] attempted to condense all the data in the literature, and Table 71 is based upon his summaries. The test meal given was 100 grams glucose in all, except a few cases whose inclusion he thought legitimate because the curves were, in each, as high as after the usual dose.

TABLE 71.—BLOOD-SUGAR STANDARDS IN CONDITIONS NEITHER NORMAL NOR DIABETIC (GRAY).

Test meal, 100 grams glucose.

Condition.	Number of curves.	Average percentage of blood sugar.				
		Fasting.	½ hr.	1 hr.	2 hrs.	3 hrs.
Hypertension without nephritis	29	0.11	0.19	0.18	0.16	0.13
Nephritis without hypertension	11	0.14	0.19	0.23	0.20	(0.24)
Renal glycosuria without nephritis	70	0.09	0.13	0.12	0.11	0.09
Pregnancy with blood sugar 0.11 per cent or less	51	0.09	0.14	0.14	0.12	0.13
Hypothyroidism, cretinism, myxedema	8	0.10	0.16	0.15	0.12	0.11
Hypothyroidism:						
Blood sugar (fast.), 0.12 or more	9	0.13	0.17	0.18	0.18	0.11
Blood sugar (fast.), 0.11 or less	58	0.09	0.16	0.16	0.14	0.11
After operation	4	0.08	0.12	0.10	0.09	0.09
Hepatic disease:						
Obstructive jaundice	7	0.13	..	0.22	0.23	
Cardiac cirrhosis	6	0.14	..	0.18	0.21	
Alcoholic or syphilitic cirrhotic	28	0.10	0.15	0.17	0.17	0.18
Catarrhal jaundice	10	0.10	..	0.15		
Bailey's case	1	0.12	0.32	0.37	0.34	0.27
Hypopituitarism or dyspituitarism	4	0.11	0.17	0.17	0.14	0.12
Acromegaly or hyperpituitarism	11	0.09	0.13	0.17	0.15	0.11

The percentage of sugar in the blood is also increased in apoplexy, pneumonia, typhoid, tuberculosis in the presence of fever, and in some cases of cancer. There is a decided increase after ether and

[1] Allen: Jour. Exp. Med., 1920, **31**, 402.
[2] Gray: Arch. Int. Med., 1923, **31**, 241.

in fact all varieties of general anesthesia and in operations on all kinds of cases. If the ether anesthesia is less than an hour, the increase is 32 to 89 per cent, but if more than an hour, the increase is greater. Pain, fear of operation or of anesthesia exert a negligible influence upon the blood sugar.[1]

Abnormal blood sugar curves in patients without glycosuria, and conversely normal curves in patients with glycosuria, have recently been studied by Ohler[2] with the following results:

In a series of 160 cases who underwent glucose tolerance tests, glycosuria was absent with 103 and 57 showed only small amounts. Of the 103 cases without glycosuria, 37 gave normal glycemic reactions, 53 definitely abnormal and 12 doubtful reactions; or in other words, 60 per cent of the cases without glycosuria gave abnormal sugar tolerance reactions. An analysis of the cases in this group shows that a very large percentage of the abnormal reactions were found in the following pathological conditions (arranged in order of frequency): Gall-bladder diseases; cirrhosis of the liver; bronchial asthma; arteriosclerosis; carcinoma; obesity; endocrine disturbances; chronic nephritis; chronic arthritis.

In the group of 57 cases in which glycosuria was found, 9 cases gave perfectly normal reactions. These 9 fulfill all the requirements of so-called renal glycosuria. The remaining 48, or 84 per cent showed definitely abnormal reactions, despite the fact that in every instance the fasting blood sugar was perfectly normal.

Blood volume in blood-sugar estimations is of significance according to Epstein and Baehr.[3] They point out that the increase in the percentage of sugar in the blood is only indicative of a relative, that is percentile, but not of absolute hyperglycemia, and suggest the advisability of studying the blood volumes and computing thereby the total blood sugar in cases of diabetes mellitus. In a later publication Epstein[4] defines "hyperglycemia as an increase in the total amount of blood sugar over the normal, and not merely an increase in concentration or percentage. Thus, it is possible to have a hyperglycemia even when the percentage of sugar is normal or below normal." Whereas such estimations would be valuable, they are at present impracticable owing to the lack of a blood volume method accepted as reliable. Fitz and Bock have recently computed the quantity of sugar in the blood. (See p. 286).

7. **Hyperglycemia (Extreme).**—The highest percentage of sugar in the blood, 1.40 per cent, was found in a case, the data for which were furnished me by W. H. Olmsted, of St. Louis.

---

[1] Epstein and Aschner: Jour. Am. Med. Assn., 1916, **56**, 1929.
[2] Personal communication.
[3] Epstein and Baehr: Jour. Biol. Chem., 1914, **18**, 21.
[4] Epstein: Proc. Soc. Exper. Biol. Med., 1916, **13**, 67.

"Hoffman, F., aged fourteen years. Onset symptoms one year previous. Two weeks before admission sore throat; five days before admission fell down stairs. Completely comatose on admission; could not be aroused for twenty hours. Moderate acetone breath; air hunger; edema of entire body and eyelids; eyeballs soft. Blood-pressure 78/34. Blood sugar 1.40 per cent. Blood CO_2 27.7 per cent. Non-protein nitrogen 140 milligrams. There was found an ulcerative stomatitis (streptococcus). Complete anuria. Catheter washing showed + sugar, insufficient for ferric chloride test. Large number of white blood cells and red blood cells; no casts. Benzidine ++; acetone, no reaction (too small amount). History of strong ferric chloride before coma. Treatment: Insulin and alkali. Died: Uremia." Is this case not similar to Case IV described by Bock, Field and Adair?[1] (See p. 85.)

Case No. 1015 of my series also deserves detailed mention. Here too, anuria was a factor. A schoolmaster, aged forty-seven years, highest weight 216 pounds. Family and past history negative. Indefinite onset of diabetes in February, 1916. Sugar first discovered March 12, 1916, and three days later the urine contained 6 per cent; albumin was reported absent. The patient came under my observation for the first time on March 18, 1916. During the preceding twenty-four hours he had been fasted except for 1 ounce of whisky in 3 ounces of black coffee, which he had taken every two hours. No other liquid had been given save about a pint of water in which a tablespoonful and a half of sodium bicarbonate had been dissolved. During this period he had vomited fluid which contained blood. He was dull, but conscious, and there was no hyperpnea. No edema. He had no fever; pulse 104; arteries not sclerotic. The systolic blood-pressure in the right arm was 60 mm. mercury, in the left arm 80 mm. mercury, and the diastolic pressure in the left arm 50 mm. mercury (Tycos apparatus). These observations were controlled by another physician. The heart was little if any enlarged and there was a systolic murmur at the apex. The liver was 2 cm. below the costal margin. During the twenty-four hours 30 cc of urine were obtained by catheter, showing a slight trace of albumin, no diacetic acid, and a positive reaction for sugar. The sediment contained many coarsely and finely granular hyaline casts, pus, and 6 to 8 red blood corpuscles to a field. Death was preceded by edema of the lungs and coma, although in nowise suggesting diabetic coma. The blood sugar taken twelve hours before death contained by the Bang method, 1.15 per cent, 1.45 per cent, and 1.49 per cent of sugar, or an average of 1.37 per cent. The accuracy of the solutions used in the test was immediately controlled with a standard solution of glucose.

[1] Bock, Field and Adair: Jour. Metab. Research, 1923.

8. Hypoglycemia.—Hypoglycemia had begun to appear as a serious factor in the treatment of diabetes even before the introduction of insulin. Four cases have developed in my own series and 4 others have come to my attention in the clinics of my friends. So serious did the problem appear in 1921 and so evident the cause that I reported the first 3 cases under the caption "The Critical Period of Hypoglycemia in Undernutrition."[1] Even in non-diabetics a prolonged undernutrition may be accompanied by hypoglycemia. This occurred with L. C., whose weight and vitality were brought low by partial pyloric obstruction extending over a period of years. When he came to the hospital for operation the blood sugar three hours after his noon meal was 0.05 per cent. At first it appeared as if prolonged undernutrition was necessary to produce a threateningly low blood sugar, but now it is apparent that this state can develop in the course of a few hours, and just as Mann's hepatectomized dogs, be relieved in a few minutes with a few grams of glucose. The condition is infrequently enough described to merit a detailed report of the cases.

Inanition in diabetes was the recorded cause of death of the first patient, but it takes little imagination to infer the hypoglycemia. Case No. 1085, a frail woman of thirty-four years with a history of diabetes of seven months' duration, became sugar-free with great difficulty, despite fasting and a low diet. After four months the sugar in the blood decreased from over 0.5 to 0.1 per cent, coincident with a fall in weight from 88 to 61 pounds of which the last 10 pounds were lost between November 3 and 10, 1916. At this time her weight represented a total loss of 95 pounds and was 56 per cent below standard. No subsequent blood-sugar determination was made, but inasmuch as a few days later, without change in treatment or in general condition at her home she died without pain or coma, there is little doubt that hypoglycemia was present. The data upon the metabolism of this patient will bear insertion. They are remarkable in three ways. (1) The metabolism was —40 per cent which was almost as much substandard as her weight, 56 per cent; (2) the respiratory quotients were high for a diabetic, 0.81, 0.81, 0.79 and 0.81 with but a single value as low as 0.70; and (3) the quotient rose after levulose to 0.86 and even 0.90. It is quite possible that the levulose, though given for another reason may have prolonged the life of this patient. Table No. 72.

A man, Case No. 1831, with onset of diabetes April, 1917, at the age of thirty-eight years and seven months, entered the hospital May 5, 1920. The details of the course of treatment with laboratory findings are shown in Table 73. Acidosis was present, sugar in

---

[1] Joslin: Med. Clin. of North America, 1921, **4**, 1923.

TABLE 72.—METABOLISM MINUS 40 PER CENT, WEIGHT MINUS 56 PER CENT IN A DIABETIC WITH FALL OF BLOOD SUGAR FROM 0.5 TO 0.1 PER CENT. CASE 1085.

Experimental conditions	Case No.	Date	Apparatus	Body weight, naked	Average pulse-rate	Carbon dioxide, per minute	Oxygen, per minute	Respiratory quotient	Heat output per 24 hours — Total	Heat output per 24 hours — Per kilogram body weight	Total heat greater (+) or less (−) than predicted (H. and B.)	NH_3	Diacetic acid	CO_2 in alveolar air	Urinary nitrogen per 24 hours — Preceding day	Urinary nitrogen per 24 hours — Experimental day	Urinary sugar per 24 hours	Carbohydrate balance
Postabsorptive	**1085**	1916 Oct. 11–12	..	34.2	—	80	98	0.81	679	20	−40	—	0	—	—	—	0	0
		19–20	..	30.4	53	82	102	0.81	707	23	−35	—	0	—	15.9	8.8	2	+50
		23–24	..	31.5	49	85	108	0.79	749	24	−32	—	0	—	14.6	5.9	5	+45
		30–31	..	32.2	56	81	115	0.70	778	24	−30	1.7	—	20	9.5	6.1	15	+60
		Oct. 31–Nov. 1	..	31.6 Av.	53	77	96	0.81	662	21	−40	—	0	34	6.1	5.2	2	0
Lev., 50 grams	··	Oct. 19–20	IV¹		53	90	105	0.86	734	24								
					51	91	113	0.81	783	26								
					51	85	99	0.86	694	23								
					52	100	111	0.90	787	26								
			Av.	30.4 Av.	52	91	107	0.86	749	25	—	—	0	—	15.9	8.8	2	+50
Lev., 50 grams	··	Oct. 23–24	IV¹		51	89	113	0.79	778	25								
					50	97	125	0.78	864	27								
					50	96	115	0.83	801	25								
			Av.	31.5 Av.	50	94	118	0.80	816	26	—	—	0	—	14.6	5.9	5	+45
Lev., 75 grams	··	Oct. 30–31	IV¹		59	104	144	0.73	979	30								
					62	99	119	0.84	835	26								
					63	110	137	0.80	950	30								
			Av.	32.0 Av.	61	104	133	0.79	917	28	—	1.7	—	34	9.5	6.1	15	+60

¹ Cot chamber.

TABLE 73.—THE DEVELOPMENT OF HYPOGLYCEMIA DURING UNDERNUTRITION. CASE NO. 1831.

Date.	Volume, cc.	Alb.	Diacetic acid.	Sodium chloride.	Nitrogen, gm.	Sugar in urine, reduction, per cent.	Diet in grams.				Naked weight, pounds.	Non-protein nitrogen.	Bloor's blood fat, per cent.	Blood sugar, per cent.	Alveolar air CO$_2$, mm. Hg.
							Carbohydrate.	Protein.	Fat.	Calories.					
1920 May															
5- 6	1600	..	+	..	..	2.3	..	..	..	..	93	..	..	..	30
6- 7	3000	..	+	..	..	2.4	23	15	3	179	93	26.1	..	0.36	30
7- 8	2000	0	+	..	..	1.8	64	33	0	388	96	..	..	..	..
8- 9	3300	..	0	6.7	..	1.7	36	27	0	252	95	..	..	..	35
9-10	3800	..	0	6.1	16.9[1]	0.7	15	5	0	80	96	..	..	..	..
10-11	2800	0	0	6.1[1]	16.9[1]	0.4	0	0	0	0	95	..	..	0.29	..
11-12	4200	..	0	6.1[1]	16.9[1]	0.4	0	0	0	0	94	..	..	..	..
12-13	4600	..	0	6.1[1]	16.9[1]	0.2	0	14	4	83	94	..	..	..	..
13-14	3800	..	0	..	19.6[1]	0.1	0	21	5	129	95	..	..	..	..
14-15	1600	..	0	..	..	0	0	35	8	212	94	..	..	..	..
15-16	3800	..	0	..	..	0	1	43	10	246	94	..	..	..	..
16-17	4700	..	0	..	19.6[1]	0	2	50	16	332	96	..	..	0.11	..
17-18	4000	..	0	..	19.6[1]	0	4	57	22	422	91	..	1.10	0.05	..
18-19	2700	0	0	..	19.6[1]	0	13	46	28	488	90	..	..	0.04	..
19	..	..			..		..	Died	1.55 P. M.		..	..	..	..	

[1] Aliquot values.

the urine amounted to 2.4 per cent, and in the blood to 0.36 per cent. After four days of undernutrition, during which the total calories consumed amounted to less than 900, followed by two days of fasting, the patient failed to become sugar-free and the blood sugar remained 0.27 per cent. Upon resumption of 14 to 35 grams of protein per day and 3 to 8 grams of fat the blood sugar dropped to 0.11 per cent. On the next day, despite a slight increase in protein and fat and 2 grams of carbohydrate, the blood sugar was 0.05 per cent. This unusually low value was assumed to be erroneous and, unfortunately, not reported, Upon the following morning the patient became irrational, disoriented, but an hour afterward again apparently normal, and was able to sit up and even walked around. Physical examination was negative. The next morning he could not be roused, coma gradually deepened, though unassociated with acidosis, and death occurred in a few hours. The blood sugar was 0.04 per cent. No marked loss of weight during hospital stay was observed though he had lost 72 pounds in the three years before admission, when his weight was 93 pounds. Quantitative examinations of the nitrogen in the urine were made and showed an average excretion of 16.9 grams from the tenth to the sixth day before death, and an average excretion of 19.6 grams on four of the five days preceding death.

Experience with these two individuals made it possible to forestall a similar outcome with Case No. 2079. This man developed diabetes in September, 1919, at the age of twenty-nine years and nine months, and came for treatment on February 5, 1921, weighing 119 pounds after a loss of 66 pounds below his maximum weight. Acidosis was severe, sugar in the urine 5.8 per cent, and blood sugar 0.27 per cent, and even after thirty days of treatment the blood sugar was 0.23 per cent. Yet two days later the patient became sugar-free, and within a week the blood sugar was 0.12 per cent, and on the forty-third day 0.09 per cent. This premonitory fall in blood sugar being noticed, the diet was at once changed to carbohydrate 19 grams, protein 59 grams, fat 62 grams. Despite the fact that this patient had required so long to become sugar-free, steady additions of carbohydrate were made to the diet until on the forty-ninth day from admission the total carbohydrate was 68 grams, the protein 71 grams, the fat 66 grams, and the blood sugar was 0.05 per cent. Even one hour after a meal two days later, when the carbohydrate was 86 grams, the blood sugar was 0.1 per cent. The patient was then discharged with carbohydrate 82 grams, protein 74 grams, fat 66 grams, calories 1234, weight 92 pounds, in contrast to a weight of approximately 110 pounds on the first day of treatment.

Two weeks later the report came that his blood sugar was 0.1 per cent, and the newly acquired tolerance was preserved. Such a

12

gain in tolerance from such a critical state had not before come to my attention. On November 20, 1921 he died from cardiac disease, but no coma.

While on the watch for insulin reactions the fourth case of hypoglycemia was discovered in an old lady of sixty-four years, Case No. 2716, whose diabetes began one year and nine months before. Her loss in weight amounted to fully 100 pounds, essentially all of which had occurred since her disease began. At no time did she receive insulin. On the morning of July 18 the blood sugar was 0.33 per cent, the plasma creamy with 3.4 per cent blood fat. Three days later following a sharp restriction of diet the percentage of blood sugar was 0.03 and this value was carefully checked by three observers. Although Mrs. L. had no characteristic reaction, she felt that she was dying and actually was too weak to feed herself. Her pulse was thin and rapid and only after frequent feedings with oatmeal gruel did she recover. The patient required 42 units of insulin daily in September, 1923.

A fifth case of hypoglycemia occurred in another hospital.[1] The patient was a man who was 65 per cent overweight when he developed diabetes. Two weeks before his death two-thirds of his weight had vanished and 31 pounds of it in the preceding forty-four days. A pound of body flesh is equivalent to about 1500 calories and consequently his calorie deficit between December 9 and January 22 was 46,500 calories or roughly 1000 calories a day. His inanition had reached 36 per cent below standard weight on January 22 and in the ensuing two weeks undoubtedly fell still lower. On December 10, 1922 the blood sugar was 0.16 per cent. On January 17, 1923 the blood sugar was 0.25 per cent, on January 18, it was 0.23 per cent, and insulin which had been given intermittently in doses of 5 and 10 units daily was omitted and the diet changed to carbohydrate 10 grams, protein 20 grams, fat 40 grams. By January 22 the blood sugar was 0.1 per cent and by January 31, 0.07 per cent, although the carbohydrate was 40 grams, protein 40 grams, and fat 100 grams. Upon the following day despite a further increase in diet to carbohydrate 80 grams, protein 65 grams and fat 120 grams the blood sugar was 0.042 per cent, and he died February 5, 1923. Autopsy showed, primary fatal lesions, hyaline degeneration of the islands of the pancreas, and secondary terminal lesions focal pneumonia, edema of the lungs, slight arteriosclerosis.

Woodyatt[2] refers to a case of hypoglycemia coming to his attention, but not on his service, who died in convulsions. Recently N. B. Herman[3] has written about a patient under his observation at the Johns Hopkins Hospital, making the eighth non-insulin case

[1] Cabot, R. C., and Cabot, H.: Case Records, Massachusetts General Hospital, April 17, 1923, vol. 9 (Case 9161).
[2] Woodyatt: Jour. Metab. Research, 1923.
[3] Personal communication, May 14, 1923.

of hypoglycemia. Dr. Herman has kindly furnished me data about this case, in connection with which he is planning to report later in detail. "In brief, the patient, a man, aged forty-six years, was told six years ago that he had diabetes and for four years lived on a diet prescribed by his physician. At the end of this time, still feeling rather weak, he broke diet and ate whatever the rest of the family ate. From 1917 to 1921 he lost about 25 pounds and from 1921 to November, 1922 about 35 pounds. In November, 1922, following the use of male fern for supposed tape worm, an intractable diarrhea started and continued to the time of death.

"On admission his weight was 93 pounds and his height 6 feet, 50 per cent below standard. After one day on calculated maintenance diet his blood sugar was 0.054 per cent. He was immediately put on ward diet and his blood sugar rose to 0.284 per cent. There was sugar in the urine, of course, at this time. His diet was modified and his blood sugar varied between 0.054 and 0.09 per cent. The diarrhea remained about the same and we were never able to be sure about the cause. There was no evidence of outspoken pancreatic insufficiency; the stool was lower than normal in diastase content. The patient seemed to be getting along a little better than usual when he suddenly went into coma and died, the intravenous injection of $6\frac{1}{2}$ grams of glucose having no effect. The blood sugar at the onset of coma was 0.017 per cent."

Marked loss of weight has characterized all of these cases for whom the data have been recorded. In 2 of the cases sudden decline in weight even from one already low took place shortly prior to the hypoglycemia. In 2 instances the excretion of urinary nitrogen per kilogram body weight was high, 0.216 grams, and from 0.523 to 0.165 grams. The metabolism in Case No. 1085, who presumably died of hypoglycemia a few days later, was −40 per cent. At the time I reported this first case no similar one had come to my attention. How easily the second case could be saved today.

9. **The Blood Sugar in Relation to Clinical Aspects of the Disease.** —The diagnosis of diabetes is aided greatly by a knowledge of the percentage of the blood sugar. When the fasting blood-sugar percentage is above 0.12 per cent, the test should be repeated, and if constantly elevated, it indicates diabetes. The same is true for a blood-sugar percentage of 0.18 per cent after a meal, and a value of 0.17 per cent is suspicious. The demonstration of a normal blood-sugar percentage coincidently with the presence of glycosuria is reassuring and suggests renal glycosuria. For exceptions, see Table 71. According to Petrén the twenty-four-hour blood-sugar curve in diabetic patients during a fasting day showed as a rule that the drop in the blood-sugar is greatest during the first six hours, a smaller decrease during the next six hours, while during the last twelve hours a very slight drop or even an increase may occur.

Estimations of the blood sugar are of great value in the treatment of diabetes. An increase in the percentage of blood sugar almost invariably precedes the appearance of glycosuria. It thus enables earlier measures to be undertaken to eradicate the cause. Though valuable, it is certain that such tests will be made in but a very small proportion of the diabetics who need treatment for some years to come.

Cases can be treated very satisfactorily without such estimations or with infrequent estimations, and in proof Table 74 is submitted, showing the course of the disease in 10 children in the first decade of life, untreated with insulin, and 8 similar children treated without any estimations of the blood sugar.

TABLE 74.—THE COURSE OF DIABETES IN CHILDREN WITH INFREQUENT BLOOD-SUGAR TESTS.

Living

With blood-sugar tests.				Without blood-sugar tests.		
Case No.	Age at onset.	No. of tests.	Duration, years.	Case No.	Age at onset.	Duration, years.
1162 . . .	5.0	3	7.8	1035 . . .	8.0	8.0
1484 . . .	9.9	3	6.0	1139 . . .	2.0	7.0
1568 . . .	8.1	9	5.3	2084 . . .	3.0	5.0
1612 . . .	10.6	5	5.9	2997 . . .	5.0	8.0
1707 . . .	6.2	9	5.4			
1753 . . .	8.8	8	6.3			

Fatal.

894 . . .	1.6	6	8.0	534 . . .	9.0	6.6
949 . . .	7.3	1	7.0	620 . . .	4.0	5.8
1151 . . .	3.6	4	8.2	750 . . .	10.0	5.2
1231 . . .	9.5	2	6.0	1202 . . .	2.0	5.8
1266 . . .	5.4	7	6.5			

The above table is inserted here not to discredit blood-sugar estimations, but to show that there is no excuse for a case to be neglected because such laboratory facilities are not available. Children will live a considerable number of years without them.

10. **The Prognosis in Relation to Blood Sugar.**—The prognosis is also aided by blood-sugar tests. In the following tables analyses of blood sugar of my cases have been correlated with the age of the patient, the duration of the disease, and glycosuria or its absence, by Gray. The relation of blood sugar to prognosis is also recorded by Gray.[1] Analyzing the records of 210 of my fatal cases he has tabulated the percentage of blood sugar when first seen in connection with the date of death. The table shows quite clearly that the higher the percentage of sugar in the blood when the patients come for treatment the shorter the duration of the disease. Thus, the 10 patients who showed a blood sugar of 0.4 per cent or above

[1] Gray: Blood-sugar Levels in Diabetics when First Seen, Med. Clin. of North America, 1923 (in press).

succumbed within two-thirds of a year. Whereas those with a blood-sugar percentage between 0.3 and 0.39 lived one and thirteen-hundreth years, those with a blood sugar 0.2 to 0.29 per cent, one and twenty-three-hundreth years, while those whose blood sugar was less, 0.19 per cent lived one and eighty-one-hundreth years. Of course it must be emphasized that these values relate purely to fatal cases of diabetes and that the causes of death in these cases may have not been directly dependent upon the diabetes but upon other factors. The table, however, does indicate that the higher the blood sugar the more serious the diabetes. It is a cautionary signal to all who use insulin and thereby allow the percentage of blood sugar to rise, because of the increased diets permitted.

TABLE 75.—BLOOD SUGAR IN FATAL CASES IN HOSPITAL SINCE APRIL 1, 1919.

Case No.	Age at onset, years.	Duration, years.	Blood sugar, per cent.		Time intervening between tests, years.	Total sugar in urine during 24 hours preceding time of blood analyses, gm.		Cause of death.
			First.	Last.		First.	Last.	
1089	55	5.0	0.17	0.36	3.7	..	31	Coma.
1305	10	5.5	0.09	0.54	5.4	0	14	Coma.
1511	52	9.6	0.21	0.50	1.0	11	35	Coma.
1545	62	0.3	0.31	0.48	0.2	..	39	Coma.
1870	13	0.8	0.35	0.31	0.7	129	..	Coma.
2218	24	1.3	0.15	0.40	1.2	0	..	Coma and pregnancy.
2595	27	12.8	0.26	0.40	4 days	61	53	Coma and gangrene.
1652	34	3.8	0.24	0.27	0.3	..	10	Inanition.
1831	38	3.1	0.36	0.04	11 days	38	..	Inanition.
1876	8	0.3	0.50	0.30	0.2	..	6	Inanition.
1907	23	0.8	0.18	0.44	0.3	6	20	Inanition.
600	46	10.7	0.21	0.33	4.7	..	72	Gangrene.
1924	23	30.2	0.27	0.55	...	0	88	Gangrene.
2479	60	9.0	0.44	0.50	0.2	107	52	Gangrene.
2523	47	14.0	0.15	0.38	11 days	0	20	Gangrene.
2339	63	7.9	0.25	0.11	0.2	..	0	Gangrene.
1722	27	1.4	0.18	0.31	0.1	10	62	Pneumonia.
2446	35	1.1	0.24	0.57	1.0	..	..	Pneumonia.
3010	25	15.0	0.32	0.36	2.5	9	..	Pneumonia.
3051	?	?	0.31	0.14	9 days	1	..	Nephritis.
2546	42	4.6	0.48	0.50	2 days	..	..	Nephritis.
2046	37	1.9	0.20	0.21	1.7	..	80	Septicemia.
3079	61	0.2	0.40	0.50	4 days	18	45	Septicemia.
866	31	8.9	0.24	0.17	5.0	0	0	Erysipelas.
705	52	14.0	..	0.18	..	..	24	Angina pectoris
2742	54	6.7	0.25	0.28	8 days	5	4	Cardiac.
870	36	17.0	0.10	0.26	2.3	0	0	Gall stones.
2116	60	5.6	0.26	0.31	15 days	117	7	Cancer of liver.
2463	30	2.7	0.23	0.28	12 days	11	45	Abscesses of liver.
2720	18	0.9	0.33	0.30	7 days	..	127	Abscess, paranephritic.
2670	25	5.0	0.26	0.12	0.2	4	0	Tuberculosis.

TABLE 76.—RELATION OF BLOOD SUGAR (FASTING, FOLIN AND WU) TO
PROGNOSIS. (GRAY.)

Blood sugar, per cent.	No. of patients.	Duration after blood sugar to death, years (average).
0.40–0.57	10	0.66
0.30–0.39	48	1.13
0.20–0.29	90	1.23
Less than 0.19	62	1.81

The method of Ivar Bang was employed in the earlier analyses, the Lewis-Benedict method in 1916 and 1917, and the Folin-Wu method from April, 1919, to date.

Petrén regards a blood-sugar percentage of 0.24 as of serious import, and when the blood sugar has once reached 0.3 per cent considers the chances for the survival of the patient for a year are rather small, while 60 per cent of his patients with a blood sugar of 0.24 to 0.29 survived more than a year.

11. **Age.**—The influence of age upon the sugar in the blood of diabetic patients is shown in Table 77. In general, the younger the patient the lower the blood sugar, but the converse is not true, and indeed the difference between different decades is slight. To our original data 100 recent cases have been added, but they simply confirm the earlier series. Four cases, all under the age of ten, showed respectively, 0.06, 0.04, 0.08 and 0.07 per cent of sugar within a few days of the beginning of treatment. Their course in the hospital was by no means as favorable as such low percentages would imply. The total duration of the disease was one year in one of these cases, two and three-tenth years in another, and six years and six and five-tenth years in the third and fourth. Death resulted from coma in 3 and from accident in the other.

TABLE 77.—THE INFLUENCE OF AGE UPON THE BLOOD SUGAR (FASTING)
IN DIABETES.

Age, years.	1916.			1922–1923.[1]		
	Cases No.	Analyses No.	Blood sugar, per cent, average.	Cases No.	Analyses No.	Blood sugar, per cent, average.
0–10 . . .	11	23	0.19	20	20	0.19
11–20 . . .	23	56	0.21			
21–30 . . .	27	131	0.24	20	20	0.19
31–40 . . .	28	145	0.23			
41–50 . . .	18	53	0.22	20	20	0.22
51–60 . . .	35	67	0.20			
61–70 . . .	18	44	0.21	20	20	0.24
71 and over .	2	2	0.27	20	20	0.22

12. **Duration.**—The duration of the disease does not bear a close relation to the percentage of sugar in the blood. In general there is a tendency to a slight rise in the blood sugar, but it is so moderate as to afford little support to the theory that diabetes

[1] Values obtained early in the course of hospital treatment, but not invariably the first day.

becomes more severe the longer it lasts. It is distinctly encouraging to see that cases with duration over ten and even fifteen years should show so little increase. One would have expected that a rising renal threshold alone would have exerted a deleterious influence. In comparing cases of long and short duration one must not

TABLE 78.—THE INFLUENCE OF THE DURATION OF THE DISEASE UPON THE BLOOD SUGAR IN DIABETES.

Duration, years.	1916.			1922–1923.[1]		
	Cases No.	Analyses No.	Blood sugar, per cent, average.	Cases No.	Analyses No.	Blood sugar, per cent, average.
Under 1 . .	54	141	0.21	20	20	0.18
1– 5 . .	81	258	0.22	20	20	0.21
6–10 . .	26	81	0.22	20	20	0.26
11–15 . .	12	19	0.23	20	20	0.21
16–29 . .	7	26	0.22	20	20	0.23

forget that in general one is comparing two types of the disease, the severest and the mildest. One would prefer to compare the effect of duration alone in each type, but that is difficult. Furthermore it would really be necessary to use the same standard diets at the different periods, because the few cases of hypoglycemia cited above show the importance of this factor.

Gray writes, "A rise in blood sugar might appear if instead of tabulating averages of groups of patients with successive durations, one either considered the same patient at different periods, or in each group considered not the average, but the relative frequency of different blood thresholds at different periods from onset."

13. **Glycosuria.**—The presence of sugar in the urine (during the preceding twenty-four hours) is almost invariably accompanied by an increase of sugar in the blood. Among 207 blood-sugar analyses, there were only 5 instances in which this did not occur. On the other hand, the sugar in the blood may be as high as 0.5 per cent without glycosuria. This is most apt to occur in nephritis.

In Table 79 is shown the range of the percentage of blood sugar in a group of my cases and the quantity of sugar excreted in the urine in the preceding twenty-four hours.

A close relation between the percentage of sugar in the blood and the severity of the disease became apparent when the cases of long duration were collected and divided into those with low and those with a distinctly high tolerance for carbohydrate (Table 79). The average percentage of sugar in the blood of the 15 patients with a tolerance for only 20 grams carbohydrate or under, as determined

[1] Values obtained early in the course of hospital treatment, but not invariably the first day.

by 37 tests, was 0.23. The average percentage of sugar in the blood of 8 patients whose tolerance was distinctly high, as determined by 11 tests, was 0.18. It is evident that, as a rule, the lower the tolerance the higher the percentage of blood sugar, and it is also evident that when the tolerance is distinctly high the blood sugar is but little above normal, although there are exceptions.

TABLE 79.—THE BLOOD SUGAR IN RELATION TO THE TOTAL QUANTITY OF GLUCOSE EXCRETED IN THE PRECEDING TWENTY-FOUR HOURS.

Excretion of glucose in preceding 24 hrs., grams.	Cases, No.	Analyses, No.	Blood sugar, per cent.		
			Lowest.	Average.	Highest.
0	135	321	0.07	0.19	0.50
1– 5	41	62	0.11	0.24	0.50
6– 10	19	29	0.09	0.24	0.35
11– 20	27	38	0.18	0.28	0.50
21– 30	18	22	0.15	0.26	0.43
31– 50	18	25	0.19	0.24	0.45
51– 70	11	12	0.11	0.28	0.45
71–100	8	9	0.24	0.32	0.40
101–150	6	6	0.19	0.31	0.38
151–200	1	1	0.13	0.13	0.13
318	1	1	0.25	0.25	0.25

Among these clinically severe cases in adults, there were 2 whose low blood sugars, 0.13 and 0.11 per cent respectively, were exceptions to the rule. Case No. 564 represented a severe type of diabetes in a boy of sixteen years who, although ultimately becoming sugar-free, remained so with strict adherence to diet. He lived for ten years when he succumbed to a gastric ulcer. Case No. 706, it is true, represents a serious form of diabetes, but in spite of this fact he eventually became sugar-free and lived until February 4, 1923, The blood sugar indicated better than the clinical impression the true nature of the case.

TABLE 80.—ANALYSES OF BLOOD-SUGAR FASTING MADE UPON DIABETIC PATIENTS DURING THE COURSE OF TREATMENT.

Treatment without insulin.				Treatment with insulin.			
		Hospital cases, blood sugar.				Hospital cases, blood sugar.	
Year.	No. of cases.	Within 3 days of admission, per cent.	At discharge, per cent.	Year.	No. of cases.	Within 3 days of admission, per cent.	At discharge, per cent.
1916	33	0.22	0.17				
1919	100	0.19	0.14	1922	30	0.27	0.19
1922	100	0.22	0.15	1923	100	0.22	0.17

No essential change has undergone the percentage of blood sugar in patients admitted to the hospital for treatment in the years 1916, 1919 and 1922 as shown by various groups of cases collected in Table 80. On the other hand the blood sugar at discharge is a trifle lower. It reached its lowest value in 1919 when undernutrition was more strenuously followed than now. For comparison two series of cases treated with insulin are added. The first series is the earlier and hence made up of more severe cases, the second series comprises both severe and moderately severe diabetics.

Coma may or may not increase the percentage of sugar in the blood. If anuria develops, the blood sugar will increase (see page 73, Case No. 1015), and the case reported by Olmsted (see page 172). If the urinary volume is well maintained the low diet of coma may lead to a fall in the blood sugar, though not to normal. The blood sugar percentage is recorded in 7 cases of coma in Table 75. It averaged 0.43 per cent. The blood-sugar percentages at the time of death from various complicating diseases are not distinctive.

B. BLOOD LIPOIDS.

1. **Blood Lipoids in Health.**—Lipoids (fat) are normally present in blood in four forms:

(a) Glycerides of the fatty acids, usually oleic, palmitic or stearic, of which an example is triolein—

$$C_3H_5 \diagdown \begin{matrix} OOC & . & C_{17}H_{33} \\ OOC & . & C_{17}H_{33} \\ OOC & . & C_{17}H_{33} \end{matrix}$$

—glyceride of oleic acid (a compound [ester] of glycerin and three molecules of fatty acid). Glycerides contain about 95 per cent of their weight of fatty acids.

(b) "Lecithin"—a compound of glycerin with two molecules of fatty acids and one molecule of phosphoric acid, which is in turn combined with one molecule of cholin. The fatty acids compose about 70 per cent of the whole compound, and the phosphoric acid about 12 per cent. In addition to various kinds of lecithin other phosphatides are present in the blood, notably cephalin, which is very nearly like it in composition and is determined along with it.

In the graphic formulæ the fatty acids are in **black-face** letters, the alcohols (glycerin, cholesterol, and cholin) in CAPITAL letters and the phosphoric acid in *ITALIC CAPITAL* letters.

Oleo-palmito lecithin contains: 1 molecule of glycerin; 2 molecules of fatty acid (oleic and palmitic acids); 1 molecule of phosphoric acid; 1 molecule of cholin.

$$
C_3H_5
\begin{cases}
OOC \quad . \quad C_{17}H_{33} \\
OOC \quad . \quad C_{15}H_{21} \\
OH \\
O\!-\!-\!P\!=\!O \\
\quad\quad O \\
\quad\quad O\!-\!-\!C_2H_4 \\
\quad\quad\quad (CH_3)_3\!=\!N \\
\quad\quad\quad\quad H\!-\!O
\end{cases}
$$

(*c*) Cholesterol—a secondary alcohol belonging to the terpene series of compounds and containing one double bond,

$$
C_{39}H_{24}
\begin{cases}
OH \\
\\
CH \quad . \quad CH \ : \ CH_2
\end{cases}
$$

About two-thirds of the cholesterol in the plasma is combined with fatty acids, thus forming esters, but in the corpuscles all of the cholesterol is free. In the cholesterol esters the fatty acids constitute about 44 per cent of the whole molecule.

(*d*) Cholesterol esters—combinations of cholesterol with a fatty acid, ordinarily oleic or palmitic acid. The formula for cholesterol oleate is as follows:

$$
C_{24}H_{39}
\begin{cases}
OOC_{17}H_{33} \\
\\
CH \quad . \quad CH \quad . \quad CH_2
\end{cases}
$$

In a discussion of the lipoids of the blood one usually refers to (1) the total fatty acids, including in this term (*a*) the fatty acids in the glycerides, (*b*) the fatty acids in lecithin, (*c*) the fatty acids in the cholesterol esters; (2) lecithin; (3) the cholesterol existing free or combined with fatty acid, as a cholesterol ester.

The total fatty acids represent the predominant form, about 50 per cent, in which fat appears in the blood. The average normal percentage of fatty acids is 0.37, range 0.29 to 0.42 per cent. The lecithin comes next and the average is 0.3 per cent, range 0.28 to 0.33 per cent. Cholesterol is least abundant, the average being 0.22 per cent, the range 0.19 to 0.25 per cent.

Analyses for the total fatty acid, lecithin, and cholesterol in the whole blood, the plasma, and the corpuscles are given in Table 81, which is based upon Bloor's figures for 19 normal individuals. The plasma affords the best index of changes in the lipoids of the blood. The lipoid content of the corpuscles varies but slightly in health or disease and little attention need be paid to it.

TABLE 81.—LIPOIDS OF NORMAL BLOOD.[1]
(Compiled from tables of W. R. Bloor, Jour. Biol. Chem., 1916, **25**, 585.)

	Total fatty acids, grams per 100 cc.			Lecithin, grams per 100 cc.			Cholesterol, grams per 100 cc.			Total lipoids, calculated.
	Whole blood.	Plasma.	Corpuscles.	Whole blood.	Plasma.	Corpuscles.	Whole blood.	Plasma.	Corpuscles.	Whole blood.
Highest normal . . .	0.42	0.47	0.45	0.33	0.26	0.48	0.25	0.31	0.24	0.76
Av. (19) normals . . .	**0.37**	**0.39**	**0.34**	**0.30**	**0.21**	**0.42**	**0.22**	**0.23**	**0.20**	**0.68**
Lowest normal . . .	0.29	0.30	0.27	0.28	0.17	0.35	0.19	0.19	0.17	0.57

[1] The results of the analyses of blood lipoids of both males and females have been combined in this table.

The analyses of the fat in the blood made upon my own patients have been performed with samples of blood obtained in a post-absorptive condition, unless otherwise stated. Usually the blood has been secured fourteen hours after the last meal. The analyses have been begun as a rule not later than two hours from the time the samples of blood were obtained.

The influence of food upon the blood fat is striking, but as yet there is no fat tolerance meal to serve as a standard. Speculation suggests that as wide a variation might exist in the blood lipoids after the ingestion of fat in diabetes as takes place in the blood sugar in diabetes after the ingestion of carbohydrate. Thus, Bloor found the blood fat to be 0.6 per cent twenty-four hours after a meal, but 0.73 per cent three hours and a quarter after 100 cc olive oil, 1.2 per cent in six hours and a quarter, and 0.87 per cent in eight hours. Surraco[1] noted that the cholesterol could be easily influenced in ascitic fluid by changes in the diet.

Fasting, hemorrhage, and narcosis cause an increase in the blood lipoids, but this is not constant, apparently depending upon the nutritional condition of the animal. In those instances without marked increase it could be obtained after a period of forcing fat food. However, in starving animals, according to Rosenfeld, the fat mobilization ordinarily produced by phosphorus poisoning in dogs was absent.

The total fatty acids of the blood are increased in nephritis, pneumonia, pregnancy, and in extremely severe anemia. In these conditions acid poisoning may be a factor.

Lecithin appears to be an intermediate stage in the metabolism of fat, and Bloor points out that the blood corpuscles, and in this instance the red corpuscles, are the principal carriers, take up the fat from the plasma, and transform it into lecithin, and that most, if not all, of the absorbed fat is so transformed. The increase of lecithin in the blood during fat absorption suggests that lecithin is a stage through which the fats must pass before they can be utilized in metabolism. Lecithin may be increased in nephritis and high values have been observed in the blood corpuscles in leukemia, but in the cachexia of carcinoma low values obtain. It has also been reported increased in experimental conditions in animals, such as in the anemia produced by continued bleeding, and in depancreatized dogs. Lecithin is destroyed upon standing by the action of an esterase in the corpuscles, and this may account for the low values occurring in the literature.

Cholesterol is a relatively well defined and stable chemical substance, and is the lipoid which can be most readily determined.

---

[1] Surraco: Jour. Am. Med. Assn., 1918, **70**, 1269.

It does not appear to increase in the blood directly after feeding fat alone, according to recent work, but is increased in narcosis, alcoholism, and pregnancy, as well as in all cases of jaundice, because of the stoppage of one of its normal paths of excretion. It is increased in nephritis, but decreased in cachexia of various origins. Cholesterol appears to play a minor part in the phenomena of fat absorption. In the blood of natives of the tropics cholesterol is very low despite the fact that infections of the liver are common. DeLangen[1] noted the rarity of gall stones in the tropics. He observed but 1 case, and that not in a native of the East Indies, among 15,000 patients, and no case was recognized among 40,000 out-patients. The rarity of diabetes was also commented upon. Luden[2] has studied the influence of diet upon cholesterol in the blood.

Cholesterol and lecithin are constituents of all living cells and probably constitute most of the "built in" or invisible fat of the tissues. Both may be synthesized in the body. Lecithin probably takes an active part in fat metabolism and is the first stage through which the fats pass in their utilization by the organism. Where the vitality was low McCrudden[3] found a relation between the severity of the condition and the low values for cholesterol and blood sugar. When the patient improved under treatment, the values for both blood sugar and cholesterol increased.

Fat gets into the blood in two ways: About 60 per cent passes into the chyle and in this way reaches the blood stream, the remainder is probably absorbed directly by way of the intestinal capillaries. Formerly it was supposed that the fats, after their hydrolysis in the intestine, were resynthesized during their passage from the intestinal wall and passed into the blood stream in essentially the form in which they were ingested—that is, as glycerides—and that alimentary lipemia was due to nothing more than the addition of these glycerides. Today it appears more likely that instead of a lipemia, a lipoidemia exists, in that, along with the increase of glycerides of fatty acids, there is also an increase of lecithin and cholesterol. Thus, it has been shown that the fat of the chyle has a somewhat different composition from that of the food fat.

Sugar falls but fat rises in the blood in starvation and an antagonism between the two exists, which has also been noted in the liver, though in depancreatized dogs treated with insulin the antagonism ends.[4] Coincident with this change in the blood

[1] DeLangen: Jour. Am. Med. Assn., 1918, **71**, 1099.
[2] Luden: Jour. Lab. and Clin. Med., 1917, **3**, 141.
[3] McCrudden: Jour. Am. Med. Assn., 1918, **70**, 1216.
[4] Loc. cit., p. 22.

acidosis appears. From this increase in fat in the blood it appears plain that the blood is mobilizing fat from its fat depots for its nutritional needs, and it is readily conceivable that in the presence of abnormal metabolism the fat of an obese subject might be more easily drawn upon and that the effect would be the same as that of ingested fat. For this reason the lipoids in the blood of fat and thin people present an interesting field for study.

2. **Blood Lipoids in Diabetes.**—With an excess of fat diabetes begins and from an excess of fat diabetics die. In 75 per cent of 1000 of my diabetic cases an increase of body fat preceded the onset of diabetes and in 66 per cent of my earliest cases, though in only 21 per cent of recent hospital patients, abnormal fat metabolism resulting in acidosis caused death.

Disordered fat metabolism was first associated with diabetes when phlebotomy disclosed a milkiness of the blood of diabetic patients. Severe diabetes was, and is, the only disease in which lipemia is frequent enough to be of special significance. The milky appearance of the serum and the "cream" which rose from it on standing indicated the fat. When bleeding fell into disuse, nothing more was learned regarding the nature of this fat until in 1903 Fischer observed that the quantity of cholesterol in diabetic blood was abnormally high, and this finding was confirmed by Klemperer and Umber, who made a similar observation with regard to lecithin.

The percentage of fat reported was extreme, and in 1 case Klemperer found 26 per cent; figures of 15 to 20 per cent were not unusual. Among my cases the highest values are 13.1 per cent as found by Bloor,[1] Case No. 786, and 16.3 per cent in the same patient as found by H. Gray, but these two analyses are based actually upon a patient undergoing treatment with restriction of fat and after fasting fourteen hours. In comparison with the extreme values of Klemperer the increase of 13.1 per cent appears only moderate, but in reality it represents an increase of twenty times the average normal value.

Lipemia (cloudiness or milkiness of the plasma) does not normally appear in the postabsorptive period, although the blood plasma contains an excess of cholesterol, lecithin, and probably some fat. The introduction of more fat into the blood by feeding or mobilization from body fat generally produces a milkiness normally lasting but a few hours, but under certain conditions for considerably longer periods. If the total fat of the plasma rises above a normal value of 0.5 per cent to 0.8 per cent, lipemia usually appears, but in diabetes values above 1 per cent with clear plasma are often found. Bloor obtained a value of 4.35 per cent total lipoid in

---

[1] Bloor: Jour. Biol. Chem., 1921, **49**, 201.

my case, H, with clear plasma. Such cases of "masked" lipemia have been frequently noted. The "masking may be an unstable condition since on standing for a time, twenty-four hours to forty-eight hours, milkiness may develop in a plasma which was clear when drawn." In one of my cases of lipemia, Case No. 786, Bloor found all the lipoids increased, but as the lipemia disappeared the total fat diminished most rapidly, the lecithin less rapidly, and the cholesterol relatively slowly, "showing that the fat is the first to decrease as it was the first to increase, the lecithin next, and the cholesterol last." In one case with a clear plasma the total lipoid content was over 4 per cent, the lecithin 1 per cent, and the cholesterol 1.4 per cent. Bloor believes that both the fat of the food and the fat stored in the body may be sources for the lipemia and that the former is the more important. The accumulation of fat in the blood which causes the lipemia, he ascribes to the difficulty which the diabetic has in removing fat from the blood in contradistinction to the lipemia following hemorrhage, which can be explained by an excess of inflow of fat into the blood. Bloor also inclines to the belief that there is a deficiency in diabetes of a hormone whose function it is to aid in the removal of fat from the blood, basing his opinion upon: (1) The lipemia which is so common with diabetics; (2) its easy production in dogs made diabetic, but the difficulty of its production in normal dogs; and (3) upon the high content of blood lipoids in diabetics.

All the lipoids are increased in diabetes. This is shown in Table 82 taken from Bloor, in which he compares the blood lipoids of normals and 28 of my diabetic patients, and Table 83, which represents analyses of 131 bloods of my cases made by H. Gray, in Bloor's laboratory. The increase is greatest in the plasma, the composition of the corpuscles remaining so nearly constant as to be disregarded.

TABLE 82.—COMPARISON OF BLOOD LIPOIDS OF NORMAL AND 28 DIABETIC INDIVIDUALS.

(Compiled from table of W. R. Bloor, Jour. Biol. Chem., 1916, **26**, 424.)

	Total fatty acids, gms. in 100 c.c.			Lecithin, gms. in 100 c.c.			Cholesterol, gms. in 100 c.c.		
	Whole blood.	Plasma.	Cor-puscles.	Whole blood.	Plasma.	Cor-puscles.	Whole blood.	Plasma.	Cor-puscles.
Diabetic extremes .	.41–.76	.46–.93	.33–.62	.26–.50	.17–.48	.32–.60	.19–.44	.16–.65	.17–.24
Diabetic average[34]	.52	.59	.43	.36	.30	.46	.29	.36	.20
Normal average[19]	.37	.39	.34	.30	.21	.42	.22	.23	.20
Normal extremes .	.29–.42	.30–.47	.27–.45	.28–.33	.17–.26	.35–.48	.19–.25	.19–.31	.17–.24

Gray's series of 131 specimens of blood fat were divided into three groups, according to whether the patients were mild, moderate,

---

[1] Joslin, Bloor and Gray; Jour. Am. Med. Assn., 1917, **69**, 375.

TABLE 83.—LIPOIDS IN DIABETES. ANALYSES BY H. GRAY.

| | No. of bloods. | Fat by Bloor's method.[1] | | Total fatty acids.[2] | | | Lecithin. | | | Cholesterol. | | | Total lipoids. | Blood sugar, per cent. |
		Whole blood, per cent.	Plasma, per cent.	Whole blood, per cent.	Plasma, per cent.	Cor-puscles, per cent.	Whole blood, per cent.	Plasma, per cent.	Cor-puscles, per cent.	Whole blood, per cent.	Plasma, per cent.	Cor-puscles, per cent.	Plasma, per cent.	
Normal	23	0.50	0.62	0.37	0.39	0.34	0.30	0.21	0.42	0.22	0.23	0.20	0.68	0.10[3]
Mild diabetes	32	0.83	0.90	0.59	0.64	0.45	0.32	0.24	0.42	0.24	0.26	0.21	0.98	0.17
Moderate diabetes	37	0.91	1.06	0.65	0.76	0.48	0.33	0.28	0.40	0.26	0.30	0.20	1.16	0.26
Severe diabetes	55	1.41	1.80	1.01	1.28	0.62	0.40	0.40	0.40	0.41	0.51	0.24	1.98	0.23

[1] Represents about 90 per cent total fat.
[2] Represents fat (Bloor) minus cholesterol.
[3] Estimated, not analyzed.

or severe in degree. All of these types of diabetes are distinguished by a marked increase in lipoids of the blood, and the general statement can be made that the increase is progressive with the seriousness of the disease. Thus, the average quantity of lipoids obtained by Bloor's method in the whole blood amounted to 0.59 per cent in 19 normal individuals, but was increased to 0.83 per cent in 32 mild diabetics, to 0.91 per cent in 37 moderately severe diabetics, and to 1.41 per cent in 55 severe cases of diabetes. The increase holds not alone for the lipoids obtained by Bloor's method, which extracts approximately 91 per cent of the total blood lipoids, but for each of the three groups of lipoids.

The patient who showed the greatest increase of total fatty acids in the plasma—save for lipemia—was Case No. 983, who was obese and developed severe acidosis upon restriction of carbohydrate and only after eighteen days of treatment became sugar- and acid-free. (See p. 228.) Eventually she was proven to be one of the mildest of diabetics, showing that *a diabetic is mild or severe as the diet and doctor make him*. On the other hand, a clinically mild case may show considerable abnormality, due probably to diet, as in Case No. 914 (p. 424, Bloor[1]) whose increase in total fatty acids was 60 per cent. His tolerance for carbohydrate was 150 grams. Between the mild and severe cases were all degrees of gradation in the blood lipoids, but in general the more severe the diabetic condition the more marked was the abnormality in the blood lipoids.

The relations between the different lipoids in diabetics were not the same in the larger group of cases examined by Gray as contrasted with the small group first examined by Bloor. Although the quantity of total fatty acids is trebled, the cholesterol is only doubled and the lecithin increased but one-third. The increase in cholesterol is significant and suggestive and seems indeed pathognomonic of the prolonged diabetic hyperlipemia, since Bloor has found it lacking in the acute lipemia of overfeeding which is characterized by an increase in the total fatty acids alone.

The occurrence of increased amounts of lecithin and cholesterol has led to the belief that the increase was due to degeneration of tissue cells, setting free their lipoids, but analyses of various tissues have shown that the lipoid content of the tissues in diabetes is not abnormal. The increased fat in the liver, rising to even more than 10 per cent does constitute an exception, because it represents storage. Increased mobilization of stored fat as the result of the partial starvation has also been offered as an explanation, but

---

[1] Bloor: Jour. Biol. Chem., 1916, **26**, 424. Other articles by Bloor are: Lipemia, Jour. Biol. Chem., 1921, **49**, 20; Fat Transport in the Animal Body, Phys. Reviews, 1922, **2**, 92.

13

here again the evidence does not bear out the assumption. In the first place the stored fat contains only traces of lecithin and cholesterol, and in the second place, though fat at onset, diabetics generally become thin later and have very little stored fat; also even complete starvation does not necessarily mean increased blood fat. A third interpretation considers the increase due merely to an accumulation of food fat which the organism can no longer burn, and in the light of the knowledge that in diabetes the fat-burning mechanism is probably deranged and of the recent discovery that lecithin and probably cholesterol (as ester) are steps in normal fat metabolism, this seems to be the most reasonable explanation.

Lecithin, however, except for lipemia, varies with the fatty acids in nearly all cases, but not as constantly as does the cholesterol. In Case No. 786, with lipemia, the values for lecithin were not greatly increased, as shown by a comparison with the lecithin values in this same patient when he did not present lipemia.

Cholesterol runs parallel with the total fatty acids in all cases, including lipemia. Therefore, the determination of the cholesterol alone in the plasma gives valuable information regarding the lipoid content of the blood in diabetes. Wishart's[1] studies revealed no especial retention of cholesterol when diabetic patients, subject to lipemia, were fed cholesterol or foods rich in cholesterol.

In the right hand column of Table 83 the blood sugar values corresponding to the fat values are inserted. Gray thus shows the greater reliability of blood fat in prognosis.

Williams examined the cholesterol in 89 cases of diabetes. In 52 of these it was under 0.25 per cent, in 11 between 0.25 and 0.3 per cent and in 26 it amounted to over 0.3 per cent, compared with Bloor's 0.23 per cent for normals.

The total fatty acids afford the surest indication of a change in the blood lipoids. It will be seen that the normal variations for lecithin and cholesterol were so great as to overlap the variations for the lecithin and cholesterol in diabetic blood. On the other hand, the lowest figure obtainable for total fatty acids in diabetic blood was at the upper normal limit for these acids in normal blood, but this held good only for the plasma.

The mild cases of diabetes were subdivided into two groups based upon the presence or absence of nephritis. The differentiation, however, showed nothing characteristic. Indeed, the uniformity for the groups was so close that it extended to all the different lipoids.

The effect of fasting upon the blood lipoids was studied by Cowie

---

[1] Wishart: Jour. Metab. Research, 1922, **2**, 199.

and Hoag[1] in a boy, aged seven years, with diabetes presenting acidosis. After four days without food, the total lipoids increased 182 per cent. Another patient showed a 64 per cent increase during three days of fasting, and this was also accompanied by acidosis. When these patients were given a diet high in fat and low in carbohydrate and protein, the lipoids decreased. This increase in the blood fat during starvation should be related to the insufficient combustion of carbohydrate. In fact, all our conclusions upon the utilization of fat by the body or the accumulation of fat in the blood must be restudied in the light of our present knowledge of the ketogenic-antiketogenic ratio. Blau and Nicholson[2] recognized this in their conclusions upon their studies of the blood fat in 26 cases of diabetes. They also call attention to the presence of another factor—namely, infection—which might easily complicate the problem.

The administration of fat in the form of cream to normal children was also investigated by Cowie and Hoag. They found that the maximum amount of lipoids in the blood was reached from the fifth to the seventh hour after ingestion and that with 3 adults the maximum was obtained in six hours. When the fat was given together with a large amount of carbohydrate, the highest point was reached with the adults during the second hour.

"The fat absorption-utilization curve of an adult diabetic patient was studied following the ingestion of 143 grams of fat, 6 grams of carbohydrate, and 16 grams of protein in a single meal. The maximum concentration in the blood was reached at the sixth and eighth hours, showing however, a rise of only 10 per cent over the first hour after ingestion. A boy, aged eleven years, with diabetes, showed at the eighth hour a 26 per cent increase over the first hour, following ingestion of 90 grams of fat, 14 grams of protein, and 11 grams of carbohydrate. These results show no gross variation from the normal curves.

"All the 8 diabetic patients examined showed an increase of total lipoids, the highest being 8.8 per cent. When these patients were fed a minimum of carbohydrate and protein, but large amounts of fat, ranging from 100 to 200 grams daily, and furnishing an adequate caloric intake for the individual, the lipoid content of the blood steadily decreased. The patient whose case is cited above had 8.18 per cent on entrance, which was reduced to 1.5 per cent before he was discharged from the hospital on a diet containing 220 grams of fat."

The high fat, low protein and low carbohydrate diet led to a

---

[1] Cowie and Hoag: Jour. Am. Med. Assn., 1921, **77**, 493.
[2] Blau and Nicholson: Arch. Int. Med., 1920, **26**, 738.

reduction of the lipemia likewise in the cases studied by Marsh and Waller.[1]

The above results are similar to those of Newburgh and Marsh[2] in their studies of high fat feeding. It should be noted that these results were obtained coincident with a decrease in the sugar in the urine and in the blood, and the explanation is offered that the decrease in fat in the blood of their cases was not on account of the large quantity of fat in the diet, but rather on account of the improvement in the diabetes brought about by the better utilization of carbohydrate. This agrees with Allen's[3] statement that the one indispensable prerequisite for diabetic lipemia is the existence of active, severe symptoms in the form of glycosuria and that severe cases whose glycosuria has been abolished by diet never exhibit any extreme grade of lipemia, however high the fat intake. In other words, the improvement in the treatment of the patient as a whole is the important factor, irrespective of the method employed. My old explanation of the decrease of fat in the blood as due to reduction of fat in the diet, though consistent with clinical facts, was likewise probably erroneous and better explained as above—namely, a better utilization of carbohydrate and the disappearance of an abnormal ketogenic-antiketogenic ratio. Although the diets of Newburgh and Marsh were high in fat, it is probable from the work of DuBois and Richardson[4] as well as McCann[5] that considerable portions of this were not burned. It is all the more striking that the fat in the blood was not increased to a greater extent. If there is a defect in the metabolism of fat in diabetes apart from that dependent upon the deranged metabolism of carbohydrate, one would expect it to show more plainly.

Cases of mild and moderate diabetes were found by Blatherwick[6] to utilize satisfactorily large amounts of fat. He determined this point by demonstrating the consistency of the blood-fat level of their patients and by the absence of acid bodies in the urine. His results, however, were during short periods.

The influence of acidosis upon the blood lipoids deserves attention, because it is from abnormalities in the fat metabolism that so great a per cent of our patients die.

However, data based upon groups of cases classified according to the severity of acidosis do not give consistent results. In Gray's series of 131 bloods, 21 severe diabetics with acidosis showed 1.81 per cent of total lipoids in the plasma while 34 cases supposed to

[1] Marsh and Waller: Arch. Int. Med., 1923, **80**, 655.
[2] Newburgh and Marsh: Arch. Int. Med., 1923, **31**, 63, also 455.
[3] Allen: Jour. Metab. Research, 1922, **2**, 219.
[4] DuBois and Richardson: See p. 235.
[5] McCann: Loc. cit., p. 202.
[6] Blatherwick: Jour. Biol. Chem., 1921, **49**, 193.

be without acidosis showed 2.07 per cent. In the smaller group of analyses of Bloor there were 3 with blood fat 0.93 per cent whose CO_2 in the alveolar air was between 14 and 24 mm. mercury, 4 analyses with blood fat 0.82 per cent whose CO_2 in the alveolar air was 26 mm. mercury, 8 analyses with blood fat 1.07 per cent whose CO_2 in the alveolar air was 29 to 33 mm. mercury, and 6 analyses with blood fat 0.92 per cent whose CO_2 in the alveolar air was 35 to 41 mm. mercury. On the other hand, if the entire series of 131 bloods examined by Gray from mild, moderate, and severe diabetics are classified according to acidosis, the evidence is clear that those cases of diabetes with acidosis exhibited a higher level of total lipoids than the cases without acidosis, but even then the patients classified as having moderate acidosis showed higher values than those with severe acidosis. To the writer the explanation possibly lies in the differentiation of the cases with and without acidosis. For such an investigation a detailed study of a few protocols under varying degrees of acidosis might furnish a clearer idea of the relation between coma, acidosis, and blood fat.

The blood of two patients dying in coma was examined for blood lipoids one day and three days before death. With these patients the lipoids were by no means high. It is true that Case No. 1004 came into the hospital in beginning coma with a history of having retained but little food for thirty-six hours. The diabetes was f short duration, and coma developed apparently with rapid change of diet outside the hospital. Case No. 1005 entered the hospital in beginning coma, having eaten almost no food for three days. A summary of a large series of blood-fat determinations in coma is desirable.

TABLE 84.—INFLUENCE OF COMA ON BLOOD LIPOIDS.

Date. 1916.	Case No.	Days before death.	Total fatty acids, gms. in 100 c.c.			Lecithin, gms. in 100 c.c.			Cholesterol, gms. in 100 c.c.		
			Whole blood.	Plasma.	Corpuscles.	Whole blood.	Plasma.	Corpuscles.	Whole blood.	Plasma.	Corpuscles.
Feb. 29	1004	0.1	0.44	0.43	0.45	0.33	0.18	0.51	0.21	0.18	0.24
July 6	1005	.3	.49	.56	.36	.32	.25	.44	.26	.30	.19
	Aver.	0.2	0.46	0.49	0.40	0.32	0.21	0.47	0.23	0.24	0.21

Cholesterol and blood-sugar values stand in close relation in the milder cases of the disease, but as the disease advances in intensity the cholesterol tends more to increase than does the blood sugar.

Ether increased the total fatty acids in the blood, whereas the lecithin and cholesterol remained unchanged. The increase in total fatty acids was followed later by a fall in the same below that of the patient's level before anesthesia.

TABLE 85.—THE COMPARISON OF THE CHOLESTEROL AND BLOOD SUGAR IN THE BLOOD OF DIABETIC PATIENTS.

Case No.[1]	Whole blood.		Case No.	Whole blood.	
	Blood sugar, per cent.	Cholesterol, gms. in 100 cc.		Bood sugar, per cent.	Cholesterol, gms. in 100 cc.
560	0.17	0.19	966	0.23	0.28
998	0.21	0.23	974	0.19	0.23
1026	0.20	0.21	821	0.34	0.23
970	0.16	0.25	1029	0.26	0.40
1007	0.13	0.20	969	0.21	0.40
1028	0.25	0.30	951	0.16	0.37
914	0.18	0.34	810	0.16	0.40
610	0.26	0.31	786	0.29	0.37
983	0.29	0.30	1004	0.41	0.21
979	0.17	0.29	1005	0.42	0.26
1008	0.35	0.31	1005	0.27	0.26
632	0.17	0.33	765	0.31	0.44
632	0.16	0.25	765	0.20	0.35
632	0.19	0.31	765	0.17	0.44
1025	Lost	0.22	1011	0.23	0.31
966	0.24	0.22	996	0.40	0.26
966	0.21	0.20			
Averages	0.21	0.26		0.27	0.33

The blood lipoids do not rise and fall with the changes in the blood sugar.

The prognosis in diabetes, to the percentage of fat in the blood is definitely related as shown by a study of 171 of my fatal cases recently made by H. Gray, who will publish his results more extensively when completed. Patients with the highest percentages of fat lived on the average but a few weeks, whereas those with percentages but slightly above normal lived for three to five years. (See Table 86.) Between the extremes of the table the values vary quite uniformly. When the statistics are examined for the same number of cases but based on twice the number of analyses of the blood, including those made both at entrance and during the course of treatment, the same results are to be seen. The table therefore shows clearly that conditions which favor an increase in the fat of the blood of diabetics are inimical to a favorable prognosis, and furthermore, that even very slight increases are distinctly harmful. However it should be emphasized that these high percentages of fat are amenable to treatment and can be made innocuous. (See Case No. 983, p. 193 and p. 228.)

[1] Cases from 560 to 996 are arranged approximately in order of severity from mild to severe.

TABLE 86.—RELATION OF BLOOD FAT TO PROGNOSIS. H. GRAY.[1]

Duration of life after blood was taken to death, years.	Admission blood fat only.		Consolidated admission and later blood fat.	
	No. fatal cases.	Average blood fat, per cent.	No. specimens on same, fatal cases.	Average blood fat. per cent,
0.0–0.1 inclusive . . .	18	1.00	46	1.17
0.2–0.5 " . . .	39	1.09	68	1.14
0.6–0.9 " . . .	37	1.03	79	1.00
1.0–1.9 " . . .	44	1.06	106	1.05
2.0–2.9 " . . .	19	0.93	29	0.91
3.0–3.9 " . . .	7	0.74	15	0.95
4.0–4.9 " . . .	4	0.75	5	0.79
5.0–	3	0.77	3	0.77
Total number . . .	171	..	351	

Cholesterol in the blood is also distinctly related to the prognosis in diabetes. (See Table 87.) The higher the percentage of cholesterol the more unfavorable the prognosis. The statistics in the table vary consistently between its extremes. Here again none of the values obtained for cholesterol with the blood of diabetics were normal, and the therapeutic indication is plain—an excess of cholesterol as well as of total fat is to be combatted.

TABLE 87.—RELATION OF BLOOD CHOLESTEROL (BLOOR METHOD, WHOLE BLOOD) TO PROGNOSIS. H. GRAY.[1]
(123 specimens obtained from patients treated in 1916 and 1917.)

Duration of life after blood was taken to death or, if alive, to June 1, 1923, years.	No. of specimens.	Cholesterol, whole blood (Bloor method), per cent.
0.8	4	0.80–1.50
1.9	27	0.43–0.79
2.4	19	0.32–0.42
4.0	73	0.31 or less

Overweight does not cause an increase in the blood fat of diabetes, because patients +11 per cent or more above actuarial standards showed the same percentage of blood fat as those diabetics within a broad zone between +10 per cent and −10 per cent of the standard. (See Table 88.) Yet these comfortably nourished diabetics exhibited average percentages of blood fat 0.81 per cent and 0.82 per cent which are 20 per cent above the normal blood fat—namely, 0.68 per cent. The differences in these percentages of blood fat are absolutely slight, but relatively considerable. An increase of 20 per cent in the blood fat is not to be disregarded. In the data of Newburgh and Marsh similar increases in the blood fat of their patients are recorded but are considered by them as normal and

[1] The statistics in this table were compiled from my cases by H. Gray. The analyses were made by Bloor's method with whole blood, oxalated.

as proof that a high fat diet does not increase the blood fat of a diabetic. Their contention is true to a greater extent than I considered possible, but one must not get the impression that their patients have a normal blood fat. When the diabetic patients showed an average weight 11 per cent or more below standard, their blood fat was increased to 1.25 per cent, which is almost twice the normal fat value. But from other tables in this section this increase can be explained as due to these diabetic patients being more severe in type rather than by an attempt to relate it to the substandard weight. However, it suggests that it would be desirable to have a series of analyses of the blood fat of non-diabetics some of whom are above and some of whom are below standard weight.

TABLE 88.—RELATION BETWEEN BLOOD FAT AND BODY WEIGHT. (H. GRAY.)[1]

Weight of patient at time of analysis expressed in per cent overweight (+) or underweight (−) compared with medical actuarial standard, per cent.	Number of specimens.	Average blood fat (Bloor's method), whole blood, per cent.
+11 or more	12	0.81
+10 to −10	36	0.82
−11 and under	116	1.25

Prognosis in diabetes may be related to the blood fat, providing the blood fat remains constantly at the level at which it was first determined. Fortunately, treatment will modify the prognosis, as shown by the results in Case No. 983, who showed the greatest increase of total fatty acids in the plasma among my early cases and yet now, seven years later, is a mild diabetic. With her the decrease in fat took place during the course of weeks. How different the condition of today. A total blood fat of 6.3 per cent in Case No. 2842 decreased with 63 units of insulin in four and a half days to 2.95 per cent. Clearly the prognosis in diabetes cannot be related to a single blood-fat value, but is dependent upon the modification of that blood value by treatment.

C. THE TOTAL METABOLISM IN DIABETES.[2]

Two equally emaciated and severe diabetic patients come for examination. When asked to disrobe, the one who is bright-eyed with flushed cheeks and red, dry lips removes his clothes to the skin, refuses a blanket, says he is thankful to cool off, and stands awaiting further orders; his pale, sallow companion slowly

[1] Gray: Unpublished data.
[2] Prior to the discussion of the effect of food upon the metabolism on page 276, various considerations upon metabolism in general are set forth, and the computation of metabolism is described on p. 400 and p. 753.

undresses, regretfully removes his underclothes, and without invitation picks up a blanket, shivers, and sits down. The pulse of the former is rapid and that of the latter is slow. If put to a physical test, the difference between the two individuals would prove to be far less than the contrast in appearance would indicate.

An observer trained in the interpretation of metabolism tests could not fail to discern that the metabolism of the one was as distinctly above normal as that of the other was distinctly below normal. The two represent the dangerous extremes reached by patients having the same disease. So frequently were instances of the former type encountered among the diabetic patients studied at the Nutrition Laboratory in Boston before June, 1914, and so commonly those of the latter type after that date, and so clearly did the transition in type of these cases correspond to the abandonment of overnutrition and the adoption of undernutrition at that time, that no more appropriate title could be found by the writer for a monograph, based upon studies of diabetics between the years 1908 and 1917, by F. G. Benedict and himself than "Diabetic Metabolism with High and Low Diets."[1]

Though it is possible by simple observation alone to infer the increased and decreased metabolism of the two individuals above described, the establishment of these facts by proof and the explanation of the causes which brought this about are far less easy and have been attained only with laborious effort. To a considerable extent this has been due to the fact that observations upon metabolism in health quite as much as in disease are of very recent development. For this reason, in what follows, an attempt will be made to bring out the salient features of the diabetic metabolism which have been encountered in studies made upon 113 of the writer's patients prior to 1917, and the more recent observations begun in 1922,[2] and to refer rather freely to certain aspects of normal metabolism. The early investigations were made possible by the constant help and participation of F. G. Benedict and his co-workers at the Nutrition Laboratory of the Carnegie Institute of Washington situated in Boston. Valuable papers upon diabetic metabolism have appeared from the Russell Sage Laboratory embodying the work of DuBois in collaboration with Allen and Geyelin, and more recently with Richardson, who has become associated with the laboratory, as well as the discerning critical comments

---

[1] Joslin: Pub. No. 323, Carnegie Inst. of Washington, D. C., 1923. See also Benedict and Joslin: Metabolism in Diabetes Mellitus, Pub. No. 136, ibid., 1910. Benedict and Joslin: A Study of Metabolism in Severe Diabetes, Pub. No. 187, 1912. The literature is given in these monographs.

[2] These latter are discussed on p. 539.

by Lusk. Falta has contributed also to our present knowledge, both by experiment and discussion. One of the most detailed investigations by Wilder, Boothby, and Beeler, came from the Mayo Clinic in 1922, and in August, 1923, appears a contribution from McCann, Hannon, Perlzweig and Tompkins[1] which unites clinical, chemical and respiratory data with a review of recent literature.

The total metabolism, or more specifically the gaseous or respiratory metabolism, of diabetes attracted the attention of Pettenkoffer and Voit in 1867. They came to the conclusion that diabetic patients gave off less carbon dioxide and consumed less oxygen than the normal individual. In 1905, Magnus-Levy, in an excellently conducted study of four diabetic patients, showed an increased consumption of oxygen by the patient per kilogram body weight. Varying results were obtained by other investigators, but these were so divergent in character that the question still remained an open one in 1908. The problem was then taken up afresh with the writer's private patients and with the coöperation of Prof. Benedict, and investigations were carried on in the course of routine hospital treatment. Recognizing that the lack of uniformity in the results of other observers might be due to the fact that different types of diabetics were studied, our attention was directed almost entirely to the metabolism of severe diabetics. The metabolism of the mild and moderately severe diabetic was early recognized to be essentially normal. As years passed on, it developed that the same diabetic patient might exhibit a metabolism at one time distinctly above normal and at another time below normal.

Between 1908 and 1912, the metabolism of 22 severe diabetics was observed. Upon comparing these individuals with 20 normal individuals of approximately the same size and weight, the conclusion was reached that the average metabolism of the diabetic group exceeded that of the normal group by from 15 to 20 per cent. At that period normal standards for estimating the metabolism were unknown and the publication of these data called forth criticism as to the propriety of comparing the metabolism of the diabetic with normal but emaciated controls. This criticism stimulated the search for normal standards of metabolism to which subject it is appropriate to refer.

1. **Normal Standards of Metabolism.**—Normal individuals are so unlike one another that it is impossible to conceive of a fixed type from which so comprehensive an expression of their vitality as is their metabolism will not swerve. *A priori*, therefore, in

---

[1] McCann *et al.:* Arch. Int. Med., 1923, **32**, 226.

the endeavor to create a normal standard of human metabolism, it should be conceded that success will be attained if the standard reached should prove to be a zone with considerable latitude rather than a line. How wide this normal zone should be is a matter for speculation, but there are few investigators in metabolism who would venture to narrow the zone to less than 10 degrees—in other words, to 5 per cent below or above a given base line. It speaks well for the accuracy of the present methods employed in the determination of the metabolism of men that the Harris and Benedict and DuBois standards for normals, the two standards commonly employed, come within this rather narrow zone; in fact, when the two standards are compared, it has been shown that a metabolism of about—5 per cent according to the DuBois standard corresponds with the Harris and Benedict base line. When the metabolism diverges greatly from the normal zone, the difference between the two methods of estimating the metabolism grows less.

The material upon which the Harris and Benedict standard is based is drawn from a large number of healthy individuals, 136 men and 103 women, such as would be accepted as good risks by any insurance company. The metabolism of these individuals was directly determined at the Nutrition Laboratory. From subsequent correlations the independent influences of age, sex, height, and weight were found and prediction formulas and standard multiple-prediction tables involving these four factors were derived. The standard for men advocated by DuBois and his associates is based upon practically the same material as that used by Harris and Benedict with a somewhat greater degree of restriction. It was made up as follows: 72 men were chosen from the large series of the Nutrition Laboratory, already mentioned, and 7 subjects added whose metabolism had been studied at the Cornell Laboratory. To these 79 individuals other subjects, also studied by DuBois, were subsequently added, these being 6 men between seventy-seven and eighty-three years of age and 8 boys twelve and thirteen years of age. From these subjects DuBois derived a measure of the normal metabolism by means of his formula for determining body surface and to this later applied corrections for sex and finally for age. (See page 754.)

Unless otherwise stated, the Harris and Benedict standards are employed throughout this book and more particularly in this chapter as a basis for the comparison of the metabolism of diabetic subjects.

The prediction of the basal metabolism according to the Harris and Benedict standard is most quickly obtained by using standard multiple-prediction tables for men and women between the ages of twenty-one and seventy years, inclusive, which have been derived from the Harris and Benedict formulas. These are inserted upon p. 755 together with the Harris and Benedict formulas.

2. **Metabolism of Diabetic Patients Before and After June, 1914.**—Comparing the results obtained with my diabetics between 1908 and 1914, with the Harris and Benedict standard, instead of with the originally selected emaciated controls, the metabolism will be found to be 12 per cent *above* normal. This was the metabolism of diabetics ten or more years ago. Similar patients with different treatment today show a metabolism nearly as much— 11 per cent—*below* standard. The comparatively constant deviation from the normal zone of individuals with hyper- or hypothyroidism can be contrasted with the marked variation in the metabolism observed in diabetes. One might say that the metabolism of the disease diabetes, even of severe diabetes, varies but little from normal, but that the metabolism of the diabetic patient, particularly the severe diabetic patient, varies greatly from normal, not from intrinsic causes as with the thyroid patient, but from extrinsic causes of which the diet is the chief cause. This is due to the fact that the methods of treatment to which the diabetic has been subjected have been so radically diverse in type. The fundamental change in treatment began about June, 1914.

The cause for a marked alteration in the aspect of the diseased patient was surely adequate. Prior to 1914, diabetic patients were overfed, all cases being treated with a low carbohydrate and high protein-fat diet. Excess of calories was encouraged, and to guard against coma, instead of limitation of fat and undernutrition, sodium bicarbonate was employed in large doses and continued for periods of months   Fat was given *ad nauseam*, and even such fatty foods as cheese and eggs were served, mixed with about equal proportions of butter. The good results of fasting days were overlooked; Naunyn's observation, von Noorden's recommendation, and Weintraud's proof that diabetic patients could subsist upon remarkably few calories, were known but unappreciated and considered more of scientific interest than of therapeutic significance. Hodgson, however, had grasped the principle and with it attained unusual success in practical treatment. It was at this time that Guelpa's conceptions of fasting and of the waning severity of diabetes in the presence of an emaciating disease were recognized, utilized, and enlarged by Allen into a system of treatment based upon a reduced caloric intake and adopted by the author in June, 1914.

Patients given the fasting treatment when this procedure was first used were almost invariably underfed to a marked degree, because the hospital period was spent in securing quick results and these were most readily obtained by extreme dietetic restrictions.

In 1915, the writer recognized that fat was largely responsible for acidosis, and its omission at the beginning of treatment was emphasized. Sodium bicarbonate was abandoned in September, 1915. The reduction of weight for therapeutic purposes was followed with some hesitancy, and lapses of treatment were more tolerated than at present.

In the presentation of the data acquired upon the metabolism the policy has been followed of studying the data on the basis of individual days rather more frequently than by grouping the results for the individual cases. This has been rendered necessary because a single case has so many phases. Thus, during the period of observation of a patient there may be changes in age, weight, and even occasionally in height, and almost certainly in degree of severity and acidosis, and with each of these factors the metabolism varies so that a single case becomes in reality many cases. The data for an experimental day means the data obtained for one patient on that day and may represent one observation of the basal metabolism or the average of several estimations, often rendered possible because the patients formerly frequently fasted for twenty-four or more hours.

If the postabsorptive metabolism of all diabetics (exclusive of the girl patients) is compared with the normal standard, it will be found that before the change in treatment in June, 1914, to fasting and a reduced diet, the metabolism was above the standard for one hundred and seven days and below it on twelve days with an average metabolism of 12 per cent above normal. (See Table 89.) In the series made after June, 1914, the metabolism was below standard on two hundred and twenty-five days and above on fifty days with an average metabolism of 11 per cent below normal. The two average variations for the observations before and after June, 1914, are so nearly equal in distance from the normal standard that the average metabolism for the two periods before and after June, 1914 is 0.

TABLE 89.—VARIATION IN BASAL METABOLISM OF DIABETICS FROM THE NORMAL STANDARD BEFORE AND AFTER INAUGURATION OF TREATMENT BY UNDERNUTRITION IN JUNE, 1914.

Period of observation.	Number of observation days with metabolism.		Average variation from standard.	Average metabolism computed from cases.		Average variation from standard.
	Above standard.	Below standard		Above standard.	Below standard.	
Before June, 1914: 29 cases . .	107	12	+12	27	2	+13
After June, 1914: 76 cases . .	50	225	−11	19	57	−7

If the results for the different cases are compared, instead of for experiments, regardless of the individuality of the diabetics, as is likewise done in Table 89, the general trend of the metabolism before and after June, 1914, is seen to be like that observed in the other comparison. Before June, 1914, 27 cases showed a metabolism above, and only 2 cases below, the normal standard, while after that date the metabolism with 19 cases was above, and with 57 cases below, standard. The average variation by cases before June, 1914, is +13 per cent, but the percentage below normal after that date is −7 per cent.

(*a*) **High and Low Metabolism in Diabetes** —The wide divergence which may be found in the metabolism of diabetics is strikingly shown in Table 90, which presents the 6 cases with the highest and the 7 cases with the lowest metabolism in the entire series, as indicated by the percentage variation from standard. With all of these cases the diabetes was severe.

For the cases with high metabolism the percentage variation ranged between +26 per cent and +33 per cent. Perhaps the best idea of the gravity of the conditions under which the subjects were living is obtained from the duration of life following the recorded observations. Case No. 1412, succumbed to the disease within three days. Cases Nos. 549, 210, and 246 lived from one to six months, Case No. 220 lived nearly a year and a half, and Case No. 983 is still alive in 1923. Comment upon the latter exceptional case is made elsewhere. (See p. 228.) It is sufficient to state here that this patient was markedly obese, being 43 per cent above normal weight. Her high metabolism and accompanying acidosis would appear to be due to sudden restriction of carbohydrate and free use of protein and fat for the week preceding entrance to the hospital.   This is an example of what occurs when such measures are adopted. The carbohydrate given for the four days before the test was 80, 55, 50 and 50 grams, and although for these same days the caloric intake amounted to but 545, 414, 321, and 240 calories, large quantities of body fat were drawn upon for active caloric needs. This case is also particularly instructive, because it shows that a marked increase in metabolism and acidosis may be temporary and not necessarily of bad prognostic import.

In contrast to the cases with high metabolism are 7 patients with an exceptionally low metabolism, these averaging 32 per cent below standard. Despite this extraordinary decrease in metabolism, the life of these patients was evidently not in so great jeopardy as those with high metabolism Of these patients with low metabolism one succumbed within a month, but the others lived between six months and two years and five months from the

TABLE 90.—HIGHEST AND LOWEST POSTABSORPTIVE METABOLISM OF DIABETICS AS EXPRESSED BY VARIATION FROM STANDARD (ALL CASES SEVERE).

Case No.	Date.	Variation of metabolism from normal standard, per cent.	Loss from maximum body weight, per cent.	Variation from normal standard of body weight,	Acidosis.	Sugar in blood, per cent.	Urinary nitrogen per kg. of body weight per 24 hours. For days preceding observation. Number of days.	Urinary nitrogen per kg. of body weight per 24 hours. For days preceding observation. Nitrogen.	Urinary nitrogen per kg. of body weight per 24 hours. On observation day, gm.	Sugar in urine on preceding day, gm.	Respiratory quotient.	Duration of life after this observation, years.
					HIGHEST METABOLISM.							
210	Aug. 2– 3, 1910	+26	24	−27	+++	..	7	0.325	0.315	268	0.71	0.3
220	Mar. 13–14, 1909	+32	24	−25	+++	..	..	..	..	..	0.69	1.4
246	June 8– 9, 1909	+28	15	+ 1	++	..	1	0.210	..	104	0.67	0.5
549	Nov. 5– 6, 1912	+30	18	−14	+++	..	2	0.370	..	185	0.69	0.1
983	Feb. 2– 3, 1916	+28	..	+43	+++	0.30	1	0.145	0.125	72	0.73	
1412	Oct. 18–19, 1917	+33	22	−23	+++	0.37	..	..	0.380	170	0.72	Living 3 days
	Oct. 19–20, 1917		22	−23	+++	..	..	..	..	167	0.76	
					LOWEST METABOLISM.							
765	Feb. 9–10, 1916	−27	23	−31	++	0.23	7	0.180	0.110	14	0.76	0.8
821	Apr. 3– 4, 1916	−30	25	−17	+	..	7	0.260	0.225	0	0.81	0.5
	Apr. 10–11, 1916		26	−19	+	0.20	7	0.285	0.210	+	0.82	
1011	Nov. 23–24, 1917	−37	49	−49	0	0.29	7	0.285	0.260	42	0.94	0.8
1085	Oct. 11–12, 1916	−40	50	−43	0	..	..	..	..	0	0.81	0.1
	Oct. 31–Nov. 1, 1916		54	−46	++	0.35	7	0.275	0.165	15	0.81	
1196	Dec. 15–16, 1916	−27	29	−22	++	0.15	6	0.255	0.115	35	0.80	1.0
	Jan. 6– 7, 1917		34	−27	0	..	3	0.415	0.380	0	0.80	
1233	Feb. 19–20, 1917	−33	30	−23	0	0.13	1	0.280	0.210	0	0.86	1.3
1378	Nov. 13–14, 1917	−29	31	−46	0	0.24	..	..	..	..	0.88	2.4

date of the observation here recorded. Evidently, therefore, a diabetic patient whose metabolism is far below normal is, on the whole, in a safer condition than the diabetic patient whose metabolism is exceptionally high, though either extreme in metabolism may be dangerous, though not necessarily of fatal significance.

The respiratory quotients are strikingly different. With the omission of Case No. 983, the 5 remaining patients with the highest metabolism had an average quotient of 0.7, while with the 7 patients with the low metabolism the average quotient was 0.84. The significance of this wide variation in the respiratory quotient is discussed on p. 258 *et seq*

The average loss in weight from maximum of 5 of the 6 patients with the high metabolism was 21 per cent. Two of the patients were respectively +1 per cent and +43 per cent above normal standard weight. The losses in weight of the 7 patients with low metabolism were decidedly greater than those above mentioned. Thus, the average loss in weight below maximum was 37 per cent, and the average variation in weight from the normal standard was −34 per cent. Three patients were 46 to 49 per cent below normal weight, and the nearest approach to normal weight was Case No. 821 who was 17 per cent under weight. The low metabolism was evidently connected with an exceptional loss of body weight, but this was not the only factor.

With one exception the cases with the highest metabolism had an extreme degree of acidosis, but of the 7 cases with the lowest metabolism 3 showed no acidosis, while with the other 4 cases acidosis was either absent in some of the tests or not more than moderate in degree in others.

A considerable number of determinations were made of the urinary nitrogen, either for the day of the observation or within one week. The average urinary nitrogen per kilogram body weight of the cases with high metabolism (omitting Case No. 983) for the days preceding the observation and also for the day of the test was 0.32 gram, and the average urinary nitrogen for the patients with lowest metabolism was 0.255 gram per kilogram body weight. The nitrogen excretion per kilogram body weight for a normal adult is about 0.165 gram. It will be observed that the highest value for urinary nitrogen per kilogram body weight was encountered with Case No. 1196, whose metabolism was −27 per cent. The significance of a high urinary nitrogen is twofold. A high urinary nitrogen implies the disintegration of much protein, usually superabundant in the diet, and this leads to a high metabolism under ordinary conditions, as is universally recognized. On the other hand, a high urinary nitrogen due to disintegration of body protein and loss of body nitrogen is an entirely different situation, because it represents the last resort of the body to preserve existence and occurs when the metabolism is at its lowest ebb. (See p. 238.)

The difference in treatment of the two groups of cases is shown plainly by the quantity of sugar in the urine for the twenty-four hours preceding the period of observation. With the omission of Case No. 983 this varied from 104 to 268 grams with the patients having a high metabolism and from no sugar to 42 grams with the cases having a low metabolism, thus affording evidence that the early cases were fed more liberally than the later cases.

(b) **Variations in the Metabolism of Individual Diabetics.**—The course of the metabolism of 5 severe cases of diabetes was noted during intervals of from one to one and eighth-tenths years. The average metabolism was lowered 12 per cent as a result of this interval. In 3 of these cases the metabolism was above normal at the first observation and below normal at the second observation. Corresponding to this lowering of the metabolism, there was an average decrease of body weight of 17 per cent. Calculating the decrease in metabolism in terms of calories instead of in standards, the fall in metabolism was exactly the same as that of loss in body weight, namely: 17 per cent. The average pulse-rate fell during the period 11 beats. In sharp contrast to this alteration of the basal metabolism is the metabolism of 6 patients studied after food at intervals of one and one-tenth to one and seven-tenth years. No loss in the response of the metabolism to food was observed.

A classic example of the marked variations in the metabolism of a single diabetic is well exemplified by a case studied by Geyelin and DuBois.[1] A young man, aged nineteen years, weight 172 pounds, began to grow thin November 1, 1915, and on November 20, weighed about 150 pounds. Before he came to the authors, carbohydrate had been greatly restricted and protein (and presumably fat) much increased with resulting severe acidosis. Between December 7 and 11 he was fasted, and 50 to 114 grams sodium bicarbonate were given daily. He was then fed (see Table 91), alkali continued, and the metabolism studied. From the table it can be seen that: (1) The metabolism varied from 73 calories per hour (31 calories per kilogram body weight per twenty-four hours) to 43 calories per hour (23 calories per kilogram body weight per twenty-four hours) in the course of a few weeks;[2] (2) that a dextrose-nitrogen ratio in excess of Lusk's 3.65:1 ration, was obtained on three successive days, to wit: 3.97:1, 4.01:1, 3.87:1; (3) that the nitrogen in the urine was extreme, being 29.8 grams on the second day of fasting and 38.27 grams even when 99 grams of protein were ingested; (4) that the acidosis was

---

[1] Geyelin and DuBois: Jour. Am. Med. Assn., 1916, **66**, 1532.

[2] Gephart, Aub, DuBois and Lusk (Arch. Int. Med., 1917, **19**, 908) discuss this case more in detail.

14

extreme, for the β-oxybutyric acid eliminated amounted on one
day to 87 grams.   The case is remarkable in all of the above par-
ticulars and will always remain a classic in diabetic metabolism,

TABLE 91.—CLINICAL AND EXPERIMENTAL DATA IN CASE OF CYRIL K.
(GEYELIN AND DUBOIS).[1]

Date.	Carbohydrate, gm.	Protein, gm.	Fat, gm.	Output, glucose, gm.	Urine nitrogen, gm.	D:N ratio.	β-oxybutyric acid, gm.	Blood CO₂, mm. Hg.	Average R. Q.	Average calories per hour.
1915–1916.										
Dec. 8– 9	0	0	0	74	27.9	2.68	43	30		
9–10	0	0	0	78	29.8	2.61	34			
10–11	0	0	0	74	24.8	2.95	...	26		
11–12	41	17	17	108	30.6	2.17	60	21		
12–13	50	50	69	112	34.5	1.80	53	22		
13–14[2]	50	55	58	118	35.4	1.92	57	22		
14–15	53	58	51	118	37.7	1.73	55			
15–16	23	118	41	167	36.6	3.97	70	19	0.687	81
16–17	0	99	5	153	38.2	4.01	75	19	0.714	76
17–18	0	39	2	140	36.2	3.87	87	35		
18–19	0	0	0	55	20.0	2.76	58	35	0.707	73
19–20	0	0	0	44	16.7	2.65	56	49		
20–21	1	10	0	35	14.0	2.44	41	52	0.721	66
21–22	1	20	0	39	14.4	2.65	26			
22–23	5	21	0	25	18.2	1.12	10	52	0.734	62
Feb. 16[3]	..	..	..	0	..	0	0	..	0.915	42
Mar. 8[4]	..	..	..	0	..	0	0	..	0.860	50

but to me it is far more interesting from other points of view, and
my interpretation of it is as follows: A fat young man develops
diabetes rather acutely.   Such cases we know now are quickly
amenable to moderate undernutrition consisting of a non-fat diet
but if placed upon a protein-fat diet with little carbohydrate, as
was this case nearly eight years ago, develop severe acidosis which
is not easily overcome unless taken early.   Fat patients are especially prone to develop such an acidosis.   (See Case No. 983 on
p. 228.)   On December 11–12 a diet with 42 grams carbohydrate,
18 grams protein, and 18 grams fat lowered the D:N ratio.   It is
true the acidosis increased, but this may be explained by large

[1] Geyelin and DuBois: Loc. cit., p. 209.
[2] Transferred to Bellevue Hospital.
[3] Transferred to Bellevue Hospital.   Liberal diabetic diet the days before these
calorimeter observations.
[4] After meals which might cause increase in metabolism of 5 to 10 per cent above
basal.

doses of sodium bicarbonate. At any rate, when protein and fat were increased on the following three days, the severity of the case increased and the phenomenon noted above occurred. Is it not probable that if fat has been decreased in the diet at the very beginning of treatment, acidosis would have been avoided? Did not the sodium bicarbonate act harmfully by setting free β-oxybutyric acid which previously was innocuously combined? Had not the case been intrinsically a comparatively mild case, as was later shown by a toleration of 169 grams carbohydrate, and a youthful individual, death from coma must have resulted. As it was, the case survived (*a*) an initial nearly non-carbohydrate diet; (*b*) the increase of fat in the diet when acidosis was well under way; (*c*) the setting free of enormous quantities of β-oxybutyric acid through the use of alkalis, and (*d*) a furuncle, which, though small, undoubtedly increased the severity of the case (see Case No. 610, p. 525) and recovered when (1) fat was eliminated from the diet and protein in moderate quantities given; (2) followed after two days by fasting. Was it not in this case, as in so many of my own in the past, though with less fortunate terminations, the hand of man that made the diabetes severe, just as later the hand of man made it mild?

(*c*) **Age.**—The influence of age upon the metabolism of the diabetic patient is distinct. All the results available indicate, that both prior and subsequent to June, 1914, in the two decades fifty-one to seventy years the metabolism varied only 1 per cent from normal. The normal diabetic metabolism for these decades corresponds to the generally accepted idea of the mildness of the disease at this epoch; in fact, of the 18 cases studied 10 were mild or moderate in severity. Greeley[1] from his experience at Hodgson's clinic several years ago emphasized the connection between the decreasing severity of the diabetes with the simultaneous decrease in normal metabolism which advance in age brings.

Both prior to and after June, 1914, the metabolism in the second decade (eleven to twenty years) varied respectively 4 per cent above and 4 per cent below normal. These are significant figures when considered in relation to each other, because they show for this decade the same tendency of rise and fall in metabolism for the two periods as the entire series. On the other hand, the data are so nearly within normal limits that they confirm the impression already furnished by Table 89, that the diabetic metabolism is essentially normal. The disease in youth is so apt to be severe and has universally been considered to be so severe that it is also important and encouraging that the metabolism should prove to

[1] Greeley: Boston Med. and Surg. Jour., 1916, **175**, 73.

be so nearly normal for these boys   In the Shattuck Lecture for 1922, it was reported that 8 children contracting diabetes even in the first decade of life lived more than five years with the disease. However, before concluding too much from this series of 8 cases, the results supplied by 6 young female diabetics, not here included but discussed in detail in Publication No. 323, p. 201, should be given due weight, particularly as the standard of comparison in that group is different.   By the Girl Scout standard the metabolism averaged +33 per cent before and +8 per cent after June, 1914, and with the Harris and Benedict standard extended for this purpose, +7 per cent and −19 per cent, respectively.   The values by the DuBois standard were −1 per cent and −21 per cent.   The girls showed greater variations in metabolism than the boys.   Does this mean they were more amenable to the high and low diets imposed?

The three decades between twenty-one and fifty years present an average increase above normal of 17 per cent before June, 1914, and an average decrease below normal of 10 per cent after that date.   Since it is chiefly for these three decades that the question of an abnormal metabolism in diabetes is raised, it is significant that these are the decades which have supplied the majority of the subjects for this study of diabetic metabolism and also the decades in which we have the most data for normals.   It may be that these peculiarities in the metabolism can be explained by the fact that in the decades with an average metabolism either notably above or below the normal standard the patients were treated most strictly and showed the effect of overfeeding or low diet, whereas the patients in the decade eleven to twenty years were less amenable to treatment, and those in the decades subsequent to fifty years did not require rigorous treatment.

(d) **Sex.**—Sex affects normal metabolism in that females have a lower metabolism than males of the same age, height, and weight, and in diabetes the same relation holds.

3. **Pulse-rate and Metabolism.**— (a) **In Health.**—A study of normal individuals such as those which furnished the basis for the Harris and Benedict standards of metabolism furnishes clear evidence that when the pulse-rate is low there is a tendency for the metabolism to be low and when the pulse-rate is high there is a distinct tendency for the metabolism to be high.   It is a matter of interest that the average pulse-rate for 121 of the 136 men in the Harris and Benedict group of normals was 61 and that the average pulse-rate for the men in the DuBois series was the same. Sturgis and Tompkins, who have investigated the relation between pulse-rate and metabolism, conclude that "there is in general an inter-relationship between the pulse-rate and metabolism when

a group of individuals are considered; that is, an extreme degree of tachycardia usually indicates a slight or moderate increase. The fact that a pulse-rate at complete rest below 90 per minute is seldom and below 80 per minute is rarely associated with an increase in metabolism is of practical importance in the recognition of the large group of nervous patients who have symptoms similar to those occurring in hyperthyroidism."

(b) **In Diabetes.**—In the course of the studies on the metabolism of diabetic subjects at the Nutrition Laboratory between 7000 and 8000 records were made of the pulse-rate. In our early observations between 1908 and 1912 it was shown that whereas the average minimum and maximum pulse-rates of the 25 normal, but somewhat similarly emaciated, male and female subjects used for comparison were 54 and 74 beats, respectively, the corresponding figures for the 24 male and female diabetics were 65 and 81. Without taking account of the sex the average pulse-rate of the normals was 63 and of the diabetics 73. It will be seen, therefore, that for the normal individuals the minimum and maximum pulse-rates and also the average pulse-rate were markedly lower than those of the diabetics studied between 1908 and 1912.

If we compare the pulse-rate of the diabetics treated since June, 1914, with values for 219 subjects from the same normal series, an entirely different picture is presented. Thus, the average diabetic pulse value, which is based upon 69 cases, was but 1 beat higher than the normal value, or 65 as compared with 64. This shows, therefore, that the average pulse-rate of diabetic subjects decreased markedly in the period subsequent to June, 1914, as compared to the period before that date.

TABLE 92.—RELATION BETWEEN PULSE-RATE AND POSTABSORPTIVE METABOLISM IN DAILY OBSERVATIONS WITH DIABETICS.

Range in pulse-rate.	Before June, 1914.		After June, 1914.	
	Heat output per kilogram of body weight per 24 hours, cals.	Variation in metabolism from standard, per cent.	Heat output per kilogram of body weight per 24 hours, cals.	Variation in metabolism. from standard, per cent.
45–49	..	....	22	−16
51–60	30	+ 2	23	−14
61–70	30	+13	24	−10
71–80	31	+13	26	− 5
81–90	32	+22	26	− 1
91–122	37	+25	33	+18[1]

[1] Range of pulse-rate in this group after June, 1914, was 98 to 101.

Coming now to the relation between the pulse-rate and the metabolism in diabetes, it is clear from inspection of the figures in Table 92, that both before and after June, 1914, the pulse-rate registers with considerable accuracy the changes in metabolism, the latter steadily rising as the pulse-rate increases. When, however, the values for the metabolism in the two periods are compared, we find that with the same range in pulse-rate the metabolism varies materially, and for a pulse-rate of 61 to 70 the calories per kilogram are 30 and 24, respectively, under the two methods of treatment, or expressed in terms of normal standard from $+13$ per cent before June, 1914, to -10 per cent after that date. Accordingly, *similar conditions of living are requisite for an interpretation of the pulse-rate as a measure of the metabolism.* Granted these similar conditions, the value of the pulse-rate in estimating the comparative change in metabolism of diabetic patients is almost as great as the measurement of the metabolism itself.

(c) **Effect of Loss in Weight on Pulse-rate of Normal Individuals.**— The losses in weight of the diabetic patients below their maximum weight were so material that the question arises how much bearing similar losses in weight might have upon the pulse-rate of normal individuals. Fortunately the pulse-rates accompanying considerable losses of body weight in a series of experiments carried out by the Nutrition Laboratory are available. The pulse-rates were determined for a group of 11 healthy young men in the International Young Men's Christian Association College at Springfield, Massachusetts, when they were upon a normal diet and also when they had lost on an average of 9 per cent of their weight as a result of a reduced diet.[1] In consequence there was an average decrease in pulse-rate of 14 beats, or 25 per cent. All of the men registered a fall in rate, but this was by no means uniform, for with 1 subject the fall was but 5 beats and with 2 others it was 21 beats. These individuals lost on the average but 9 per cent of their initial weight, whereas 111 of the 113 diabetics under observation had an average loss in body weight from maximum of 25 per cent. From these data acquired with normal subjects it would therefore appear that in view of the marked loss in weight of the diabetics, a decrease in the pulse-rate should be very considerable. Before considering the relationship between the loss of weight with diabetics and their pulse-rate, however, various factors should be mentioned which may have an influence upon this relationship.

(1) *Factors Influencing Relation Between Pulse-rate and Loss in Weight.*—At the present moment it is prudent to state that the changes in pulse-rate observed with the normal subjects studied

[1] Benedict, Miles, Roth and Smith: Carnegie Inst. of Washington, D. C., Pub. 280, 383.

at Springfield *accompanied* the 9 per cent loss in weight rather than were *dependent* upon it. This is necessary, because while these normal individuals were losing weight, they were also losing large amounts of body nitrogen, since 10 of the 11 men lost, on the average, 175 grams of body nitrogen between October 4, the initial day of the reduced diet, and January 27, inclusive. It is yet to be determined whether the changes in pulse-rate and also in metabolism which were observed were due: (1) To the loss in weight which had already taken place; (2) to the loss in body nitrogen; or (3) what appears to be the most probable cause, to the continued underfeeding. Loss in weight and loss in nitrogen apply equally well to the diabetics, but the continued underfeeding with constant loss in weight was probably less marked with them than with the Springfield students.

The losses in weight above described with normal individuals took place during a few months, whereas the losses in weight with the diabetic patients usually occurred during a few years. It is possible that the greater loss in weight of the diabetic patients might be counterbalanced to some extent by the greater length of time during which it occurred. With the diabetics, however, there was a fourth factor, namely: The growing weakness due to the progress of the disease which accompanied their loss in weight. This, however, is not so simple a factor as would appear at first thought, because this weakness is manifestly of at least two types. The first type of weakness develops rather rapidly in the diabetic who has been living upon a stimulating protein-fat diet, is associated with and perhaps dependent upon acidosis, and is most evident as he is about to pass into coma preceding death. It is akin to the weakness of the patient with hyperthyroidism and high metabolism. Then there is the second type of weakness due to inanition. For the former type of weakness there are few comparable data upon the pulse-rate with normal individuals, though perhaps exhaustion after strenuous exertion might serve, and strangely enough the same may be said of the latter, since inanition seldom occurs in uncomplicated form. In the inanition of tuberculosis and sometimes in pernicious anemia, fever is present. The inanition of cardiac and renal disease is caused by organic disease of the heart itself and thus invalidates pulse records Complications are less frequent in cancer, yet what data exist upon the pulse-rate in the successive months of cancer? Here is a field for research.

(2) *Effect of Loss in Weight on Pulse-rate of Diabetics and Comparison with Normals.*—That diabetics, whose body weight has suffered so great a loss from their maximum body weight, should have a pulse-rate as high or even higher than normal, must be of significance. In the Springfield series of experiments in which

the pulse-rate averaged rather low, even with normal diet, the subjects were normal, healthy men who maintained their muscular vigor, as was proved by physical tests, despite the loss of weight. The loss in weight of the diabetics, on the other hand, can be considered to have been accomplished by a greater loss of muscle as well as of fat. This was a *fait accompli* and in the period before June, 1914, they were actually being overfed, though the food was not wholly utilized and showed an increased pulse-rate; in the period after June, 1914, they were underfed and the pulse-rate was far lower.

Both before and after June, 1914, the diabetic subjects were markedly underweight. Before that date the loss in weight of 30 diabetics from their maximum was, on an average, 21 per cent, yet in spite of this loss the average pulse-rate was 73 beats, or 31 beats (74 per cent) greater than the average pulse-rate of 42 beats found with the group of normal men on reduced diet after a loss in weight of approximately half as much, or 9 per cent. This brings out strikingly the increased pulse-rate of the diabetics before June, 1914. Subsequent to June, 1914, the loss in weight from maximum of 66 diabetics averaged 27 per cent. Notwithstanding that this loss in weight was three times that of the normals, the average pulse-rate of this group of diabetics was reduced only to 65 beats in contrast to the undernourished normals whose average pulse-rate was 42 beats. It is thus seen that both groups of diabetics, with a much greater loss in weight than the undernourished normals, had higher pulse-rates than the latter and that the highest pulse-rates were obtained with the diabetics before June, 1914, when they were overfed. Despite the fact that the loss in weight of the group of diabetics after June, 1914, was greater than that of the normal subjects and despite the fact that their intake of food was low, the diabetic still maintained a higher pulse-rate than the normals. The evidence is not sufficient to show that the difference in the pulse-rate of 42 of the normals with 9 per cent loss of weight and of 65 of the diabetics with 27 per cent loss of weight can be entirely explained on the ground that the normals were still losing, but the diabetics had lost their weight. At present, therefore, we are forced to conclude that an increased pulse-rate is characteritic of diabetes.

(*d*) **Relation of Severity of Diabetes to Pulse-rate.**—If the pulse-rate in diabetes is characteristic of the disease, one would anticipate a variation with the degree of severity. Tabulation of the data discloses that with increasing severity before June, 1914, the pulse-rate rose, but after June, 1914, it fell. The force of severity cannot act in opposite directions. Obviously these changes in pulse-rate are either not due to severity *per se*, or the effect of severity is overcome by stronger influences, *e. g.*, acidosis and difference in the quantity of food administered.

(*e*) **Relation of Acidosis to Pulse-rate.**—The average pulse-rate for 45 cases without acidosis was 63 beats and for 24 cases with severe acidosis 73 beats. Two cases on the verge of coma had pulse-rates of 98 and 101. Excellent examples of increases in pulse-rate associated with rising acidosis are also to be found in the publications of Allen and DuBois[1] and Gephart, Aub, DuBois, Lusk.[2]

4. **Edema.**—Perhaps no one gross observation made during the course of diabetes mellitus is of greater significance and causes greater alarm, both to the patient and to the physician, than the persistent loss in body weight. On the other hand, slight changes in body weight which may accompany dietetic alterations or the ingestion of sodium chloride and sodium bicarbonate are looked upon as material gains and are thus liable to be misunderstood by the patient. To interpret intelligently these changes, it is necessary both for the physician and for the patient to realize the factors affecting the body weight of normal as well as pathological cases. Few realize that the normal individual is continually undergoing changes in body weight throughout the twenty-four hours. Even during sleep it has been shown that a man of 85 kilos loses 30 grams per hour, and a woman of 65 kilos 29 grams per hour. With exercise this is, of course, greatly increased and may amount to 6.4 kilos for a foot-ball player during one hour and fifteen minutes of active exercise.

Edema is a common source of error and it is important to recognize it as a cause of gain in weight in diabetes. Patients may seem to be gaining when in reality they are losing weight because of insufficient diet. The edema occurred most frequently in former years following oatmeal days and the administration of alkalis, but now is common with fasting diabetics of severe type and is apparently related to the large quantity of salt which they ingest with broths and vegetables.

The edema may become extreme and one of my patients (Case No. 922), whom I had not seen for months, called in a laryngologist and barely escaped tracheotomy for edema of the larynx. This quickly disappeared with the omission of salt and a diet of water and a few oranges. The patient later entered the hospital, became sugar-free and developed a tolerance for 49 grams carbohydrate, 69 grams protein and 143 grams fat.

Diabetic patients should be weighed, preferably naked, before breakfast, and after the urine has been voided, for a patient frequently voids a pound at a time.

[1] Allen and DuBois: Arch. Int. Med., 1916, **17**, 855.
[2] Gephart, Aub, DuBois and Lusk: Arch. Int. Med., 1917, **19**, 908.

(a) **Water Content of the Body.**—A factor which should be taken into consideration in interpreting changes in body weight is the fluctuation in the water content of the body. It should be realized that the average man at rest without food oxidizes per day about 75 grams of protein, 25 grams of glycogen and 200 grams of fat—a total of 300 grams of water-free, organized body tissue. It can readily be seen, therefore, that with the subjects at rest, large and rapid changes in weight must be due not to the oxidation of organic material, which amounts to only 300 grams per day, but to large excretions of water. Under certain conditions it is possible for the body to retain considerable quantities of water, and conversely, to be deprived of considerable amounts of water that would normally be retained. Since about 60 per cent of the body is water, any change of water content may result in material gains or losses in body weight. A man, weighing, for example, 65 kilos, may have an absolute water content of 39 kilos, so that a relatively small change in the percentage of water in the body may produce a change in body weight of 1 kilo.

(b) **Influence of Fat and Carbohydrate Diets upon Weight.**—Remarkable changes in the weight of normal individuals will also occur, if the proportion of fat to carbohydrate is altered, although the caloric value of the diet remains constant. A diet rich in carbohydrate brings about an increase in weight, whereas a diet of exactly the same number of calories, though chiefly made up of fat, lowers the weight. These changes undoubtedly are due simply to the retention of water by the tissues upon a carbohydrate diet and loss of water upon a fat diet. Such changes appear reasonable because the storage of 1 gram carbohydrate in the body demands the retention of 3 grams of water,[1] 1 gram of protein would appear to require the same amount, and 1 gram of fat requires only 0.1 gram of water. These changes are well illustrated by the following table:

TABLE 93.—CHANGES IN WEIGHT WITH FAT AND CARBOHYDRATE DIETS.
CARBOHYDRATE DIET.[2]

| Date, 1904. | Food and drink. | | | Body weight, kg. | Gain (+) or loss (−), gms. |
	Solid matter, gms.	Water, gms.	Total gms.		
Apr. 16 . . .	...		..	75.086	
16–17 . .	970	3577	4547	75.443	+357
17–18 . .	966	3553	4519	75.414	− 29
18–19 . .	966	3491	4457	75.269	−145

FAT DIET.

Apr. 19–20 . .	750	3108	3859	74.319	−950
20–21 . .	745	4150	4896	73.480	−839
21–22 . .	747	4152	4899	72.528	−952

Average gain per day, carbohydrate diet, +61 gms.
Average loss per day, fat diet, −914 gms.
Water stored per day, carbohydrate period, +165 gms.
Water lost per day, fat period, −906 gms.

[1] Zuntz: Biochem. Ztschr., 1912, **44**, 290.　　　[2] Carnegie Pub. No. 176, p. 93.

It is important to bear in mind the effect upon weight which must occur when a carbohydrate-free diet is prescribed, for otherwise the loss of the few pounds which is bound to ensue might cause undue apprehension or be interpreted as loss of tissue.

An increase in weight following a marked increase of carbohydrate in the diet is strikingly illustrated in severe diabetic patients under the oatmeal treatment. Under these conditions the weight may rise 4.5 kilos during one or two days. It is not uncommon to observe that edema develops during the course of an oatmeal cure. It is significant that some of these cases show little or no carbohydrate in the urine. There will probably be general agreement to the statement that the gain in weight following the sudden introduction of large quantities of carbohydrate is to be explained by the storage temporarily, perhaps, of carbohydrate in the body, and along with this, as has been pointed out, marked quantities of water will be retained. That this storage or delay of excretion is accentuated in the case of the presence of diseased kidneys is common knowledge. Barrenscheen[1] showed that excretion of lactose was delayed upon the day following an oatmeal cure.

(c) **Influence of Sodium Chloride upon Weight.**—The quantity of salt in the diet also affects the weight. For example, in the study of an individual upon a salt-free diet consisting of the whites of 18 eggs (216 calories), 120 grams olive oil (1080 calories) and 200 grams crystallized sugar (800 calories), total 2096 calories, or 30 calories per kilogram body weight, the weight fell from 70.2 kilograms on the first day to 64.9 kilograms on the thirteenth day, as will be seen from the following table:

TABLE 94.—LOSS OF WEIGHT COINCIDENT WITH A SALT-FREE DIET.[2]

Day.	Intake of H_2O. c.c.	Urine, c.c.	Urinary analysis. Sp. gr.	P_2O_5, gms.	Cl., gms.	Weight, kg.
1	1470	1720	1012	1.29	4.60	70.2
2	1550	1810	1010	1.29	2.52	
3	1560	1430	1012	1.28	1.88	
4	1290	930	1017	1.20	0.87	67.4
5	1290	1100	1013	1.43	0.69	
6	1545	1170	1012	1.04	0.48	66.6
7	1200	850	1015	1.15	0.46	
8	1125	1000	1013	0.78	0.40	66.1
9	1290	1160	1011	0.95	0.26	
10	1200	860	1015	0.89	0.22	
11	1260	650	1018	0.76	0.22	
12	1215	510	1023	0.79	0.17	65.1
13	1170	560	1023	0.86	0.17	64.9
15 Diet unrestricted.		940	1029	..	3.50	
16	..	..	..	..	..	69.0
17	..	4090	1017	..	25.76	

[1] Barrenscheen: Biochem. Ztschr., 1912, **39**, 459.

[2] Goodall and Joslin: Experiments with Ash-free Diet, Arch. Int. Med., 1908, **1**, 615.

The subject was then put upon a free diet and three days later the weight had risen to 69 kilograms.

(d) **Influence of Sodium Bicarbonate upon Weight.**—The administration of sodium bicarbonate is frequently followed by a gain in weight. Thus, in Case No. 220 the changes in weight during the administration of sodium bicarbonate were as follows:

TABLE 95.—GAIN IN WEIGHT COINCIDENT WITH ADMINISTRATION OF SODIUM BICARBONATE.

Date.	Sodium bicarbonate gms.	Body weight, kilos.	Date.	Sodium bicarbonate gms.	Body weight, kg.
Nov. 2 . . .	0	48.1	Nov. 7 . . .	20	50.7
3 . . .	0	48.6	8 . . .	20	51.5
4 . . .	0	49.0	9 . . .	20	52.4
5 . . .	0	48.6	10 . . .	20	53.3
6 . . .	20	49.3	11 . . .	20	53.3

In order to show that this gain in weight was not directly due to the alkali but rather to retention of salt, the weights of another diabetic patient, Case No. 135, were taken while upon a salt-free diet.

TABLE 96.—ABSENCE OF GAIN IN WEIGHT COINCIDENT WITH ADMINISTRATION OF SODIUM BICARBONATE WHEN THE DIET IS SALT-FREE (CASE No. 135).

	Diet. Salt-free.						Urine.								
Date, 1908.	NaHCO₃, gms.	Carbohydrate, gms.	Protein, gms.	Fat, gms.	Alcohol, gms.	Liquids, c.c.	Vol., c.c.	N, gms.	NH₃, gms.	Acetone and diacetic acid, gms.	β-oxybutyric acid, gms.	P₂O₅ gms.	Cl., gms.	Sugar, gms.	Weight, lbs.
Jan. 26	0	135	110	185	..	3500	3720	21.8	4.2	7.9	20	4.4	8.2	160	88¼
27	0	135	110	185	..	3500	3940	19.6	4.3	7.8	29	4.5	6.3	165	89¼
28	0	135	110	185	..	3500	3210	20.5	4.4	7.3	24	4.6	5.9	160	86¾
29	0	135	90	155	..	3500	3210	19.2	4.1	7.3	26	4.2	4.8	163	85¾
30	25	135	70	185	..	3500	3190	16.3	3.5	8.7	33	4.1	1.6	146	85
31	25	120	60	95	23	5370	4600	19.1	4.3	12.6	51	5.1	2.3	146	83¼
Feb. 1	37	130	100	130	45	5250	4050	18.7	3.3	10.7	39	4.3	2.0	137	82¼
2	52	70	60	95	45	5370	3510	16.0	3.5	10.2	37	3.9	2.1	121	81¾
3	..	15	15	30	45	800	360	15.0	..	..	..	..	..	86	

It will be seen that while upon the salt-free diet the weight steadily fell and, despite the administration of sodium bicarbonate later, no increase in weight occurred. This observation has been confirmed by Levison.[1] The explanation of the usual gain in weight of diabetic patients following the use of sodium bicarbonate was

[1] Levison: Jour. Am. Med. Assn., 1916, **64**, 326.

pointed out by Goodall and Joslin[1] some years ago. Apparently the administration of sodium bicarbonate, by favoring the excretion of large quantities of retained acid bodies, leads to irritation of the kidneys, resulting in their inability to excrete salt in the normal manner. If the salt in the diet is restricted, there is less to be retained and consequently no gain in weight results.

The explanation of the edema which is found in severe diabetics is by no means simple. Falta[2] has recently shown that if sodium bicarbonate is replaced by potassium bicarbonate the edema will disappear although the salt in the body and in the diet are low. Labbé[3] explains the edema by the retention of the sodium and not of the chlorine. Atchley, Loeb and Benedict[4] have removed the edema of a diabetic with the use of 20 to 35 grams of calcium chloride a day.

I might here make the clinical observation that a salt-free diet in diabetes is inadvisable. It is noteworthy that patients during the period of coma markedly lose weight. Edema, which may be present just prior to coma, disappears during coma; in fact, I remember to have seen but one patient in coma who showed edema.

The severe diabetic during coma utilizes apparently all possible liquid in the tissues to aid in the excretion of toxic bodies. The importance of maintaining sufficient fluid in the body deserves emphasis. Hodgson[5] has thoroughly appreciated it for years and endeavored to make his patients retain large quantities of fluid.

(*e*) **Weights and Losses of Weight in Diabetic Patients.**—During a series of observations upon a single diabetic individual the variations in weight were sometimes considerable. Not infrequenly these were due in large measure to the increase or decrease of water in the body, which was often demonstrated by the presence of edema. As a result conclusions based upon the metabolism of diabetics are especially liable to error. This is evident in the case of Freda, a little girl of sixteen years, Case No. 1012. She weighed 26.3 kilograms on September 22, 33.2 kilograms on October 2, on which date the salt was excluded from the diet, and on October 25 the weight had again fallen to 26.3 kilograms. The transitory gain in weight in early October was obviously due to edema and represented a gain in weight of 26 per cent. (!) If the actual body weights are employed for the period from October 9 to December 1, the variation in the metabolism from standard would range from +7 to +31 per cent, but if the weight of September 22 is accepted

[1] Goodall and Joslin: Jour. Am. Med. Assn., 1908, **51**, 727.
[2] Falta: Wiener Arch. f. inn. Med., 1922–23, **5**, 581.
[3] Labbé and Cumston: Diabetes Mellitus, New York, 1922, p. 115.
[4] Atchley, Loeb and Benedict: Jour. Am. Med. Assoc., 1923, **80**, 1643.
[5] Hodgson: Jour. Am. Med. Assn., 1911, **57**, 1187.

as the correct weight for the entire period, the metabolism oddly enough would vary in just the reverse manner: that is, from $+31$ to $+7$ per cent.

The percentage of loss in body weight of some 200 of my cases was computed for me by the Nutrition Laboratory. The average loss previous to the first visit was 16 per cent. and between this time and the last observation a further loss of 3 per cent occurred. This is good evidence that these cases came almost uniformly late for treatment.

(*f*) **The Loss of Weight Prior to and during Coma.**—The loss of weight of patients immediately prior to and during coma has always appeared to me to be great, but from the nature of the case it has been difficult to determine this point. A hint of this was afforded by noting the marked loss in weight which occurred in Case No. 135, from whose diet salt was excluded, but a still better example was that of Case No. 513, referred to on page 631, who lost 35 pounds in the eleven days preceding the third day before death in coma. Further observations of this character should be made.

(*g*) **The Caloric Value of a Kilogram of Body Weight and Hypothetical Estimations Connected Therewith.**—L., the Nutrition Laboratory subject, in the course of his thirty-one day fast, lost 13.2 kilograms, or an average of 0.7 per cent of his original body weight each day. Each kilogram lost represents a metabolism of 3258 calories if the estimated total metabolism of each day of L's. fast is used for the computation. If the first four days of the fast are excluded, when the loss was somewhat rapid, and the remaining twenty-seven days, when the loss was more gradual, are employed for the calculation, *each kilogram of body material lost would represent 3766 calories and the average loss of body weight each day would be 0.62 per cent.*

In computing the metabolism of a patient the factor of the error introduced by edema should be borne in mind. If the actual weight of Case No. 1012, is taken for October 9, 1917, it varies $+40$ per cent from standard as compared with $+7$ per cent if the computed weight is taken. Here, therefore, is a difference of 33 per cent in computing the variation from standard metabolism for one day according to whether the recorded weight of the patient is taken or the calculated true weight independent of edema.[1]

(*h*) **Relation of Loss in Body Weight to Metabolism in Diabetes.**—The loss in body weight of the diabetic patients from their maximum was considerable, but most of this loss occurred before these individuals came under observation. Information was sought which would disclose the result of similar marked losses in weight upon the metabolism of normal individuals.

---

[1] In the Carnegie Monograph Pub., No. 323, p. 65, the subject is discussed in more detail and more facts presented.

Inasmuch as data are lacking for a series of normal individuals with losses in weight as considerable as those found with the diabetics, the computed standard metabolism of a group of 20 male and 20 female diabetics at the time of their maximum weight was learned and compared with the metabolism actually observed after marked losses in weight. Similarly, the metabolism of 20 normals was compared with their metabolism computed for a loss like that of the diabetics of 35 per cent in weight.

From such computations the conclusion was reached that the 19 per cent decrease in metabolism of the Y. M. C. A. normals, who lost 10 per cent in weight in contrast to the 22 per cent decrease in metabolism of the diabetics who lost 35 per cent in weight, was probably to be explained by the normals losing weight more rapidly.

TABLE 97.—DECREASE IN BODY WEIGHT AND METABOLISM COMPARED.

Group.	Number of individuals.	Decrease in weight, per cent.	Decrease in metabolism, total, per cent.	Decrease in metabolism per kilogram, per cent.	Time.
Y. M. C. A. series . .	11	10	19	1.90	3 mos.
Diabetic	20	35	22	0.63	5 yrs.
Normals, comparable to diabetics at their maximum and minimum weights	20[1]	35	18	0.51	

(*i*) **Diabetic Variations from Standard in Metabolism and Weight Compared.**—It has generally been the custom in discussions of the weights of diabetics to record the weight of the individual below maximum. In our computations at the Nutrition Laboratory we have employed quite extensively loss of weight below the normal standard for age, height, and sex. It seems desirable to introduce this custom more generally, and I have noted its use by the Ann Arbor clinicians.

Prior to June, 1914, no relation is apparent between the variation of the metabolism from standard and the percentage variation of the body weight from standard, when the metabolism was more than 10 per cent above standard. But, when the metabolism was 10 to 5 per cent above standard, the average variation of the weights of the patients from normal was −2 per cent and when the metabolism was 35 to 40 per cent below standard, the average variation from standard weight was the most subnormal in the series, namely: −48 per cent. Between these extremes mentioned almost uniform gradations are registered.

[1] Minimum weights computed at 35 per cent reduction from maximum and metabolism predicted for these weights.

5. **Relation of Severity of Diabetes to Metabolism.**—The relation of the degree of severity of the diabetes to the postabsorptive metabolism is shown in Table 98. As heretofore the experiments are classified according to whether they took place prior to or subsequent to June, 1914. Before June, 1914, the mild cases showed a normal metabolism in the daily observations, the few moderate cases a metabolism of 14 per cent above normal, and the severe cases a slightly less variation, +12 per cent. After June, 1914, the metabolism in most of the daily observations with mild cases and with moderate cases as well was lower than standard, but the average in each group was still within the normal zone. The daily observations with severe cases averaged 13 per cent below standard. In general, prior to June, 1914, the severer types of diabetes gave a higher metabolism than the mild, while subsequent to that date, on the contrary, the severest type of the disease exhibited a lower metabolism than the mild and moderate forms.

TABLE 98.—RELATION OF SEVERITY OF DIABETES TO BASAL METABOLISM BEFORE AND AFTER 1914.

Percentage variations from standard metabolism.	Daily observations before June, 1914.			Daily observations after June, 1914.		
	Mild diabetes.	Moderate diabetes.	Severe diabetes.	Mild diabetes.	Moderate diabetes.	Severe diabetes.
Above standard:						
35–30 . . .	..	1	1	..	..	2
30–25 . . .	..	..	8	..	..	2
25–20 . . .	..	1	12			
20–15 . . .	..	7	15	..	1	1
15–10 . . .	..	5	18	..	3	6
10– 5 . . .	3	3	15	1	6	1
5– 0 . . .	1	3	14	5	13	12
Below standard:						
0– 5 . . .	1	..	7	7	13	25
5–10 . . .	1	..	2	5	9	19
10–15 . . .	..	..	1	3	20	22
15–20 . . .	..	..	..	1	6	33
20–25 . . .	..	..	..	..	1	34
25–30 . . .	..	..	..	..	..	18
30–35 . . .	..	..	..	..	..	6
35–40 . . .	..	..	..	..	..	4
Aver. percentage variation, all experiments .	+4 (6 days)	+14 (20 days)	+12 (93 days)	−4 (22 days)	−5 (72 days)	−12 (185 days)

That the increasing severity of diabetes in and of itself will at one time raise the metabolism and at another lower it is inconceivable, for, as was brought out in discussing the relationship between the pulse-rate and severity, the force of severity cannot act in opposite directions. It is, therefore, reasonable to conclude that one or more extraneous influences must have been present before and after June, 1914, to bring this about.

Of four extraneous factors which might influence metabolism— drugs, exercise, diet, and acidosis—little need be said regarding the first two. Drugs were never given to either group of patients with the exception of sodium bicarbonate, and this was discontinued after September, 1915. There is no evidence that sodium bicarbonate exerts the slightest influence upon the metabolism in health, and a critical study of the protocols of these diabetic patients bears out the same conclusion.

Exercise played no rôle, because the experiments were basal, and exercise was not a part of the routine. Furthermore, there were no essential differences in the amount of exercise at other times of the day before and after June, 1914.

The change in the character of the diet is of far more importance in determining the cause of the change in the metabolism of these patients after June, 1914. The severe cases underwent strenuous overfeeding before June, 1914, and strenuous underfeeding after June, 1914, and the quantitative changes in the diet appear nearly adequate to account for this phenomenon of changing metabolism.

6. **Relation of Acidosis to Metabolism of Diabetics.**—Of the intrinsic causes which might affect the metabolism of the diabetic, none would appear to be more potent than acidosis, for acidosis is a complication of diabetes rather than a symptom. It may occur in all types of the disease and can easily be made extreme in a mild case, just as it can with a healthy individual. During the years that these experiments were in progress, acidosis was undoubtedly responsible for two-thirds of all the deaths from diabetes in the community and possibly for three-fourths of these deaths. Of the fatal cases studied at the Nutrition Laboratory before June, 1914, 86 per cent of those who later died succumbed to coma, and of those studied from that date to the end of the research, December 5, 1917, 72 per cent of the deaths were due to coma.

What effect has acidosis upon the metabolism of a diabetic? Is it responsible to a considerable degree for the wide swing of the metabolic pendulum previously discussed?

The relation of the acidosis to the total metabolism is exhibited in Tables 99 and 100 in which the result of 398 observations upon 106 cases of diabetics are recorded. These indicate that with the development and increase of acidosis there is a steady rise in the metabolism.

15

TABLE 99.—ACIDOSIS AND METABOLISM WITH 106 DIABETICS ON FOUR HUNDRED DAYS.

Degree of acidosis.	Number of observation days.	Average variations of metabolism from standard, per cent.
+++	61	+10
++	144	− 5
+	82	− 5
0	111	− 9

TABLE 100.—ACIDOSIS AND BASAL METABOLISM OF DIABETICS BEFORE AND AFTER JUNE, 1914.

Percentage variations from standard metabolism.	Before June, 1914, variation with acidosis.				After June, 1914, variation with acidosis.			
	+++ per cent.	++ per cent.	+ per cent.	0 per cent.	+++ per cent.	++ per cent.	+ per cent.	0 per cent.
Above standard:								
35–30	+32	+31	..	..	+33	..	..	..
30–25	+29	+27	..	..	+28	..	..	..
25–20	+22	+22	+22	+23	..	..	..	..
20–15	+18	+18	+16	+17	..	+19	+16	..
15–10	+14	+13	+13	+13	..	+12	+12	+12
10– 5	+ 8	+ 9	+10	+ 9	..	+ 8	+ 8	+10
5– 0	+ 4	+ 3	+ 5	+ 5	+ 1	+ 3	+ 2	+ 3
Below standard:								
0– 5	− 2	− 2	− 1	− 3	− 5	− 2	− 3	− 3
5–10	..	− 7	..	− 9	− 6	− 8	− 8	− 8
10–15	..	−12	..	..	−13	−14	−12	−13
15–20	..	..	..	..	−18	−18	−18	−18
20–25	..	..	..	..	−23	−23	−23	−23
25–30	..	..	..	..	..	−28	−29	−28
30–35	..	..	..	..	..	−32	..	−33
35–40	..	..	..	..	..	−38	..	−39
Av. variation for all daily observations	+13	+13	+12	+10	+1	−12	−8	−13

Prior to June, 1914, acidosis was of frequent occurrence. Of the one hundred and nineteen experimental days included in Table 100 for this period there were but eighteen on which no acidosis was found, but after June, 1914, of the two hundred and seventy-nine experimental days on only thirteen experimental days was the acidosis severe.

In the earlier period there was a tendency for the metabolism of the diabetic with acidosis to be higher than that of the diabetic without severe acidosis, and the same relation holds after June, 1914. Since June, 1914, acidosis has had less opportunity to exert an influence upon the metabolism, (*a*) **Variations in the Same Individual of Acidosis and Metabolism.**— The relation between acidosis and metabolism would admit of more exact analysis if the metabolism of the same individual during different stages of acidosis could be determined. By this means the error introduced by the difficulty in classifying the acidosis would be lessened, because it is manifestly easier to decide upon the relative degree of acidosis for the same individual at two different periods than to compare the degree of acidosis in one patient with that of another.

Observations upon 12 patients before June, 1914, and upon 24 patients after June, 1914, are available whose metabolism was observed, in each instance, during at least two stages of acidosis. Prior to June, 1914, the average metabolism of those individuals without acidosis was 8 per cent above standard with slight and moderate acidosis, 14 per cent above standard, and with severe acidosis, 15 per cent above standard. After June, 1914, during the period of undernutrition, the group with no acidosis showed the lowest metabolism, 17 per cent below standard, and the group with the most severe acidosis the highest metabolism, 5 per cent below standard.

Confining our attention to severe cases of diabetes, the effect of acidosis upon the metabolism is still more clearly evident. With 22 cases in various stages of acidosis observations were made on ninety-three days prior to June, 1914. On only nine of these days was the metabolism below normal. On two days with cases without acidosis the average metabolism was 9 per cent above standard. On five days with slight acidosis the metabolism was 12 per cent above standard, on thirty-eight days with moderate acidosis likewise 12 per cent, and on forty-eight days with severe acidosis 13 per cent above standard.

After June, 1914, experiments were made on one hundred and eighty-five days with 41 cases of severe diabetes. The lowest average metabolism was found on forty-nine days with diabetics having no acidosis, namely: 19 per cent below standard. On thirty-seven days with mild acidosis present, the metabolism was 14 per cent below. The experiments on eighty-seven days with moderate acidosis indicated a metabolism 12 per cent below standard. On the twelve days with severe acidosis the metabolism was 2 per cent above standard. In conclusion, therefore, it can be said that an examination of the influence of acidosis upon the metabolism of diabetics of different degrees of severity supports the view that acidosis raises the metabolism of severe cases.

(*b*) **Acidosis and Metabolism of Individual Diabetics.**—Certain cases are worthy of special discussion because of the opportunity they present for a comparison of acidosis and metabolism. The experimental data of Case No. 983, show clearly such association in a fat diabetic. This patient stated that she had eaten little for a week preceding January 29. How true this is one cannot say, but the presence of acidosis, despite 6.3 per cent of sugar in the urine, leads one to infer that presumably the relations for the carbohydrate, protein, and fat in the diet at least may have been altered. The effect of the caloric content of the daily diet upon the acidosis and metabolism is brought out by the data in Table 101. From these records it is seen that the postabsorptive metabolism of this woman in the course of six days decreased from 28 per cent to 12 per cent above normal, the urinary nitrogen per twenty-four hours for the experimental days fell from 13 grams to 5.3 grams, and the sugar in the urine disappeared. The decrease in the excretion of nitrogen, sugar, and ammonia, and the fall in the metabolism were coincident with the marked reduction in the total diet, namely: a change from a diet so abundant as to allow 6.3 per cent of sugar on January 29, 1918, to a diet so low that it averaged but 76 calories a day for the six days preceding the last metabolism test. The decrease in the metabolism of protein, which amounted to but 46 grams (13 −5.3 =7.7 x 6) for a woman weighing 90 kilograms, appears insufficient to explain the change in metabolism.

Despite the fact that the patient was fat, that she was upon a very low diet, and was ultimately given a total fast, the acidosis decreased. This behavior is absolutely different from that of the fat women reported by Folin and Denis[1] when fasted for two four-day, and one five-day periods, whose acidosis continually advanced in each period from day to day, though the total acidosis decreased in successive periods. In the diabetic the acidosis decreased upon fasting, whereas with the normal individual it developed. The explanation is found by computing the actual values of carbohydrate, protein, and fat burned at the beginning and end of the period. This has been done in the usual way with the use of the non-protein quotient and by having added 20 per cent to the heat output per twenty-four hours as computed from the basal metabolism. On February 2–3 the carbohydrate in the diet was 50 grams, but the carbohydrate actually burned by the patient was 7 grams, whereas on February 8–9, the carbohydrate ingested was 5 grams, but the carbohydrate burned by the patient was 38 grams. Using Shaffer's formula (see p. 459) the theoretical quantity of carbohydrate sufficient to prevent acidosis upon the first day would have been 25 grams. As the patient only actually burned 7 grams, the deficiency of carbohydrate was 72 per cent corre-

[1] Folin and Denis: Jour. Biol. Chem., 1915, 21, 183.

TABLE 101.—THE METABOLISM OF A DIABETIC (CASE NO 983, FEMALE) WITH HIGH ACIDOSIS.

(Age, fifty-five years; average weight, 90.4 kg.; height, 160 cm.; diabetes, severe. All experiments postabsorptive.)

Date	Blood sugar, per cent.	Acidosis			Urinary nitrogen per 24 hours.		Urinary sugar per 24 hrs., gm.	Diet.			Respiratory quotient.	Heat output per 24 hours, (Basal).		Body materials, katabolized.			Carbohydrate. (Shaffer).	
		CO_2 in alveolar air, mm. Hg.	Diacetic acid.	NH_3, gm.	Total, gm.	Per kg., gm.		Carbohydrate, gm.	Protein, gm.	Fat, gm.		Total calories.	Variations from H. and B. standard, per cent.	Carbohydrate, gm.	Protein, gm.	Fat, gm.	Required to prevent acidosis, gm.	Deficiency in metabolism of Case 983, per cent.
1916.																		
Jan. 30-31	0.39		++				130[1]	80	35	10								
Jan. 31–Feb. 1		24	+++	4.3	13.0	0.145	86	55	25	10								
Feb. 1-2	0.30	23	+++	4.4	11.2	0.125	72	50	20	5								
Feb. 2-3		26	++++	4.3	11.7	0.130	56	50	10	0								
Feb. 3-4			+++++	4.6	7.7	0.085	42	40	10	0								
Feb. 4-5	0.25	28	+++++	3.3	5.8	0.065	10	0	0	0	0.73	1989	+28	7	67	216	25	72
Feb. 5-6			+++++	3.1			0	0	0	0								
Feb. 6-7			+++++					0	0	0	0.72	1858	+19	8	35	214	33	76
Feb. 7-8	0.20	29	+++	2.2	5.3	0.060	0	0	0	0								
Feb. 8-9	0.18	29	++	2.0	5.4	0.060	0	5	25	15	0.73	1757	+12	38	32	189	31	0

[1] Six and three-tenths per cent of sugar was determined in specimens of urine on January 29, preceding the night urine of January 29-30, 1916. Sugar in urine for twelve hours on night of January 29-30, 1916, was 126 grams.

sponding to the severe acidosis which she showed on that day. On the last day the theoretical quantity of carbohydrate sufficient to prevent acidosis would be 31 grams. On this day 38 grams were actually burned which would be as much as required. Corresponding to this improvement in the oxidation of carbohydrate, the acidosis decreased but was still present, and is explainable, as Shaffer has stated, on the ground that each ketogenic molecule does not meet its antiketogenic molecule in the body. This led him to advise giving twice the theoretically sufficient carbohydrate.

Case No. 1026, a fat man with a mild type of diabetes, was also treated upon a low diet quite similar to that given to the fat woman, Case No. 983. In contrast he at no time showed more than a slight to moderate acidosis. His metabolism changed from −8 to −15 per cent in seven days. This is again in contrast to Case No. 983, who, with marked acidosis, presented a metabolism of +28 per cent and six days later, with far less acidosis, a metabolism of +12 per cent. With the decrease in acidosis the metabolism fell twice as rapidly with Case No. 983, as with Case No. 1026, who had no acidosis. The difference in the metabolism of these two cases is not to be explained by the diet, for Case No. 983, during the first six days of treatment received 3.2 (0.3 net) calories per kilogram body weight per twenty-four hours.

With Case No. 1181, there was a gradual and consistent decrease in the metabolism as compared with the standard from −1 per cent to −24 per cent, as determined in postabsorptive experiments on nine days in the course of a period of sixteen days. The body weight and urinary nitrogen remained essentially constant during these sixteen days. The energy in the diet on successive days ranged from 40 to 575 calories with six fasting days in all. In this instance it is plain that the decrease in metabolism occurred during a period of continual undernutrition. The acidosis gradually decreased and eventually disappeared.

With Case No. 765, the metabolism decreased between January 22, and February 12 from −1 per cent to −25 per cent and coincidentally the acidosis which was originally high disappeared. The urinary nitrogen for the first three days varied between 0.175 and 0.150 gram per kilogram body weight and for the last two days between 0.130 and 0.135 gram per kilogram body weight. The fall in metabolism and the disappearance of acidosis are independent of marked changes in the urinary nitrogen.

Table 102 is a recomputation of an exhaustive study of the metabolism of a case of diabetes by Wilder, Boothby, and Beeler.[1] It shows that the metabolism is definitely related to the degree of

---

[1] Wilder, Boothby and Beeler: Jour. Biol. Chem., 1922, **51**, 312.

acidosis, for when the metabolism is highest, the acidosis is highest, and when the metabolism is lowest, the acidosis is least. In the following table three other factors are introduced which, singly or together, may be of importance in this supposed relation. These are the nitrogen excreted and the fat and total calories ingested. From Table 103 it will be seen that with each of these factors the metabolism varied as with the acidosis. Shall one ascribe the entire cause of the variation to the nitrogen or in part to the acidosis which the fat and excessive diet caused? From evidence already submitted, and to be submitted, the latter alternative appears as the more reasonable explanation. It is not for a moment denied that protein increased the metabolism of this individual, but that 40 grams of protein raised the metabolism of this patient to so great an extent as here shown appears improbable. In their own study of Bessie B., Wilder, Boothby, and Beeler believe they can demonstrate that the change in metabolism preceded the change in acidosis.

TABLE 102.—VARIATIONS IN BASAL METABOLISM AND ACIDOSIS (COMPUTED FROM WILDER, BOOTHBY AND BEELER.)

Variation from DuBois standard, per cent.	Metabolism.		Acidosis.		
	Blood.		Urine (preceding day).		
	Carbon dioxide, vol., per cent.	Acetone bodies (as acetone), gm.	NH_3, gm.	$\dfrac{NH_3 - N}{\text{Total N,}}$ per cent.	Acetone bodies (as acetone), gm.
− 1 to −10 . .	38	0.057	1.58	10	8.1
−11 to −20 . .	49	0.028	1.19	13	4.2
−21 to −30 . .	52	0.020	0.50	7	2.0

TABLE 103.—COMPARISON OF BASAL METABOLISM WITH FAT AND CALORIES IN THE DIET AND NITROGEN EXCRETED (COMPUTED FROM WILDER, BOOTHBY AND BEELER).

Variation of metabolism from DuBois standard, per cent.	Urinary nitrogen of preceding day, gm.	Fat in diet of preceding day, gm.	Total calories in diet of preceding day.
− 1 to −10	13.7	127	1587
−11 to −20	9.4	104	1225
−21 to −30	7.0	95	1074

7. Relation Between Metabolism and Percentage of Sugar in the Blood.—(a) The percentages obtained for the blood sugar secured before breakfast from diabetics of all types of severity when compared with the metabolism indicate no general relationship between the two. If the comparison is limited to severe cases,

a different picture is presented inasmuch as the metabolism rose as the blood sugar increased. The data are sufficiently numerous to warrant some significance being attached to this mutual change, though the extreme values are both based upon only two experiments. The lowest percentages of blood sugar (0.05—0.11) are associated with an unusually low metabolism of −21 per cent, of (0.12—0.20) per cent with −15 per cent, (0.21—0.30) per cent with −14 per cent (0.31—0.40) per cent with −11 per cent, and the highest (0.41—0.43) with an average metabolism of +5 per cent. This definite relation for the severe cases of diabetes between the increasing percentage of blood sugar and increasing metabolism has further interest in view of the reverse relationship found between the blood sugar and the respiratory quotient, which will be subsequently discussed. (See p. 273.) The low blood sugar in diabetes, like the low metabolism, may be an expression of inanition.

(b) **The Relation Between Blood Fat and Metabolism.**—The relation between the fat in the blood and the metabolism was noted in a few patients and indicated that the metabolism decreased as the percentage of blood fat increased. The patients with the lowest percentage of blood fat had an average metabolism of −5 per cent, but when the blood fat was highest, that is, over 2 per cent, the average metabolism was −25 per cent. It is possible that this association of low metabolism with high blood fat simply results from some common cause and is not in direct connection. Investigations along this line should be further pursued. In passing it may be stated that the patients whose blood-fat values average nearest the normal had a body weight 8 per cent below standard, and as the blood fat increased in quantity there was a steady loss in body tissue. These three factors, therefore, are in some relation: high blood fat, low metabolism, and loss in body weight.

(c) **Relation Between Non-protein Nitrogen in the Blood and Metabolism.**—The 17 instances in which the non-protein nitrogen was determined at the time the metabolism was estimated are so few as to merit but brief notice and are recorded simply to indicate the desirability of further study. In this limited series the metabolism varied inversely with the non-protein nitrogen, the average variation of the metabolism from standard for the group with low non-protein nitrogen being −6 per cent, for the group with normal non-protein nitrogen values −17 per cent, and for the group with the highest non-protein nitrogen values the average variation was −22 per cent. In this series the non-protein nitrogen rose as the body weights successively fell below the normal standard.

The respiratory quotient directly followed the course of the non-protein nitrogen. With the lowest values it averaged 0.77, with the normal values it averaged 0.81, and with the group with the highest non-protein nitrogen values it was 0.83. While not wishing to attach undue importance to this limited series of cases, the facts herewith brought out regarding the non-protein nitrogen and its various relations suggest that the high values obtained were due to an unusual activity in protein metabolism with retention not attributable to diseased kidneys. The evidence is consistent with one explanation of the high respiratory quotients observed with some of the patients and described later. (See p. 265.) According to this theory, such quotients might be due to the katabolism of the protein molecule, the oxidation of the carbohydrate portion, and the retention of the non-carbohydrate portion, the latter condition presumably being connected with the need of the body for new protein synthesis.

Finally, it must be mentioned that in cases of diabetes with acidosis shortly before death high non-protein nitrogen values are often encountered. Such values are in all probability simply an evidence of retention of non-protein nitrogen. Thus, Case No. 3079, Case No. 1924, and Case No. 2595 had non-protein nitrogens of 60 to 75 mgm. shortly before death.

(*d*) **Relation Between Urinary Sugar and Metabolism.**—Freedom of the urine from sugar was associated with lowering of the metabolism, both before and after June, 1914. Between the extremes of sugar-free urine and a content of over 100 grams of sugar the transitions from low to high metabolism are not uniform, but it can be stated that the metabolism of a patient voiding over 100 grams of sugar is usually increased.

8. **Nitrogen Excretion.**—How dependent the nitrogen excretion of diabetic patients is upon the diet is evident when one notes the quantity present in the urine of an untreated severe diabetic. Occasionally values of 25 to 30 grams nitrogen are obtained in contrast to half this quantity for the normal individual. Under modern treatment the nitrogen excretion of a diabetic patient falls to the neighborhood of 8 to 12 grams per day.

An abnormal nitrogenous excretion in diabetes has always seemed to me to be lacking, but one of my own cases disproves it. Case No. 513, p. 631, while ingesting 11 grams protein daily, excreted an average of 33.8 grams nitrogen daily for five days ending the second day prior to coma. This patient had multiple abscesses originating in a carbuncle. Another similar case is that of Geyelin and DuBois, already cited on p. 209, who excreted an average of 33.2 grams nitrogen daily between December 8–9 to December 17–18, inclusive, while the average of the protein intake during this period was 44 grams daily. He had an infection.

Münzer and Strasser report the nitrogen in the urine of a man, fasting, during the first day of coma to be 32 grams; the patient died the next day.

Case No. 1196 is remarkable because he differs from all the above in that he showed no acidosis, although he excreted a daily average of 25.5 grams nitrogen for eight days, losing much in weight and becoming so weak as to be barely able to raise his hand. The case later began to improve and is described in full under the discussion upon inanition. He had no infection. At the time it did not seem possible that broths could account for the high nitrogen.

Prior to June, 1914, the nitrogen excretion based upon 37 cases is known for four hundred and fifty-eight days, and subsequent to June, 1914, for 75 cases for one thousand and fifty days. The data, therefore, are so extensive that they give a clear picture of the diabetic nitrogenous metabolism, both before and after June, 1914. Approximately one-fourth of the nitrogen values obtained were for days upon which observations of the metabolism were made. The balance of the values were largely for the day immediately preceding the metabolism test. In a way these values serve as a better indication of the nitrogenous metabolism at the time of the metabolism test, because they represent the dietary conditions in the twenty-four hours immediately preceding the observations of the metabolism. The diabetic patients vary so much in weight that the nitrogenous excretion will be discussed as grams per kilogram body weight per twenty-four hours.

Prior to June, 1914, the diabetic patient excreted on the average 0.265 gram of urinary nitrogen per kilogram body weight. After June, 1914, the excretion averaged about one-third less or 0.185 gram per kilogram body weight. This latter quantity computed as protein would amount to a little over 1 gram of protein per kilogram body weight. This is generally considered as an ample allowance of protein for a normal individual, though it is possible to exist with even a third less.[1] Perhaps the fact that the nitrogen excretion was not further reduced after June, 1914, is due not so much to the character and the amount of the food ingested as to the undernourishment of the patients during this period which obliged them to draw upon body protein for energy. If more calories are supplied, either in carbohydrate or fat, the quantity of nitrogen metabolized and, in consequence, excreted may be decreased. The recent work of Marsh, Newburgh, and Holly[2] suggested that the general belief that, unless a considerable proportion (10 per cent) of the total calories is supplied in the form of carbohydrates the protein metabolism is not greatly decreased,

[1] Sherman: Jour. Biol. Chem., 1920, 41, 97.
[2] Marsh, Newburgh and Holly: Arch. Int. Med., 1922, 29, 97.

was incorrect. These writers based their conclusion on observations upon their patients, which appeared to show that nitrogen balance can be maintained when the carbohydrate is but 3.8 per cent of the total caloric intake the remainder of the diet being made up of 0.68 gram of protein per kilogram body weight and of fat sufficient to bring the total energy of the diet up to 33 calories per kilogram body weight. Recent work of DuBois and Richardson, however, makes it clear that it is inaccurate to compute the carbohydrate burned from that ingested and it is probable the Newburgh and Marsh patients oxidized more carbohydrate than supposed. It is surely very important for diabetic patients to be kept in nitrogen equilibrium save for temporary periods, particularly if by analogy protein loss is regained with as great difficulty as loss in weight.

CALORIES OF CARBOHYDRATE, PROTEIN AND FAT IN DIET AND METABOLISM COMPARED. (DUBOIS AND RICHARDSON.)

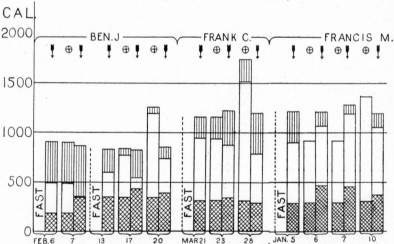

FIG. 8.—The columns indicate calories per twenty-four hours, the lowest portion indicates protein, the middle, fat, the upper, carbohydrate. The circles ⊕ indicate calories in diet, the arrows, ↓ calories metabolized. The diet was given, divided into two-hour intervals, and the calorimeter observations were made after the last meal.

In the chart comparison may be made between calories metabolized on different days under different conditions of diet, or between the calories of the diet and those metabolized on any given date. Ben. J. was a boy with severe emaciation and a high respiratory quotient.

The influence of the character of the food given and the food metabolized is shown by a chart placed at my disposal by Dr. DuBois and Dr. Richardson. When the same quantity of food was given on February 7, to Ben. J., as he had metabolized fasting February 6, (1) his metabolism decreased, (2) the protein burned doubled and (3) the quantity of carbohydrate rose, while (4) the metabolism of fat was almost eliminated. On February 20, when the fat in the diet was greatly increased, the metabolic record shows that not even one-half of it was burned and the total metabolism remained unaffected. These results were duplicated with Frank C. With Francis M., although carbohydrate was withheld from the diet, an appreciable quantity of carbohydrate was burned. Therefore, the food given is by no means an indication of the food burned on the same day.

(a) **Errors in the Interpretation of the Urinary Nitrogen Excretion.** —Strange figures are often encountered for the urinary nitrogen with diabetic patients. It is desirable to call attention to such instances because the nitrogen excretion is more and more employed in planning the treatment of a patient.[1] Thus, Case No. 1673, once a patient at the New England Deaconess Hospital and later cared for elsewhere, according to Dr. A. A. Hornor, presented the anomaly of a minus nitrogen balance amounting to 8.7 grams daily for a period of six days. When, however, the nitrogen was quantitated in the broths and bouillon cubes which the boy surreptitiously received, the explanation was found, because this amounted to 8 grams and thus offset the nitrogen loss. This same boy also voided between 19 and 24 grams of sodium chloride daily, and the source of this large excretion was likewise found in the broths and bouillon cubes.

(b) **Individual Variations in Excretion of Urinary Nitrogen.** — Individual variations in the nitrogen excretion were considerable, both before and after June, 1914. Prior to June, 1914, the lowest excretion of urinary nitrogen per kilogram body weight per twenty-four hours was 0.08 gram (Case No. 707) and the highest excretion was 0.835 gram (Case No. 550), representing a total excretion for the twenty-four hours of 4.1 grams and 48.1 grams, respectively, when calculated according to the patients' weights, or 4.8 grams and 50.1 grams when calculated for an individual with a body weight of 60 kilograms.

The nitrogen excretion for Case No. 550 was not only the highest value obtained before June, 1914, but was the highest value noted for the entire series of patients. This patient was an Italian, the only one of the 113 cases not finally traced, who just before commencement of treatment voided in twenty-four hours 7000 cc of urine containing 48.3 grams of nitrogen. This illustrates the large quantity of protein food which an untreated diabetic consumes.

---

[1] Shaffer: Jour. Biol. Chem., 1922, **50**, 26.

After June, 1914, the lowest excretion of nitrogen per kilogram body weight was that of Case No. 1207, amounting to 0.05 gram, and the highest was 0.515 gram for Case No. 1011. It is of particular interest that the latter case showed upon another occasion a nitrogen excretion of 0.055 gram per kilogram body weight.

(*c*) **Low Nitrogen Excretion.**—The very low excretion of urinary nitrogen of the boy, Case No. 707, mentioned above; namely, 0.08 gram per kilogram body weight, took place in May, 1914. At that time he was receiving a diet containing a large number of calories which were chiefly in the form of fat. Various tests were being made with vegetable days and oatmeal days, and on May 16–17, he was given a diet consisting of 3 eggs and 180 cc of olive oil. The case is mentioned to illustrate that with a large caloric intake, even though the amount of carbohydrate is extremely small or temporarily absent from the diet, the nitrogen excretion can be depressed to a very low degree, in this instance to 4.1 grams in the twenty-four hours or 0.08 gram per kilogram body weight. This value, however, is by no means as low as those obtained by Newburgh and Marsh[1] and Petrén.[2] Frequently in their cases with high fat diets for long periods, the daily quantity of urinary nitrogen excreted was under 3 grams.

The low values for urinary nitrogen after June, 1914, were due to other causes. (1) They were associated with obese patients who had been placed upon a very low diet or even fasted, and (2) they were obtained with diabetic patients in a stage of extreme inanition, often combined with a diet actually low in calories or whose net caloric value was low for the patient in question because unassimilated. Thus Case No. 1026, whose weight was 98 kilograms or 59 per cent above normal, voided 0.055 gram nitrogen per kilogram body weight upon April 24–25, 1916, having taken but 6 calories per kilogram body weight per twenty-four hours for the preceding sixteen days. Case No. 983, was another obese woman, weighing 91 kilograms or 44 per cent above normal. Following an average caloric intake per day of 1 calorie per kilogram body weight for five days, she excreted upon a fasting day 0.06 gram nitrogen per kilogram body weight. Case No. 1207, a woman with a body weight of 88 kilograms, or 43 per cent above normal, excreted upon a fasting day 0.05 gram nitrogen per kilogram body weight. These three individuals, excreting a low quantity of nitrogen, may be placed in comparison with Case No. 707, just cited, who also had a low nitrogen excretion. The three fat women protected their body protein by their endogenous fat, while the

---

[1] Newburgh and Marsh: Arch. Int. Med. 1920, **26**, 647.

[2] Petrén: See foot note therein. A review of a paper by Petrén is given by Allen: Jour. Metabolic Research 1922, **1**, 421.

latter (the thin boy) protected his body protein by the excessive quantity of fat which he ingested.

Examples of a low urinary excretion of nitrogen due to inanition may also be cited. Case No. 1011, on March 26–27, 1916, excreted 0.055 grams of nitrogen per kilogram body weight. At that time her weight was 30 per cent below normal. *In the preceding ten days she had received a total of 750 calories, or approximately 2 calories daily per kilogram body weight.* This in itself would appear to be a sufficient example of the extremes to which treatment by undernutrition was carried in the early days of its use, were not other still more striking evidences at hand based upon analyses of the urinary nitrogen of this patient and of that of Case No. 1085, already described and mentioned later. (See p. 175 and p. 239.)

(*d*) **High Nitrogen Excretion.**—A high excretion of urinary nitrogen may simply reflect the diet as has already been noted in the instance of Case No. 550, or may reflect exactly the opposite condition, namely: the extreme state of inanition reached just before death in which a so-called prelethal rise of nitrogen takes place. This prelethal rise was found with Case No. 1011, the patient just described as having shown an extremely low value for urinary nitrogen in the spring of 1916. She returned for treatment in the fall of 1917. Her diet was low at this time also and her weight had fallen to 26.4 kilograms or 52 per cent below normal in contrast to 38.8 kilograms or 30 per cent below normal in March, 1916. The diet varied from day to day, but for the days immediately in the neighborhood of the date on which the high nitrogen excretion of 0.515 gram per kilogram body weight was observed, it consisted of carbohydrate 10 grams, protein 40 grams, fat 27 grams, and alcohol 23 grams. The high nitrogen excretion on this day was not exceptional for this patient. Thus, upon eleven days in the two weeks before the day cited the average nitrogen excretion was 0.305 gram per kilogram body weight. Her basal metabolism varied between 878 and 686 calories and the calories in her diet varied bweteen 1213 and 210.

Criticism may rightly be raised that Case No. 1011 did not exhibit a true prelethal nitrogen, as she did not die until October of the following year, 1918. This is readily explained. The patients who died of inanition, and they were fortunately few in number, by no means proceeded to death in a mathematical fashion, but irregularly. High feeding was interspersed with low feeding. This patient was undoubtedly near her end when this high value was obtained, but she left the hospital, broke her diet, ate liberally, and it would appear thereby prolonged her life for upward of one year, though eventually she succumbed to diabetic coma as a result of excessive food. For the severe diabetic in 1918, it was Scylla or Charybdis, but it is not so today.

Case No. 1085, represents still more clearly a prelethal high nitrogen. This patient on October 18–19, 1916, excreted 0.51 gram of nitrogen per kilogram body weight. A few days later, on November 10, the blood sugar had fallen to less than 0.1 per cent. This was the first case of inanition with low blood sugar which had come to the writer's attention, and the need of carbohydrate feeding was not recognized. The patient, realizing her desperate condition, desired to go home, and left the hospital. Five days later she succumbed to inanition. Attention is directed to the sudden fall in weight of this patient from 34.2 kilograms to 30.4 kilograms in the course of eight days during the period when the high nitrogen value was obtained. This loss in weight was apparently only in part due to the removal of edema and was accompanied by an extreme loss of strength. The relationship between high excretion of urinary nitrogen, reduction in weight, extremely low metabolism, and high respiratory quotient will be considered in detail later. (See p. 240 and p. 265.)

The relative excess of nitrogen in the urine prior to June, 1914, goes a long way toward explaining the increased metabolism found for the patients in that period and is probably the best confirmatory evidence at hand that these patients were overfed. It is not meant to imply that the increased metabolism was due alone to the excessive amount of protein consumed, but rather that the excessive nitrogen was an index of an excessive protein and, by inference, excessive caloric intake. Following June, 1914, undernutrition was the practice, and these nitrogen values are very likely high in comparison with the intake, because the body tissues of the subjects were more frequently called upon to supply calories, and these were often obtained at the expense of body protein as well as of body fat. The fact that metabolism is lowered on an undernutrition diet served to keep these patients as well as they were.

If one examines the values from the point of view of the severity of the disease, it will be found that the mild cases invariably showed a lower nitrogen excretion than the severe cases. The conclusion may be drawn from the values for both periods that the excretion of nitrogen increased with the severity of the disease. It is not yet proved, however, that the severity of the diabetes was due to the high nitrogen excretion in that it represented a high protein intake, but the evidence is strong that the severe cases, both before and after June, 1914, were undergoing an unusually active protein katabolism. Before June, 1914, a high protein intake must be admitted, but after June, 1914, the protein given was not above the normal quantity taken in health and usually it was far less, and yet the cases of greatest severity in this period showed the very high nitrogen excretion to be explained only by the katabolism of body protein. Manifestly it would be of the greatest importance if it could be proved that patients would be safer if they were fed either 10, 20, or even 30 per cent less than the customary 1 or 1.5 grams of protein per kilogram daily or 10, 20 or 30 per cent more than this amount. This is not readily demonstrated, because such special diets should be continued for years; in fact, essentially during the remainder of the life of the patient.

A relation between the nitrogen excretion and acidosis was not found. After June, 1914, the highest nitrogen excretion was found usually when the acidosis was absent and the loss of weight was greatest.

(e) **Relation of Excretion of Urinary Nitrogen to Basal Metabolism.** —The relation of the urinary nitrogen to the basal metabolism of the diabetics under observation, both before and after June, 1914, is shown in Table 104. The average nitrogen excretion of 21 diabetics prior to June, 1914, was 0.24 gram per kilogram body weight per twenty-four hours and for 69 diabetics after June, 1914, 0.15 gram per kilogram body weight per twenty-four hours. Oddly enough this latter figure corresponds rather closely with the average excretion of the subject L., during his thirty-one days of fast at the Nutrition Laboratory, which was 0.17 gram per kilogram body weight per twenty-four hours, and with that of a healthy young woman, later described, undergoing the routine treatment of a severe case of diabetes during twenty days, which was 0.14 gram per kilogram body weight per twenty-four hours.

Prior to June, 1914, the nitrogen excretion followed the course of the metabolism, both above and below standard. Thus, when the metabolism was 35 to 30 per cent above the basal standard, the nitrogen excretion was 0.38 gram per kilogram body weight, and when the metabolism was 5 to 10 per cent below standard the nitrogen excretion was 0.095 gram per kilogram body weight. After June, 1914, a radical change is noted in the relation of the basal metabolism and the urinary nitrogen. When the metabolism was within 10 per cent of the normal standard, the nitrogen excretion was constant, but when the metabolism was decreased to 10 to 15 per cent below standard the nitrogen excretion was 0.13 gram per kilogram body weight and thereafter progressively rose as the metabolism decreased until the highest value for the nitrogen excretion, namely, 0.215 gram, was reached with a subnormal metabolism of 35 to 40 per cent.

Prior to June, 1914, the excretion of urinary nitrogen decreases with the metabolism, but after June, 1914, when the metabolism is 10 to 15 per cent below standard, the nitrogen excretion rises as the metabolism decreases further. *A rising nitrogen excretion at one time associated with increasing metabolism and at another with decreasing metabolism certainly suggests that the nitrogen metabolism in and of itself does not control the metabolism of the diabetic.*

TABLE 104.—RELATION OF URINARYNITROGEN TO BASAL METABOLISM OF DIABETICS BEFORE AND AFTER JUNE, 1914.

Percentage variation in metabolism from standard,	No. of observation days.	Before June, 1914.			No. of observation days.	After June, 1914.		
		Nitrogen excretion per kg. of body weight per 24 hours, gm.	Variation in the body weight from normal standard, per cent.	Average respiratory quotient.		Nitrogen excretion per kg. of body weight per 24 hours, gm.	Variation in the body weight from normal standard, per cent.	Average respiratory quotient.
Above standard:								
35–30 . . .	1	0.380	− 5	0.73	1	0.380	−23	0.72
30–25 . . .	3	0.290	−27	0.71	1	0.125	+43	0.73
25–20 . . .	10	0.255	−26	0.73				
20–15 . . .	12	0.250	−18	0.72	2	0.105	+18	0.75
15–10 . . .	11	0.245	−20	0.73	8	0.150	− 9	0.74
10– 5 . . .	13	0.240	−16	0.74	4	0.165	− 2	0.76
5– 0 . . .	12	0.245	−20	0.74	23	0.145	−11	0.77
Below standard:								
0– 5 . . .	4	0.135	−19	0.76	38	0.145	−14	0.75
5–10 . . .	2	0.095	−16	..	27	0.140	−17	0.77
10–15 . . .	..	..	..	..	38	0.130	−14	0.78
15–20 . . .	..	..	..	..	31	0.145	−23	0.77
20–25 . . .	..	..	..	..	29	0.145	−23	0.79
25–30 . . .	..	..	..	..	18	0.185	−31	0.80
30–35 . . .	..	..	..	..	6	0.205	−39	0.82
35–40 . . .	..	..	..	..	2	0.215	−48	0.88
Average . . .	68[1]	0.240	−20	0.73	228[2]	0.150	−18	0.77

Prior to June, 1914, the high nitrogen excretion would seem to indicate the large quantity of protein food which the patients consumed, this being an index also of the total quantity of food in the diet. After June, 1914, the occurrence of the highest excretion of nitrogen was associated with rare exception with those patients having the lowest metabolism and must be explained in an entirely different manner. All these patients were free from acidosis, yet their diabetes was of the severest type. The more severe the diabetes, the less the food administered. Accordingly, the tissues

[1] The metabolism was above standard on fifty-two days, below standard on six days.
[2] The metabolism was above standard on thirty-nine days, below standard on one hundred and eighty-nine days.

16

of these diabetics must have been taxed severely to provide not only calories but protein. Furthermore, as has been pointed out already, the body fat of these patients was largely exhausted, and so to supply calories it was all the more necessary for body protein to be drawn upon.

Evidence of the extreme degree of inanition which these patients with subnormal metabolism had reached is also supplied by Table 104, for the data show that in the period of undernutrition after June, 1914, the body weight was likewise subnormal and followed the course of the decreasing metabolism. Thus, when the average metabolism of 31 patients was 15 to 20 per cent below standard, the average weight was 23 per cent below normal, and when the lowest metabolism was reached, namely, 35 to 40 per cent below standard, the weight was −48 per cent. The high nitrogen excretion of these extremely emaciated diabetics with the lowest metabolism clearly indicates a prelethal rise of urinary nitrogen.

TABLE 105.—UNUSUALLY LOW EXCRETION OF URINARY NITROGEN UPON A HIGH-FAT, LOW-PROTEIN AND LOW-CARBOHYDRATE DIET.

(Case No. 707, male, aged seventeen years; height, 176 cm.).

| | | Urine per 24 hours. | | | | | | Diet. | | | | |
| | | | | | Nitrogen. | | | | | | | Variation of basal metabolism from normal standard, per cent. |
Date.	Body weight naked, kg.	Volume, cc.	Diacetic acid.	NH₃, gm.	Total.	Per kg. of body weight, gm.	Sugar, gm.	Carbohydrate, gm.	Protein, gm.	Fat, gm.	Calories.	
1914												
May 15–16	51.8	900	+ +	..	5.9	0.115	18	50	30	185	1985	
16–17	51.7	570	+++	..	4.1	0.080	5	0	20	200	1880	− 8
17–18	51.7	570	+++	2.7	4.8	0.095	Trace	15	20	115	1175	− 4
18–19	51.7	900	+++	3.1	7.5	0.145	7	35	45	145	1625	0
19–20	52.2	900	+++	3.8	7.8	0.150	7	0	0	0	0	+ 1
20–21	51.6	720	+ +	2.2	6.7	0.130	29	115	40	105	1565	− 3
21–22	52.5	540	..	3.1	5.5	0.105	..	35	20	100	1120	− 6
22–23	52.8	..	..	..	..	..	..	..	..	..	..	−12

The independence of the nitrogen excretion and the metabolism is well shown by 2 cases of extreme inanition, Cases Nos. 1011 and 1085. With Case No. 1011 the nitrogen excretion was almost the lowest in the series, i. e., 0.08 gram per kilogram body weight, with the metabolism 19 per cent below standard, while at another time it was 0.445 gram per kilogram body weight, or nearly at the highest mark, with the metabolism 18 per cent below standard. With Case No. 1085, the nitrogen excretion was 0.51 grams per kilogram body weight, with the metabolism 35 per cent below standard, and later it was 0.19 grams per kilogram body weight, with the metabolism 40 per cent below standard. Furthermore, when the nitrogen excretion was extremely low as a result of the oxidation of large quantities of fat, either exogenous (see Case No. 707 in Table 105) or endogenous, (see Cases Nos. 983, 1026, and 1207) the metabolism with different individuals varied to a great degree and to a considerable degree with the same individual. Case No. 591, see p. 302, furnishes evidence upon the relative importance of protein and acidosis in raising the metabolism.

The relation of urinary nitrogen, as an index of protein katabolism to the metabolism, has been extensively discussed by Bernstein and Falta.[1] They, as well as Wilder, Boothby, and Beeler,[2] believe the protein katabolism an all controlling factor in regulating the metabolism of the diabetic. The data of the latter admit of various interpretations, and to the writer the evidence does not seem to warrant this assumption.

(*f*) **Dextrose-nitrogen Ratio.**—The relation between the excretion of dextrose and that of nitrogen—the dextrose-nitrogen ratio—is considered of great importance by Lusk.[3] [4] [5] He has reached the conclusion, based upon many observations with dogs following injections of phlorhizin and by one case of diabetes coming under his personal observation, and others selected from the literature, that in the severest diabetic the dextrose-nitrogen ratio is 3.65 : 1. By this he means that when the patient is on an exclusively fat-protein diet 3.65 grams of dextrose appear in the urine for 1 gram of nitrogen, or the 6.25 grams of protein which it represents. In other words, 60 per cent—actually 3.65 divided by 6.25 equals 58.4—of the protein burned by the body appears in the urine in the form of sugar. Lusk considers that this is the greatest possible amount of sugar which can appear in the urine on a carbohydrate-free diet, and he assumes that it comes wholly from protein. He has collected in a table notable illustrations of such ratios. A dextrose-nitrogen ratio in the neighborhood of 3.65 : 1 Lusk showed to be of very serious prognostic import.

TABLE 106.—D : N RATIOS. (AFTER LUSK.)

Phlorhizin.			Diabetes mellitus in man.			
In dog.	In man.					
		Mandel and				
Lusk.	Benedict, S. R.	Lusk.	Grünwald.	Foster.	Mosenthal.	Joslin.
3.65	3.58	3.60	3.75	3.58	3.75	3.69
3.66	3.82	3.65	3.56	3.38	3.85	3.67
3.62	3.66	3.66	3.70	..	3.44	3.67
3.64	3.68	3.64	3.64	3.48	3.66	3.68

[1] Bernstein and Falta: Deutsch. Arch. f. klin. Med., 1916, **121**, 95.
[2] Wilder, Boothby, and Beeler: Loc. cit., p. 230.
[3] Mandel and Lusk: Deutsch. Arch. f. klin. Med., 1904, **81**, 479.
[4] Lusk: Arch. Int. Med., 1909, **3**, 1; also Harvey Lectures, J. B. Lippincott Company, Philadelphia, 1908–1909, Metabolism and Diabetes.
[5] For a full discussion of the subject see Lusk, The Science of Nutrition, Philadelphia, 1917, 3d Edition.

To this table it is not easy to add other examples. For the last few years it has been the custom in the presence of acid intoxication to omit all fat from the diet and to treat the patient without alkalis. Under these circumstances high dextrose-nitrogen ratios quickly vanish.

Unfortunately one cannot be sure that in the disintegration of the protein molecule the nitrogen and carbohydrate leave the body hand in hand. As a rule, the nitrogen loiters behind, greatly to our annoyance in estimating the source of the sugar in the urine. Mendel and Lewis[1] were able to show that this delay was increased if either indigestible substances or cotton-seed oil formed a prominent part of the diet—just the sort of foods which our diabetic patients eat. Even the amount of water taken can markedly influence the rate of digestion. Consequently in attempting to determine the quantity of carbohydrate derived from protein, this irregularity in the excretion of nitrogen must be considered. Tileston and Comfort[2] found the non-protein nitrogen normal in uncomplicated cases of diabetes, but there was retention in 2 cases examined during coma. In the series of non-protein nitrogen determinations made upon my cases it was evident that these were by no means always normal and might even be considered high if the preceding diet was taken into account. In Case Nos. 2595 and 1305, both proved to have good renal function before the onset of acidosis. The non-protein nitrogen of the blood rose to 61 and 48 milligrams per 100 cc during coma. There is good ground, therefore, for the supposition that retention of nitrogen might easily complicate a dextrose-nitrogen ratio. When one adds to this difficulty that of determining what share the quantity of residual carbohydrate in the body bears to the total sugar excreted the complexity of the problem increases. Case No. 1213, with apparently no tolerance for carbohydrate, excreted only 10 per cent of the 60 grams levulose given, and her weight was but 31 kilograms.

In Table 107, are collected a series of dextrose-nitrogen ratios in excess of that of 3.65 : 1. Hitherto a patient who showed dextrose-nitrogen ratio above 3.65 : 1 has frequently stood convicted of larceny if not of perjury. The reputation of these workers will allow no such interpretation. No one believes today that the human D : N ratio exceeds 3.65 : 1. Higher ratios are illustrations of irregularities in excretion of the two substances. That 4 cases should have recovered with such ratios is confirmatory of this conclusion.

[1] Mendel and Lewis: Jour. Biol. Chem., 1913–1914, **6**, 19, 37.
[2] Tileston and Comfort: Arch. Int. Med., 1914, **14**, 620.

TABLE 107.—DEXTROSE-NITROGEN RATIOS IN EXCESS OF 3.65 TO 1.

Author.	D : N ratios upon successive days.							Immediate outcome.
Murlin and Craver[1] .	4.20	4.00	4.00	3.50	3.10	..	..	Recovery.
Geyelin and DuBois[2] .	1.73	3.97	4.01	3.87	2.76	..	..	Recovery.
Christie[3]	3.18	2.40	3.93	2.51	3.27	..	..	Recovery.
Allen and DuBois[4] .	2.28	3.93	3.14	3.10	3.44	..	3.82	Recovery.

Light upon the D : N ratio has been offered by Janney,[5] who has worked out an exact method for the determination of the formation of glucose in the animal body. By feeding various forms of animal protein to fasting phlorhizinized dogs, he demonstrated that 58 per cent of these proteins went over into glucose. By these direct experiments and other proofs which cannot be entered into here, he concludes that the actual D : N ratio is 3.4 : 1.

If one would determine the dextrose-nitrogen ratio accurately in patients, the following requisites should be fulfilled: (1) An exclusive fat-protein diet or fasting; (2) surroundings which make errors in diet impossible; (3) a period of observation of at least seven days to exclude the washing out of stored carbohydrate; (4) a constant (not falling) D : N ratio of 3.65 : 1 for the last three of the seven days.

9. **Heat-production per Kilogram of Body Weight as Index of Caloric Needs of Diabetics.**—Since for years it has been customary to express the metabolism of an individual in calories per kilogram body weight, and most physicians still treat their diabetic patients on this basis, the data for the metabolism per kilogram body weight of this series of diabetic patients when they were at rest have been grouped in this manner. With 18 patients the basal metabolism ranged between 15 to 20 calories per twenty-four hours, and the average heat-production was 19 calories. The largest group of subjects, namely, 61—gave a range of basal metabolism of 21 to 25 calories and averaged 23 calories per kilogram body weight. A third group nearly as large comprised 45 patients whose basal metabolism ranged between 26 and 30 calories with an average of 28 calories. Another group of 25 patients showed a range in basal metabolism of 31 to 35 calories and averaged 32 calories per kilogram body weight. The metabolism of 5 cases ranged from 36 to 40 calories with an average of 38 calories per kilogram body

[1] Murlin and Craver: Jour. Biol. Chem., 1916, **28**, 301.
[2] Geyelin and DuBois: Jour. Am. Med. Assn., 1916, **66**, 1532.
[3] Christie: Jour. Am. Med. Assn., 1917, **68**, 170.
[4] Allen and DuBois: Arch. Int. Med., 1916, Part II, **17**, 1010.
[5] Janney: Am. Jour. Med. Sci., 1917, **153**, 44.

weight. Case No. 295, showed a basal metabolism of 41 calories per kilogram body weight. This was the highest metabolism per kilogram body weight recorded in this series and corresponded to 22 per cent above standard by the Harris and Benedict method. The lowest value on this basis was obtained with Case No. 1207, and it amounted to 15 calories per kilogram body weight, or for this patient 15 per cent below standard. The highest basal metabolism, as compared with the Harris and Benedict standard, was with Case No. 1412, who showed 33 per cent above normal on two days, and the lowest was with Case No. 1085, who showed 40 per cent below standard on two days.

These data are of clinical importance inasmuch as with this large group of diabetics examined in periods of treatment of both over- and undernutrition but one-sixth of the observations indicated a need for more than 30 calories per kilogram body weight to maintain the basal metabolism. It is equally of clinical importance to observe that in only 1 out of every 12 observations was there a basal metabolism of 20 calories or less per kilogram body weight. By the method of beginning the treatment of diabetic cases with undernutrition, the energy intake per kilogram body weight for days and weeks was often below 20 calories. Such procedures are temporarily justifiable if a gain in tolerance for carbohydrate or for a larger amount of food is achieved, but it is almost as bad practice for a physician to keep his patient sugar-free by requiring him to live permanently upon a diet below the caloric needs as it is, through carelessness, to allow the presence of glycosuria and thus bring the net caloric intake below the necessary minimum. The treatment of the diabetic should be planned for a period of years rather than of months.

In this connection it should be remembered that the normal individuals studied by the Nutrition Laboratory who were subjected to a loss in body weight of approximately 10 per cent presented a reduction in metabolism per kilogram of 15 to 20 per cent.[1] Subsequent to this loss of weight the diet necessary for maintenance represented a reduction of nearly 40 per cent from that in the pre-experimental period. The evidence afforded by the studies upon diabetic patients, however, does not show that they could subsist upon a correspondingly lowered ration despite a loss in weight even greater than that of the normal subjects referred to. Indeed, if comparison is justifiable between these two groups, it is plain that although the metabolism of the diabetic was, as a rule, subnormal, it was actually increased relatively in comparison to that of other undernourished individuals, a conclusion also reached

[1] Benedict, Miles, Roth and Smith: Carnegie Inst., Washington, Pub. No. 280, 1919, p. 525.

by Lusk in his discussion of the metabolism of Cyril K.[1] It is safe to say that diabetic patients who receive less than 20 calories per kilogram body weight are almost certainly drawing upon their own tissues for energy even if they keep perfectly still in bed, and furthermore, that this is likely to be the case even if they receive as much as 26 calories per kilogram body weight. If any activity at all is attempted, about 20 per cent more calories are necessary. Such activity would be represented by hospital life, including sitting up, reading, and an occasional slow walk.

10. **Fasting and Undernutrition in Health.**—Undernutrition plays such an important part in the treatment of diabetes that its significance, both with a healthy individual and with a diabetic patient, should be kept clearly and constantly in view. As a basis for a true understanding of the effects of undernutrition upon diabetic patients, it is, therefore, desirable to study first the results of observations with individuals during prolonged fasting or undernutrition when living under conditions similar to those of the diabetic patients.

(*a*) **Metabolism of a Healthy Individual During a Prolonged Fast.** —No data are better fitted for studying the metabolism during a long fast than those obtained with the subject L., with whom observations were made at the Nutrition Laboratory during a fast of thirty-one days in the year, 1912. These are recorded in Table 132, p. 306.

It is a curious coincidence that the range in metabolism of this individual from 5 per cent above to 14 per cent below standard as determined before the beginning of his fast and again at the end of the fasting period closely approximates that of the diabetic patients +13 per cent before June, 1914, when they were in a state of overnutrition and −7 per cent after June, 1914, when they were in a state of undernutrition.

In the averages above cited a comparison is drawn between the metabolism of a healthy man at the conclusion of a prolonged fast and that of diabetic patients and also the comparison of the metabolism of a healthy man before and at the end of his fast compared with the standard for normal individuals in normal nutrition at both periods. This, however, tells but part of the story. The actual metabolism of L. at the end of his fasting period should be compared with his metabolism immediately preceding the beginning of the period. If this is done, it will be observed that his basal metabolism decreased during the thirty-one days of fasting from 1526 to 1118 calories per twenty-four hours or 27 per cent. The loss in weight of L. during his period

---

[1] Lusk: The Science of Nutrition, Philadelphia, 1917, 3d edition, p. 477.

of fast was 13.2 kilograms, his original weight being 60.6 kilograms and his final weight 47.4 kilograms. Comparing this loss in body weight of 22 per cent with the decrease in metabolism of 27 per cent, it is evident that L's. decrease in metabolism proceeded more rapidly than his loss in weight. If one should select two individuals from the prediction tables corresponding to the weights of L. at the beginning and end of the fast, the metabolism of the lighter would be 12 per cent less. Thus, to the fast must be attributed the 15 per cent greater decrease in L's. metabolism. *This illustrates the importance of not only considering the metabolism of a given individual on a given day, but also of considering what the diet has been in the preceding period.*

If one accepts the current view that 3 per cent of the body weight is due to nitrogen, the body of L., with an initial weight of 60.6 kilograms, would contain 1818 grams of nitrogen. As he lost 277 grams of nitrogen during the fasting period, this loss amounted to 15 per cent of the original amount of nitrogen in the body. This decrease in body nitrogen of 15 per cent was distinctly less than the decrease in the body weight, which was 22 per cent, and considerably less than the decrease in the basal metabolism of 27 per cent. The tissue lost by this subject amounted to 13.2 kilograms, and each kilogram of body tissue thus lost contained 2.1 per cent of nitrogen which is a third less than the 3 per cent of nitrogen per kilogram body weight which body tissue has been assumed to contain. The body, therefore, conserved its nitrogen. On the other hand, the percentage of nitrogen being katabolized per kilogram body weight at the beginning of the fast was more than that being katabolized at the end of the fast. It is not justifiable, however, to assert that the lowering in metabolism was a result of diminished nitrogenous katabolism exclusively and not due to the total loss in weight represented by carbohydrate protein, and fat. The point was evidently not reached by this individual when there was insufficient body fat to supply the metabolic needs, requiring in consequence that an excessive amount of protein be drawn upon to make up the deficiency. In contrast to this normal individual who fasted thirty-one days and maintained a proper proportionate excretion of nitrogen at the end of the period are certain of the diabetic patients whose proportionate nitrogen excretion after prolonged undernutrition was much greater.

1. *Calorie Equivalent of each Kilogram Body Weight Lost.*— The number of calories represented by each kilogram body weight lost by L., may be determined since his activities were somewhat definitely estimated, thus giving the material for computing with a fair degree of accuracy his total metabolism for each twenty-

four hours. The total metabolism for the thirty-one days, when computed in this way, amounted to 43,010 calories,[1] or 1387 calories per day. This would be equivalent to 3258 calories for each kilogram body weight lost. Knowing the loss in body nitrogen for the period, the total metabolism for the twenty-four hours can be apportioned to the carbohydrate, protein, and fat oxidized daily by using the proper factors involved in the method.[2]

The computations of the body material lost show that, on the basis of per kilogram body weight lost, the average amount of carbohydrate oxidized during the thirty-one days was 15 grams per kilogram,[3] of protein 125 grams, and of fat 277 grams. The remaining 582 grams of each kilogram body weight lost must, therefore, be attributed to a loss of water and, to a slight extent, of salts.

The calories lost by L. for each kilogram decrease in body weight probably represent with a fair degree of accuracy the calories lost by a diabetic subject with the loss of each kilogram body weight. These amounted to about 3258 calories per kilogram or 1500 per pound. All clinicians are in practical agreement today that overnutrition must be avoided in diabetics. It is seldom that more than 5 or 10 per cent of extra food can be taken by a diabetic patient without injury to his carbohydrate tolerance. This being true, it is evident that the loss of a kilogram body weight, or the equivalent of 3200 calories, by an individual whose ordinary metabolism is 1500 calories, would require twenty-two days for replacement, providing he could take an excess of 10 per cent of calories per day, and forty-four days if he could bear but 5 per cent excess. Is it therefore strange that a loss of a kilogram body weight by a diabetic patient is seldom regained?

(*b*) **Metabolism of a Healthy Young Woman Undergoing the Routine Undernutrition Treatment of a Diabetic.**—Whereas thousands of diabetic patients are placed upon a diet which radically departs from the normal, it is almost unique for a healthy individual to undergo the same regime. On this account it was decided in 1916 to observe the effect upon a normal individual of methods then commonly employed in the treatment of diabetes: namely, fasting, followed by a progressively increasing diet.

---

[1] Benedict: Carnegie Inst., Washington, Pub. No. 203, 1915, p. 403.

[2] In these computations no allowance is made for the loss of nitrogen in feces, as the bowels did not move during the fasting period. It is, of course, incorrect to assume that no feces were formed during these thirty-one days and that no nitrogen was thus lost to the body, for the feces, though subsequently proved to be small in amount, simply accumulated in the intestinal tract, but for these somewhat gross compilations the nitrogen lost in this way may be disregarded.

[3] The oxidation of carbohydrate, however, occurred wholly in the first thirteen days of the fast.

TABLE 108.—THE METABOLISM OF A HEALTHY YOUNG WOMAN SUBJECTED TO THE TREATMENT OF A DIABETIC PATIENT.

(Age, twenty-five years; height, 170 cm. All experiments were postabsorptive.)

Day	Weight, kg.	Blood sugar, per cent.	Acidosis CO_2 in blood, vols., per cent.	Acidosis CO_2 in alveolar air, mm. Hg.	Acidosis Diacetic acid.	NH₃ Total gm.	NH₃ Total nitrogen, per cent.	Urinary nitrogen Total gm.	Urinary nitrogen Per kg, gm.	Diet Carbohydrate,[1] gm.	Diet Protein, gm.	Diet Fat, gm.	Diet Calories.	Pulse-rate.
1	57.2	0.12	60.9	41	0	..	..	4.9	0.085	0	0	0	0	
2	56.8	0.11	..	..	0	..	..	7.7	0.135	0	0	0	0	
3	55.8	0.10	..	41	++	1.2	11	8.8	0.155	0	0	0	0	
4	55.0	0.10	..	36	++	1.9	17	9.4	0.170	10	5	0	60	62
5	54.0	0.09	36.2	29	++	2.7	25	8.9	0.165	20	10	0	120	78
6	53.1	0.11	..	31	++	2.8	30	7.7	0.145	30	15	0	180	76
7	..	..	..	32	++	2.5	31	6.5	0.120	40	20	0	240	
8	53.1	0.08	..	34	++	2.5	31	6.9	0.130	40	35	20	480	68
9	53.5	..	..	36	++	2.1	29	6.0	0.110	50	50	30	670	65
10	53.2	0.09	52.2	39	+	2.0+	25	6.6+	0.120+	55	60	45	865	60
11	53.1	..	..	40	++	1.7	20	7.2	0.135	55	75	70	1150	
12	53.2	0.09	..	43	++	1.4	18	6.5	0.120	55	60	60	1000	63
13	53.8	..	..	41	+	1.4	15	8.0	0.150	55	75	85	1285	
14	..	..	..	41	Sl.+	1.4	12	9.7	0.180	55	70	105	1445	
15	54.0	0.09	59.4	41	0	1.1	11	7.7	0.145	55	75	115	1555	
16	54.2	..	..	40	0	0.9	9	7.9	0.145	55	85	120	1640	
17	53.6	0.09	..	39	0	..	..	9.2	0.170	55	75	130	1710	57
18	53.5	..	63.8	43	0	..	..	11.2	0.210	60	75	145	1845	
19	53.2	0.11	..	39	0	..	..	7.5	0.140	155	90	145	2285	59
20	53.1	..	..	43	0	..	..	6.2	0.115	200	75	140	2360	61
22	53.6	0.13	..	44	0	..	..	5.3	0.100					

Day	Metabolism[2]								Materials katabolized per 24 hours			
	Heat output per 24 hours							Protein (N × 6.0), gm.	Carbohydrate and fat.			
									Method I[3]		Method II[4]	
	CO_2 per min., cc.	O_2 per min., cc.	Respiratory quotient.	Total calories.	Per kg., calories.	H. and B., per cent.	Non-protein respiratory quotient.		Carbohydrate, gm.	Fat, gm.	Carbohydrate, gm.	Fat, gm.
1	149	180	0.83	1254	22	−10	0.83	29.4	137	83	137	83
2	159	202	0.79	1393	25	0	0.79	46.2	99	110	99	110
3	152	193	0.79	1331	24	−4	0.78	52.8	81	107	81	107
4	138	179	0.77	1228	22	−11	0.76	56.4	53	105	53	105
5	138	184	0.75	1256	23	−8	0.74	53.4	35	118	10	129
6	141	180	0.78	1238	23	−9	0.78	46.2	76	101	20	126
7								39.0				
8	141	189	0.75	1290	24	−5	0.73	41.4	27	131	40	126
9	152	177	0.86	1243	23	−9	0.87	36.0	176	62	40	123
10	144	185	0.78	1272	24	−7	0.77	39.6	70	111	50	120
11	132	173	0.76	1184	22	−13	0.75	43.2	44	110	55	105
12	148	179	0.80	1237	23	−9	0.84	39.0	141	75	55	114
13	142	187	0.76	1280	24	−6	0.75	48.0	47	118	55	115
14								58.2				
15	130	158	0.82	1098	20	−20	0.83	46.2	111	68	55	93
16	142	186	0.76	1273	24	−7	0.76	47.4	57	113	55	115
17	138	175	0.79	1207	23	−12	0.79	55.2	81	90	55	103
18	140	178	0.79	1228	23	−10	0.78	67.2	70	92	60	98
19	151	199	0.76	1362	26	0	0.75	45.0	51	128	155	84
20	147	175	0.81	1213	23	−11	0.85	37.2	150	69	200	50

[1] The experiments were made for the most part between the hours 9 A.M. and 12 NOON.

[2] An increase of 20 per cent over metabolism for the twenty-four hours is assumed as the effect of food and exercise.

[3] In Method II the non-protein respiratory quotient is used as obtained from the morning experiment on the first four days.   For the remaining days it is assumed that the carbohydrate burned is represented by the carbohydrates in the food for the day and that the remainder of the estimated heat production was from protein and fat.

[4] Does not represent the complete volume of urine for this day.

Miss L., a healthy nurse, long familiar with diabetic patients, volunteered to undergo such a test. Her age was twenty-five years, body weight without clothing 57.2 kilograms, and height 170 centimeters. The observations began June 5, 1916, (first day), and were concluded June 24, 1916 (twentieth day), covering a period of twenty days.

For the first four days of the period of study, Miss L. fasted, save for small quantities of weak bouillon, Thereafter the carbohydrate in the diet was steadily increased from 10 grams on the fifth day to 155 and 200 grams on the nineteenth and twentieth days. The protein, which was 5 grams on the fifth day, amounted to 90 grams on the nineteenth day, and 75 grams on the twentieth day. The fat, which was begun on the ninth day with 20 grams, reached 145 and 140 grams on the nineteenth and twentieth days. The ultimate diet reached represented an intake of 2360 calories, or 44 calories per kilogram body weight.

The body weight of this normal subject while taking the diabetic diet decreased 4.1 kilograms. The body weight was the same on the sixth and twentieth days of the experiment, although on the days between there were fluctuations upward of 0.1 to 1.1 kilograms. For the entire period of twenty days the net deficit in calories computed from the basal metabolism plus 20 per cent for hospital activity after deducting the caloric value of the food taken was 13,000 calories, or 3.17 calories for each kilogram body weight lost, which corresponds quite closely to the 3258 calories per kilogram of reduction in body weight of the subject L. in his fast of thirty-one days.

The heat output per kilogram body weight was 22 calories at the beginning of the observation and 23 calories on the last day.

The urinary nitrogen for the first day of fasting was 0.085 gram per kilogram body weight, but thereafter steadily rose until at the end of the fourth day of fasting it was 0.17 gram per kilogram. Thereafter it dropped to between 6 and 7 grams daily, an average of 0.125 gram per kilogram body weight, and increased but slightly when additional food was given, an obvious nitrogen retention taking place. Each kilogram body weight lost contained less nitrogen and more water than body tissues.

Upon the nineteenth and twentieth days of the experiment Miss L. was given 2285 and 2360 calories, representing 43 and 44 calories per kilogram body weight. Upon this diet she failed to gain weight, but there was marked retention of body nitrogen, the excretion for the two days being but 7.5 and 6.2 grams, respectively. The average metabolism upon these two days was actually less than the average metabolism for the first four days when the patient was fasting. In other words, *fasting does not immediately lower the basal metab-*

olism nor does an excess of food following a period of restricted diet immediately raise it. The organism does not at first decrease metabolism with sufficient rapidity to save body tissue. Conversely, feeding does not immediately raise the metabolism, for the surplus food is utilized to replace body tissue lost.

The postabsorptive blood sugar decreased from 0.12 per cent at the beginning of the experiment to 0.08 per cent on the eighth day. During the preceding seven days the subject had taken a total amount of food containing carbohydrate 60 grams, protein 30 grams, and fat none. Thereafter the blood sugar gradually rose, until upon the second morning after the conclusion of the experiment, when the patient was on full diet, it had reached 0.13 per cent, essentially the same as at the beginning of the experiment.

Evidence of acidosis appeared after two days of fasting. This sufficed to produce a positive reaction for diacetic acid and an ammonia excretion of 1.2 grams, but the carbon dioxide in the alveolar air remained unchanged. All tests appeared or were more marked following the third day of fasting, and if the subject had been a diabetic, she would have been said to exhibit mild acidosis. This became great enough during the fifth to eighth days to be classified as moderately severe. This did not begin to subside until the subject had taken 30 grams of carbohydrate, representing 15 per cent of the calories of the total basal metabolism plus 20 per cent additional for effect of food and exercise. The acidosis did not entirely disappear until the carbohydrate, with gradually increasing protein and fat, had risen to 55 grams and had been continued for an additional five days.

The basal metabolism varied between 1393 calories (for the second day) and 1098 calories (for the fifteenth day), or from 26 to 20 calories per kilogram body weight. The striking feature of the metabolism is that upon all but two of the eighteen days on which it was determined, it was subnormal. If the average is taken for the entire period, it was 8 per cent below the normal standard. These observations, therefore, show that a normal individual who lived for twenty days upon a diet similar to the routine diet advised for diabetics had a metabolism which was 8 per cent subnormal. As the diabetics frequently have a smaller diet and for a portion of the period while under treatment in addition lose calories in the form of sugar, it is readily understood why their metabolism should be somewhat more subnormal than that of Miss L.

The respiratory quotient fell steadily from 0.83 to 0.75 during the four days of fasting. It was the same upon the morning of the eighth day as might be expected, since the carbohydrate in the diet of the preceding day was 30 grams and the protein 15 grams. From this point onward, however, the respiratory quotient was higher.

The average respiratory quotient for the ten days during which the subject was taking but 40 to 55 grams of carbohydrate daily was 0.79, which differs but slightly from the average respiratory quotient of 0.81 for 68 female subjects whose postabsorptive metabolism was observed when they were on a full diet.[1]

The materials katabolized were computed from the non-protein respiratory quotient. Obviously it is inaccurate thus to estimate the materials katabolized for the entire day, because the experiments in this case were in the morning and they approximated only two hours in duration. A suggestive picture of the kind of katabolism which was taking place may be gained, however, and although the defects are realized, it is presented.

The loss of carbohydrate for the first four days of fasting was marked, amounting to 370 grams, an amount similar though larger than that usually observed by others in fasting experiments. Even though the actual figures might be somewhat less, if based on longer calorimetric periods, it presents vividly the enormous drain upon the glycogen reserves of the body which fasting entails. The fasting subject, L., at the Nutrition Laboratory lost 154 grams glycogen in the same space of time and other subjects studied in this laboratory have katabolized amounts between 119 and 259 grams. Even in the following two days the katabolism of carbohydrate averaged over 50 grams per day. This quantity of carbohydrate would appear to have come almost exclusively from carbohydrate as such, because the nitrogen excretion remained low.

The protein katabolized gradually increased from 29.4 grams on the first day to 56.4 grams on the fourth. This may be compared with L's. values, which were 42.6 and 71.2 grams on the first and fourth days, respectively. His weight on these days averaged but 2 kilograms more than that of our subject.

The quantity of fat metabolized varied between 83.3 grams on the first day and 104.8 grams on the fourth, rising to 109.9 grams on one of the intervening days. These values are but slightly below L's., which were 135, 142, 130 and 136 grams.

11. **The Respiratory Quotient in Health and Diabetes.**—The relation which the volume of carbon dioxide produced by an individual bears to the volume of oxygen required during the same interval of time constitutes his respiratory quotient. This has been found to be dependent upon the character of the material in the body which is oxidized or burned at this time. An examination of the composition of the carbohydrate molecule will show that it contains sufficient hydrogen to unite with all the oxygen present during its oxidation. Consequently, for each volume of oxygen

---

[1] Benedict and Emmes: Jour. Biol. Chem., 1915, **20**, 253.

used in the oxidation of carbohydrate a volume of carbon dioxide will be produced and the respiratory quotient of such a carbohydrate as glucose ($C_6H_{12}O_6$) will therefore be 1. It matters not whether the oxidation takes place rapidly outside of the body in a flame, or less obtrusively in the body during twenty-four hours. Protein, on the other hand, does not contain sufficient oxygen for the oxidation of the hydrogen atoms contained in its molecule. As a result, in the burning of protein, oxygen must be used not only for the carbon in the molecule, but for the hydrogen as well. The denominator of the fraction is thus increased, and the final quotient of protein must be less than 1 and is 0.81. The protein molecule is made up of many component parts and while the respiratory quotients of these parts vary greatly, yet for protein as a whole the above quotient (0.81) holds. With fat a similar condition exists to that in protein, only there is still more hydrogen present to require oxygen, so that the amount of oxygen necessary for the combustion of fat is still greater, and as a result the respiratory quotient falls to 0.71. The respiratory quotient of alcohol is still lower, and is 0.67. β-oxy-butyric acid, which can be taken as the chief one of the group of acid bodies formed in diabetes, has a respiratory quotient of 0.89, diacetic acid of 1 and acetone of 0.75, so that one will not go far astray to take 0.89 as a common respiratory quotient for these three acid bodies.

TABLE 109.—THE RESPIRATORY QUOTIENT (R. Q.) OF A FOOD IS OBTAINED BY DIVIDING THE VOLUME OF CARBON DIOXIDE PRODUCED DURING ITS OXIDATION BY THE VOLUME OF OXYGEN ABSORBED.

Carbohydrate: $C_6H_{12}O_6 + 6O_2 = 6CO_2 + 6H_2O$ R. Q.
  Oxygen is required for oxidation of the carbon alone

$$\frac{\text{Volume} \quad 6CO_2 \text{ produced}}{\text{Volume} \quad 6O_2 \text{ absorbed}} = \quad \ldots \ldots \ldots \ldots \quad 1.00$$

	R.Q.
Fat: Oxygen required for carbon and a large quantity of hydrogen	0.71
Protein occupies an intermediate position	0.81
Alcohol (C_2H_6O)	0.67
B-oxybutyric acid ($C_4H_8O_3$)	0.89
Diacetic acid ($C_4H_6O_3$)	1.00
Acetone (C_3H_6O)	0.75

The respiratory quotient of an individual can be determined by measurement of the quantity of carbon dioxide exhaled and the oxygen absorbed. When this is done information is obtained concerning the character and total amount of the combustion taking place in the body. Since the urinary nitrogen gives us a definite idea of the quantity of protein metabolized, if we calculate what this represents in terms of carbon dioxide and oxygen, and subtract it from the total carbon dioxide exhaled and the total oxygen absorbed we have left the combustion derived simply from fat and carbohydrate. Knowing the respiratory quotient produced when fat and carbohydrate are oxidized as well as that of the individual, it is possible, by computation, to determine the share which these two variables have taken in the total metabolism.

There is always a temptation to calculate the body materials burned when the values for the O_2 intake, CO_2 output, and nitrogen excretion are known. Such calculations are not warranted unless the measurements of the metabolism occur throughout many of the hours of the twenty-four. Even under such circumstances an allowance for the increased metabolism due to muscular exercise is problematical. Recently Krogh[1] has advanced the hypothesis that fat is formed from carbohydrate when the available supply of carbohydrate is in excess of that of fat. This formation is distinct when the respiratory quotient rises above 0.90. When the total quotient has risen above unity, the katabolic quotient has only reached 0.95. This transformation takes place with a loss in energy, and, in consequence, there is a slight rise in metabolism. When fat is in excess of the available carbohydrate, then carbohydrate is formed, and though the total quotient may reach 0.71, the katabolic quotient would be 0.74. This process likewise takes place with a loss of energy and consequent rise in metabolism. Therefore, not alone is carbohydrate needed for the oxidation of fat, but, what has not been previously contended, fat is needed for the oxidation of carbohydrate. Extremes in respiratory quotient are thus theoretically disadvantageous. Already extremes in metabolism have been shown to be disadvantageous clinically, and the next few pages will show also by clinical evidence that this is true of extremes in the respiratory quotient.

The respiratory quotient of normal individuals twelve hours after a meal has been determined by Benedict, Emmes, Roth and Smith, and is summarized in Table 110.[2]

TABLE 110.—RESPIRATORY QUOTIENT AND TOTAL METABOLISM OF NORMAL INDIVIDUALS AT REST AT A PERIOD TWELVE HOURS OR MORE AFTER THE LAST MEAL.

Individuals.	Average respiratory quotient.	Calories per kilo per twenty-four hrs.
89 men	0.83	25.5
68 women	0.81	24.9

If the fast is prolonged the respiratory quotient will fall because the individual is forced to draw upon fat and protein for nutritive material, and it will be remembered that these have a respiratory quotient of 0.71 and 0.81 respectively, in comparison with carbo-

[1] Krogh and Lindhard: Biochem. Jour., 1920, **14**, 290.
[2] Benedict, Emmes, Roth and Smith: Jour. Biol. Chem., 1914, **18**, 139.

hydrate, which is 1. The respiratory quotients of the individual studied at the Nutrition Laboratory[1] who fasted for thirty-one days, are shown in the following Tables 111 and 112.

TABLE 111.—THE RESPIRATORY QUOTIENTS OF A MAN DURING A PROLONGED FAST.

Period.	Time.	Respiratory quotient.	Calories per kg. body weight per 24 hours.
Preliminary period	Days 1–4 before fast	0.85 (av.)	30
Period of fast	Days 1–5 of fast	0.77 (av.)	29
	Days 6–31 of fast	0.72 (av.)	26
After period {	Second day after breaking fast .	0.78	
	Third day after breaking fast[2] .	0.94	

TABLE 112.—QUANTITIES OF PROTEIN, CARBOHYDRATE AND FAT OXIDIZED BY FASTING MAN AT NUTRITION LABORATORY.[3]

Period of fast.	Respiratory quotient. Actual.	Non-protein.	Quantities oxidized. Protein, gms.	Carbo-hydrate, gms.	Fat, gms.	Calories per kilo per twenty-four hours.
1st day . . .	0.78	0.76	43	69	135	30
2d day . . .	0.75	0.74	50	42	142	30
3d day . . .	0.74	0.74	68	39	130	29
4th day . . .	0.75	0.71	71	4	136	28
5th day . . .	0.76	0.72	63	15	133	28
6th to 31st day av.	0.72	0.70	53	0[4]	114	26

It will be seen that the respiratory quotient became approximately that of fat within six days and remained there for the balance of the period; that it rose sharply within two days after breaking the fast, and upon the third day reached 0.94, showing that the individual must have taken an extraordinarily large quantity of carbohydrate food.

The respiratory quotient differs little from that of normal individuals in mild cases of diabetes when the urine is free from sugar and the carbohydrate in the diet large. The respiratory quotient of these same mild cases of diabetes will be lowered by fasting or by the withdrawal of carbohydrate, as shown above in the case of the normal fasting man. Evidence is thus afforded that the limited quantity of carbohydrate in the diet in cases of severe diabetes is responsible to a large degree for the low respiratory quotient which such patients exhibit. Magnus-Levy called attention to this, and so have other observers.

The problem of drawing inferences from the respiratory quotient

[1] Benedict: A Study of Prolonged Fasting, Carnegie Inst. of Washington, No. 203.
[2] Twelve hours after food.
[3] Determined from the daily metabolism, the urinary nitrogen and the calculated non-protein respiratory quotient.
[4] Actually a total of 32 gms. carbohydrate were burned during the sixth to thirteenth day inclusive, and later none.

17

in diabetes is further complicated by the fact that much of even the little carbohydrate which is given to a diabetic patient is lost in the urine. The patient really approaches the condition of the fasting man in that he is living largely on fat and protein, although in this case not necessarily that of his own body. If all the carbohydrate ingested is lost in the urine, his respiratory quotient has been computed to be 0.72 upon the assumption that 15 per cent of the metabolism is due to protein and 85 per cent to fat. But there are other complications. Occasionally cases of diabetes are seen where the sugar in the urine exceeds that of the diet, and speculation at once arises as to the source of this excess of sugar. Magnus-Levy has pointed out that if the sugar in the urine amounted to 60 grams and the protein in the diet to 100 grams, the additional quantity of oxygen which would be demanded to form this amount of sugar out of protein would lower the respiratory quotient to 0.7. The situation is still further complicated by the presence of unoxidized acid bodies in the urine, amounting frequently to 20 to 40 grams and occasionally to 60 grams calculated as β-oxybutyric acid. The amount of oxygen consumed in the formation of these bodies, for β-oxybutyric is far richer in oxygen than are protein and fat— would again lower the quotient, and it has been calculated again by Magnus-Levy[1] that the respiratory quotient of a case of diabetes presenting 60 grams of sugar in the urine for 100 grams of protein in the diet, and excreting 20 grams of β-oxybutyric acid, would fall as low as 0.69.

TABLE 113.—THEORETICAL RESPIRATORY QUOTIENTS (FROM MAGNUS-LEVY).

Diet.		Calories.	Respiratory quotient.
Protein, 100 gm. Carb., 567 gm.	$\begin{cases} 100 \times 4.1 = 410 \\ 567 \times 4.1 = 2325 \end{cases}$ . . .	2735	0.97
Protein, 100 gm. Fat, 250 gm.	$\begin{cases} 100 \times 4.1 = 410 \\ 250 \times 9.3 = 2325 \end{cases}$ . . .	2735	0.72
Loss in urine			
Sugar, 60 gm.	$(60 \times 4.1 = 246)$ . . .	2489	0.70
Sugar, 60 gm. B-oxy. acid, 20 gm.	$\begin{cases} 60 \times 4.1 = 246 \\ 20 \times 4.7 = 94 \end{cases}$ . . .	2395	0.69

(*a*) **Low and High Respiratory Quotients.**—The respiratory quotient represents the proportions of fat and carbohydrate burned at any given moment. It cannot be expected to change unless there is a change in this proportion. In general, if carbohydrate is being burned, the quotient will remain high, but if carbohydrate is not being burned, the respiratory quotient will fall.

[1] Magnus-Levy: Ztschr. f. klin. Med., 1905, **56**, 83.

There are two sources of carbohydrate which the individual can burn, the exogenous and the endogenous, and from each source carbohydrate may be obtained in three forms: (1) From carbohydrate, 100 per cent; (2) from protein, 58 per cent; and (3) to a slight extent from fat, 10 per cent. So far as the quotient is concerned, save in exceptional instances, one deals only with carbohydrate obtained from carbohydrate, as starch and sugar in the diet, or glycogen and sugar stored in the body. If the diet contains no starch and sugar and if there is no storage of glycogen or sugar in the body, then the only methods by which the quotient can continue high or rise are: (1) By the liberation and oxidation of carbohydrate derived from the excessive katabolism of protein and the non-oxidation of the protein residue, or (2) what has hitherto been undemonstrated with the severe diabetic, though an everyday occurrence in normals, by the transformation of carbohydrate into fat. By the former method it is theoretically immaterial whether the protein so metabolized is supplied from without the body or from the body itself, but so far as is known the oxidation of protein from without the body has never raised the respiratory quotient above the characteristic protein quotient of 0.81. On the other hand, some observations upon our diabetic patients appear to indicate that when an excessive amount of body protein is oxidized, as is evidently the case when the body has reached a stage of extreme inanition with almost complete exhaustion of its storage of fat, the quotient will then rise above the respiratory quotient of protein.

Then, too, the possibility exists of the conversion of carbohydrate into fat, for which hypothesis evidence will be submitted in the discussion of high respiratory quotients in diabetes, following the administration of levulose.

The factors which influence the respiratory quotient in diabetes are therefore many. Not only are we dealing with the standard quotients for carbohydrate, protein, and fat, of 1, 0.81 and 0.71, respectively, and already mentioned, but with many other quotients. If the glucose derived from protein is not burned, the quotient for protein reverts to 0.632,[1] but if the amino-acid molecules in protein, which are producers of fat, are not burned, a different quotient results. During periods of acidosis ammonia is formed and excreted. The nitrogen thus removed from the body does not require oxygen, and in consequence the quotient tends to rise to 0.88 if all the nitrogen of protein metabolism is eliminated as ammonia.[2] Nor does the metabolism of fat run smoothly with the diabetic. Imperfect oxidation may take place and β-oxybutyric acid, diacetic acid, and acetone be formed which have very different quotients from that

---

[1] Lusk: Arch. Int. Med., 1915, **15**, 939.
[2] Grafe: Ztschr. f. physiol. Chem., 1910, **65**, 48.

of the mother molecule. The formation of these bodies from fat tends to lower the respiratory quotient, their oxidation to raise it. Magnus-Levy[1] calculated that from 100 grams of fat it is possible to form 36.2 grams of β-oxybutyric acid. If this should take place, the respiratory quotient for fat would be 0.669, instead of 0.707. In the light of all these variations taking place in the diabetic organism, one may expect strange quotients, and their explanation at present is fraught with difficulties.

(*b*) **Relationship Between the Respiratory Quotient and the Metabolism of Diabetics.**—The metabolism, not only of diabetics but of normal individuals as well, has been considered quite unrelated to the respiratory quotient, the belief being general that the latter merely registered the quality and not the quantity of material burned. Inasmuch as great variations have been seen to take place in the metabolism of these 113 diabetics, it is especially worth while to investigate this supposed non-relationship between their metabolism and respiratory quotients. The data for such a comparison have therefore been gathered together in Table 114.

It will be seen from Table 114, based upon severe diabetics, that before June, 1914, the average respiratory quotient for 94 observations was 0.73, and after June, 1914, the average respiratory quotient was 0.77 for 199 experiments. The average metabolism in these same observations was 14 per cent above standard prior to June, 1914, and 13 per cent below standard after June, 1914. The respiratory quotient in diabetes, therefore, appears to bear a definite relation to the metabolism in that it is low when the metabolism is high and high when the metabolism is low. This is in striking contrast to the universally accepted idea that the respiratory quotient is independent of the metabolism.

TABLE 114.—RELATION BETWEEN RESPIRATORY QUOTIENT AND BASAL METABOLISM IN SEVERE DIABETES.

	Before June, 1914.			After June, 1914.	
Respiratory quotient.	Number of observations.	Average variation of metabolism from standard, per cent.	Respiratory quotient.	Number of observations.	Average variation of metabolism from standard, per cent.
0.68	16	+17	0.68	7	− 1
0.72	63	+13	0.73	75	− 7
0.76	11	+12	0.77	51	−14
0.80	1	+10	0.81	47	−19
0.86	3	+12	0.85	18	−23
....	..	....	0.94	1	−37
0.73	**94**	**+14**	**0.77**	**199**	**−13**

Prior to June, 1914, the lowest average quotient of the series, 0.68, was accompanied by the highest average metabolism of the

---

[1] Magnus-Levy: Ergeb. d. inn. Med., 1908, **1**, 384.

series: namely, 17 per cent. With the higher respiratory quotients the metabolism fell to as low as 10 per cent, but with the highest average quotient, it increased again to 12 per cent. After June, 1914, the metabolism steadily fell from a variation of 1 per cent to 37 per cent as the average respiratory quotient rose from 0.68 to 0.94.

The inferences to be drawn from this table as to the relationship between the respiratory quotient and the metabolism are of the utmost clinical importance. With the low carbohydrate diet of the diabetic a low respiratory quotient is to be expected, and was found, as evidenced by the average quotient of 0.73 for the cases before June, 1914. The low quotient is in contrast to the average quotient of 0.83 found with 236 of the 239 normal individuals in the Harris and Benedict series.[1] After June, 1914, the average quotient for the diabetics was higher than previous to that date, namely, 0.77, which is still somewhat below the normal. In looking for a cause for the difference in the quotients in these two periods, we have not the usual recourse to variations in the amount of carbohydrates in the diet because in both epochs this was low, certainly averaging less than a fourth of the normal quota, with a difference between the two periods of probably less than 25 grams. Moreover, after a postabsorptive period of fourteen hours, the small amount of carbohydrate taken would have but little influence upon the quotient. Some other cause, therefore, than the usual oxidation of carbohydrate must be found for these varying quotients, and it is not easy to explain them by the normal metabolism of protein and fat.

Associated with this change in respiratory quotient between the two periods is a change in the metabolism of 27 per cent (from +14 to −13 per cent) with the severe cases. A high metabolism with diabetic patients is found to be associated with a low respiratory quotient. As the respiratory quotient approaches that of normal individuals, the metabolism tends toward the normal level. When the metabolism attains a very low level, the respiratory quotient rises to a level abnormally high for a severe diabetic.

With the cases of severe diabetes we find that both excessively low and excessively high respiratory quotients are usually associated with an abnormal metabolism, so that, although a high respiratory quotient is welcomed in such a disease as diabetes because it suggests the ability of the patient to burn carbohydrate, one must not lose sight of the fact that it is obtained only through a metabolism of threateningly low degree. The causes of the low respiratory quotients and the accompanying high metabolism and the high respiratory quotients and low metabolism must be eradi-

---

[1] Harris and Benedict: Carnegie Inst. Washington, Pub. No. 279, 1919, pp. 40 and 44, Tables C and D. The respiratory quotients are not printed in these tables, but have been calculated.

cated for successful treatment of a case. The data here set forth
show that an added significance can be attached to the respiratory
quotient in diabetes. Our observations are quite in line with the
opinions expressed by Krogh.

In the arrangement of the diet for the diabetic, therefore, one
must bear in mind that a diet which produces a low quotient in its
utilization is a diet which calls for a higher metabolism than a diet
which produces a high quotient.

(c) **Low Respiratory Quotients in Diabetes.**—The studies of Means,[1]
upon fat individuals also show unusually low quotients. His Case
No. 1 gave respiratory quotients of 0.69, 0.69, 0.68 and 0.74, respectively, during four days of fasting. Corresponding to this low
quotient the metabolism itself was below standard rather than
above, amounting to 2 per cent. In a second period of fasting,
about ten days later, the respiratory quotients were 0.75, 0.75, 0.72,
0.71 and 0.73, with which rise of quotient the metabolism was −8
per cent, thus corresponding to the general relation between respiratory quotients and metabolism observed with diabetics. Also,
during the third period, when the respiratory quotients were practically the same as in the second period, the metabolism was correspondingly low: namely, −10 per cent. His other observations upon
the same case are significant in that they confirm the accuracy of
the data given, because they show that, as the respiratory quotient
rose with this normal obese individual, not only the metabolism fell,
but also, incidentally, the acidosis lessened.

Extremely low respiratory quotients have been noted in the past
in the literature, but usually have been looked upon with suspicion
and often considered the result of poor technic. Such quotients,
however, have been obtained far too frequently in health and disease and by too many authors to be disregarded. A study of the
literature indicates that the diabetic patients who gave these low
quotients were living upon a fairly strict non-carbohydrate diet or
upon a diet with high protein and fat.

Magnus-Levy[2] reports quotients in a series of studies upon diabetics of 0.654, 0.657 and 0.651. His patient excreted about 100
grams of sugar in the urine daily and the diet contained carbohydrate
about 40 grams, protein 100 to 150 grams, and fat 200 to 300 grams.

In Leimdorfer's[3] series following the periods of non-carbohydrate
diet the patients were placed upon a diet of vegetables with fat in
the form of butter, or bacon and eggs, or egg yolks and some alcohol.
Still later he gave three oatmeal days during which the oatmeal
amounted to 250 grams, but 250 grams of butter were also given,

[1] Means: Jour. Med. Research, 1915, **27**, 121.
[2] Magnus-Levy: Ztschr. f. klin. Med., 1905, **56**, 83.
[3] Leimdorfer's: Biochem. Ztschr., 1912, **40**, 326.

as well as alcohol. As a result the above patients showed quotients respectively of 0.655, 0.655 and 0.691.

The Russell Sage Laboratory, in all of their publications, report but one low respiratory quotient with a diabetic.[1] With Cyril K., a quotient of 0.687 was obtained, the quotient in one of the periods being 0.656.

In contrast to this one quotient below 0.69 from the Russell Sage Laboratory are 17 such quotients ranging as low as 0.65 recently reported by Wilder, Boothby, and Beeler[2] in the course of 44 experiments with a single case of diabetes. The case was not exceptionally severe. This is shown by the absence of glycosuria for four successive days (May 15–18) with a diet containing approximately 1 gram of protein and 30 calories per kilogram body weight with carbohydrate amounting to 14.7 grams, and again later for seven days (June 4–10) upon a diet of $\frac{2}{3}$ gram of protein and 33 calories per kilogram body weight. At the end of these periods D:N ratios ceased to exist and the respiratory quotients were respectively 0.72 and 0.73. By placing these patients upon diets containing 57 calories per kilogram (April 30–May 4) and 51 calories per kilogram (May 30–June 2), containing respectively 138 and 126 grams of fat and 3 and 4 grams of carbohydrate, D:N ratios of 3.65 : 1 were obtained, though not obtained when larger quantities of carbohydrate (43 grams), less protein, and larger quantities of fat (151 grams) were given. None of the low quotients were obtained when the patient had received upon the preceding day over 20 grams of carbohydrate, save with one exception. The protein and fat in the diet shortly preceding the tests were comparatively high. Thus, the fat with these quotients varied between 83 and 151 grams, save on May 30, which was but three days after an eight-day period of the ingestion of 151 grams of fat daily. At no time were quotients below 0.69 obtained when the energy in the diet was less than 30 calories per kilogram body weight upon the preceding day, save in three instances when one or two days of lower diets or fasting intervened between periods of the administration of 51 to 57 calories per kilogram for four to seven successive days.

1. *Extremely Low Respiratory Quotients at the Nutrition Laboratory.*—Among the 113 patients studied at the Nutrition Laboratory between 1908 and 1917, respiratory quotients of 0.69 or below were observed on 21 occasions with 9 patients in the postabsorptive state. The data for these observations are given in Table 115. Fifteen of these occurred in the period before June, 1914, and 6 before May, 1915, thus showing their relation to the period of overfeeding. Save for the 6 exceptions above noted, such low quotients were absent

---

[1] Gephart, Aub, DuBois and Lusk: Arch. Int. Med., 1917, **19**, 908.
[2] Wilder, Boothby and Beeler: Jour. Biol. Chem., 1922, **51**, 311.

with the 80 patients studied since June, 1914, when they were in the postabsorptive condition. The hall-marks of overnutrition in the early period are apparent with these patients, and the over-feeding was chiefly in the form of fat, though to a considerable extent in protein as well. It was not uncommon for patients to receive 200 or more grams of fat upon the day preceding the metabolism test. Case No. 786 was given alcohol freely upon admission to the hospital, but otherwise was upon a low diet for the intervening time. This was the patient with whom Bloor found 13.1 per cent total lipoids in the blood plasma some months later, on June 15, 1916.

TABLE 115.—LOW RESPIRATORY QUOTIENTS (0.69 AND BELOW) IN POSTABSORPTIVE EXPERIMENTS WITH DIABETICS.

Case No.	Date.	Respiratory quotient	Variation from standard metabolism per cent.	Variation of body weight from standard, per cent.	Severity.	Acidosis	Urinary nitrogen per kilogram of body weight, gm.	Urinary sugar on preceding day, gm.
220	Mar. 13–14, 1909	0.69	+32	−25	S	+++		
246	June 8– 9, 1909	0.67	+28	+ 1	S	++	0.211	104
"	" 15–16, 1909	0.67	+22	+ 1	..	++	0.348	122
"	" 25–26, 1909	0.69	+14	+ 1	..	++	0.357	123
"	Oct. 25–26, 1909	0.69	+17	−10	..	+++	0.391	89
"	" 28–29, 1909	0.66	+15	− 8	..	+++	0.349	134
"	" 29–30, 1909	0.68	+ 8	− 8	..	+++	0.345	107
"	" 31–Nov. 1, 1909	0.69	+ 7	− 8	..	+++	0.291	93
441	Oct. 9–10, 1911	0.68	+ 6	−31	S	+++	0.277	54
549	Nov. 5– 6, 1912	0.69	+30	−14	S	+++	0.312	185
"	" 12–13, 1912	0.69	+16	−17	..	+++	0.155	92
591	Apr. 14–15, 1913	0.65	+15	−21	S	+++	0.144	77
"	" 15–16, 1913	0.69	+10	−20	..	+++	0.140	48
740	Apr. 15–16, 1915	0.69	+ 1	−13	S	+++	0.276	
773	Oct. 10–11, 1914	0.69	+64[1]	−22	S	+++	0.216	52
786	Nov. 9–10, 1914	0.66	− 1	−25	Mo.	+	—	0
"	" 12–13, 1914	0.68	−10	−25	..	+	0.144	0
806	Dec. 22–23, 1914	0.68	− 1	−14	S	++	0.135	0

Respiratory quotients of 0.69, or below, were obtained also in 24 instances after the ingestion of food. These occurred almost exclusively before January, 1915. The acidosis was severe or moderate with one exception. All cases were severe in type. Like the low quotients secured by other observers, ours were almost without exception found with patients who had ingested many calories, much fat, and occasionally alcohol.

With 1 patient, Case No. 707,[2] so many low quotients were obtained that they were originally rejected, but upon reëxamination of the protocols it appeared that the cause for rejection was inadequate and that the quotients of 0.65 which were obtained were well

---

[1] Case No. 773 was a girl diabetic. Variation in metabolism on this day was +64 per cent by the Girl Scout Standard.

[2] Case No. 707 is described in detail in the Carnegie Pub. No. 323, p. 176.

substantiated. These occurred after large meals of oatmeal and fat in an exceptionally severe diabetic. Moreover, with this patient there is no evidence that he was asleep, a factor which must be considered in the interpretation of low quotients, because Carpenter[1] has shown that there is a lowering of the quotient in sleep amounting to from 0.05 to 0.07.

Low quotients, and to a certain extent it can be said of dextrose-nitrogen ratios of 3.65:1, are *forced quotients* and *forced ratios*. They are not inherent in the ordinary metabolism of diabetes. The undisturbed diabetic has no such quotients. They are analogous to the condition produced by an overdose of digitalis in an individual with a moderately decompensated heart. When administered in moderate doses, digitalis, like fat and protein, does good, but in excessive doses auricular fibrillation results on the one hand, low quotients and dextrose-nitrogen ratios of 3.65:1 on the other, and the patients are brought to the verge of death. Low respiratory quotients and dextrose-nitrogen ratios of 3.65:1 are evidence of poor medical treatment. In the past these were frequently obtained through ignorance, but their occurrence today demands explanation.

(*d*) **High Respiratory Quotients in Diabetes.**—High respiratory quotients, when obtained with mild or moderately severe cases of diabetes, are readily explained by the combustion of carbohydrate in the diet or by the combustion of carbohydrate previously stored in the body. On the other hand, the explanation of high respiratory quotients found in observations with cases of severe diabetes is by no means simple, since carbohydrate as such is not available for combustion, either from the diet or from the body. Some evidence exists to show that the high respiratory quotients appear when the body is compelled to draw upon protein owing to a lack of available fat, and there is also some evidence which will be presented in the discussion of the experiments which followed the ingestion of levulose that there is a transformation of carbohydrate into fat which would also sufficiently explain this unlooked for phenomenon. (See Tables 116 and 127.) Examination of the case histories of the severe type of patients whose experiments gave these high quotients shows that they were most often obtained when the individuals were *in extremis* and without acidosis. This precludes the explanation of the high respiratory quotients on the theory of oxidation of acid bodies which have high quotients, because, though this explanation would hold for a few days when the patient was free from acidosis, it would hardly explain the phenomenon for long periods when no evidence of acidosis exists.

Respiratory quotients of 0.84 or over may be considered as

---

[1] Carpenter: Am. Jour. Physiol., 1922, **59**; Proc. Am. Physiol. Soc., 440.

unusual with severe cases of diabetes in the postabsorptive state. The average respiratory quotient for the 94 observations before June, 1914, was 0.73, and the average respiratory quotient for the 199 observations after June, 1914, was 0.77. (See Table 114). These same averages were found likewise for cases of all degrees of severity in 122 observations before, and in 292 observations after, June, 1914. Among these observations there were 35 tests with severe cases in which the respiratory quotient was 0.84 or over.

There was but 1 patient among the severe cases (Case No. 1011) with a respiratory quotient as high as 0.94. The metabolism at the time of this observation was −37 per cent, and a study of the protocols proves that this value was well supported by other data obtained with this young girl. She was, at that period, in a state of extreme inanition, with a body weight 49 per cent below normal, and was, moreover, free from acidosis. A feature possibly contributing to the explanation of this high quotient and low metabolism was her high nitrogen excretion at this time, which on the day preceding the observation amounted to 0.285 gram of urinary nitrogen per kilogram body weight. Three and four days after the experiment the excretion per kilogram body weight was 0.41 and 0.515 gram, respectively, with the protein in the diet during the six days between November 22 and 27, varying from 0 to 51 grams per day, or on the average 1.1 grams per kilogram of body weight.

The average respiratory quotient for all of these specially selected severe cases, including the girl diabetics, was 0.86. How unusual these quotients are is shown by noting the dates of the observations, there being but 3 of these quotients which were obtained before June, 1914. In fact, these 35 high quotients with severe cases represent but a little over 10 per cent of the respiratory quotients obtained with the 67 severe cases for whom postabsorptive quotients were secured.

The high quotients in the 3 tests before June, 1914, were accompanied by a metabolism above standard, but those obtained after June, 1914, for the remaining 19 experiments with the adult group of severe cases were accompanied in most instances by an extremely low metabolism, the average variation from standard in these 19 observations being −24 per cent.

A marked loss of weight also characterized the cases represented in this group of high quotients. Whereas the average greatest loss of weight from maximum during the experimental period for all of the diabetics was 25 per cent, the average loss of weight from maximum of the severe cases in Table 116, as shown by the records for these dates, was 33 per cent for the adult group, and 28 per cent for the girl diabetics. That this loss of weight actually

TABLE 116.—HIGH RESPIRATORY QUOTIENTS OBSERVED IN POSTABSORPTIVE EXPERIMENTS WITH SEVERE DIABETICS.

Case No.	Date.	Respiratory quotient.	Variation of metabolism from standard, per cent.	Acidosis.	Body weight naked, kg.	Variation in body weight from normal standard, per cent.	Urinary nitrogen per kg. of body weight per 24 hours.	Calories per kg. of body weight per 24 hrs. in diet for 7 to 10 days preceding observation day.	Carbohydrate balance of preceding day, gm.	Date of death.
226	Dec. 6- 7, 1913	0.86	+8	++	64.4	-13	0.175	0	- 5	Nov. 26, 1915.
289	Sept. 30-Oct. 1, 1909	0.88	+12	++	52.3	-15	..	..	-40	Sept. 17, 1912.
610	Oct. 4- 5, 1909	0.85	+16	+	52.3	-15	..	40	-40	April, 1918.
	Mar. 22-23, 1917	0.84	- 7	0	51.2	-24	0.195	11	+ 5	
786	Apr. 18-19, 1917	0.85	- 2	0	52.6	-22	..	19	+ 5	Mar. 31, 1917.
1011	Jan. 19-20, 1916	0.84	-23	++++	48.6	-33	0.350	3	+60	Oct. 1, 1918.
	June 28-29, 1916	0.85	-24	++++	51.0	-30	0.160	27	+20	
	Oct. 8- 9, 1917	0.84	-26	+	28.6	-48	0.245	28	+10	
	16-17, 1917	0.84	-31	0	28.0	-49	0.265	36	+30	
	24-25, 1917	0.94	-30	++	27.3	-50	0.230	31	+40	
1069	Nov. 23-24, 1917	0.85	-37	0	27.6	-49	0.285	14	+15	Jan., 1916.
1070	Nov. 25-26, 1914	0.84	-11	0	33.7	-39	0.190	17	+30	Oct. 11, 1917.
1233	Mar. 17-18, 1917	0.86	-23	0	50.9	-11	..	22	0	June, 1918.
	Feb. 19-20, 1917	0.87	-33	0	48.3	-22	0.280	27	+10	
	26-27, 1917	0.85	-28	0	48.3	-22	0.220	27	+30	
	Mar. 5- 6, 1917	0.84	-29	0	51.3	-18	0.185	26	0	
	12-13, 1917	0.86	-24	0	50.1	-20	0.245	29	+45	
	19-20, 1917	0.87	-24	0	50.1	-20	0.225	20	+35	
	26-27, 1917	0.86	-27	0	47.2	-24	0.160	22	+30	
1259	Mar. 31-Apr. 1, 1917	0.90	-22	0	49.4	-33	0.185	19	+ 5	Nov. 19, 1917.
1378	Nov. 9-10, 1917	0.88	-21	0	30.6	-45	..	26	0	April, 1920.
	13-14, 1917	0.85	-29	+	30.6	-45	..	22	..	
1012[2]	Oct. 23-24, 1917	0.84	..	0	27.0	-36	0.165	29	+ 5	Jan. 22, 1919.
	Dec. 1- 2, 1917	0.85	..	+	25.7	-39	..	29	..	
1213[3]	Feb. 7- 8, 1917	0.91	..	0	31.2	-45	0.250	28	0	Feb., 1920.
	Mar. 1- 2, 1917	0.84	..	0	32.2	-44	0.240	..	+55	
	14-15, 1917	0.84	..	0	32.7	-43	0.230	..	+10	
	Apr. 4- 5, 1917	0.91	..	0	32.5	-43	..	..	+20	

[1] Two observations averaged 57 per cent below maximum weight, yet only 24 per cent below standard weight.

[2] Metabolism of Case No. 1012, when compared with metabolism of a series of Girl Scouts studied at the Nutrition Laboratory shows an almost steady fall from +22 per cent on October 23–24 to +15 per cent on December 1–2.

[3] Metabolism of Case No. 1213 varied on the same basis from 0 on February 7–8 to –8 per cent on March 1–2, rising to +12 per cent on March 14–15, with remaining values between these extremes.

represented emaciation is better evidenced by the percentage variation from the normal standard. The diabetics included in this research had an average minimum weight of 18 per cent below the normal standard, but the adults with high quotients in Table 116 were 29 per cent below standard and the girl diabetics 41 per cent below standard.

In this connection one might also refer to Table 104 in which it is shown that after June, 1914, progressive lowering of the body weight was accompanied by a progressive lowering of metabolism and a progressive rise of the respiratory quotient and excretion of urinary nitrogen. From observations made upon mild, moderate, and severe cases before and after June, 1914, it was found that the quantity of nitrogen in the urine upon the day preceding the observation, and upon the observation day as well, was comparatively large. The average quantity of nitrogen in the urine for all the diabetics after June, 1914, for both days was about the usual normal figure, 0.175 gram per kilogram body weight, but in this series (Table 116) of experiments with high quotients, the nitrogen in the urine was notably in excess, especially for the severe cases.

Acidosis was usually absent. In 8 of the observations with the severe cases it was present in moderate degree, and in 4 to a slight degree.

The energy in the diet preceding the observations was low in contrast to the high diets which preceded the very low quotients. With only 3 of the 18 observations with adult severe cases, for which the data regarding the preceding diet are available, did the energy exceed 30 calories per kilogram body weight during a period of several days before the experimental day. The loss of weight and the condition of these cases, however, is not so much to be attributed to the diet at this particular period as to the prolonged low diets or unselected diets during earlier stages of the disease.

The carbohydrate balances for the preceding day were positive, as a rule, but with the adult severe cases and the girl diabetics no instance occurred in which the positive balance exceeded 60 grams, and it was usually but half this amount. These meager balances rule out the possibility of explaining the high quotients by the carbohydrate intake.

Regrettably few observations were made of the non-protein nitrogen in the blood, and they are therefore omitted from Table 116, but the few values obtained indicate an excess. As there was no reason for nitrogen retention, evidence favors the theory that excessive protein katabolism was going on and that the nitrogenous portion of the molecule was being retained instead of excreted. It is, however, inconceivable that these high quotients should continue for long if due to protein katabolism, because this would result in an excessive retention of non-protein nitrogen and would terminate in early death from toxemia. If death did not occur, it would mean that the respiratory quotient had fallen and the patient was taking a diet with fat which in such severe diabetes would eventually end in death from coma. Clinically, the above reasoning is borne out by the subsequent histories of these patients. Therefore, it should not be considered that a low quotient alone is of grave significance in diabetes, for an extremely high quotient may be equally hazardous for the patient.

The values obtained for the blood fat, although meagre in number, show that an excessive quantity was present in the circulating blood. The meaning of this is not clear. It is true that unusual quantities of fat have been reported in the blood of fasting individuals, and perhaps these large amounts signify no more than this. On the other hand, the body fat is constantly being drawn upon for body needs. Bloor[1] writes:

"In fasting it (the lipoid level) may or may not be disturbed, depending apparently on the nutritional condition of the subject, or rather perhaps on the availability of the stored fat, since it is apparently the case that fat may be more or less loosely stored, with the result that the stimulus of hunger may produce an excessive or merely adequate outflow, depending on the nature of the storage. It is significant that the increase in blood lipoids in fasting takes place only in the first days, and after that the lipoid content remains constant or slowly diminishes till the death of the animal."

Under such circumstances the passage of fat from the tissues into the blood is constantly taking place and not intermittently as after a meal, yet such high values for blood fat as those here recorded are seldom found. This explanation is, therefore, hardly satisfactory. Neither is the evidence satisfactory that the sugar in the blood of these patients is being transformed into fat. The data, however, so far as they go, supply some support to this latter idea, for while the blood fat is high, the blood sugar for this type of case is comparatively low. There is just enough hint of these two possibilities, namely, the oxidation of the carbohydrate portion of the protein molecule with the retention of the nitrogenous portion and the conversion of carbohydrate into fat, to warrant seriously pursuing the study of other cases along these lines.

A mild case of diabetes may have a high respiratory quotient without any loss of body weight. A severe case of diabetes can have a high respiratory quotient only when the loss of weight is marked, but an extremely severe case of diabetes presents a high respiratory quotient only when the loss of weight is extraordinary,

---

[1] Bloor: Physiol. Reviews, 1922, **2**, 92.

and even then the respiratory quotient will not rise quite so high as that of the other groups. A high postabsorptive respiratory quotient in an extremely severe case of diabetes is only attained when the caloric intake is extremely low.

(e) **The Respiratory Quotient in Relation to the Different Types of Severity.**—In the earlier period the diabetics of mild and moderate severity had an average respiratory quotient of 0.76, while those of the severe type had the lower average quotient of 0.73. On the other hand, with the diabetics after June, 1914, in the three groups of mild, moderate, and severe, the average quotient was the same for all degrees of severity; i. e., 0.78. These figures are significant, because they show the profound difference in the condition of the patients before and after June, 1914. While all three types of severity were observed in both epochs, yet after June, 1914, something took place which prevented the patients of a severe type from having a lower quotient than those of the milder types.

An explanation of the difference in the average respiratory quotient of 0.73 for all cases before, and 0.78 for all cases after June, 1914, may be the character of the diet, or perhaps we may better say the character of the diet and its utilization. Prior to June, 1914, it is possible that less carbohydrate was given, but at any rate less carbohydrate was utilized than after June, 1914. Conversely, prior to June, 1914, a much greater quantity of fat was given which, like the carbohydrate, was not well utilized, a considerable proportion being excreted as β-oxybutyric acid. With Case No. 344, 25 to 50 grams or more of β-oxybutyric acid were excreted almost daily for weeks.[1] The formation of this acid, therefore, would tend to lower the quotient more than even the fat alone. After June, 1914, the smaller quantity of fat consumed, the lesser quantity of β-oxybutyric acid formed, and the greater quantity of carbohydrate oxidized, would all tend to raise the quotient. The data in this table, therefore, may be interpreted as showing that it was not so much the severity of the case which influenced the quotient as the relative quantities of carbohydrate and fat ingested and also oxidized by the patients irrespective of severity.

(f) **The Respiratory Quotient in Relation to the Degree of Acidosis.**—It has been shown in the previous discussion that the principle appears to hold in diabetes that the lower the respiratory quotient falls the higher the metabolism will rise and *vice versa*. Support of this principle should be afforded by a study of the relation of acidosis to the respiratory quotient, because acidosis indicates

---

[1] Benedict and Joslin: Carnegie Inst. Washington, Pub. No. 176, 1912, Table 65, p. 57 *et seq.*

primarily an abnormal fat metabolism, and this is of such a nature that it tends to lower the quotient.

The relationship between the respiratory quotient and acidosis is very plainly shown. With patients free from acidosis (0), there were no records of respiratory quotients below 0.70, and patients with severe acidosis $(+++)$ supply none of the respiratory quotients above 0.83 and but one above 0.79. In general the intermediate quotients of the table also bear out the conclusion that experiments upon patients free from acidosis gave high respiratory quotients, and that as the acidosis increased the respiratory quotient decreased. It is thus seen that although the metabolism varied markedly in the two periods before and after June, 1914 and the respiratory quotients were notably higher after June, 1914, yet the relation between acidosis and the respiratory quotient holds for both epochs. Increasing acidosis was always accompanied by a falling respiratory quotient. It is also significant that 49 observations upon patients with severe acidosis before June, 1914, gave a respiratory quotient of 0.72, and that this is exactly the average quotient of the 17 observations upon patients after June, 1914, with similar acidosis. The definite relation between acidosis and respiratory quotient is thus very clearly demonstrated and incidentally the dependence of acidosis upon the fat metabolism.

TABLE 117.—RELATIONSHIPS BETWEEN RESPIRATORY QUOTIENT, METABOLISM AND ACIDOSIS IN POSTABSORPTIVE EXPERIMENTS WITH DIABETICS BEFORE AND AFTER JUNE, 1914.

Range in respiratory quotient.	Before June, 1914. No. of experiments with acidosis.				After June, 1914. No. of experiments with acidosis.			
	0	+	++	+++	0	+	++	+++
All cases:								
0.64–0.69 . .	..	..	6	10	..	2	5	5
0.70–0.75 . .	8	9	31	34	10	25	57	11
0.76–0.79 . .	9	2	6	5	25	21	36	2
0.80–0.83 . .	2	..	2	..	36	20	14	1
0.84–0.90 . .	..	1	2	..	27	6	6	
0.91–0.94 . .	..	..	..	..	7			
Average respiratory quotient:								
All cases . .	0.76	0.75	0.73	0.72	0.81	0.77	0.76	0.72
Percentage variation in metabolism of severe cases[1] . . .	+9	+12	+15	+12	−19	−14	−11	+2

[1] Group confined to cases compared with H. and B. standard.

Shaffer[1] has clarified the whole subject of acidosis both in normals and diabetics. He has calculated the respiratory quotients for total glucose and fatty acid by subtracting from the total CO_2 and O_2 the amounts corresponding to the metabolism of the non-carbohydrate quota of protein during the respiration period. He has constructed a table which exhibits these fatty acid: glucose respiratory quotients. Along with these he gives the per cent of calories from glucose and fatty acid and the molecular ratio of the mixture burned. According to his calculations: "*A total respiratory quotient of 0.76 indicates the oxidation of a metabolic mixture made up of approximately equimolecular amounts of ketogenic substances (fatty acids or ketogenic amino-acids), and of antiketogenic derivatives of amino-acids, glycerol, or carbohydrate, expressed in terms of glucose.* Expressed in the same terms, a respiratory quotient of 0.73 indicates approximately 2 molecules of ketogenic to 1 of antiketogenic substance in the mixture; while a quotient of 0.8 indicates only 0.5 molecule of ketogenic to 1 of antiketogenic glucose equivalent.

"With these values in mind we may inspect any respiratory data and provided we assume that the latter are truly representative of metabolic reactions, the ketogenic ratio of the subject may be determined. . . .

"After an examination of many experiments by others as well as by ourselves there appears to be no doubt that the mixture in all subjects, *at the threshold of ketonuria* is, according to respiratory data, that which corresponds to *equimolecular* mixtures of ketogenic and antiketogenic substances, *the latter being calculated in terms of glucose equivalents.*"

Shaffer has analyzed the data accumulated for Case No. 740, of our series and previously published as an example of acidosis disappearing during fasting, and has added to our data the calculations of the ketogenic ratio. These are shown in Table 118.

TABLE 118.—SEVERE DIABETIC WITH DECREASING ACIDOSIS ON FASTING (CASE 740).

Date.	Total R. Q.	Ketogenic ratio.	Total hydroxy-butyric acid excreted, gm.	Harris and Benedict.[2]	Nitrogen.
April 15–16	0.72	3.2	24.9	− 3	16.5
16–17	0.73	2.1	18.9	− 1	16.2
17–18	0.72	3.2	11.8	− 4	9.6
18–19	0.74	1.9	11.0	− 8	8.1
19–20	0.76	1.0	7.9	−10	6.7
21–22	0.75	1.2	6.5	−14	7.9
24–25	0.74	1.9	5.4	−16	9.1
27–28	0.75	1.4	4.7	−13	7.4
May 1	0.76	1.0	4.1	−19	7.6

[1] Shaffer: Jour. Biol. Chem., 1921, **49**, 143.
[2] Added to Shaffer's table by E. P. J.

The acidosis decreased but did not entirely disappear with the rising quotient, since when a respiratory quotient of 0.76 was reached the total β-oxybutyric acid excreted still amounted to 4.1 grams. Shaffer explains this with the assumption that the actual metabolic quotient of the subject was really below 0.76. This is possible, but perhaps it may be explained by the fact that the 4.1 grams hydroxybutyric acid represented acid for the twenty-four hours immediately preceding the experiment. At the actual moment of the experiment the acidosis might have been absent or nearly so. Shaffer continues:

"It is evident from an analysis of Joslin's data (not included in our table) that the gradual rise of the respiratory quotient, the lowering of the ketogenic ratio which that rise indicates, and the decline of the acidosis, were not caused by any increase in sugar burning power but were caused by the decrease in total metabolism resulting from the fast, and in the amount of ketogenic material (fat and protein) in the metabolic mixture. The metabolism of ketogenic substances was merely slowed down by undernutrition to the point where it no longer markedly overbalanced the already low rate at which the body was able to provide antiketogenic substance for 'neutralization.' This appears to the writer to be the probable explanation of the beneficial effect of fasting and undernutrition in causing a decrease of diabetic acidosis."

The variations in metabolism and the nitrogen values of the day of the observation are added to this table as abstracted by Shaffer. The fall in metabolism with fasting is well shown. It would be easy to ascribe it to the nitrogen alone.

(*g*) **The Respiratory Quotient in Relation to Pulse-rate of Diabetics.** —Like the metabolism, the pulse-rate in diabetes varies with the respiratory quotient. This is evident for the entire period of the research. As the respiratory quotients rise, the pulse-rates successively decrease. With quotients of 0.91 and over, the lowest average pulse-rate (60) was encountered. When the pulse-rate averaged 70, the range in respiratory quotient was 0.64 to 0.69.

(*h*) **The Respiratory Quotient in Relation to the Glycosuria of the Preceding Twenty-four Hours.** —When the sugar in the urine amounted to 26 grams or more in the twenty-four hours, the respiratory quotient was approximately 0.73; when the urine was sugar-free, or nearly sugar-free, the average respiratory quotient was 0.76 to 0.79; but with quantities of urinary sugar of 200 grams or more, the respiratory quotient was sometimes 0.75 or above, indicating that a great excess of carbohydrate in the diet was accompanied by the oxidation of at least a portion of it.

(*i*) **The Respiratory Quotient in Relation to Blood Sugar and Blood Fat.** —It would be easy to give undue importance to the relation

18

brought out between blood sugar and the respiratory quotient. The blood sugar is an index of the severity of the disease, and with increasing severity there is usually an increase in the percentage of sugar. On the other hand, after prolonged inanition there may be a terminal stage in which the blood sugar falls.

TABLE 119.—RELATION OF AMOUNT OF SUGAR IN URINE TO RESPIRATORY QUOTIENT OF DIABETICS IN POSTABSORPTIVE EXPERIMENTS.

Sugar in urine of preceding 24 hours, gm.	Before June, 1914.		After June, 1914.		Before and after June, 1914.	
	No. of experimental days.	Average respiratory quotient.	No. of experimental days.	Average respiratory quotient.	No. of experimental days.	Average respiratory quotient.
0	5	0.76	161	0.79	166	0.79
1– 5	4	0.77	30	0.78	34	0.78
6– 25	9	0.74	40	0.76	49	0.75
26– 50	11	0.73	11	0.76	22	0.74
51–100	33	0.73	18	0.76	51	0.74
101–452	38[1]	0.73[1]	5[2]	0.75[2]	43	0.73

With the severe diabetics when the respiratory quotient was low (0.69 to 0.73), the blood sugar averaged 0.27 per cent. When the respiratory quotient was high (0.80 to 0.83) the percentage of blood sugar had fallen to 0.22. When it was still higher, *i. e.*, between 0.84 and 0.94, the average percentage of blood sugar was even lower, or 0.2. Although certain exceptions to this general relationship can be found in each group, the study of the blood sugar in severe cases of diabetes confirms the conclusions regarding all cases of diabetes in showing that a low respiratory quotient is accompanied by a high percentage of blood sugar, and a high respiratory quotient by a significantly lower, though not normal, percentage of blood sugar.

These data give no encouragement to the practise sometimes followed of administering carbohydrates to diabetics when the blood sugar is high.

When carbohydrate is burned in the body, the respiratory quotient approaches 1, but when fat is consumed it falls toward 0.71. One would naturally expect, therefore, a tendency toward a high quotient with a high percentage of carbohydrate in the blood and a low quotient with a high percentage of fat in the blood. It has already been found that, so far as carbohydrate is concerned, the reverse is true, for the higher the percentage of sugar is in the blood, the lower is the respiratory quotient. A like reversal is found in the relation between the quotient and the blood fat.

When the blood fat was essentially normal (between 0.59 and 0.75 per cent) the average respiratory quotient was 0.77, but when

[1] Range of sugar values in this group before June, 1914, was 102 to 452 grams.
[2] Range of sugar values in this group after June, 1914, was 102 to 170 grams.

the blood fat was above normal and between 1.26 and 2 per cent in 10 analyses, the average respiratory quotients were 0.88, 0.85 and 0.85. An exception to the general trend is the average quotient for 6 analyses when the fat in the blood was 2.01 per cent or over, for here the respiratory quotient fell again to 0.78.

TABLE 120.—RELATION BETWEEN RESPIRATORY QUOTIENT IN POSTABSORPTIVE EXPERIMENTS AND PERCENTAGE OF SUGAR IN THE BLOOD OF DIABETICS.

Range in respiratory quotient.	Number of experiments with percentage of sugar in the blood ranging from:					Total number of experiments.
	0.05–0.11	0.12–0.20	0.21–0.30	0.31–0.40	0.41–0.43	
0.64–0.69 . .	0	2	1	0	0	3
0.70–0.75 . .	2	23	33	17	2	77
0.76–0.79 . .	2	31	31	3	0	67
0.80–0.83 . .	2	24	19	4	0	49
0.84–0.90 . .	2	13	14	2	0	31
0.91–1.00 . .	0	3	3	0	0	6
All experiments .	8	96	101	26	2	233
Average respiratory quotient .	0.80	0.79	0.78	0.76	0.71	

An increased amount of fat in the blood accompanying a high quotient, therefore, implies that the fat is being transported rather than burned. The questions now arise for investigation whether the increased fat in the blood is due to the intake of fat in the food, whether it comes from the tissues, or whether it is being formed from carbohydrate or even protein. Inconsistencies appear in the table which studies arranged with design should clear away. The investigation of the respiratory quotient when the blood fat is high is a fruitful field for work. As a rule increased fat in the blood signifies acidosis and with acidosis the respiratory quotient is low.

TABLE 121.—RELATION OF FAT IN THE BLOOD TO RESPIRATORY QUOTIENT IN POSTABSORPTIVE EXPERIMENTS WITH DIABETICS (AFTER JUNE, 1914).

Percentage of fat in the blood.	No. of observations.	Average respiratory quotient.
0.59–0.75	16	0.77
0.76–1.00	26	0.78
1.01–1.25	23	0.79
1.26–1.50	5	0.88
1.51–1.75	3	0.85
1.76–2.00	2	0.85
2.01+	6	0.78
All determinations of blood fat	81	0.79

12. **General Factors Influencing the Normal Metabolism.**—
Before the presentation of various data obtained with diabetic
patients upon their metabolism after the ingestion of food, certain
considerations are here recorded upon metabolism in general which
will help in their interpretation.

The knowledge acquired regarding metabolism is of such recent
origin that the most fundamental facts relating to it are often overlooked.   Among these is its extraordinarily labile character.   When
one considers the varying circumstances which occur in the waking
hours of a man, it is inconceivable that the metabolism with any
two individuals should be exactly alike.   Even in sleep[1] the metabolism varies with the individual.   More influences tend to raise
the metabolism under normal conditions than to depress it.   The
chief of these are exercise and food.

(*a*) **Factors Increasing Metabolism.**—(1) *Exercise.*—Although re-
clining in an easy chair[2] may not appreciably increase the heat-
production of the human organism over that obtained with the
body in a horizontal position, yet the simple maintenance of an
upright position will raise the metabolism 10 per cent.   This
statement is likewise applicable to diabetics as was shown in the
two previous monographs on metabolism in diabetes.   Walking
raises the metabolic rate still more, the increase, as demonstrated
in the Nutrition Laboratory,[3] varying between 100 and 800 per
cent according to the rate of walking.   Experiments also conducted in the Nutrition Laboratory upon a professional bicycle
rider have shown that under extreme conditions the increase due
to muscular effort might amount to more than ten times the normal
metabolism, or 1000 per cent.[4]   The total metabolism of a normal
individual engaged in a sedentary occupation may be estimated
as 25 to 30 per cent above the basal level and for the inactive
diabetic at 20 per cent above his basal metabolism.

(2) *Increase in Metabolism Due to Ingestion of Food*—The changes
in the metabolism produced by food are not so sensational as those
just cited as a result of exercise.   They are, however, very considerable and, furthermore, continue for a relatively longer period.
This last consideration is one of no mean importance.   Whereas,
following exercise the metabolism returns to essentially a normal
(basal) level in a comparatively few minutes, hours are required
before the normal is reached after food.   For this reason the total
caloric excess above the basal metabolism produced by a meal of
600 to 800 calories may be the equivalent of a climb up the Washing-

---

[1] Benedict: Carnegie Inst., Washington, Pub. No. 203, 1915, p. 343.
[2] Soderstrom, Meyer and DuBois: Arch. Int. Med., 1916, **17**, 872.
[3] Benedict and Murschhauser: Carnegie Inst., Washington, Pub. No. 231, 1915.
Smith: Carnegie Inst., Washington, Pub. No. 309, 1922.
[4] Benedict and Cathcart: Carnegie Inst., Washington, Pub. No. 187, 1913.

ton Monument (168 meters high, with a requirement of 80 calories), and the excess of calories following a light breakfast might suffice to carry the subject to the top of the monument on Bunker Hill, 67.1 meters high. The effect of the ingestion of protein upon the metabolism may not cease for twelve or more hours,[1] that of fat continues for a somewhat shorter period, while with a meal of carbohydrate food, the metabolism usually reaches its maximum within two hours, and then rapidly falls.[2]

Two dimensions, as it were, must, therefore, be considered in estimating the effect of food, namely, the average height which the metabolism reaches above the basal metabolism and the length of time during which the increase persists. From these data the total accrual of heat may be determined. The heat due to basal metabolism subtracted from the total heat obtained in the period of increment after the ingestion of food gives the *total heat increment*. If this total heat increment is compared with the caloric value of the meal, *i. e.*, fuel value—the resulting percentage represents the *cost of digestion*. The highest point which the metabolism reaches after the administration of food is known as the *peak effect* of that food, and this same term is sometimes applied to the change in respiratory quotient. For example, the total heat production following the ingestion of 100 grams of levulose by a healthy subject[3] was 379 calories, covering a period of about five and a half hours. The basal metabolism for this length of time was 343 calories and the difference between the two, or 36 calories, represents the *total heat increment*. The energy of the levulose was 379 calories. Dividing the total heat increment of 36 calories by the caloric value of the meal (379 calories), one obtains 9 per cent, which represents the *cost of digestion* of the meal. The metabolism reached its highest point, or 18 per cent above the basal metabolism, two hours after the ingestion of levulose, and this maximum increase therefore represents the *peak* effect of the meal. About one hour after the ingestion of the food, the respiratory quotient attained a maximum of 1.03, or the *peak* effect.

The results obtained in a study[4] of the increase in the metabolism of healthy individuals following the ingestion of different classes of food materials are summarized in Table 122. A number of the

[1] Benedict and Carpenter: Carnegie Inst., Washington, Pub. No. 261, 1918.
[2] The rate of decrease is to a considerable extent dependent upon the rate of absorption from the stomach. Even with a pure carbohydrate like glucose, this is most variable, as Fitz reported at the American Society for Clinical Investigation, May, 1922.
[3] Benedict and Carpenter: Carnegie Inst., Washington, Pub. No. 261, p. 212, 1918, Table 141.
[4] Ibid., 1918, Pub. No. 261.

experiments, especially those with protein foods, were not continued long enough to obtain the full period of increment. The figures may, therefore, be considered in some cases as below the actual percentage increases.

TABLE 122.—EFFECTS OF FOOD UPON THE METABOLISM IN HEALTH.

Kind of food.	Energy (fuel value) of food.		Period of increment observed in experiment, hours.	Increase in heat production over basal.		Cost of digestion, per cent.
	Average, calories.	Range, calories.		Average, per cent.	Average maximum, per cent.	
Carbohydrate foods .	526	280–1562	1½–8	10	16	6
Protein	434	168–1305	2–8	12	19	13
Fat	956	666–1362	3–8	6	11	3
Mixed diets:						
Mixed meals . .	998	468–1731	3½–4	16	26	5
Beefsteak, bread .	431	399– 480	5	10˙	17	10
Beefsteak and pota-						
to chips . . .	518	425– 676	3–4½	10	16	5
Milk	392	358– 444	4–6	9	14	8
Specific foods:						
Carbohydrate:						
Starch:						
Bananas . .	406	403– 409	3–4	11	19	6
Pop-corn . .	822	796– 847	8	8	13	7
Rice (boiled) .	432	432	4	1	6	2
Sugars:						
Dextrose . .	354	286– 385	2–5	7	14 .	5
Levulose . .	359	280– 384	1½–5½	9	15	7
Sucrose . .	384	295– 756	1½–6	11	18	6
Lactose . .	380	374– 385	3–4½	9	14	5
Maltose-dex-						
trose mixture	992	449–1382	3–8	12	19	6
Protein:						
Beefsteak . .	486	221–1305	2–8	14	21	12
Fat:						
Cream . . .	956	666–1362	3–8	6	11	3

From these data it would appear that an ordinary sized meal of carbohydrate food may increase the heat production over basal on the average 10 per cent, with an average maximum increase of 16 per cent. As the result of a meal of protein the heat production was increased on the average 12 per cent with an average maximum of 19 per cent, while after a meal of fat the average and maximum increases were 6 and 11 per cent. With the specific foods studied, the metabolism increased with starches from 1 to 11 per cent with a range in average maximum from 6 to 19 per cent. With pure carbohydrates (sugars) the average increase was from 7 to 12 per cent and the average maximum increase from 14 to 19 per cent. Beefsteak increased the metabolism on the average 14 per cent with an average maximum of 21 per cent, while the average increment following the taking of cream was 6 per cent and the average maximum 11 per cent. Ordinary mixed meals raised the heat production on the average 16 per cent with an average maximum of 26 per cent; beefsteak and bread or beefsteak and potato chips gave an average increase of 10 per cent with an average maximum of 16 and 17 per cent. With milk these increases were 9 and 14 per cent, respectively. If the amounts ingested are limited to an energy content of 1000 calories, no great variation is found in these percentages.

The estimated cost of digestion for the pure carbohydrates (sugars) ranged from 5 to 7 per cent, for starches from 2 to 7 per cent, for protein foods 13 per cent, for fat 3 per cent, for milk 8 per cent, and for mixed meals 5 per cent.

The mechanical act of eating is in itself an expense. Thus, the drinking of more than 500 cc of cold water may affect the metabolism, which has been known to rise in consequence as much as 16 per cent, though the average increase in 11 observations was but 3 per cent. Chewing may cause a rise of 17 per cent. Beef-tea and coffee increase the metabolism, coffee increasing it considerably.

The ingestion of a *large* cupful of *strong* coffee increases the metabolism about 8 per cent for several hours.

(*b*) **Factors Decreasing the Metabolism.** — A decrease in the metabolism is known to take place normally as a result of undernutrition and is considerable. A decrease also occurs during normal sleep. In the experiments upon a fasting man, conducted by the Nutrition Laboratory, the basal metabolism at the end of the thirty-one days of fasting had been lowered to 14 per cent below standard.[1] The actual decrease in calories was 408 calories, or 27 per cent. Subsequent observations by the Nutrition Laboratory upon two groups of students (Squad A and Squad B) in the International Young Men's Christian Association College at Springfield,[2] who were subjected to a loss in body weight of 10.5 per cent for Squad A, and 6.5 per cent for Squad B in eighteen weeks, and three weeks, respectively, showed a decrease in metabolism of 19 per cent for both groups.

The metabolism of a neurasthenic man studied by Magnus-Levy[3] was 33 per cent below standard, an actual fall of 44 per cent. His weight was 30 per cent below normal. Undernutrition with coincident loss of weight, therefore, is a very important factor in

[1] Benedict: Carnegie Inst., Washington, Pub. No. 203, 1915.

[2] Benedict, Miles, Roth and Smith: Carnegie Inst., Washington, Pub. No. 280, 1919, p. 228.

[3] Magnus-Levy: Ztschr. f. klin. Med., 1906, **60**, 177.

the lowering of the metabolism. This has already been considered. (See p. 222.)

(c) **Variations in Metabolism Due to Pathological Conditions.**— Under pathological conditions the most notable example of increased metabolism is in hyperthyroidism.[1] Here the increase may reach 100 per cent and is frequently as great as 50 per cent. Fever may also cause an increase, as is shown by the report of Carpenter and Benedict[2] on cases of probable mercurial poisoning and by the studies upon typhoid fever patients conducted by Coleman and DuBois.[3] These latter investigators observed that at the height of the fever there was an average increase in the basal metabolism of about 40 per cent above the normal, but in some cases it rose to more than 50 per cent. In malaria Barr and Du Bois[4] found that the heat production increased 100 to 200 per cent during the chill; immediately after the chill it fell to within 20 to 38 per cent of the average basal level. McCann and Barr[5] found the basal metabolism of tuberculous patients may be normal or very slightly above that of normal men of the same size. In 10 cases the variation from average normal was from −3 to +15 per cent. DuBois refers to experiments conducted at the Russell Sage Laboratory which show an increase in metabolism in erysipelas, arthritis, and the fever produced by intravenous injections of protein. Leukemia causes a marked rise in metabolism. This has been observed in lymphatic leukemia by Murphy, Means, and Aub[6] and in myelogenous leukemia by Gunderson.[7]

A lowering in metabolism occurs chiefly in myxedema, and at times the metabolism may fall to 33 per cent below normal. In chronic anemia, when it is profound, the metabolism may sometimes be reduced to 26 per cent below normal.

Aub,[8] in a recent paper upon the relation of the internal secretions to metabolism, has shown that following removal of the thyroid gland the metabolism is lowered. He points out the predominating influence of the thyroid and the adrenal glands upon the total metabolism, considers the mechanism of their action independently, and probably due to thyroxin and adrenalin, respectively.

Attention has already been directed to the decrease in metabolism of the average diabetic since the introduction of undernutrition in 1914. In a patient recently under observation at the New Eng-

---

[1] DuBois, Means and Aub: Arch. Int. Med., 1916, **17**, 915; ibid., 1919, **24**, 645.
[2] Carpenter and Benedict: Am. Jour. Physiol., 1909, **24**, 203.
[3] Coleman and DuBois: Arch. Int. Med., 1915, **15**, 887.
[4] Barr and DuBois: Arch. Int. Med., 1918, **21**, 627.
[5] McCann and Barr: Arch. Int. Med., 1920, **26**, 663.
[6] Murphy, Means and Aub: Arch. Int. Med., 1917, **19**, 890.
[7] Gunderson: Boston Med. and Surg. Jour., 1921, **185**, 785.
[8] Aub: Jour. Am. Med. Assn., 1922, **79**, 95.

land Deaconess Hospital, the metabolism reached the lowest level
I recall for a diabetic; namely, −43 per cent. This patient, Case
No. 866, was 185.9 cm. in height, weighed 90 to 92 pounds, was
thirty-nine years of age. His basal metabolism in the course of
two weeks varied between 765 calories and 930 calories. (See
p. 97.)

(*d*) **Food and the Respiratory Quotient of Normal Individuals.**—
A study of the effect of food upon the total metabolism is incomplete unless the influence which it exerts upon the respiratory
quotient is also given. The average postabsorptive respiratory
quotient of 236 of the 239 individuals upon whom the Harris and
Benedict prediction tables are based was 0.83.[1] Presumably the
diets of these subjects for the previous day were the usual average
diet, namely, carbohydrate 400 to 300 grams, protein 100 to 75
grams, and fat 100 to 50 grams, which when expressed in proportion of calories for each food material would be carbohydrate
58 per cent, protein 14 per cent, fat 28 per cent. The ingestion
of additional carbohydrate immediately before a test would raise
this quotient, because the respiratory quotient of carbohydrate
is 1. Whether the addition of more fat would tend to lower it,
since the respiratory quotient of fat is 0.71 is yet to be proved
for normals, but for diabetics it seems probable. An increase or
decrease in the proportion of protein in the diet would make little
change, since the characteristic quotient for protein is 0.81.

The effect upon the respiratory quotient the morning following
a hearty evening meal, rich in carbohydrate as compared with one
low in carbohydrate, was studied by Benedict, Emmes, and Riche.[2]
In a series of experiments with 7 subjects they found that with an
excessive carbohydrate diet the average respiratory quotient was
0.88, while with a low carbohydrate diet the respiratory quotient
was 0.81. It is seldom, however, that such great changes in the
diet are encountered as were employed by these experimenters with
their subjects.

On the other hand, there is no doubt that Bernstein and Falta
were right in emphasizing the importance of standard diets before
metabolism tests and in recommending that these be continued
for several days. This criterion was fulfilled at the Russell Sage
Laboratory in the observations with Cyril K. One of the chief
values of the recent work of Wilder, Boothby, and Beeler[3] is that
this procedure was carried out in their 44 tests made with Bessie
B., a diabetic. (See Table 123.) Between May 19 and May 26,

---

[1] Harris and Benedict: Carnegie Inst., Washington, Pub. No. 279, 1919, pp. 40–47,
inclusive. Quotients can be calculated from data for carbon dioxide and oxygen.
[2] Benedict, Emmes and Riche: Am. Jour. Physiol., 1911, **27**, 383.
[3] Wilder, Boothby and Beeler: Loc. cit., p. 230.

the patient was upon a constant diet of carbohydrate 43 grams, protein 27 grams, fat 151 grams, equivalent to 55 calories per kilogram of body weight. The metabolism at the beginning of this period was −22 per cent as compared with the DuBois standard, the carbon dioxide in the blood 49 and 50 volumes per cent, and the acidosis slight. In the middle of the period the average metabolism had risen to −12 per cent with an increase in acidosis as shown by the carbon dioxide in the blood of 45 volumes per cent. At the conclusion of the period the metabolism was −11 per cent and the acidosis again, higher for the carbon dioxide in the blood was 41 volumes per cent. If the tests after the first two days of dieting were alone considered, the influence of acidosis in raising the metabolism in this patient would have been overlooked.

TABLE 123.—THE ADVANTAGE OF CONSTANT DIETS OF SEVERAL DAYS' DURATION IN METABOLISM EXPERIMENTS. COMPILED FROM WILDER, BOOTHBY AND BEELER.[1]

Date.	Carbo-hydrate, gm.	Protein, gm.	Fat, gm.	Calories per kg.	Acidosis.				Variation of metabolism from DuBois standard, per cent.
					Urine.		Blood.		
					Acetone bodies as acetone, gm.	Ammonia nitro-gen, gm.	Acetone bodies as acetone per 100 cc mgm.	Carbon dioxide, vol., per cent.	
May 10–14	16	10	83	28	2.0	0.6	19	59	−22
15–18	15	31	109	38	3.2	0.5	26	49	−20[2]
19	43	27	151	55	5.3	0.6	..	..	−22
20	43	27	151	55	3.0	0.6	..	..	−20
21	43	27	151	55	2.4	0.6	..	..	−17
22	43	27	151	..	4.4	0.6	30	50	
23	43	27	151	55	3.5	0.6	..	..	−10
24	43	27	151	55	6.2	0.6	25	45	−12
25	43	27	151	55	6.5	0.8	..	..	−14
26	43	27	151	55	6.5	1.1	..	..	−15
27	0	0	0	0	0.6[3]	0.7	38	41	−11

In the discussion of the series of observations upon food with diabetics one must remember the many opportunities for unusual

[1] Wilder, Boothby and Beeler: Loc. cit., p. 230.

[2] For computing this average, the basal metabolism (−22 per cent) for May 19 is included because the value represents the result for the diet of this period.

[3] This is a decrease of 91 per cent in twenty-four hours and a value lower than that obtained on any day between March 31 and July 12. (I am assured it is correct.)

quotients which have previously been mentioned. (See p. 254.) The respiratory quotient of an individual will rise when (1), an additional proportion of carbohydrate is burned in the metabolism; when (2), β-oxybutyric acid and its derivatives are burned, if the basal respiratory quotient is below 0.75; and when (3), the quotient is under 0.81, it will rise when additional protein is oxidized; the respiratory quotient will also rise, even if the carbohydrate is not burned, provided (4) the carbohydrate is changed into fat, because in this process an excess of carbon dioxide is set free and the numerator of the respiratory quotient fraction $\dfrac{CO_2}{O_2}$ is thereby increased; the conversion of protein to fat (5), will accomplish the same result, though in much smaller degree; it is also conceivable that (6), a rise of the respiratory quotient above 0.81 would take place if the carbohydrate portion of the protein molecule was burned and the non-carbohydrate portion retained in the body. There are but two possibilities by which the respiratory quotient may rise above 1. These are by the conversion of carbohydrate into fat, or of protein into fat.

The respiratory quotient will fall when the percentage of carbohydrate in the diet which is oxidized decreases, and also when there is incomplete oxidation of fat. For further discussion of this question see p. 262.

Finally, great caution must be exercised in the interpretation of respiratory quotients. An uncertain element is introduced into the computations of the respiratory quotient when the carbohydrate ingested is not oxidized immediately but is stored as glycogen to be drawn upon later from time to time for oxidation. The mere storage of carbohydrate, however, would not affect the respiratory quotient. Fat may also be stored and not immediately burned. The storage capacity for protein is most uncertain.

This question of the storage of carbohydrate, protein, and fat in the body, particularly in the liver, greatly complicates the problem. This organ, which contains about one-half to one-fifth of the glycogen in the entire body, may vary in its content of glycogen from a negligible amount to 10 per cent,[1] even upon a protein diet, and this percentage is as great as after feeding carbohydrate alone. These figures relate to the dog. The liver normally contains less than 6 per cent of fat; in starvation the quantity may amount to 10 per cent. When Pflüger[2] fed a dog for thirty days exclusively on large quantities of fat, at the end of this period the liver contained 45 per cent of fat and no glycogen.

[1] At the annual meeting of the New York State Medical Society, May 25, 1923, Macleod stated that in the depancreatized dog with carbohydrate feeding and insulin even 20 per cent of glycogen had been found in the liver.

[2] Pflüger: Arch. f. d. ges. Physiol., 1907, **119**, 123.

The antagonism in the liver between glycogen and fat, formerly supposed to exist, vanishes before Macleod's statement that following the administration of insulin both exist together. The metabolism of protein is well known to be in large measure affected by the storage of fat in the body. When the fat in a fasting organism is abundant, protein metabolism is spared and the influence upon it of the ingestion of 100 to 300 grams of fat has been shown to be slight. This is, however, in the healthy animal, not in the diabetic. On the contrary, when the store of fat is very, very greatly reduced in the body, protein is drawn upon to excess.

Finally, if carbohydrate and fat are both available to the organism for combustion, the carbohydrate is burned first. Even when the metabolism has been raised by the ingestion of fat, it will be still further raised by the ingestion of carbohydrate.

(e) **The Storage of Carbohydrates in Diabetes.**—It is well known that following a period of fasting large quantities of carbohydrate can be administered to a diabetic without immediately appearing in the urine. The best illustration of this is von Noorden's oatmeal treatment. Thus, Case No. 344 (see p. 574) showed a positive carbohydrate balance of 520 grams when undergoing an oatmeal cure under the direction of Prof. von Noorden, although he never after this cure became sugar-free, despite a rigorous diet, save for occasional days. A more spectacular demonstration is the severe diabetic of Klemperer[1] who took 100 grams of glucose in divided portions during twenty-four hours without its appearing in the urine. More impressive are the observations recorded with levulose in which severe diabetics are shown to assimilate practically all the carbohydrate administered. Our severe cases excreted but 12 per cent of the quantities ingested. Here another problem enters into the situation, because the levulose may or may not be stored as carbohydrate, since transformation into fat is quite probable.

How large a quantity of carbohydrate it is possible for the body to store is really unknown, but its importance is none the less evident. Unless the amount of stored carbohydrate is known, it is unjustifiable to say that the carbohydrate excreted represents a part of that ingested during the same twenty-four hours. All data with reference to the D : N ratio are confused by our ignorance of stored carbohydrate. The influence of carbohydrate so stored in the body upon carbohydrate assimilation or retention, but not necessarily utilization, is also great. Whatever virtue the oatmeal cure possesses, all agree that it depends in major part upon preceding starvation which has tended to exhaust the carbohydrate depots

---

[1] Klemperer: Therapie der Gegenwart, 1911, **52**, 447.

of the body. On the other hand, it is quite possible that the storage of carbohydrate as glycogen in the body may activate the process by which further carbohydrate may be utilized. Roger[1] emphasizes the importance of a storage of glycogen in the liver and the intimate part it takes in the prevention of acidosis. He cites Chevrier as authority for the usefulness of 150 grams of carbohydrate the night before and morning of an operation for the protection of the liver from anesthetics. See Figs. 13 and 14 for illustration of the abnormal storage of glycogen and fat in the diabetic kidney and spleen.

(1) *As Glycogen.*—Carbohydrate is stored in the body in various ways, but most of it is supposed to be in the form of glycogen, and this is divided between the liver and muscles. An old estimate of Bunge that the body contained 400 grams carbohydrate, is roughly approximated by experiments upon fasting men and professional athletes doing severe work without food. This figure may be taken as a fair average, but there are enormous variations. This statement is based upon glycogen which has been shown to be burned in calorimetric experiments; it does not exclude the possibility of some glycogen still remaining in the body. Experiments of fasting men show that they may burn from 93 to 232 grams of glycogen in the first three days of a fast.[2]

In diabetic patients the quantity of glycogen is universally considered to be far below this amount, but Frerichs[3] found, upon puncturing the liver of 2 diabetics, a small amount of glycogen in 1 and a considerable amount in the other, and Külz found 10 to 12 grams glycogen in the liver of a diabetic who had been for a long time on a diabetic diet. Examinations of the tissue removed from the livers of living diabetic patients also show appreciable quantities of glycogen, and it is the experience of pathologists that the organs of diabetic patients contain more than traces of glycogen. It is most unfortunate that no data exist which enable us to determine what this minimum is. It is quite conceivable that although it might be extremely small at any one moment, a small quantity might be continuously formed and destroyed, and the sum of these small quantit es reach a substantial amount in twenty-four hours.

The work of Helly[4] throws light upon the problem. He points out the striking contrast between the constant presence of glycogen in the liver of human diabetes and the very small quantity which

[1] Roger: Presse Medicale, 1922, **30**, 345.

[2] Benedict: The Influence of Inanition on Metabolism, Carnegie Inst., Washington, Pub. 77, 1907, p. 464; A Study of Prolonged Fasting, Carnegie Inst., Washington Pub. 203, 1915, p. 251.

[3] Cit. Nehring and Schmoll: Ztschr. f. klin. Med., 1897, **31**, 59; Pflüger's Archiv, 1876, **13**, 267.

[4] Helly: Ztschr. f. exp. Path. u. Therap., 1914, **15**, 464.

is found in the severe diabetes of depancreatized dogs, yet even in the latter the power of the liver to form or deposit glycogen is shown when levulose is administered. If a milder form of diabetes is produced in the dog more glycogen remains in the body and there is a closer resemblance to human diabetes. Whereas with total removal of the pancreas there was only 0.065 per cent of glycogen in the liver; with partial removal there was 0.3 per cent of glycogen, even though 8 to 10 per cent of sugar remained in the urine. By microscopical examination so considerable a quantity as this appeared small.

2. *As Blood Sugar.*—Sugar is also stored in the body in the form of blood sugar. The normal quantity of sugar in the blood of healthy individuals varies between 0.07 and 0.11 per cent, and for convenience in calculation may be considered 0.1 per cent. This rises quickly after a meal rich in carbohydrates, but soon falls to its former level. Of 191 observations upon 72 of our diabetic patients the percentage of blood sugar varied from 0.45 to 0.07.[1] The percentage of sugar rapidly increased in the blood of diabetics following a carbohydrate meal, but it does not fall as rapidly as in normals.

Certain types of diabetic patients—namely, those with disease of the kidneys—are especially prone to maintain high percentages of sugar in the blood for many days after their urines have become sugar-free. It is impracticable to consider that the percentage of blood sugar is maintained independently of the other tissues in the body because: (1) The percentage is so unstable; (2) there is no constant relation between the sugar in the blood serum and the sugar in the total blood; and (3) because the capacity of the blood for storage of sugar is so slight. Confirmation of the above statements has been afforded by the ingenious experiments of Woodyatt and his co-workers later to be described (see p. 428). If we assume an individual of 70 kilograms body weight and consider that 7 per cent of his weight is made up of blood, we have 4.9 kilograms of blood of which the sugar content is 0.1 per cent. This would amount to 4.9 grams, even taking the highest for the normal individual. Fitz and Bock[2] determined the total sugar in the blood of normal individuals. It varied, but did not exceed 7.5 grams. With 9 diabetics the highest blood sugar content was 15 grams and the highest plasma sugar was 10.78 grams, and should we take a high figure such as that encountered in some diabetics after the administration of food—namely, 0.45 per cent—the total quantity of sugar stored in the blood could not be far from 22 grams. Falta[3]

[1] In a later case, No. 1015, it amounted to 1.37 per cent. (See p. 173.)
[2] Fitz and Bock: Jour. Biol. Chem., 1921, **48**, 313.
[3] Falta: Med. Klinik., 1914, **10**, 9.

has called attention to the slow return of the blood sugar of diabetic patients after a carbohydrate meal to the former sugar level. Kleiner and Meltzer[1] have also beautifully shown this same difference to exist between normal and depancreatized dogs. Whereas the sugar in the blood of normal dogs increases fourfold, namely, from 0.2 per cent to 0.79 per cent, following the injection of 4 grams of dextrose per kilogram body weight, and of depancreatized dogs threefold, from 0.38 per cent before to 1.19 per cent after the injection, the blood sugar of the former returned nearly to normal at the end of an hour and a half, while diabetic dogs then showed 0.86 per cent. It is significant that in these experiments the quantities of sugar excreted in the urine were practically the same.

3. *Other Possible Storehouses for Carbohydrate.*—The small amount of glycogen in the body and the still smaller quantity of blood sugar represent an amount of carbohydrate far too low to account for the phenomena above described in diabetes. Other sources for storage of sugar in the body must be sought, and this has been emphasized by Ivar Bang.[2] If we should assume that the percentage of sugar was the same for all the fluids in the body as in the blood, certain amounts of sugar might be stored in this manner. While such an assumption is not wholly justifiable, it has some basis, for we know that sugar exists in the spinal fluid of diabetes as well as in other fluids. In normal individuals Dr. Jacobsen affirms that he has not found it to follow the blood so closely, but that the opposite was true in his cases of diabetes mellitus. Hopkins[3] has observed in diabetic patients that the reducing substances in the spinal fluid were but slightly less than the blood sugar of the same individuals. These varied from a minimum of 0.074 to a maximum of 0.623 for the spinal fluid and the corresponding values for the blood were 0.077 and 0.66. Notable percentages of sugar, not very different from those in the blood, have been found in pleuritic and ascitic fluids, and Husband[4] found even 0.7 per cent in the amniotic fluid. Yet granted that the assumption of uniform distribution of sugar in the fluids of the body is correct, we cannot increase our storage capacity very much in this way. For example, assuming the total quantity of fluid in the body as 60 per cent of the body weight of 70 kilograms, we have 42 kilograms of body fluid from which we must deduct 4.9 kilograms already reckoned as blood. This leaves us a remainder of 37.1 kilograms of fluid in the body, and using the high figure (0.45 per cent) for blood sugar, the quantity of sugar in this mass of fluid would be only 167 grams.

[1] Kleiner and Meltzer: Proc. Soc. for Exp. Biol. and Med., 1914, **12**, 58.
[2] Ivar Bang: Wiesbaden, 1913.
[3] Hopkins: Am. Jour. Med. Sci., 1915, **150**, 837.
[4] Husband: Loc. cit., Naunyn, p. 190.

This is not enough, relatively, to explain Kleiner and Meltzer's experiment and far less those of Woodyatt.

(f) **The Ingestion of Carbohydrate and the Respiratory Quotients of Normals.**—Before taking up the consideration of the effect of carbohydrate upon diabetics, it will be advantageous to note the influence rather more specifically of carbohydrate upon normal individuals. For this purpose Benedict and Carpenter[1] studied the effect of various sugars upon the respiratory quotient when given to healthy subjects. The amount of carbohydrate administered was 100 grams, or on the average 1.6 grams per kilogram body weight. The average maximum increase in the respiratory quotient for the series of experiments with each sugar follows: The increase in the respiratory quotient with levulose was 0.18, and with sucrose 0.21, in contradistinction to the increase for lactose 0.14, and dextrose 0.12. Such figures suggest that levulose, derived by inversion of the sucrose molecule, may be responsible for the high quotient obtained with sucrose. The actual quotients obtained both with levulose and sucrose rose above 1, this in each instance rising much higher than those obtained with dextrose and lactose. Almost invariably, four hours elapsed before the quotient returned to the basal value, and in some of these experiments it had not returned in six hours. Both Dürig[2] and Lusk[3] have also noted the greater increase in metabolism after levulose than after glucose.

Benedict and Carpenter state: "It is clear that there is a specific property of levulose that is markedly different from dextrose in its effect on the metabolism, both quantitatively and (as is now seen) qualitatively. To what extent this is determined by direct and rapid combustion, intermediary processes in transformation to glycogen or fat, or to the stimulating action of intermediary products may not at present be stated with surety."[4]

It has been pointed out that a rise in respiratory quotient may be due to the substitution of the combustion of carbohydrate for that of protein and fat, and second to the formation of fat from carbohydrate as a result of excessive carbohydrate feeding. The rapid ingestion of 100 grams of carbohydrate makes immediately available 400 calories with which to offset a basal requirement of perhaps 70 calories per hour. The taking of this moderate quantity of carbohydrate would, therefore, logically suffice for the basal requirement during a period of five or six hours. In normal individuals, therefore, whether carbohydrate is oxidized or changed to

[1] Benedict and Carpenter: Carnegie Inst., Washington, 1018, Pub., No. 261, p. 256, Table 183.
[2] Tögel, Brezina and Dürig: Biochem. Ztschr., 1913, **50**, 296.
[3] Lusk: Jour. Biol. Chem., 1915, **20**, 555.
[4] Benedict and Carpenter: Carnegie Inst., Washington, 1928, Pub. No. 261, p. 243.

fat, additional carbon dioxide is being produced and the quotient should be raised for about five hours. If this does not take place, one is forced to conclude that the carbohydrate is being stored as glycogen or, what is equally important, the carbohydrate is being excreted. The only other alternative for an increase in carbon dioxide would be an increase in the total intake of food, but in this event the respiratory quotient would remain the same.

From what has been said in the foregoing pages concerning the administration of food to *normal* individuals and the many possibilities which must be considered in the interpretation of results, it is evident that the problem will become far more intricate when it is desired to learn what takes place when food is given to a patient with so complicated a disease as diabetes. That investigator is over-sanguine who expects to unravel more than a few of the tangled threads by any one series of experiments.

13. **The Ingestion of Levulose by Diabetics.**—Minkowski[1] discovered that levulose diminished the protein metabolism in a diabetic dog, but Mandel and Lusk,[2] as well as von Noorden,[3] were unable to confirm this with a diabetic man. On the other hand, Verzar[4] demonstrated that levulose, when given to a depancreatized dog, raised the respiratory quotient for a considerable period after glucose had failed to do so, though eventually it, too, lost the power.

Tögel, Brezina and Dürig[5] observed that levulose increased the metabolism to a greater degree than glucose, that the increase began earlier, and in their opinion, led more to the formation of fat than glucose. With a patient to whom they gave 30 grams of levulose, in hourly doses, the respiratory quotient was kept at 1 for a long time. They also observed that the respiratory quotient fell for the first few minutes after carbohydrate was given. Külz[6] was apparently the first clinician to advocate seriously the therapeutic use of levulose in diabetes.

Lusk[7] used the oxygen as well as the carbon dioxide in the study of the effect of 50 grams of various sugars, glucose, sucrose and levulose, which he gave to a dog. He noted increases in metabolism, in the order named, of 30 per cent, 34 per cent, and 37 per cent, but only with levulose did any considerable increase persist throughout the fifth and subsequent hours. The respiratory quotients rose to

[1] Minkowski: Arch. f. exp. Path. u. Pharm., 1890, **26**, 371, or 1893, **31**, 85.

[2] Lusk: Science of Nutrition, Philadelphia, 3d Edition, 1917, p. 485.

[3] Cited by Lusk, loc. cit., p. 486.

[4] Verzar: Biochem. Ztschr., 1914, p. 75.

[5] Tögel: Biochem. Ztschr., 1913, **50**, 298.

[6] Külz: Diabetes Mellitus, Marburg, 1874, p. 130. For a summary of the earlier literature see von Noorden, "Metabolism and Practical Medicine," Chicago, 1907, **3**, 635.

[7] Lusk: Jour. Biol. Chem., 1915, **20**, 555.

19

1, 1.02, and 1.02, respectively. There was no increase in the
metabolism and respiratory quotient with lactose and but little
with galactose. Levulose (2.8 grams) appeared in the urine as such
in the levulose experiment and 0.25 gram appeared as sucrose after
the sucrose experiment, but the urine was sugar-free following
glucose. In the light of Folin and Berglund's[1] recent studies upon
blood sugar (see page 297), the question arises whether the particular
dog used in Lusk's investigation might not have had a low levulose
threshold.

Bernstein and Falta[2] gave 100 grams of levulose on three successive days to a diabetic patient. No rise in respiratory quotient is
recorded, but from the text it would appear that the metabolism
tests made were postabsorptive tests and upon the mornings *after*
the levulose was given, too late a period to show results.

The most extensive investigations with levulose have been made
by Johansson. In 1904 he, with Billström and Heijl,[3] gave 100
grams of dextrose, sucrose and levulose to normal individuals and
determined the rise in carbon dioxide expelled as compared with
basal values for succeeding hours. They observed that glucose
increased the carbon dioxide 7 per cent, sucrose 14 per cent and
levulose (93 grams) 15 per cent. They noted that the rapidity of
oxidation of levulose was greater and the rapidity of storage as
glycogen less than for glucose.

In a subsequent article Johansson[4] confirmed the results just
cited. Incidentally, he noted that the increase in carbon dioxide
varied with the rapidity of absorption of the sugars from the gastro-
intestinal tract, and thought he demonstrated quite definitely that
the increase in carbon dioxide varied with the amount of glycogen
stored in the body at the beginning of the experiment. Levulose
increased the excretion of carbon dioxide twice as much as glucose.

He performed several experiments with diabetic patients. In
some instances the ingestion of sugar increased the carbon dioxide
and in others did not, or increased it to a less extent than with
normals. In one diabetic dextrose brought about an increase of
7 per cent in the carbon dioxide elimination, whereas levulose
increased the carbon dioxide elimination 13 per cent. In other
words, the same relation between glucose and levulose was obtained
with this diabetic as with normals.

Loeffler[5] gave 100 grams of levulose to a diabetic patient and at
an interval of seven hours repeated the dose. He observed an
increase in the metabolism with an increase in the respiratory

[1] Folin and Berglund: Jour. Biol. Chem., 1922, **51**, 213.
[2] Bernstein and Falta: Deutsch. Arch. f. klin. Med., 1916, **121**, 95.
[3] Johansson, Billström and Heijl: Skand. Arch. f. Physiol., 1904, **16**, 263.
[4] Johansson: Skand. f. Arch. Physiol., 1908, **21**, 1.
[5] Loeffler: Ztschr. f. klin. Med., 1919, **87**, 309.

quotient, both of which were greater after the second feeding. The increases were not more marked than with glucose but less of the levulose was excreted in the urine.

Fifty-one tests with levulose were carried out with diabetic patients at the Nutrition Laboratory and New England Deaconess Hospital between March 31, 1911, and June 25, 1917, only 3 of these being previous to January 11, 1916. Since that date 17 other tests have been made.

At the time of taking the food the patients were in the post-absorptive state in all instances, except that in 1 case 90 grams of oil had been taken earlier in the day. The total quantity of levulose ingested varied between 28 and 100 grams, and per kilogram body weight between 0.9 gram and 2.5 grams.

(*a*) **Utilization.**—The quantities of levulose ingested were well utilized by the patients. In the two experiments with the mild cases no sugar appeared in the urine after the administration of 1 gram of levulose per kilogram body weight. Almost equally good results were obtained with the 5 moderate cases who received, on the average, 1.2 grams of levulose per kilogram body weight. In the severe group there were 41 experiments with 19 cases. The urines remained sugar-free for the twenty-four hour period in only 9 of these 41 experiments. The average quantity of levulose given in the various experiments with the severe cases was 1.55 grams per kilogram body weight, and 88 per cent of this carbohydrate was assimilated. Thus it is seen that the levulose was nearly all utilized and, if not oxidized, must have been retained in the body in some form. These results help to explain how certain mild cases of diabetes may be able to take foods rich in levulose, such as honey and raisins, with impunity.

(*b*) **Effect Upon the Metabolism.**—The administration of levulose to this series of diabetic patients increased the metabolism in 51 observations on the average by 17 per cent. An increase in the metabolism occurred in each experiment, the least increase being 5 per cent and the greatest increase 32 per cent. This rise in metabolism of the diabetic patients is remarkable, as it was plainly greater than the rise (9 per cent) found in the Nutrition Laboratory with normal subjects under similar conditions. Furthermore, it persisted at a higher level for a greater period of time than with the normal individuals.

In seeking for an explanation of the wide variation in the response of the diabetics to levulose, it was found that it was in part due to the difference in the quantities of levulose given per kilogram body weight. With the lowest amount of levulose, namely, 0.9 to 1.25 grams per kilogram body weight, the average rise in metabolism was 14 per cent, but when 1.8 to 2.5 grams per kilogram body weight were taken by the patient, the average rise in metabolism was 20 per cent.

For the severe cases of diabetes the response to levulose was also directly proportional to the quantities given. With the largest quantity of levulose, 2.5 grams per kilogram body weight, in 9 out of 18 experiments the increase of metabolism varied between 21 and 32 per cent. Thus the severe cases reacted more energetically with a rise in metabolism to levulose than did the normals, and also more than did the moderate or mild diabetics. This might be made of diagnostic value in the differentiation of renal glycosuria from diabetes.

Acidosis is not a factor in the effect which the administration of levulose produces upon the metabolism of diabetic patients. (See Table 124.) This suggests that acidosis itself does not exert as deleterious an influence upon the metabolism of carbohydrate, or at least of levulose, as has generally been thought, and that some other method must be sought to explain the harmful effect of acidosis clinically.

TABLE 124.—EFFECT OF ACIDOSIS UPON THE METABOLISM OF DIABETICS AFTER THE ADMINISTRATION OF LEVULOSE.

Acidosis.	Levulose per kilogram of body weight, gm.	No. of observations.	Increase in heat production, per cent.	Respiratory quotient.		Observations showing.		
				Basal.	After levulose.	Increase.	Decrease.	No change.
+++	1.95	5	17	0.74	0.73	0	4	1
++	1.55	13	19	0.75	0.78	10	2	1
+	1.45	13	15	0.78	0.80	9	3	1
0	1.50	20	16	0.82	0.86	16	2	2
Average	1.55	51	17	0.79	0.81			

(c) **Effect Upon the Respiratory Quotient.**—The wide variation in basal respiratory quotients of the patients who took the levulose afforded opportunity to study its effect under these varying conditions. So far as the observations in this series went, the rise in respiratory quotient after levulose was independent of whether the basal quotient was low or high. Likewise, the increase in heat production over basal after the ingestion of levulose was practically the same at all quotient levels. This is contrary to an analogous line of investigation pursued by Staub. He showed in his work on the blood sugar that a protein fat diet represented by a low respiratory quotient presented an unfavorable substratum for the action of carbohydrate, since the storage of glycogen in the body was depleted. Of course it is possible that in the present series of experiments the amount of glucose formed from levulose was so great that it not only sufficiently filled the reservoirs but afforded sufficient for oxidation, too, but if this were the case one would not expect a rise in the respiratory quotient with small quantities of levulose, but such did take place. All these difficulties are avoided if one assumes that the levulose is first transformed into fat, because in that event the quotient would rise to an equal degree independently of the basal respiratory quotient.

Even if the levulose were not transformed into fat, but burned directly without transformation into glycogen, the rise in respiratory quotient would be explained. An argument against this immediate oxidation, however, is the general depletion of the body in levulose or rather the great capacity which exists in the body for storing levulose, which makes immediate oxidation unnecessary. Apparently, however, immediate oxidation or change into fat does take place even though the capacity for storing more levulose is present.

The average respiratory quotient in the basal control experiments with the diabetics preceding the ingestion of levulose was 0.79 and for the interval during which the metabolism was tested after the ingestion of levulose was 0.81, a rise of but 0.02.

The slight increase in the respiratory quotient after levulose appeared peculiar. This is explained in part because of the different quantities of levulose given per kilogram body weight. When these were investigated, it was found that when the quantity of levulose ingested was below 1.25 grams, the quotient rose 0.02; when between 1.3 and 1.75 grams, it rose 0.03; and when 1.8 grams or more, it rose 0.04. One must remember that only a certain amount of carbohydrate can be absorbed in an hour from the alimentary tract, and this may in part explain the comparatively slight differences for the rise in quotients after varying quantities of levulose. In fact, the normal individuals in the Nutrition Laboratory showed analogous phenomena. The important factor, however, in the elucidation of this apparently slight increase in quotient is that the *quotients above mentioned were average quotients for the entire duration of the experiments and not for individual periods immediately following the ingestion of levulose.* Our data do not show what took place for the first thirty or thirty-five minutes, but they do indicate the results in subsequent half hour periods. In the second half hour these are shown in Table 125, and it will be noted that the chief rise in the respiratory quotient took place in the second[1] half hour and then

---

[1] In Tables 126 and 127 this is more clearly shown than in Table 125.

declined, reaching the basal level in the fifth half hour and thereafter falling below it in subsequent periods. With normals the basal level was not quite reached even at the end of the tenth half hour. The maximum rise followed by a steady fall in the respiratory quotient after the ingestion of levulose is the best proof of its utilization by the body.

TABLE 125.—THE AVERAGE RESPIRATORY QUOTIENT AND THE PERCENTAGE INCREASE IN HEAT-PRODUCTION BEFORE AND AFTER INGESTION OF LEVULOSE ARRANGED IN SUCCESSIVE PERIODS OF TIME.

Kind of experiments.	Average respiratory quotient in,								
	2d half hour.	3d half hour.	4th half hour.	5th half hour.	6th half hour.	7th half hour.	8th half hour.	9th half hour.	10th half hour.
Diabetics:									
Basal[1] . . .	0.79	0.79	0.79	0.79	0.76	0.76			
After levulose .	0.84[2]	0.83[3]	0.81[3]	0.79[3]	0.74[4]	0.72[5]	0.70[6]	0.72[6]	0.69[6]
Percentage increase in heat production .	16	16	18	18	16	9	13	10	10
Normals:									
Basal experiment averages . .	0.88	0.87	0.86	0.85	0.85	0.82	0.86	0.85	0.83
After levulose .	1.04	1.00	0.98	0.97	0.94	0.86	0.93	0.90	0.84
Percentage increase in heat production .	12	14	13	11	7	−2	5	3	1

The increase in heat production after levulose persisted not only for six half hours, which is the customary length of duration of the increase in heat-production with normals under similar conditions, but continued even until the tenth half hour. This marked increase was found to persist throughout the fifth half hour in the average of 47 experiments. In considering the action of levulose with diabetics, therefore, one must bear in mind its prolonged effect in raising the metabolism for even five hours.

The metabolism of Case No. 1196 after levulose rose 41 per cent in the second half hour and 40 per cent in the third half hour. In the subsequent three half hours the increases were, respectively, 20, 36, and 25 per cent. Even to the tenth half hour the metabolism was 10 per cent above the average basal metabolism for this day. An increase in heat production of 41 per cent after the ingestion of

[1] Basal experiments secured preceding 44 of the 51 levulose experiments.
[2] Drawn from 45 experiments.
[3] Drawn from 47 to 51 experiments.
[4] Drawn from 7 experiments.
[5] Based on 2 experiments.
[6] Individual quotients. Case No. 1196.

carbohydrate is an anomaly in health and hitherto unreported in diabetes.

TABLE 126.—THE AVERAGE RESPIRATORY QUOTIENT AND THE PERCENTAGE INCREASE IN HEAT PRODUCTION BEFORE AND AFTER THE INGESTION OF LEVULOSE IN EXPERIMENTS CONTINUING BEYOND THE FIFTH HALF-HOUR.

Kind of experiments.	Average respiratory quotients, basal and for each half-hour after levulose.[1]								
	2d half hour.	3d half hour.	4th half hour.	5th half hour.	6th half hour.	7th half hour.	8th half hour.	9th half hour.	10th half hour.
Diabetics:	4	6	8	8	7	2	1	1	1
Basal, experiment averages . .	0.74	0.77	0.76	0.76	0.76	0.72	0.80	0.80	0.80
After levulose .	0.83	0.83	0.79	0.74	0.74	0.72	0.70	0.72	0.69
Percentage increase in heat production .	29	18	19	20	16	9	13	10	10
Case No. 1196. Dec. 15–16, 1916:									
Basal in half-hours . . .	0.83	0.81	0.77						
After levulose .	0.91	0.85	0.91	0.69	0.74	....	0.70	0.72	0.69
Percentage increase in heat production .	41	40	20	36	25	....	13	10	10

1. *High Respiratory Quotients Obtained after the Administration of Levulose and Their Explanation.*—Two diabetic patients showed extraordinary increases in the respiratory quotient after levulose, and with each of these patients duplicate experiments on subsequent days confirmed the observations noted. Case No. 1213 received 1.9 grams levulose per kilogram body weight when the basal respiratory quotient was 0.87, and the resulting quotients, beginning with the second half hour, were 0.98, 1.01, 1.04, 0.86. Case No. 1233 with a basal quotient of 0.86 gave a quotient in the second half hour of 1 and in succeeding half hours 0.96, 0.93, 0.90, and upon a subsequent day, with a basal quotient of 0.87, gave a quotient of 0.93 in the second half hour and quotients of 1.08, 0.99, and 0.82 on subsequent half hours. With the first case there was a third experiment in which levulose and fat, each in quantities of 1.85 grams per kilogram body weight, were administered. Here, too, the respiratory quotient rose to above 1, and, in fact, was maintained at a higher level throughout the four half hour periods than in any of the other experiments.

[1] The figures in the upper row of the table represent number of observations.

TABLE 127.—METABOLISM AND CLINICAL STATISTICS OF FIVE SEVERE DIABETICS SHOWING HIGH RESPIRATORY QUOTIENTS AFTER LEVULOSE.

Case No.	Date.	Variation in weight from normal standard.	Urinary nitrogen per kilogram per 24 hours.	Blood sugar.	Average respiratory quotient in basal experiment.	Respiratory quotient for each half-hour after levulose.				Average respiratory quotient after levulose.	Variation of basal metabolism from H & B standard.
						2d.	3d.	4th.	5th.		
		%	gm.	%							
755	May 7- 8, 1917	−20	0.135	0.14	0.81	0.88	0.81	0.79	0.83	0.83	−23
	" 14–15, 1917	−21	0.110	0.12	0.81	0.90	0.84	0.82	0.83	0.85	−18
	" 21–22, 1917	−22	.....	0.10	0.81	0.92	0.88	0.85	0.78	0.86	−17
.	" 27–28, 1916	−30	.....	0.22	0.82	0.91	0.94	0.85	0.81	0.88	−18
1049	May 19–20, 1916	−26	0.185	0.21	0.80	0.82	0.86	0.80	0.72	0.80	−20
1196	Dec. 14–15, 1916	−27	0.185	0.15	0.76	0.88	0.88	0.77	0.72	0.81	−19
	" 15–16, 1916	−23	0.115	....	0.80	0.91	0.85	0.91	0.69	0.78	−27
	" 16–17, 1916	−23	0.125	0.37	0.72	0.92	0.93	0.83	0.71	0.83	−22
1213	Feb. 7- 8, 1917	−45	0.185	0.21	0.85	0.95	0.90	0.80	0.74	0.85	
	" 14–15, 1917	−45	0.120	0.23	0.80	0.94	0.83	1.02	0.73	0.88	
	" 21–22, 1917	−45	0.150	0.15	0.87	0.98	1.01	1.04	0.86	0.97	
	" 28–Mar. 1, 1917	−42	0.240	0.28	0.91	0.96	0.95	0.87	0.91	0.92	
	Mar. 28–29, 1917	−43	0.140	0.19	0.91	0.90	0.82	0.90	0.93	0.89	
1233	Feb. 19–20, 1917	−22	0.210	0.13	0.86	1.00	0.96	0.93	0.90	0.95	−33
	" 26–27, 1917	−22	0.090	0.14	0.87	0.93	1.08	0.99	0.82	0.95	−28

The patients with the highest respiratory quotients have various points in common. Paradoxical as it may seem, the case most below standard weight, Case No. 1213, had the highest basal respiratory quotients. Three other patients also had very high quotients. All the 5 cases were considered severe cases of diabetes, all were free from severe acidosis, the average loss in weight below the reported maximum weights was 31 per cent, while the average loss in weight below standard weight was 30 per cent. Excluding the 1 girl diabetic for whose basal metabolism there are not entirely satisfactory comparisons, the remaining 4 of the 5 cases agreed in having a low basal metabolism. The values for blood sugar were also distinctly low for diabetics, and in only 6 of 15 analyses were distinctly above normal. Save with 1 patient, sugar was absent from the urine.

It is impracticable to explain the exceptionally high quotients above cited in any other way than by a conversion of carbohydrate to fat, strange as this may seem to be in diabetes. Morgulis and Pratt[1] demonstrated in a dog, extremely reduced in weight as a result of partial extirpation of the pancreas, that a change of carbohydrate to fat could go on undisturbed, as shown by the respiratory quotient of 1.06. Perhaps this result took place all the more readily because the dog was emaciated. It is certainly significant that the Russian investigators whom they cite obtained similar results with dogs which had first been subjected to a fast for several days. It would be desirable to observe whether in the presence of under-

[1] Morgulis and Pratt: Am. Jour. Physiol., 1913, **32**, 200.

nutrition carbohydrate given in temporary excess might be transformed to fat with especial readiness, and, particularly, if levulose were the carbohydrate used. If this were the case, Morgulis and Pratt's emaciated "Flora" would help explain the high quotients obtained with emaciated diabetics after levulose administration.

The average rise in the respiratory quotient for 8 cases receiving levulose on three days, though in only 1 instance on successive days, in the first levulose experiment amounted to 0.03 on the first day, 0.04 on the second, and 0.08 on the third. This indicates a progressive gain in tolerance for carbohydrate while under treatment. A further increase is to be seen with 1 of the 2 cases receiving levulose for a fourth time, Case No. 755, showing a progressive rise in the quotient of that case of 0.01, 0.02, 0.04 and 0.07. Hitherto reports have not come to my attention of demonstration of improvement in toleration of carbohydrate with diabetics by observations of the respiratory quotient subsequent to test meals. Their occurrence with these 8 cases of diabetes illustrate the inherent possibilities for improvement in the disease which is not widely enough recognized, but also another means by which such improvement can be measured.

(d) **Levulose, Respiratory Quotient and Acidosis.**—When the acidosis was absent, the increase in the respiratory quotient above basal within a period of two hours was 0.05 with moderate acidosis from 0.03 to 0.05, and there was no increase when acidosis was severe. Although the total metabolism after levulose was apparently unaffected by the presence or absence of acidosis, it is evident that acidosis had a very definite influence upon the change in respiratory quotient.

(e) **Effect of Levulose Upon the Blood Sugar.**—Folin and Berglund[1] noted that levulose produced no hyperglycemia in a normal individual to whom they gave 200 grams. Unfortunately we have few data upon the change in the blood sugar soon after the administration of levulose. For 30 experiments with 17 of the subjects the blood sugar was determined early in the morning of the experimental day before levulose was given and again twenty-four hours later. On both days the blood sugar averaged 0.19 per cent. Eight observations were made upon the percentage of the blood sugar within two and a half to four hours after levulose was given. Before administration the average per cent of sugar in the blood was 0.23 and two and a half to four hours after it was given was 0.3 per cent. In 2 instances the blood sugar percentage returned to approximately the basal value during this period. In several the rise in blood sugar was 0.1 per cent or more and in 1 experiment 0.21

---

[1] Folin and Berglund: Jour. Biol. Chem., 1922, **51**, 213.

per cent. The increases in blood sugar after levulose with diabetics are in marked contrast to what Folin and Berglund report with normal individuals.

The fact that there may be no hyperglycemia after the administration of levulose to normals as demonstrated by Folin and Berglund can be explained by a transformation of the levulose into fat. This is in line with the unusually high respiratory quotient found with normal individuals and diabetics after its administration. If the levulose were transformed into glycogen, the respiratory quotient would not rise, and if into glucose and was burned, it would give an increase in the blood sugar which they have shown does not take place normally. The possibility should be entertained that the increased metabolism following the administration of levulose, which continues after the respiratory quotient has fallen to the basal value, might be due to the levulose continuing to be burned as fat; and for this theory there is some support because, after this period the respiratory quotient falls even below the basal value.

14. **The Ingestion of Orange Juice, Dextrose, and Sucrose and the Metabolism of Diabetics.**—(a) The effect of orange juice was determined in several experiments. The quantity of carbohydrate in orange juice was accepted arbitrarily as 10 per cent. There are three different sugars found in orange juice—sucrose, dextrose and levulose. Sucrose usually makes up a little over one-half of the total sugar. After the fruit is removed from the tree, there is a gradual decrease in the amount of sucrose with a corresponding increase in the other two sugars, indicating that sucrose is changed into the other two. One group of analyses of California oranges shows variation in content of sucrose, 4.93 to 5.35 per cent, of invert sugar (dextrose and levulose) 4.36 to 6.8 per cent.

Acid is present in oranges almost entirely as citric acid. In the group of analyses above cited it varied between 1.26 and 1.51 per cent. Since citric acid is oxidized in the body, it is desirable to remember that its respiratory quotient is 1.33. Fortunately its percentage and quantity in orange juice is so low as not to interfere with our experiments.

In the 4 experiments with orange juice the average amount of carbohydrate per kilogram body weight administered was estimated at 1.2 grams. The increase in heat production varied from 1 to 21 per cent, an average of 12 per cent. The increased respiratory quotient was distinct, and although the average increase was but 0.03, the *peak* increase was considerable and the average maximum increase above the basal, 0.09.

(b) In a single experiment with dextrose the increase in heat production was less than after orange juice and the increase in respiratory quotient distinctly less.

(*c*) A single experiment with sucrose in a mild case of diabetes gave an increase in metabolism of 3 per cent, but the respiratory quotient behaved like that of a normal individual, rising on an average to 1.02 per cent and as a maximum to 1.05. As in the levulose experiments, here, too, the suggestion is near that with the burning of the sucrose some transformation of carbohydrate to fat may have taken place.

15. The Ingestion of Levulose and Fat on the Metabolism of Diabetics.—Eight observations upon 4 severe cases of diabetes free from acidosis were obtained after the patients had taken levulose and fat. As a result the metabolism rose on an average of 16 per cent. Comparing this increase with that observed when levulose was given alone to these 4 patients (19 per cent), it will be seen that despite the addition of fat, the metabolism rose slightly less during the actual period of experimentation. The average basal respiratory quotient in the 8 experiments was 0.83, and during the test this was increased on the average to 0.88, which corresponds closely with the values observed when levulose was given alone. The average maximum quotient was 0.92, thus indicating that even the peak effects of these levulose and fat meals correspond with the levulose meals without fat.

TABLE 128.—EFFECT OF INGESTION OF CARBOHYDRATE, FAT AND OLIVE OIL BY DIABETICS.

Variety of food given in experiment and Case No.	Total calories in meal per kilogram body weight of subject.	Increase in heat production over basal per cent.	Respiratory quotient.		
			Basal.	After carbohydrate and fat. Average maximum.	
Levulose and fat:					
610	11	23	0.84	0.82	0.84
"	10	12	0.82	0.84	0.88
"	10	19	0.83	0.83	0.86
"	10	16	0.85	0.85	0.88
1213	24	14	0.84	1.01	1.08
"	24	17	0.84	0.92	0.97
1233	19	16	0.85	0.93	0.97
1259	13	13	0.80	0.80	0.84
Average	15	16	0.83	0.88	0.92
Orange and fat:					
1213	16	15	0.91	0.88	0.95
1233	10	9	0.86	0.84	0.89
"	8	8	0.87	0.86	0.89
Average	11	11	0.88	0.86	0.91
Olive oil 1213	17	0	0.91	0.86	0.94

These experiments show beautifully the selective action of the body for carbohydrate when carbohydrate and fat are ingested simultaneously, the respiratory quotient rising as high when the two food elements were given as when carbohydrate was given alone; in one instance the respiratory quotient rose even above unity.

On the other hand, there was no increase in the metabolism over those experiments in which levulose was given alone, although the blood must have contained a far greater number of food molecules. In these experiments only good effects, so far as the metabolism and respiratory quotient were concerned, came from the addition of the fat to the levulose, and the patients obtained additional calories.

These data regarding the levulose and fat experiments are of service in another direction in that they offer a comparison of the effect of variation in the number of calories given in the food at one time per kilogram body weight. If one examines the table from this point of view, it will be seen that when the number of calories was lowest, *i. e.*, 10 calories per kilogram body weight, the increase in metabolism varied between 12 and 19 per cent, and when the number of calories was over twice as large per kilogram body weight, the increases in the metabolism were 14 and 17 per cent. A variation in the number of calories per kilogram body weight caused no change in the metabolism. Attention is again called to the large number of calories per kilogram body weight given in a brief period. In the course of a few minutes 1 patient (Case No. 1213) received 24 calories per kilogram body weight, a quantity sufficient to supply the basal needs of the body for twenty-four hours.

Corresponding to these experiments with levulose and fat, 3 experiments with 2 of the same patients were made after the ingestion of orange juice and fat. The comparative results are strikingly similar. The average increase in metabolism was 11 per cent, and this is essentially the same as when orange juice was given alone. In these 3 experiments the respiratory quotient did not show a rise save for the maxima, which were on the average 0.03 above the basal level. The total amount of carbohydrate given was but 30 to 40 grams, corresponding to 0.65 to 1.25 grams per kilogram body weight.

A single experiment was made with Case No. 1213 after 60 grams of olive oil had been given, or 1.85 grams per kilogram body weight. No change was noted in the metabolism as a result of the oil, thus supporting the results already noted when fat was added to levulose or orange juice. This lack of increase in the metabolism is the more noteworthy because the patient received 17 calories per kilogram body weight in the course of one or two moments, a quantity of food sufficient to supply the basal needs for eighteen hours. The average respiratory quotient *fell* 0.05, though in the first period there was a rise of 0.03 with successive decreases thereafter.

16. **The Ingestion of Protein in Diabetes.**—Small quantities of protein raise the metabolism of diabetics in a striking manner as in the case of normals. Diabetic patients are often so thin that trifling

quantities of protein really amount to more than one would think, because they are relatively large per kilogram body weight. Thus the increase in heat production when the protein per kilogram body weight amounted to from 1.55 grams to 1.70 grams varied between 20 and 32 per cent. It is noteworthy that the average respiratory quotient in the protein experiments was essentially unchanged following the ingestion of the protein. The administration of moderate quantities of fat with the protein in another series of 10 experiments brought about similar results. Thus, the average increase in metabolism was 23 per cent. In fact, these experiments with protein and fat bear the same relation to the experiments with protein as do the experiments with carbohydrate (levulose or orange juice) and fat to the experiments with pure carbohydrate. In other words, so far as the limits of these experiments go, there appears to be no tendency for fat to increase the metabolism, either when given with carbohydrate or with protein. The ingestion of fat in these experiments, therefore, produced as little effect on the metabolism as the oxidation of body fat did in the experiments with the overweight normals and diabetics.

TABLE 129.—EFFECT OF INGESTION OF PROTEIN AND FAT BY DIABETICS.

Body weight (naked) kg.	Food ingested. Protein, gm.	Fat, gm.	Increase in heat production over basal, per cent.	Basal respiratory quotient.	Average respiratory quotient in experiment.
39.6	13	..	20	0.80	0.81
36.4	18	16	23	0.82	0.81
49.7	75	54	16	0.71	0.71

In comparison with the protein experiments just cited is another group of experiments after the ingestion of beefsteak, during the years 1908 and 1918, when the basal metabolism of the cases thus studied averaged 17 per cent *above* standard in contrast to the protein experiments above mentioned in which the average basal metabolism was 17 per cent *below* standard. The observation showed that the increase was similar, being 16 per cent.

A study was made of the increases in heat production in the various food experiments at different levels of basal metabolism. Although it might be supposed that the stimulus of food would be less on an already stimulated body metabolism (*i. e.*, with acidosis and high metabolic state) it would appear from these results that there is no especial relation between the level of the basal metabolism and the degree of reaction of the body to food.

17. **Oatmeal and the Metabolism of Diabetics.**—The effect of oatmeal taken alone and with fat and in divided portions through the day was likewise investigated. When oatmeal was combined with fat, the increase in the metabolism of a series of moderate and

severe diabetics amounted to 18 to 26 per cent if the observations
were confined to the two or three hours following the ingestion of
the food. No change in respiratory quotient was observed.

TABLE 130.—METABOLISM AFTER INGESTION OF OATMEAL AND OATMEAL WITH FAT
IN EXPERIMENTS WITH DIABETICS.

Diet and No. of observa- tions.	Body weight (naked) kg.	Time elapsed since eating hrs.	Food ingested.			Metabolism. Increase in heat production over basal, per cent.	Respiratory quotient.	
			C. gm.	P. gm.	F. gm.		Average of experiment.	Basal.
Oatmeal 3	51.5	½–4	48	12	5	3	0.77	0.76
Oatmeal with fat 7	54.6	1½–3¾	83	23	53	22	0.75	0.74
Oatmeal day 6	58.0	1¾–2	57	13	44	17	0.71	0.71

The effect of oatmeal divided in 1 to 7 meals was studied.
After the first meal there was an average rise of the metabolism in
9 experiments of 14 per cent. The rise, in general, varied according
to the quantity of all the food given. After the second feeding an
increase in metabolism above basal was noted, amounting to 19
per cent. After the third meal the rise in metabolism amounted to
24 per cent and in 2 observations the increases in metabolism were
as great as 37 and 40 per cent. The respiratory quotient as after
the first and second meals was unaffected. After the fourth meal
in 5 experiments the average rise in metabolism was maintained
at 20 per cent. As a result of four successive meals of oatmeal and
fat (1) there was no clear tendency to a rise in quotient; (2) very
low quotients were secured on two successive days and are supported by similar quotients; (3) they were secured after the patient
had taken 220 and 260 grams of fat, respectively; (4) making with
carbohydrate and protein total calories equivalent to 56 and 67
calories per kilogram body weight in the preceding seven and a
half and nine and three-quarter hours, although the patient was
taking no active exercise; (5) the rise in metabolism varied from 14
to 40 per cent.

Following the fifth meal the average rise in metabolism was 26
per cent. The respiratory quotient fell notably in this series and
is chiefly to be attributed to the single experiment with Case No.
591, discussed under low respiratory quotients. (See p. 264). This
subject was an ideal one, a severe diabetic with severe acidosis.
He was given carbohydrate 35, protein 10, and fat 55 at each of
five successive meals. The rise in this patient's metabolism after
the third oatmeal feeding was 40 per cent and after the fifth meal
42 per cent. The respiratory quotient fell to 0.58. The rise in
metabolism appears hardly explainable by the protein given but

rather by the acidosis. See p. 243, as well as my Carnegie Monograph, p. 174, for further discussion of this case.

There was a single experiment after the sixth feeding of oatmeal and but one after a seventh feeding. The rise in metabolism was essentially the same: that is, 13 and 14 per cent, respectively, with an increase in the respiratory quotient in both of 0.03.

18. **The Effect of Mixed Meals of the Diabetic Diet Upon the Metabolism of Diabetics.**—A series of observations was made following the ingestion of routine diabetic mixed meals at the New England Deaconess Hospital. The increase in the metabolism after the first meal of the day was 15 per cent. This represents a period of approximately two hours beginning between one and two hours after the meal. If the metabolism observations were begun earlier after the ingestion of food, the metabolism would probably have risen to a higher level, and if continued longer the metabolism would have gradually diminished and the figures would have been reduced. In these observations it was again notable that acidosis did not prevent a rise in metabolism after food. The increase in metabolism varied chiefly with the quantity of protein, and also was associated with the calories per kilogram body weight. When the metabolism was determined after the second meal of the day, the average increase was found to be 25 per cent. This corresponds with the quantity of protein administered and would appear to be directly connected with it, because the caloric value of the meal was decidedly lower than that given in the previous series of experiments. When the metabolism was determined after two and three meals the average increase was found to be, respectively, 19 and 28 per cent. In all of these experiments after meals the change in respiratory quotient was negligible.

D. THE NATURE OF DIABETIC ACIDOSIS AND ITS RELATION TO COMA.

1. **Acidosis in Normal Individuals.**—If a healthy individual lives for three successive days upon a carbohydrate-free diet, the urine voided upon the subsequent morning will show the presence of diacetic acid and acetone. This is evidence of the intoxication which was termed by Naunyn "acidosis." Experiments and debates have taken place all these years to prove *pro* or *con* that the acid responsible for the condition was β-oxybutyric acid and its derivatives or a group of acids. At the present moment it appears as if this acid is by far the more abundant and important, but in certain states of diabetic acidosis Bock[1] and Fitz and their

---

[1] Bock: Jour. Metab. Research. To be published.

co-workers believe another organic acid is sometimes present too, though the nature of the acid is as yet unknown.

Acidosis is still more simply produced in normal individuals by fasting, but it is of a milder type. Thus Benedict's subject at the Nutrition Laboratory constantly showed an acidosis during his fast of thirty-one days. When the fasting subject is obese, Folin and Denis[1] found the acidosis still more marked. (See Table 133, page 308.)

Exercise, even without fasting, leads to acidosis and the extent of it varies with the strenuousness of the exercise.[2]

Examples of acidosis due to a non-carbohydrate diet, to fasting in an obese subject, and to exercise are shown in Tables 131, 132, 133 and 134. (See pages 306, 307 and 308.)

TABLE 131.—ACIDOSIS OF A NORMAL INDIVIDUAL UPON A FAT-PROTEIN DIET.

Day.	Acetone.	β-oxybutyric.
1	0.062	0.84
2	0.660	0.73
3	2.550	3.56
4	3.110	14.70

Prerequisite for the acidosis in all these states is the diminution of the combustion of carbohydrate in the body no matter whether caused by withholding food or the exhaustion of glycogen stores, or its failure to be burned as in diabetes. Benedict's experiment showed that so soon as the percentage of carbohydrate in the combined carbohydrate and fat metabolized fell below 12 per cent, acidosis was marked. My experiment upon the healthy nurse, Miss L., (see p. 250) showed the same phenomenon just as Ladd and Palmer[3] showed it for diabetics.

"Fat burns in the flame of carbohydrate, but without it, it smokes."[4] Signs and symptoms disappear as if by magic when the subject begins to take and burn carbohydrate. Conversely, if carbohydrate is withheld and excessive fat administered or through exercise drawn upon for energy, the acidosis is intensified. This is beautifully shown in diabetes by the falling respiratory quotient and the rising acidosis as recorded in Table 117. As the metabolism of fat replaced the metabolism of carbohydrate the ketone bodies appeared and hence it was natural to look for their source in fat.

[1] Folin and Denis: Jour. Biol. Chem., 1915, 21, 183.
[2] Landergren: Nord. med. Ark., 1910, 2, 1; Barach (reprint) Physiological and Pathological Effects of Severe Exertion (The Marathon Race) from the Dept. of Phys. Research of the Pittsburgh Athletic Assn.
[3] Ladd and Palmer: Proc. Soc. Exper. Biol. Chem., 1921, 47, 433; also Am. Jour. Med. Sci., 1923, 166, 157.
[4] Woodyatt: Jour. Am. Med. Assn., 1916, 66, 1.

The acid or ketone bodies which have been demonstrated to be present in the acidosis of fasting and, as will be seen later, of diabetes are represented by three bodies: β-oxybutyric acid ($CH_3.-CHOH.-CH_2COOH$), diacetic acid ($CH_3.CO.CH_2COOH$), and acetone ($CH_3.CO.CH_3$) all of which are excreted in the urine, and the latter in the breath as well.

(*a*) **The Source of the Acid Bodies.**—The source of these bodies is in the animo-acids found chiefly in fat, but also in protein, though not at all in carbohydrate. They develop as readily from body fat and protein as from exogenous fat and protein, so far as is known. Each molecule of a higher fatty acid, as it is broken down to a lower, provided it has an even number of carbon atoms, leads to the production of one molecule of β-oxybutyric acid. As a matter of fact, the only fatty acids which are present in the body are those containing an even number of carbon atoms. It has been extimated by Magnus-Levy that out of 100 grams of fat, 36 grams of hydroxybutyric acid may be produced.[1] Starting with this assumption, Shaffer[2] has computed the ketogenic-antiketogenic derivatives from fat, protein and carbohydrate. Taking 874 as the molecular weight of the mixed body fat one may calculate that 1 gram of such mixed fat can give rise to $\frac{1}{874} \times 3$ (molecules of fatty acid in 1 molecule fat) = 0.00343 gram molecule of ketogenic fatty acid $\times$ 102 (molecular weight of aceto-acetic acid) = 0.35 gram of aceto-acetic acid. Notable quantities of β-oxybutyric acid, however, can also be formed from protein, since leucine, phenylalanine, and tyrosine have been found to be convertible into acetone bodies. Each gram of urinary nitrogen according to Shaffer is equivalent to approximately 0.01 gram molecule of ketogenic substance, or if multiplied by 102 to 1.02 grams of aceto-acetic acid. It is interesting that those amino-acids of the protein molecule which lead to the production of β-oxybutyric acid do not produce sugar, and conversely, that those which lead to the formation of sugar produce no β-oxybutyric acid.

To offset these ketogenic factors are the antiketogenic derivatives of the diet. These are the carbohydrates par excellence. Shaffer writes "until the active derivative of glucose is known we may assume that 1 molecule of monosaccharide is equivalent to 1 molecule of the active derivative, and on this basis the antiketogenic value of carbohydrate in terms of molecules of glucose. Each gram of glucose would thus be equivalent to $\frac{1}{180}$ = 0.00556 gram molecule; and each gram of starch to $\frac{1}{162}$ = 0.00618 grams molecule.

[1] Magnus-Levy: Spez. Path. u. Therap. inn. Krank., Kraus u. Brugsch, Berlin, 1913, **1**, 30.
[2] Shaffer: Jour. Biol. Chem., 1921, **47**, 456.

20

Table 132.—Tabular Presentation of Metabolism Results Obtained in an Experiment with a Man Fasting for Thirty-one Days at the Nutrition Laboratory of the Carnegie Institution of Washington in Boston. Age, Thirty-nine Years, Eleven Months. Height, 170.7 Cms.

Observations.	April 10-11	April 11-12	April 12-13	April 13-14	April 14-15	April 15-16	April 16-17	April 17-18	April 18-19	April 19-20	April 20-21	April 21-22	April 22-23	April 23-24	April 24-25	April 25-26	April 26-27	April 27-28	April 28-29	April 29-30
					1	2	3	4	5	6	7	8	9	10	11	12	13	14	15	16
Body weight naked, kg.	60.13	60.53	60.95	60.64	59.60	58.68	57.79	57.03	56.37	55.89	55.5	55.08	54.63	54.13	53.88	53.56	53.45	53.15	52.84	52.29
Insensible perspiration per day, gms.					1086	1188	1059	779	727	606	603	569	578	672	573	691	436	540	442	578
Pulse-rate, night	82	76	78	70	68	66	62	65	63	60	59	61	59	57	57	58	56	53	53	53
Morning	72	73	72	73	74	73	70	68	67	64	59	65	63	63	61	61	59	58	57	53
Blood-pressure, lying: Systolic, mm.	122	123	124			134	113	111	113	112	112	111	110	108		103	106	104	102	94
Diastolic, mm.	90	92	93			100	80	85	85	82	85	80	81	82		78	80	80	76	75
Alveolar CO₂ tension, mm.	31.7	36.0	36.5	37.5	32.8	31.3	32.1	31.9	31.4	31.6	32.3	32.1	32.3	31.5			28.4	29.1	28.9	27.5
Volume of urine per day, cc	1485	1521	1528	1441	660	468	565	713	667	610	524	587	607	565	564	517	561	647	758	889
Total nitrogen in urine: gms.	17.02	15.92	14.48	11.54	7.10	8.40	11.34	11.87	10.41	10.18	9.79	10.27	10.74	10.05	10.19	10.13	10.35	10.43	8.46	9.58
Per kilo body weight (Kjeldahl), gms.	0.283	0.264	0.238	0.19	0.118	0.142	0.195	0.207	0.184	0.181	0.176	0.186	0.196	0.185	0.19	0.189	0.193	0.196	0.16	0.182
Ammonia-N, Folin method, original, gms.					0.41	0.60	0.95	1.4	1.6	1.67	1.52	1.62	1.7	1.57	1.56	1.51	1.57	1.51	1.43	1.91
Chlorine (Cl) in urine, gms.		0.67	0.65	0.59	0.41	1.02	0.79	0.59	0.41	0.4	0.55	0.32	0.31	0.28	0.36	0.31	0.32	0.26	0.16	0.14
β-oxybutyric acid (determined), gms.					3.77		2.1	3.5	2.1	3.5	2.8	1.6	3.5	3.5	1.4	2.4	4.2	4.7	1.6	5.2
Respiratory quotient: night	0.81	0.88	0.86	0.81	0.78	0.75	0.73	0.74	0.75	0.68	0.71	0.73	0.75	0.72	0.72	0.73	0.74	0.72	0.71	0.71
CO₂ produced per 24 hrs. (partly estimated), liters					286.3	281.1	271.8	255.2	252.4	237.9	237.9	235.1	233.3	222.9	218.1	220.8	212.1	214.5	204.2	201.5
O₂ consumed per 24 hrs. (partly estimated), liters					374.7	373.8	363.8	349.8	344.9	330.6	331.1	323.2	317.3	306.3	297.8	303.2	290.5	299.9	286.3	283.8
Carbohydrate katabolized per 24 hrs., gms.					68.8	42.1	38.5	4.3	15.1			4.0	13.5	3.8	3.8	3.8	3.5			
Fat katabolized per 24 hrs., gms.					135	142	130	136	133	133	134	127	119	120	115	118	111	117	116	112
Protein katabolized per 24 hrs., gms.					42.6	50.4	68.0	71.2	62.5	61.1	58.7	61.6	64.4	60.3	61.5	60.8	62.1	62.6	50.8	57.5
Flesh equivalent of protein, gms.					213	252	340	356	312	306	294	308	322	308	308	304	311	313	254	287
Loss of preformed water from body: Not combined with fat and flesh, gms.					585	448	350	225	166	11	-65	-47	-34	48	-202	-128	-339	-154	-80	155
Total loss, gms.					769	664	635	524	429	268	183	212	236	301	56	127	-80	108	135	396
Total calories, computed per 24 hrs.					1769	1756	1702	1626	1609	1537	1540	1503	1481	1426	1385	1410	1349	1394	1331	1319
Calories per kilo, per 24 hrs.					29.4	29.7	29.2	28.3	28.4	27.4	27.6	27.2	27.0	26.2	25.6	26.2	25.2	26.2	25.1	25.1
Total energy loss per 24 hrs., calories					1834	1845	1820	1760	1732	1653	1644	1619	1605	1537	1495	1515	1463	1505	1426	1442
Heat production per 24 hrs.: Computed from gaseous met.	1577	1541	1572	1526	1615	1555	1524	1433	1394	1349	1380	1378	1289	1277	1262	1262	1291	1222	1202	1226
Predicted from H. & B. — cal.	1478	1483	1490	1485	1471	1459	1446	1435	1427	1420	1415	1409	1402	1395	1393	1389	1387	1383	1378	1371
+ % H. & B.	+7	+4	+6	+3	+10	+7	+5	0	-2	-5	-2	-2	-8	-8	-9	-9	-7	-12	-13	-11

Beginning of Fast. (noted between April 13-14 and April 14-15.)

Partial table of metabolism results (subject L). Columns give dates (and numbered days of observation).

Observations.	Apr. 30 / May 1. 17	May 1-2. 18	May 2-3. 19	May 3-4. 20	May 4-5. 21	May 5-6. 22	May 6-7. 23	May 7-8. 24	May 8-9. 25	May 9-10. 26	May 10-11. 27	May 11-12. 28	May 12-13. 29	May 13-14. 30	May 14-15. 31	May 15-16.	May 16-17.	May 17-18.
Body weight naked, kg.	51.79	51.50	51.11	50.93	50.49	50.13	49.96	49.62	49.33	49.02	48.70	48.46	48.10	47.69	47.39	47.05	47.12	48.17
Insensible perspiration per day, gms.	509	521	550	371	623	465	504	480	468	473	557	477	554	530	625	68	64	90
Pulse-rate, night	52	52	52	52	54	53	56	59	60	61	62	59	58	58	57			
Morning[1]	57	56	57	58	59	59	58	59	55	56	58	61	63	59	60			
Blood-pressure, lying: systolic, mm.	101	104	96	100	98	97	97	98	99	106	100	98	103	98	101*	92	98	124
Diastolic, mm.	78	79	75	77	75	73	75	80	75	79	78	75	82	79	80*	74	82	102
Alveolar CO_2 tension, mm.	28.5	28.7	27.6	26.9	28.7	27.9	27.8	26.8	27.3	28.1	27.5	27.9	28.1	27.8	31.8*	32.0	35.1	
Volume of urine per day, cc	848	657	728	699	708	785	556	750	713	728	653	655	697	771	566	414	1262	241
Total nitrogen in urine, grns.	8.81	8.27	8.37	7.69	7.93	7.75	7.31	8.15	7.81	7.88	8.07	7.62	7.54	7.83	6.94	4.83	3.81	2.75
Per kilo bodyweight (Kjeldahl), grns.	0.169	0.160	0.163	0.151	0.156	0.154	0.146	0.164	0.158	0.160	0.165	0.157	0.156	0.163	0.146	0.102	0.08	0.058
Ammonia-N, Folin method, original, gms.	0.12	0.15	0.16	0.15	0.18	0.21	0.18	0.10	0.18	0.16	0.16	0.14	0.12	0.14	0.13	0.68	0.36	0.35
Chlorine (Cl) in urine, gms.	1.90	1.80	1.76	1.58	1.57	1.51	1.49	1.52	1.51	1.42	1.36	1.28	1.32	1.14	1.25	0.23	0.26	0.18
β-oxybutyric acid (determined), grns.	3.6	4.4	7.0	4.4	5.0	3.1	6.0	6.9	4.4	6.1	4.0	4.9	5.6	5.4	4.5	0.8	0.5	0.5
CO_2 produced per 24 hrs. (partly estimated), liters	199.0	192.5	191.1	191.1	196.1	189.1	189.1	190.9	193.2	190.3	193.3	198.0	192.0	189.6	195.5			
Respiratory quotient; night	0.72	0.72	0.71	0.71	0.73	0.72	0.72	0.69	0.72	0.70	0.72	0.71	0.72	0.72	0.72		0.80	0.97
O_2 consumed per 24 hrs. (partly estimated); liters	279.5	270.5	271.2	269.1	274.4	265.5	264.2	269.7	269.0	267.8	269.9	276.9	268.0	266.3	275.0			
Carbohydrate katabolized per 24 hrs., gms.																		
Fat katabolized per 24 hrs., gms.	112	109	109	110	112	108	109	109	109	109	109	114	110	108	115			
Protein katabolized per 24 hrs., gms.	52.9	49.6	50.2	46.1	47.6	46.5	43.9	48.9	46.9	47.3	48.4	45.7	45.2	47.0	41.6			
Flesh equivalent of protein, gms.	265	248	251	231	238	233	220	245	235	237	242	229	226	235	208			
Loss of preformed water from body: Not combined with fat and flesh, gms.	67	-91	7	-180	69	-2	-179	-34	-73	-55	-52	-122	4	49	-43			
Total loss, gms.	290	118	219	15	270	195	8	173	126	145	153	72	196	248	135			
Total calories, computed per 24 hrs.	1300	1257	1261	1252	1276	1235	1230	1254	1251	1246	1255	1289	1247	1239	1281			
Calories per kilo per 24 hrs.	25.0	24.3	24.6	24.5	25.2	24.5	24.6	25.2	25.3	25.3	25.7	26.5	25.8	25.9	26.9			
Total energy loss per 24 hrs., calories	1417	1361	1366	1343	1371	1328	1318	1349	1342	1336	1345	1374	1334	1326	1361			
Heat production per 24 hrs.:[1] Computed from gaseous met.	1226	1159	1183	1157	1162	1142	1116	1126	1128	1133	1164	1118	1142	1109	1118			
Predicted from H. & B., cals.	1364	1360	1354	1351	1346	1340	1339	1334	1329	1325	1321	1318	1313	1307	1303			
+% H. & B.	-10	-15	-13	-14	-14	-15	-17	-16	-15	-14	-12	-15	-13	-15	-14			

End of Fast. (noted between May 14-15 and May 15-16.)

The above is a partial presentation of metabolism results obtained with subject L. during four days prefasting period, thirty-one days fasting, and three days postfasting period. In order to bring together comparative data for every day of the fast, it has been necessary to place in each column results which represent in the aggregate a total of thirty-six hours, each single result, however, being either taken at the end of twenty-four hours or representing a total for twenty-four hours. The results recorded on the thirty-first day, to which an asterisk has been affixed, were as a matter of fact, obtained a short time after the first food had been taken. In no series of derived tables is it possible to draw complete comparisons of the various factors of metabolism, and this can be done satisfactorily only when all of the data are grouped together. All of the data obtained with this subject have therefore been summarized in one large table. From Publication No. 203 of the Carnegie Institution of Washington.

[1] Observations on morning following each designated day.

TABLE 133.—THE ACIDOSIS OF A FAT WOMAN DURING THREE PERIODS OF FASTING (FOLIN AND DENIS).

Day.	Acetone, gms.	Diacetic acid, gms.	β-oxy-butyric acid, gms.	NH_3N, gms.	Titrated acidity, c.c.	Acetone in expired air per hr., mgms.	Remarks.
1	0.04	0.27	0	0.41	230	0	Feeling well.
2	0.08	1.42	2.90	0.73	250	5.2	Slight headache.
3	0.10	1.57	17.94	1.87	508	24.0	Severe headache.
4	0.88	2.46	18.47	2.50	695	49.5	Headache, nausea, and dizziness.
15	0	0	0	0.31	180	0	Feeling well.
16	0.02	0	0	0.37	290	0	Feeling well.
17	0.03	1.17	0.17	0.53	335	30.0	Feeling well.
18	0.35	1.16	5.44	1.01	595	32.0	Slight headache, nausea.
19	0.40	1.15	13.54	1.50	655	45.0	Headache, nausea, and dizziness.
24	0	0	0	0.50	145	0	Feeling well.
25	0	0	0	0.37	160	0	Feeling well.
26	0.04	0.37	0.18	0.51	210	66.0	Feeling well.
27	0.20	1.36	17.34	0.81	300	24.0	Headache, nausea.

TABLE 134.—CHANGES IN CO_2-COMBINING CAPACITY, CO_2 TENSION, AND REACTION OF ARTERIAL BLOOD AFTER EXERCISE. BARR, HIMWICH, AND GREEN.

Subject.	Date.	Amount of work.	CO_2 capacity at 40 mm.			CO_2 tension of arterial blood.			pH.		
			Before.	After.	Difference.	Before.	After.	Difference.	Before.	After.	Difference.
(1)	(2)	(3)	(4)	(5)	(6)	(7)	(8)	(9)	(10)	(11)	(12)
	1922	kgm.	vol. per cent.	vol. per cent.	vol. per cent.	mm. Hg.	mm. Hg.	mm. Hg.			
M. L.	Apr. 7	3,285	46.2	31.9	14.3	47.5	44.5	3.0	7.28	7.11	0.17
N. P. L.	Nov. 15	3,595	46.3	34.7	11.6	43.2	40.2	3.0	7.30	7.17	0.13
J. McL.	" 30	3,605	48.4	32.6	15.8	45.2	39.5	5.7	7.30	7.15	0.15
P. R.	Dec. 10	3,695	45.0	26.2	18.8	41.3	40.0	1.3	7.29	7.04	0.25
J. E.	Nov. 2	3,700	42.7	27.9	14.8	42.0	30.5?	11.5?	7.28	7.12?	0.16?
H. B. R.	Apr. 12	3,500?	46.8	35.7	11.1	43.0	36.5	6.5	7.30	7.22	0.08
D. P. B.[2]	Aug. 8	3,770	49.2	32.9	16.3	36.5	23.0	13.5	7.36	7.27	0.09
H. E. H.	Mar. 29	3,055	48.4	40.9	7.5	46.0	40.7	5.3	7.29	7.25	0.04
H. E. H.[2]	Aug. 25	3,545	47.9	39.3	8.6	46.5	44.0	2.5	7.28	7.21	0.07
H. E. H.	Apr. 5	3,954	50.2	32.5	17.7	49.0	38.3	10.7	7.29	7.15	0.14

Protein is known to be converted into glucose by the diabetic organism to the extent of approximately 3.6 grams for each gram of nitrogen. . . .One gram of urine nitrogen would then correspond to $\frac{3.6}{180} = 0.02$ grams molecule of glucose.

A third probable source of antiketogenic substance is the glycerol

[1] Barr, Himwich and Green: Jour. Biol. Chem., 1923, 55, 495.
[2] Sodium fluoride, 0.1 per cent, used to protect blood against acid changes.

of fat, though the evidence is perhaps not conclusive. Its antiketogenic value, calculated in terms of glucose, is as follows: One gram of fat $= \frac{1}{874} = 0.00114$ grams molecule fat $\div 2 = 0.00057$ grams molecule of glucose from glycerol.

The above calculations are summarized below:

Ketogenic substance expressed as gram molecules of precursors of aceto-acetic acid.

(a) 1 gram of fat $= \frac{3 \times 1}{874} =$ 0.00343 mol.

(b) 1 gram of urine nitrogen $=$ 0.01 mol.

Antiketogenic substance expressed as gram-molecular equivalents of glucose.

(c) 1 gram of urine nitrogen $= \frac{3.6}{180} =$ 0.02 mol.

(d) 1 gram of glucose from carbohydrate $= \frac{1}{180} = 0.00556$ mol.

(e) 1 gram of fat $= \frac{1}{874} \div 2 =$ 0.00057 mol.

The sum of the values of (a) and (b) divided by the sum of the values of (c), (d) and (e) gives the ratio of ketogenic to antiketogenic substance for the mixture metabolisms, and if the general conception is correct, this ratio should determine whether or not the subject will form and excrete acetone bodies."[1]

The amount of acid formed is considerable and far more than physicians realize. Benedict's fasting subject did not excrete in the thirty-one days of the fast over 7 grams β-oxybutyric acid in any twenty-four hours, but the fat subject of Folin and Denis excreted 18.4 grams on the fourth fasting day, and Forsner[2] by forcing up the limits of fat in the diet obtained an excretion of 42.8 grams of acid bodies in one day. S. R. Benedict[3] obtained 32 grams when he depleted glycogen storage with phloridzin. It is in diabetes, however, that the excretion of ketone bodies reaches extremes. Thus, Case No. 4, male, onset at fifteen years of age, without diabetic heredity, excreted three years and two months later, during three successive days of coma, 437 grams β-oxybutyric acid as calculated from β-oxybutyric acid and diacetic acid extracted from the urine. This large quantity is nearly the maximum found in the literature. It is equivalent to the elimination of 3 grams β-oxybutyric acid per kilo body weight daily for three days for an individual weighing 50 kilograms, or if the acidity is expressed in terms of hydrochloric acid, approximately 1 gram of hydrochloric acid per kilo each twenty-four hours. It is, therefore, not strange that the kidneys which bear the brunt of excretion of this acid show "showers of casts." Naunyn estimates the quantity of β-oxybutyric acid in the tissues of a patient near coma at between 200

---

[1] Shaffer: Jour. Biol. Chem., Loc. cit., p. 305.

[2] Forsner: Arch. Skandin. f. Phys., 1910, **23**, 305.

[3] Benedict: Proc. Soc. Exp. Biol. and Med., 1914, **11**, 134.

and 300 grams and Bock, Field and Adair[1] the total acid in the form of diacetic acid in one patient recovering from coma at 103 grams.

(*b*) **The Percentage Relation of Acid Bodies to One Another.**— The interrelation of acetone, diacetic acid, and β-oxybutyric acid to one another must be very intimate. Neubauer[2] considers that there is a reversible action between diacetic acid and β-oxybutyric acid, and that these readily change back and forth with one another. It is thought by some that there is a fixed proportion between these acids, varying with different patients but constant in the same patient. Folin[3] is inclined to doubt the existence of pre-formed acetone in the body, but explains its presence in the urine as a decomposition product of diacetic acid. At any rate, acetone seldom constitutes over a small percentage of the total acidosis, and acetone and diacetic acid combined not over 30 per cent.

(*c*) **Mode of Elimination of Acid Bodies.**—Practically all the acid bodies of the β-oxybutyric acid are eliminated by the kidneys. Only one of these—acetone—is excreted by the lungs, and the amount must be small. In experiments upon a healthy man following the feeding of oleic acid, I obtained an excretion of 0.847 gram acetone calculated for the twenty-four hours in the breath. The method of estimation of the acetone in the breath was not very satisfactory, and it would be advantageous to institute a series of experiments of this nature on a larger scale. The other two bodies are excreted as salts and even as free acid in the urine. Magnus-Levy[4] found that the concentration of these acids in the urine seldom rose above 1.5 per cent, and except in coma he never encountered values greater than 0.6 per cent. It is evident, there-fore, that the elimination of the acid bodies is closely connected with the quantity of water excreted. β-oxybutyric acid circulates in the blood combined with alkali as a salt, but the acid is excreted in the urine to a large extent as free acid and the base retained in the body. It is only when much alkali is given that the large quantities of β-oxybutyric acid, such as were excreted by Case No. 4 during coma, are found.[5] I do not, however, remember data in the literature which show an increased elimination of acid bodies following the administration of alkalis to a normal individual with experimental acidosis. Such would be valuable.

It would be wrong to consider, however, that the only means the body has by which to free itself of acid is by the kidneys. The body has a most efficient pathway in the lungs through which

[1] Bock, Field and Adair: Jour. Metab. Research, 1923.
[2] Neubauer: Verhard. d. Kong. f. inn. Med., 1910, **27**, 566.
[3] Folin: Jour. Biol. Chem., 1907, **3**, 177.
[4] Magnus-Levy: Arch. f. exp. Path. u. Phar., 1899, **42**, 200.
[5] Joslin: Jour. Metab. Research, 1921, **1**, 306.

carbonic acid is constantly removed from the body. In fact, so soon as this acid begins to increase in the tissues, being displaced by the stronger β-oxybutyric acid, it also rises in the blood; this stimulates the respiratory center with resulting hyperpnea and the excess of carbonic acid is removed by the increased ventilation. The total quantity of carbon dioxide for the twenty-four hours is not increased save for the increase due to the increased metabolism which accompanies acidosis, and indeed the percentage of carbon dioxide in the alveolar air is actually diminished because it is diluted in consequence of the increased ventilation.

(*d*) **Safeguards of the Body Against Acidosis.**—The body is admirably protected against danger from acidosis. First and foremost should be placed its storage of glycogen which can make carbohydrate available for a few days to offset the acidosis of the ketone variety. Since in diabetes there is little carbohydrate in the body, and that which is eaten is often lost to the metabolism, one should never cease to strive to furnish it and to arrange treatment so that some of it will be burned.

If the diet of the diabetic individual is unrestricted, he often eats so large a quantity of carbohydrate-forming material that enough of it is oxidized to prevent the occurrence of these bodies. Thus Case No. 295, male, onset at sixteen years, seven years later excreted 10,000 cc of urine containing 680 grams of sugar, and yet failed to show a positive reaction for diacetic acid. When the carbohydrates in his diet were restricted to even 280 grams, acidosis appeared; when the diet was still further restricted, the acidosis became extreme. By devices such as this the diabetic may survive for a time, but the disease advances. In this way, Case No. 1887 and Case No. 1456 have kept alive, but I know of few others. The whole aim of diabetic treatment, both formerly and now, is to protect the patient by promoting by every means in our power the combustion of carbohydrate.

Other factors of safety are available to thwart acidosis and these factors are of a more general type since they offset acidosis of any origin. For their proper understanding a discussion of the maintenance of the normal alkalinity of the body is desirable.

"Any modification of the normal equilibrium between acids and bases within the organism whereby the power to neutralize acid is diminished is to be regarded as a condition of *acidosis*."[1] The formation of acid never goes on to such a degree that the blood shows an acid reaction. Such a condition is incompatible with life. In fact, so constant is "the reaction of the blood that a change from the reaction of ordinary tap water, which is more

---

[1] Henderson: Trans. Assn. Am. Phys., 1916.

alkaline than the blood, to that of distilled water, which is much more acid than blood, would be fatal." If the blood were acid, the carbonic acid would be displaced from its combination with an alkali by the stronger β-oxybutyric acid and set free in every cell of the body, and no alkali would be available to combine with it and take it back to the lungs for elimination. The normal blood and respiratory exchange is represented by the following formula: $2NaHCO_3 = Na_2CO_3 + CO_2 + H_2O$.

The above formula clearly shows how easy it is for β-oxybutyric acid, which is stronger than carbonic acid, to seize upon free alkali and thus hamper the removal of carbonic acid from the tissues.

"What is essential and common to all conditions of acidosis is a depletion of the alkali of the body. This involves at least a diminution of the bicarbonates of the blood, and in severe cases it probably involves the draining away of very large quantities of alkali from many sources.

"Nothing is simpler than the process by which this condition is established. If an acid is poured into an aqueous solution of carbonic acid in equilibrium with the air, to which a certain amount of a bicarbonate has previously been added, the acid will react, according to its concentration and avidity for base, to a greater or less degree with the bicarbonate, forming in due amounts its own salt and free carbonic acid, which must escape into the air, since the solution is already in equilibrium with the carbonic acid of the atmosphere. Thus, for instance, a solution of sodium bicarbonate to which half of the equivalent amount of hydrochloric acid has been added will in the course of time contain just as much free carbonic acid as it did before and just half as much bicarbonate. Now the laws governing the equilibria between acids and bases determine the fact that it is in like manner *chiefly bicarbonates which react with acids introduced into the blood,* and when the resulting carbonic acid has been liberated by the lung the result is very similar to that of the simple chemical experiment. It is to be observed, however, that the respiratory process tends, under these circumstances, to eliminate more than the newly liberated carbonic acid; the tension of carbonic acid in the blood is thus diminished nearly in proportion to the diminution of bicarbonates, and since the hydrogen-ion concentration is proportional to the ratio of the free carbonic acid to the bicarbonates, the degree of alkalinity of the blood is unchanged by the introduction of acid—hence the theory that the hydrogen or hydroxyl ion is the hormone of respiration—*but the equilibrium is changed.*

"Carbonic acid is constantly being formed in the tissues and being removed from the tissues where its concentration is highest by the bicarbonates of the blood as shown by the above formula and is taken to the pulmonary alveoli where it is set free. If the CO_2 accumulates too rapidly in the tissues and blood, hyperpnea or increased pulmonary ventilation appears as a result of the stimulation of the respiratory center, which is extraordinarily sensitive to decreased alkalinity. Hyperpnea is the best clinical sign of acidosis. As a result of the hyperpnea the CO_2 may be reduced. By this process of removal of CO_2 by the lungs alkali is left available to neutralize the offending β-oxybutyric or other acid which can then be eliminated through the kidneys. $NaHCO_3 + CH_3.CHOH.CH_2.COOH = CH_3CHOH.CH_2COONa + H_2O + CO_2$. The β-oxybutyric can then be removed by the kidneys and the CO_2 by the lungs, but in the process considerable alkali is lost.

Howland[1] describes admirably another phase of the maintenance of normal blood alkalinity. "If the bicarbonates of the plasma were the only method of defense of the body the organism would succumb to acidosis as soon as the bicarbonate was depleted by the excretion of neutral salts through the kidneys; every molecule of an acid would rob the body of a molecule of bicarbonate." This involves another mechanism "by which acids may be removed, leaving behind part of the base with which they have been combined, this base being available for further neutralization. The elimination is by the way of the kidneys. These have the capacity to excrete an acid urine from a nearly neutral blood. They remove acid phosphate and save base with each molecule of acid phosphate that they excrete. Thus, although alkali is eliminated in the urine, it is much less than would be the case without this specialized kidney activity, and can readily be replaced under normal circumstances by the alkali of the food. For instance, with the introduction of a foreign acid $-Na_2HPO_4 + HCl = NaCl + NaH_2PO_4$ —the hydrochloric acid is neutralized, the sodium chloride and acid sodium phosphate are excreted by the kidneys or the following reaction may take place $-Na_2HPO_4 + H_2O + CO_2 = NaH_2PO_4 + NaHCO_3$. By his method the sodium bicarbonate reserve of the body is renewed.

"Henderson and Palmer showed the magnitude of alkali sparing very prettily by titrating with alkali the acid urine back to the normal reaction of the blood. The alkali spared was found in normal subjects to vary in terms of tenth-normal alkali, between 200 and 800 cc. This is equivalent to saying that the kidneys eliminate from 200 to 800 cc of tenth-normal acid in twenty-four hours."

The large amount of alkali stored in the body is another safeguard against acidosis. Not only are sodium and potassium present in considerable quantities, but in emergency the organism

---

[1] Howland: Johns Hopkins Hospital Bull., 1916, **27**, 63.

can fall back upon the calcium and magnesium of the bones. Gerhardt and Schlesinger[1] originally pointed out that these alkalis met
an attack of severe acidosis by changing their path of excretion
from the bowels to the kidneys, in this manner removing β-oxybutyric acid. In a study of the urine of Case No. 4 during coma,[2]
McCrudden found unusually large quantities of calcium and
magnesium excreted in the urine. Whereas 40 per cent of the
magnesium is normally excreted in the feces, in Case No. 4 during
three days 0.55 gram was found in the urine, but only 0.15 in the
feces. Similarly, 2.03 grams calcium appeared in the urine, but
0.75 gram were eliminated by the intestinal tract.

The elimination of nitrogen in the form of ammonia instead of
urea, as in health, is still another important, and indeed a most
remarkable means of defense of the body against acidosis. How
efficiently Nature works is evident when it is realized that 1 gram
of ammonia (NH_3 molecular weight 17) can neutralize five times
as much β-oxybutyric acid as 1 gram sodium bicarbonate ($NaHCO_3$
molecular weight 84). The formation of ammonia has been shown
by Nash and Benedict[3] to take place in the kidney. One wonders
how affectively the kidney can act when damaged by acidosis.

Finally, the proteins constitute a means of protection. They
have the power to unite with both acids and alkalis. Their part
in the prevention of acidosis needs further investigation.

2. **Acidosis in Diabetes.**—(a) **Extent of Acidosis in Mild, Severe,
and Extreme Cases.**—A moderate acidosis represented by the
excretion of 5 to 10 grams β-oxybutyric acid, the elimination of
2 grams ammonia, or a fall of carbonic acid in the alveolar air to
4 per cent, or 29 mm. mercury may or may not be harmful to an
individual, but it is a sign of danger. When the quantity of acid
is present in double this amount, diabetic patients invariably show
that they are burdened with disease, but it would be unfair to
attribute this state to the acidosis alone, and not to the neglected
disease itself. In former days, when the acidosis of patients was
not controlled, over and over again I saw diabetic cases who carried
an acidosis of 4 grams ammonia for years, with only gradually
declining health. Even so extreme a case of diabetes as Case
No. 344, eight years after onset showed 51.5, 52, and 54.8 grams
β-oxybutyric acid respectively on four different days, and yet
travelled safely for thousands of miles, dying of tuberculosis without coma four months later. But it may be considered that the
acidosis is very severe whenever β-oxybutyric acid reaches an
excretion of 30 grams in twenty-four hours, the ammonia 5 grams,

[1] Gerhardt and Schlesinger: Arch. f. Path. u. Phar., 1899, **42**, 106.
[2] Joslin: Jour. Med. Research, 1901, **1**, 306.
[3] Nash and Benedict: Jour. Biol. Chem., 1921, **48**, 463.

or when the carbon dioxide tension of the alveolar air is 3 per cent the equivalent of a pressure of 22 mm. Hg or the volume per cent of CO_2 in the blood under 30.

(*b*) The danger from acidosis varies according to the rapidity of onset, the age of the patient and the condition of the kidneys. It is my impression that fatal coma may result from an acidosis of only moderate degree which has come on suddenly, whereas in another individual the gradual development of an acidosis of equal severity has been borne with comparative ease. The cases of coma which are relieved by prompt treatment are generally cases in which a moderate acidosis has suddenly appeared as the result of some temporary cause, such as excess in food or exercise.

Children and adults under the age of forty years withstand acidosis better than older patients. Goodall and Joslin[1] found that the former group of patients tolerated an acidosis estimated in terms of ammonia of 4 or 5 grams far better than the latter group bore an acidosis represented by 2.5 to 4 grams ammonia. This was due, in our opinion, to the greater vulnerability of the kidneys of older people. The sound kidneys of young people readily excreted the acid, but the kidneys of the elderly or diseased kidneys in any individual excreted the acid with difficulty, and a trifling acidosis in such individuals might lead to serious results. Tileston and Comfort have shown from investigations upon the non-protein nitrogen in the blood of children and the phenol-phthalein test that the secreting capacity of the child's kidney was better than that of an adult.[2] Harmful acidosis occurred in Case No. 347, first seen in 1910, male, aged fifty-one years, with an onset sixteen months before. He was discharged from the hospital sugar-free with no acidosis, but the urine contained a little albumin, the blood-pressure was 175 mm. mercury, and the heart extended half-way to the anterior axillary line, the liver three fingerbreadths below the costal margin and the spleen palpable. The patient, as is often the case with diabetic adults on diet, upon his own initiative still further restricted the quantity of carbohydrate which he was allowed, an acidosis developed, and with it marked albuminuria; both rapidly increased. Cardiac weakness ensued and coma gradually developed from which he was unable to recover.

(*c*) **Culmination of Acidosis in Coma.**—The effects of extreme acidosis artificially induced in normal individuals are very suggestive of the beginning symptoms of coma in diabetic patients. Such experiments show the relation of acidosis to coma quite as effectually as the coma which Walter[3] originally produced in animals

---

[1] Goodall and Joslin: Boston Med. and Surg. Jour., 1908, **158**, 646.

[2] Tileston and Comfort: Am. Jour. Dis. Child., 1915, **10**, 278.

[3] Walter: Arch. f. exp. Path. u. Pharm., 1877, **7**, 148.

by the injection of hydrochloric acid. It is impossible to state how much β-oxybutyric acid and its allied bodies are necessary to produce coma. There are probably wide variations depending on the storage of carbohydrate, protein, alkalis and water, as well as upon the ability of the cardio-renal system to excrete the acid when formed. In some cases, like Case No. 4, large quantities of acid are excreted, but undoubtedly more often large quantities are retained.

Diabetic coma usually creeps on so insidiously that unless one is in the habit of treating diabetic patients it may be overlooked until all at once its spectacular features—anxiety and exaggerated respiration with the absence of cyanosis—stare one in the face. The onset can be traced to some change by which less carbohydrate, but more protein and, especially, more fat, is burned, by design or accident. In one instance, marked nervous excitement on the part of the patient appeared to play a great rôle, but I think the accompanying refusal of food and later vomiting made this case, also, one of sudden carbohydrate restriction. Typical examples of the onset of coma are Cases Nos. 310, 252, 220, 836 and 729. Case No. 310, who had had diabetes twenty-one years, showed a moderate acidosis over a period of months, then sailed for Europe, became seasick, was unable to retain food, and in three days died of coma. Case No. 252, while upon a rather more restricted diet than usual, nine years after onset, underwent exceptional exertion and coma developed. Case No. 220, having lived comfortably for years despite a severe acidosis, had a gastro-intestinal attack, was much debilitated, the diet was disarranged, and coma followed. Case No. 836 after suffering with diabetes for only three months, travelled several thousand miles, and during the latter part of the journey acquired diphtheria; on my first visit (eight hours before death) this was discovered, and along with it diabetic coma. Case No. 729, a severe diabetic, three months after her last visit to me, without my knowledge, was taken to a dentist's office, given ether[1] by her physician, and had all her teeth extracted. This was on Monday; she was taken home, became unconscious Wednesday and died on Friday.

E. CAUSES OF DEATH.

1. **Needless Diabetic Deaths.**[2]—The needless mortality in diabetes is, unfortunately, greater than we realize. All classify as accidental the death of the little boy, Case No. 1266, following

---

[1] The blood sugar is increased during the administration of ether, according to Atkinson et al. Atkinson et al: Jour. Biol. Chem., 1922, **52**, 5.

[2] In what follows, pp. 316 to 319, I have quoted freely from my Shattuck Lecture of 1922, Boston Med. and Surg. Jour., 1922, **186**, 833.

collision with an automobile while sliding down hill, but it is not so well understood that there are many other accidental deaths. Patients who have pneumonia, tuberculosis, and cancer usually die of pneumonia, tuberculosis, and cancer, but diabetics seldom die of their disease *per se,* but of complications which are universally recognized as largely preventable—coma, gangrene, infections.

Coma is the chief complication, and coma cannot be otherwise than largely preventable. Indeed, I do not hesitate to repeat, despite von Noorden's[1] criticism of the original statement, that *the diabetic who dies of coma uncomplicated by infections dies needlessly.* Between August 7, 1922, and August 7, 1923, there have been over 400 diabetic cases admitted to the New England Deaconess Hospital and Mrs. Leatherbee's Home under my care, and there have been 2 deaths from coma, Thomas D., Case No. 1305 (see p. 38) and Mary C., Case No. 3240. Between April 1, 1919, and July 10, 1923, 33 patients have died in the hospital and of them 21 per cent of coma. Outside of the hospital the majority of diabetics succumb to it. When coma does occur in a hospital it is seldom *de novo* as Petrén has emphasized; the patients enter either with it or in a stage of severe acid poisoning. The marked reduction in the diabetic death-rate in hospitals is almost entirely due to the prevention of coma. That nearly all diabetics who die in the first year of their disease die of coma is good proof that it is avoidable, because the first year of the disease should be the safest.

Anyone who sees or has reported to him many deaths from diabetic coma becomes appalled at their needlessness. A boy, Case No. 2090, is told to eat everything and in two days is in coma. A diabetic, Case No. 44, goes on a drunk, and as he emerges from alcoholic coma he lapses into diabetic coma. Deaths like these are not far removed from manslaughter and suicide. Another diabetic boy, Case No. 1870, amenable to treatment, drops out of medical supervision, coma appears, and he dies in the tenth month of the disease, though from other cases it is reasonable to conclude he could have lived years. Two young adults, Cases Nos. 2389 and 2401, refuse to submit to dietetic treatment and die respectively in seven and six months after the onset of the disease. Deaths like those just recounted can be traced to the advice of the laity or irregular practitioners, and often to the patients themselves. For all such deaths one feels regret, but not the keen concern excited by deaths under trained supervision, yet not quite free from errors of judgment. All these deaths most commonly occur when the diet of a patient is suddenly changed. When the

---

[1] Von Noorden: Loc. cit., p. 325.

carbohydrate is restricted and protein and fat simultaneously increased, death from coma may take place the same week. How many such cases! Nearly all of us have one or more such sorrowful deaths to our discredit. It is therefore well to hold to the rule in severe, long-standing, complicated, obese and elderly cases, as well as in all cases with acidosis, to make changes in the diet gradually and not suddenly or radically.

Nearly all cases of coma following alterations in diet can be traced to overfeeding with fat, combined with diminution of carbohydrate. Sometimes the fat is taken in obvious excess, as happened when a diabetic, Case No. 1511, of long duration, living with little dietetic restriction, went to a fashionable hotel, suddenly decreased carbohydrate and made up by indulging to the limit in *larded* mushrooms. The same result occurred when a fairly well-nourished but severe diabetic, Case No. 310, who had frequently shown acidosis, was taken seasick on a steamer, retained no food, lived on her own fat and secured insufficient carbohydrate from the breakdown of body protein to prevent coma. Remember that a little carbohydrate as such goes a long way toward preventing coma in a mild or moderately severe case of diabetes, because it is helped by that other carbohydrate formed from protein; but in a severe case when even carbohydrate from protein is not well tolerated, and the high protein is also contraindicated because of its stimulating action on the metabolism and its content of ketones as well, beware before you expose a diabetic to a high-fat diet, whether endogenous or exogenous.

Then there are the cases of coma resulting from operations with ether as an anesthetic. If ether is used, it is a good plan to be as rapid and as skilled as the Mayos and to use as little ether as their anesthetists. Gas and oxygen and spinal anesthesia have been shown to be so superior to ether that in the larger hospitals in Boston it is not the custom to employ it in operations upon diabetics.

Case No. 729, a severe diabetic, three months after her last visit to me, without my knowledge, was taken to a dentist's office, given ether by her physician, and all her teeth extracted. This was on a Monday. She was taken home, became unconscious Wednesday, and died on Firday. It is hard to believe that her death represented the culmination of diabetes, or was even accidental. Case No. 348, before an operation for removal of a prostate, was free from acid and sugar and tolerated 20 grams of carbohydrate. After light etherization followed by three days' fasting, 33 and 41 grams of sugar appeared in the urine on the second and third days respectively, and the ammonia was 3.3 grams. It is true that he recovered, just as 82 per cent of my patients formerly, 91 per cent recently have also done, but the ether lowered his tolerance and made his diabetes temporarily worse. This does not mean that diabetics should not be operated upon, but it demonstrates that ether anesthesia is a burden which a light case of diabetes may easily bear, which may change a moderate to a severe case, and to a severe case may be fatal.

Diabetic patients will live untreated for many years without the appearance of coma. They suffer from complication after complication. They are tormented with sepsis, neuritic pains and pruritus; yet they still live. Their diet is atrocious. Along comes an enthusiastic young doctor, and immediately fat is increased, carbohydrate diminished, and the patient goes into coma. Out of carbohydrates it is impossible to form the acid bodies. When, therefore, carbohydrate is suddenly replaced with fat, we deliberately furnish our diabetic patients with material which though it acts partly as a food, acts far more as a poison. Diabetic patients need fat; it forms the chief constituent of their diet; but they must not be poisoned with it, they must be allowed only what they can assimilate.

Next to coma as a preventable cause of death stands gangrene. The chiropodists know the dangers of infections in diabetic feet quite as well as, if not better than the physicians, but the unfortunate patients do not. In the first place, injuries to the feet should not occur. A diabetic should keep his feet as clean as his face and protect them with equal care. Never allow one of your diabetic patients to develop gangrene ignorantly. Warning and admonition should penetrate so deeply the minds of your cases that if such a catastrophe should ever occur the unhappy patient will feel compelled to say: "Doctor, you warned me about injury to my feet, about the dangers in cutting corns, toe nails, about blisters from new shoes or old shoes with poor linings, about nails in my shoes, flatfoot plates and hot water bags. You are not to blame for my present condition." The time spent upon such homely advice yields fabulous returns in gratitude from patients and in peace of mind when patients coming for treatment of gangrene are found not to have been those formerly under one's own care.

Pneumonia, tuberculosis, cancer, heart disease, nephritis, and old age, all occur with diabetics as with any group of patients, and it is true resistance to disease, which is undoubtedly lessened in the diabetic individual, but such causes of death should not distract our attention from the main causes—coma and gangrene.

The causes of death in diabetes for a group of von Noorden's cases and for various groups of my own cases are shown in Table 135.

TABLE 135.—CAUSES OF DEATH IN DIABETES.

	Von Noorden.		Author. 1894– Dec. 1915.		1894– Jan. 1918.		1894– Mar. 16, 1922.		Aug. 1921– Jan. 1923.		Apr. 1, 1919– July 10, 1923.[3]	
	Cases.	%	Cases.	%	Cases.	%	Cases.	%	Cases.	%	Cases.	%
A. Coma present	169	58	273	66	346	62	454	51	48	48	7	21
B. Coma absent	123	42	139	34	215	38	433	49	52	52	26	79
1. Cardiorenal, vascular, total	40	14	62	15	91	16	155	17	22	22	4	12
Cardiac	11	..	28	..	42	..	81	..	14	..	2	
Nephritis	9	..	14	..	17	..	29	..	..	..	2	
Apoplexy	19	..	14	..	26	..	33	..	6			
Arteriosclerosis	1	..	6	..	6	..	12	..	2			
2. Infections, total	18	..	36	9	63	11	141	16	17	17	15	45
Pneumonia	8	..	15	..	26	..	52	..	8	..	3	
Influenza	..	..	3	..	3	..	23					
Erysipelas	..	..	1	..	1	..	1	..	..	..	1	
Pertussis	..	..	..	..	..	..	1					
Meningitis	..	..	..	..	..	..	1	..	..	..	1	
Dysentery	..	..	..	..	..	..	..	..	1			
Tonsillitis	..	..	1	..	1	..	1	..				
Acute abdominal	..	..	..	..	2	..	2					
Gall stones	..	..	1	..	1	..	2	..	..	..	1	
Appendicitis	..	..	2	..	5	..	4					
Carbuncle	3	..	4	..	7	..	9					
Abscess: Mastoid	..	..	..	..	..	..	1					
Lung	..	..	..	..	1	..	1					
Empyema	..	..	..	..	..	..	1	..	1			
Liver	..	..	..	..	..	..	2	..	1	..	1	
Gall-bladder	..	..	..	..	1	..	3					
Paranephritic	..	..	..	..	..	..	1	..	1	..	1	
Gangrene, sepsis	7	..	9	..	15	..	36	..	5	..	7	
3. Tuberculosis, total	14	5	16	4	24	4	51	6	6	6	2	6
Pulmonary	..	..	16	..	22	..	49	..	6	..	2	
Peritoneal	..	..	..	..	1	..	1					
Meningeal	..	..	..	..	1	..	1					
4. Cancer, total	12	4	17	4	23	4	35	4	1	1	1	3
Brain	..	..	..	..	..	..	1					
Face	..	..	1	..	1	..						
Breast	..	..	..	..	1	..	1					
Esophagus	..	..	1	..	1	..	2					
Stomach	..	..	4	..	6	..	7					
Intestine	..	..	..	..	1	..	3					
Rectum	..	..	1	..	1	..	1					
Liver	..	..	6	..	6	..	8	..	..	..	1	
Pancreas	..	..	..	..	..	..	4					
Kidney	..	..	..	..	1	..	1					
Bladder	..	..	2	..	3	..	5	..	1			
Penis	..	..	..	..	..	..	1					
Bones, sarcoma	..	..	1	..	1	..	1					
Location?	12	..	1	..	1							
5. Inanition	..	..	..	..	3	1	21	2	..	..	4	12
6. Miscellaneous,[1] total	39[2]	13	8	2	11	2	30	3	6	6		
Pernicious anemia	1	..	1	..	1	..	1					
Ulcer: Gastric	1	..	..	..	..	..	..	..	1			
duodenal	..	..	..	..	..	..	..	..	1			
Cirrhosis	3	..	2	..	3	..	3	..				
Enlarged prostate	..	..	..	..	2	..	2	..	1			
Suicide	..	..	2	..	2	..	2	..	1			
Accidental	..	..	1	..	1	..	9	..	2			
Old age	..	..	2	..	2	..	8					
Hyperthyroidism	..	..	..	..	..	..	1					
Insanity	..	..	..	..	..	..	4					

[1] Coma excluded.
[2] Detailed diagnosis of 34 of von Noorden's non-coma cases in this group omitted.
[3] Hospital deaths.

(*a*) **Deaths With Coma.**—It may be said in passing that of the diabetics one sees in a year the mortality during that same year is considerable. In 1916 it was 10.3 per cent for my cases and between August 7, 1922, and August 7, 1923, it was 6.7 per cent for the 293 cases treated with insulin. This percentage would undoubtedly be lowered if all the diabetic cases, 447, treated were included, because the cases receiving insulin were the more severe.

Coma was the cause of death in 66 per cent of the total deaths up to December 18, 1915. In the next compilation, ending January 1, 1918, it was 62 per cent, and in the third compilation of all of the deaths ending March, 1922, it was 51 per cent. In order to determine whether the percentage was still falling, the causes of death are recorded for 100 cases between August, 1921, and January 1, 1923. Here coma was responsible for 48 per cent of the deaths. Of 33 patients dying in hospitals between April 1, 1919, and July 1, 1923, the percentage of deaths due to coma was 21.

(*b*) **Deaths Without Coma.**—1. *Cardiorenal and Vascular.*—Cardiorenal and vascular changes, uncomplicated by coma, caused the death of 155 cases, evidence that diabetes is a disease of old age and thus is sure to increase in frequency as life is prolonged. Of these 81 died of heart disease; 18, suddenly with angina pectoris; 29 died of chronic nephritis; 33, from a cerebral hemorrhage; 12 of general arteriosclerosis. The average age at death of these patients was sixty-three years. If the methods we employ in the treatment of these same arteriosclerotic conditions in non-diabetic patients are correct, it is difficult to see how modern treatment with restricted instead of forced feeding can fail to prolong the life of these individuals.

It is really surprising that in diabetes under the age of sixty, one so seldom meets with evidence of valvular disease or failure of the heart. All recognize the frequency of arteriosclerosis in old diabetics, but the rarity of heart disease in young diabetics may not be simply a coincidence. Among my fatal cases of diabetes under the age of fifty, so far as I am aware, not one has died of a valvular disease of the heart. Of the 14 deaths from heart disease in 100 deaths preceding January 1, 1923, 4 were due to angina pectoris. These were Case No. 355, whose lower extremities had been amputated on account of gangrene four years before (see p. 641); Case No. 499, who died at the age of sixty-two years, duration of diabetes seven years; Case No. 759, described in detail on p. 128, and Case No. 705, (see pp. 58 and 181). Case No. 1019 died of acute cardiac dilatation two days after simple drainage of a distended bladder, due to an enlarged prostate. Case No. 870 died of chronic myocarditis twenty days after a successful removal of gall stones.

2. *Infections.*—The advent of an infection lowers the tolerance of a diabetic for carbohydrate and thus increases the severity of the disease. This is an old and reliable clinical fact. Case No. 813, aged eight years, sugar-free for eighteen days, developed tonsillitis and without change of diet a positive carbohydrate balance of 50 grams dropped to 14 grams, with reappearance of acidosis. An infection is an additional load for the diabetic to carry, and to it he often succumbs. If those cases are excluded in which coma was an element, the number of deaths from infections is comparatively small. With insulin medication infections are infinitely better borne, but the decrease in tolerance is still manifest.

Of general infections, pneumonia heads the list with 52 deaths, influenza claims 23, and tonsillitis and erysipelas each 1. A considerable number of patients have passed through pneumonia successfully, *e. g.*, Cases Nos. 8, 19, 36, 46, 131, 352, 358, 435, 844, 895, 911, 1274 and 1350. Of local infections, septic and gangrenous legs account for 36, carbuncles for 9, and acute fulminating appendicitis for 4 deaths. Coma was a terminal event in some of the cases of appendicitis, though the abdominal condition appeared to be sufficiently severe without it to cause a fatal issue; 2 patients died of gall stones without coma; 2 died of acute abdominal infections and of these the physician thought pancreatitis probably in 1; 1 patient died of an abscess of the lung. In every case of carbuncle or gangrene one should have a blood culture before operation. It will frequently be found to be positive.

A considerable percentage of the cases of coma occurred in connection with either general or local infectious processes. Prof. John P. Peters of the Yale Medical School writes:

"In the course of the last eighteen months 9 cases of diabetes were admitted to this hospital with diabetic coma or severe acidosis; but in only 1 instance were we unable to find obvious evidences of severe infection."

It not infrequently happens that the infection is not recognized. Better statistics upon this point and in general about the circumstances attending coma should be accumulated. Thus, Case No. 836, seen in consultation one evening, was found to be in partial coma, but I was able to demonstrate to the physician a membrane in the throat, and three hours after the patient's death the following morning, the Board of Health reported a positive culture for diphtheria.

But what I consider of far more importance is the number of procrastinating cases of mild infections in mild diabetics, chiefly in their lower extremities, which frequently prove fatal. There have been but 8 cases of gangrene of the legs in diabetics under fifty years of age in my personal experience. In other words, these conditions develop at a time of life when diabetes is mild, and why should they so frequently be fatal? Consider with what these mild cases of diabetes have to contend. Handicapped by a lingering infection, which only too often is allowed to continue for months, with kidneys less efficient for throwing off the attack of acidosis; deprived of exercise—that proved stimulus to sugar consumption—for whoever heard of a poor old gangrenous diabetic taking exercise—these pitiful patients frequently meet a fourth enemy in ether anesthesia. Is it any wonder that a formerly innocent disease becomes virulent and the victim dies of coma? There is no doubt in my mind but that if such cases had been treated vigorously, even with the dietetic methods of a few years ago, a large percentage of the legs amputated might have been saved. All are very well aware that if a diabetic patient has gall stones to be removed he instantly commands the services of the leading surgeon on the senior staff, but if a diabetic patient has a sore toe there is no house officer too young to dress it, until a few weeks later, if the patient survives that long, the surgeon in the amphitheatre amputates the thigh. No matter how trivial the ailment, secure the very best surgical skill for a surgical diabetic.

3. *Tuberculosis.*—Pulmonary tuberculosis was responsible for the death of 49 cases, 6 per cent. This is significant, for so far the predictions which followed the introduction of treatment by undernutrition have not been fulfilled. The medical profession has altogether too pessimistic a view about this complication. When the treatment of the diabetes is faithfully carried out, these patients do quite well. The trouble in the past has been that consumption was usually advanced when diagnosed. In a diabetic temperature, pulse, and respiration may give no clue to the diagnosis, and the loss of weight is attributed to the diabetes. One patient died of meningeal tuberculosis, the pulmonary symptoms having subsided in large measure, and another of tuberculosis of the peritoneum.

4. *Cancer.*—Thirty-five of the patients died of cancer. The primary growths were in the breast, face, esophagus, stomach, intestines, rectum, liver, pancreas, kidney, bladder, and I include 1 case of probable sarcoma of the pelvic bones. The average age at death of these patients was sixty-five years. Cancer apparently developed after the diabetes in 20 cases and may have developed before or coincident with the diabetes in 5 others. Several cases of cancer which have been operated upon are alive; 1 of the uterus, Case No. 2524, 1 of the breast, Case No. 1088; 1 of the bladder, Case 2057; 1 of the pancreas, Case 2034; 1 of the stomach, Case 1789. Of 2 patients with cancer of the bladder 1 died suddenly of pulmonary embolism nine days after its removal, and the other with recurrence in the abdominal scar.

5. *Inanition.*—Inanition first appeared as a cause of death in my mortality tables in 1916, but to it should be ascribed other deaths. One should not be oblivious to the effects of undernutrition which underlie and are responsible in large degree for the non-resistance of diabetic patients in infections. Few individuals ever die from pure starvation. They succumb before this is reached because their general nutrition is lowered. Occasionally a patient with diabetes died from undernutrition, and there were more such in 1917 than heretofore, simply because formerly patients died at an earlier stage of the disease Probably closer observation of the symptoms at the time of death of these cases of inanition would show one which was predominant, such as hypoglycemia, as in the case of Case No. 1085 (see p. 174). Since insulin has been introduced there has been no death from inanition, just as the deaths from coma have been reduced.

6. *Miscellaneous.*—The small number of deaths from cirrhosis of the liver is always notable in any diabetic morta'ity statistics. Of the 3 deaths from suicide, 1 patient was mentally unbalanced and another took her life after becoming pregnant a second time soon after an abortion. Her marriage had been of short duration. In this particular case today an abortion would not be necessary. Indeed, I should not advise an abortion in any diabetic unless vigorous and prolonged treatment failed to render the urine sugar- and acid-free. But 1 death has resulted from pregnancy since this patient took her life in October, 1914. I have not had an opportunity to test the effect of insulin in a pregnant diabetic.

7. *Imperfect Supervision.*—It is not customary in the tabulation of causes of death to include what is quite as important, namely, imperfect medical supervision. More deaths I believe to be caused by imperfect medical supervision than in any other way. This is a reproach and an encouragement at the same time. It has radically affected my own treatment of diabetic patients; it shows the necessity first for better education of the patient, so that when not doing well the advice of a physician shall be sought; it shows also the need for closer coöperation between the family physician and the physician who sees the patient in consultation or at the hospital, and, above all, it shows the necessity for simplification in methods of treatment. Closer supervision of the cases demands an enormous amount of time, but time so spent will be repaid by lives saved. All of us must devote more time to our cases, and we must run the risk of the opprobrium of forcing ourselves upon patients by calling to their attention and to the attention of their physicians the need of constant supervision. Patients must understand the facts and be made to realize that lack of supervision often means needless death. Each physician has in his own hands the protection of the lives of his diabetic patients,

Coma killed 94 per cent of 50 cases of diabetes treated by von Noorden[1] in the first three decades of life, but only 25 per cent of 112 cases after the age of fifty years. Coma was responsible for 86 per cent of 139 deaths in my own series for the age period birth to fifteen years; for 72 per cent of 159 deaths between sixteen and thirty years; for 52 per cent of 267 deaths between thirty-one and fifty years, and 25 per cent of 322 deaths between fifty-one and eighty-three years. Of 49 fatal cases reported by Muryama and Yamaguchi death was due to coma in only 10 per cent.

TABLE 136.—CAUSES OF DEATH IN DIABETES ARRANGED ACCORDING TO DECADE OF ONSET (VON NOORDEN).[2]

Decade.	Cases.	Coma.	Cardiorenal.	Apoplexy.	Arteriosclerosis.	Pneumonia.	Tuberculosis.	Carbuncle.	Gangrene.	Cancer.	Pernicious anemia.	Gastric ulcer.	Cirrhosis of liver.	Misc., not coma.
0–10	10	9	..	..	..	1								
11–20	14	14												
21–30	26	24	..	..	..	..	2							
31–40	64	52	..	..	1	..	3	..	..	..	..	..	..	8
41–50	66	37	8	1	..	2	4	..	..	..	1	1	..	12
51–60	61	19	7	8	..	1	5	3	1	7	..	..	3	7
61–70	49	14	5	8	..	4	..	..	6	5	..	..	..	7
71–80	2	..		2										
Total cases	292	169	20	19	1	8	14	3	7	12	1	1	3	34
Per cent	..	58	7	7	0.3	3	5	1	2	4	0.3	0.3	1	12

TABLE 137.—PERCENTAGE OF DEATHS DUE TO COMA AT DIFFERENT AGE PERIODS. JOSLIN.

Age period.	Total deaths.	Coma No.	Per cent.
0–15	139	119	86
16–30	159	114	72
31–50	267	140	52
51–83	322	81	25

F. PATHOLOGY.

The present generation has seen the transfer of diabetes from a symptom associated with multitudinous clinical states to a disease with a definite pathological basis in the islands of Langerhans of the pancreas. Beginning with Cawley in 1788, the connection between gross lesions of the pancreas and diabetes was noted and

[1] Die Zuckerkrankheit, Berlin, 7th edition, 1917, p. 342.
[2] von Noorden: Ibid.

similar observations were repeated with increasing frequency as time went on. The removal of the pancreas of dogs by von Mering and Minkowski in 1889 with resulting diabetes established the relation between the gland and the disease and opened a field for experimental study. It was not, however, until 1900 and 1901, when Opie localized the morbid process in the islands of Langerhans, and Weichselbaum and Stangl described the hydropic degeneration and vacuolation of the island cells, that the pathologist could diagnose the disease without the help of the clinical records.

The pancreas is man's protection against diabetes. Destroy it by disease or remove it by experiment, and diabetes results. The annihilation of the gland is the essential feature; the means by which this is produced is immaterial. Pathologists, however, would not have been baffled so many years did not another factor enter into consideration.

A small remnant of healthy pancreas will suffice to prevent diabetes. This explains why fairly extensive destruction of the gland by necrosis, infection, or the inroads of malignant disease frequently is unaccompanied by diabetes. Minkowski's extirpation experiments proved this point when he showed the disease was averted if the remnant amounted to one-tenth of the gland. This would be equivalent to 5 or 10 grams. These pathological and experimental observations, however, almost added to the difficulty of explaining diabetes in the presence of an apparently normal pancreas until Opie's discovery.

The islands of Langerhans,[1] embedded in the pancreas, derived from the epithelium of the ducts, independent of the acinous tissue[2] and constituting about 3 per cent of its weight, Opie showed to be the seat of its protective agency against diabetes. Homans proved that this function belongs especially to the beta cells of the islands. Clark[3] has shown the number of islands in a healthy human pancreas may vary from 250,000 to 1,750,000. In serial sections of the pancreas in 12 cases of diabetes Conroy[4] found the average number of islands per cross-section to be 74 as compared with 184 in 12 normal controls. Given enough healthy islands, either in a small remnant or scattered throughout a gland quite generally diseased, no symptoms of diabetes appear. Microscopical as well as macroscopical evidence from the pancreas is therefore necessary before a decision can be reached as to whether a given pancreas had been associated in life with diabetes.

Fairly extensive removal or destruction of the pancreas does not

[1] See pages 26 and 37 for literature.
[2] Jackson: Jour. Metab. Research, 1922, **2**, 141.
[3] Clark: Anat. Anzeiger, 1913, **43**, 81.
[4] Conroy: Jour. Metab. Research, 1922, **2**, 367.

produce diabetes provided the islands of Langerhans or a sufficient number of them are left intact. This is shown by the absence of diabetes following experimental removal of less than a certain minimum amount of tissue and by partial destruction of the glands, but not of the islands, in infections and other lesions and by ligation of the ducts which results in atrophy of the acini, but not of the islands, a procedure utilized by Banting in his preparation of insulin. In a positive way it is proved by Macleod's[1] experiments with the angler fish and the sculpin. In these fish the islands are collected in a principal islet distinct from the balance of the pancreas.

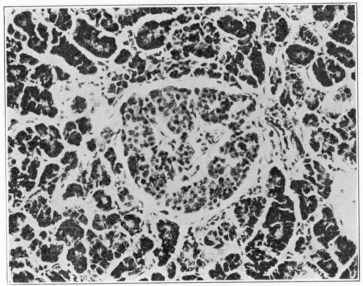

Fig. 9.—Normal island of Langerhans whose cells produce the insulin required by the body. × 250. (Mallory.)

Extracts of the principal islet act powerfully in lowering the percentage of sugar in the blood in contrast to extracts of the remaining zymogenous tissue which are inert.

Two totally distinct processes take place in the pancreas in diabetes and are to be found at autopsy. The first of these constitutes the lesions causing diabetes and represents changes resulting from an acute, subacute, or chronic pancreatitis. This appears evident from the formation of increased fibrous tissue throughout the pancreas, but especially in the islands. The experimental evidence produced by Mallory in his study of bronze diabetes furnished the

[1] Macleod: Loc. cit., page 26.

key to this process, but the more common result of inflammation is associated with the formation of hyaline material. Both of the processes result in fibrosis and atrophy of the gland in general and the islands in particular.

So-called bronze diabetes is readily explained. A yellow pigment, hemofuscin, derived from hemoglobin, is deposited in the cells of the islands and of the glands. It is quickly changed by their metabolic activity into another pigment, hemosiderin, which gives the chemical reactions for iron. The gradual accumulation of pigment in the cells leads eventually, as in the liver where pigment cirrhosis

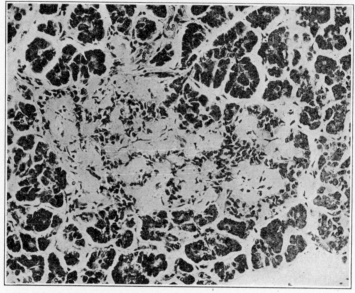

Fig. 10.—Island of Langerhans showing moderate hyaline thickening of stroma with atrophy and disappearance of the insulin-producing cells.   × 250.   (Mallory.)

is produced, to their destruction followed by more or less regeneration. The process is chronic and terminates in time in sclerosis of the pancreas. When enough of the islands have disappeared, diabetes develops. Mallory has been able to produce pigment cirrhosis and jaundice in rabbits in six to twelve months by means of chronic poisoning with copper, but only one pigment, hemofuscin, is formed. With smaller doses and longer time it may be possible to produce sclerosis in the pancreas also. The diabetes produced in hemochromatosis cannot be of nervous origin and corresponds to the type of diabetes produced by the removal of the pancreas.

Hyaline material (which sometimes gives the reaction for amyloid) is found in the islands in many cases of diabetes. This was first adequately described by Weichselbaum and Stangl. Mallory believes that this is probably produced by the fibroblasts and leads by pressure to atrophy and disappearance of living cells. In consequence, diabetes is produced in a manner analogous to that which occurs when hemosiderin is deposited.

In some cases of diabetes nothing abnormal is found in the pancreas, or, at most, only slight changes in the cells of the islands which may be interpreted as the result rather than the cause of the diabetes. Are these early cases in which our present methods do not allow the detection of abnormalities? And in the presence of

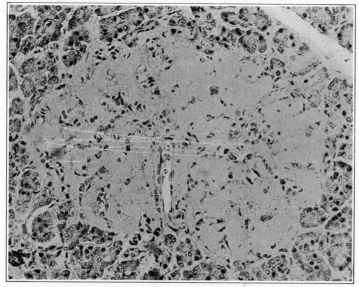

Fig. 11.—Marked hyaline thickening of stroma in island of Langerhans with complete disappearance of the functioning cells. × 250. (Mallory.)

such a lack of pathological changes should the clinician reproach himself on the ground that his treatment of the case was unskillful and that his patient should have lived for a much longer period, until the reserve power of the pancreas was more nearly exhausted?

The second process which characterizes the pancreas in diabetes is that of hydropic degeneration. This type of change can also be shown experimentally when dogs have been rendered diabetic by the removal of the larger portion of the gland. In sequence the changes are disappearance of the granules in the cells of the islands, swelling of the cells with fluid, and eventually disappearance of the islands. These changes are the result, not the cause, of the diabetes.

These susceptible animals, according to Allen, develop diabetes if overfed. This takes place irrespective of the quality of the food, carbohydrate, protein, or fat, only the time required for the effects of fat feeding is longer. Overfeeding is gradually followed by an increasing disease of the islands, and, in consequence of this, the diabetes is aggravated. The dogs are potentially diabetic, but free from symptoms on limited diets. Overfeeding causes active diabetes, which causes the hydropic changes. Allen concludes that hydropic degeneration of the islands in partially depancreatized dogs is a specific diabetic phenomenon produced solely by overstrain of the function of the cells by diets in excess of weakened assimilative power, that the condition begins within four to seven days, and attains a maximum in a month, and that by six to eight weeks all beta cells are gone. With restriction of diet the hydropic change is probably reversible within certain limits and recovery may take place.

The demonstration of hydropic change is important because it renders possible the microscopical diagnosis of active diabetes, furnishes proof that the internal secretion resides in the islands, is additional evidence of the identity of experimental and clinical diabetes, explains the lowering of assimilation in diabetics when upon excessive diets, and is a proved example of anatomical lesion resulting from overstrain of cells producing an internal secretion.

In partially depancreatized dogs the islands of Langerhans undergo various changes; (1) the stage of swelling of the beta cells caused by thinning out of the granular contents; (2) the stage of vacuolation of the beta cells as the granules disappear; (3) the stage of degeneration marked by the shrinkage of the nuclei in conjunction with the breakdown of the cell-body; and (4) the stage in which the beta cells have disappeared, leaving the islands composed only of alpha cells. This last stage is found only in animals; it has not been found in human diabetes. Hydropic degeneration according to Allen is not due to hyperglycemia, *per se*.

In the study of the pathology of the pancreas in human diabetes, Allen found no specimen of the pancreas which did not show marks of some damage or infection as the presumable cause of diabetes. In some cases a quantitative loss of islands and visible signs of their injury were to be seen. In others, the explanation of the diabetes must be attributed to functional deficiency in normal appearing island cells. Hydropic degeneration was present when the diabetic symptoms had been sufficiently intense and prolonged, but in mild cases it was ordinarily absent. In most cases of diabetes the disease can be diagnosed by decrease in the number of the islands or by hydropic degeneration. One can predict that when a patient dies with intense diabetic symptoms, hydropic changes will be found.

When a case has been treated long, and succumbs to inanition, one can feel certain that the number of islands will be few. When death occurs from some intercurrent cause in early stages, while the tolerance is high, there may be an abundance of normal islands. Allen sees in hydropic degeneration the chief or sole cause of the aggravation of the diabetes. In his opinion this interpretation alters the former conception of diabetes as an inherently progressive disease, and affords ground for regarding the average case as a consequence of the damage of the function of a vital organ, chiefly or solely from overstrain.

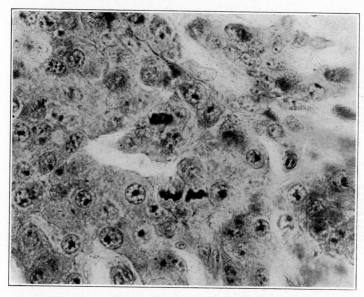

Fig. 12.—Three mitotic figures in an island of Langerhans in one microscopic field; four others were present in other parts of the same section through the island. (From a case of lobar pneumonia.) The section illustrates the great regeneration of island cells which may occur and suggests that in diabetes, if the island cells are rested by the use of insulin, regeneration may to some extent at least take place. × 1000. (Mallory.)

The complete imitation in the dog of a human diabetes is due to the work of Allen who thus rounded out Minkowski's and von Mering's original discovery. Allen demonstrated that severe acidosis could be produced in dogs by high-fat diets, which made them obese while heavy glycosuria was present. Coma can thus be produced if failure of the digestive power can be avoided. Former investigators had worked with thin rather than with fat animals, and so had not succeeded in producing acidosis. The external secretion of the pancreas exerts no influence upon the etiology of diabetes.

The influence of insulin thereby upon the condition of the pancreas has been noted by Allen[1] who reports upon a case of coma treated with 270 units. In the pancreas of this patient hydropic changes in the pancreatic islands were so slight that they were discovered only by long search. "The relative absence of such changes under insulin treatment is suggestive, but requires confirmation before any theoretical application is made. If infection be assumed as the chief cause of death, there is a previous observa-

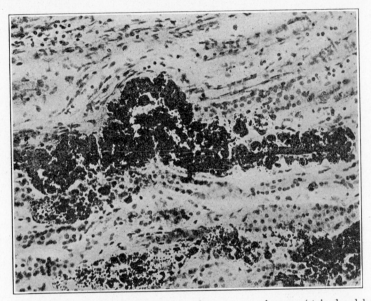

Fig. 13.—Kidney: The dark droplets and masses are glycogen (stained red by Best's carmine solution) in Henle's tubules where they make their appearance characteristically in diabetes. × 250. (Mallory.)

tion of almost as slight vacuolation of island cells in a case of diabetes with carbuncle, apparently explainable by the fact that the terminal severe stage of the previously mild diabetes was too short for the production of advanced hydropic degeneration, which requires at least several days."

A possible regeneration of the islands is suggested by the remarkable improvement in the condition of Miss M., Case No. 1542, who was treated for nine months with insulin (see p. 76), and temporarily enabled to reduce the dose from 35 to 15 units.

[1] Allen: Jour. Metab. Research, 1922, **2**, 803.

Bliss, working at the Physiatric Institute in 1922, noted that the pancreatic remnant in a partially depancreatized dog had doubled in size by the end of a year.

In a conversation with Prof. F. B. Mallory, he stated that "In various acute infectious processes, such as lobar pneumonia and diphtheria, mitosis and regeneration of the cells in the islands are of common occurrence." Macleod also states "It is at least significant in this connection that the islet tissue develops considerable powers of regeneration after much of it has been destroyed as a result of ligation of the secreting ducts of the pancreas, as

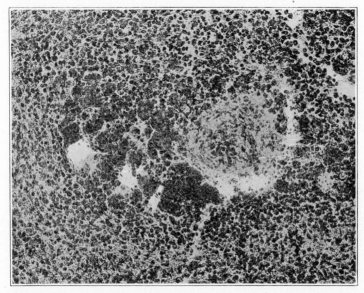

Fig. 14.—Spleen: The dark masses are groups of endothelial leukocytes containing fat (stained red by Scarlet R). They collect in large numbers in the spleen when the blood contains fat (lipemia). × 250. (Mallory.)

has been shown by R. R. Bensley to be the case, at least in the rabbit and guinea-pig. Arising, as it does in these cases, from outgrowths of the duct epithelium, may it not be possible in man, in whom the pancreas has not been completely destroyed by disease, that new islet tissue will become regenerated when, by administration of insulin, the strain to produce this hormone endogenously is removed?"[1] (Fig. 12.)

The diabetic autopsy presents by no means a barren field for investigation apart from the pancreas. The deposits of glycogen

---

[1] Macleod in Edinburgh lecture, July 24, 1923.

in the renal tubules and the deposits of fat in the spleen are in themselves phenomena of sufficient distinction. Why do these deposits occur in diabetes? What is their significance? To what amount is glycogen stored in this unusual fashion? Why this peculiar deposit of fat? It is a source of great regret that I was unable to secure colored drawings of Prof. Mallory's beautifully stained sections. However, Fig. 13 indicates the considerable amount of glycogen in the kidney and Fig. 14 the fat in the spleen. Prof. Mallory's sections of the diabetic kidney and spleen of Case No. 1305 dying in coma only heighten our curiosity.

SECTION IV.

THE EXAMINATION OF THE URINE, BLOOD AND RESPIRATION IN DIABETES.

A. THE EXAMINATION OF THE URINE.

1. **The Desirability of Routine Examinations of Urine of All New Patients, and of All Old Patients Annually.**—An early diagnosis in diabetes is as important as in tuberculosis. The diagnosis is made from the examination of the urine. How infrequent such examinations are has been shown from an analysis of groups of cases in which, prior to the examination at which the diagnosis was made, there was no history of an earlier urinary test in more than one-third of the series. The disease usually begins insidiously and its prompt detection depends upon the routine examination of the urine of all patients, rather than upon the examination of the urines of patients who present symptoms of the disease. In fact John[1] found that over two-thirds of a series of diabetics were without symptoms pointing to the disease. In all acute illnesses urinary examinations should be made for albumin and sugar, and invariably at the last medical visit the doctor should secure a specimen of urine for his own protection. Never allow a new patient to leave the office without obtaining a specimen of urine. Do not trust to the patient's sending a twenty-four-hour specimen. Each has its own value. Gray has emphasized the great advantages which may accrue from examinations of single specimens of urine and has shown that often these are of more service than twenty-four-hour specimens. It is especially desirable to secure specimens of urine within two hours after a hearty meal. Such a sample from one of my patients showed 3 per cent sugar, while the specimen only two hours later was sugar-free by Benedict's qualitative test. "Dilution is a dangerous mask. By testing separate voidings one can assure that more complete sugar-freedom which is the obvious desideratum. Hence the best method alike for early diagnosis, for

---

[1] John: Texas State Jour. of Med., February, 1923.

treatment, and for the doctor's periodic study, is to test every single specimen throughout twenty-four hours. Intermittent glycosuria often occurs at unexpected hours. Casts also are far more constantly found in fresh single specimens than in twenty-four-hour specimens, particularly in diabetic urines. When it is impracticable for the physician to study every sample, it is desirable to investigate a specimen one hour after a hearty meal. . . . For patients about to take insulin, single specimens seem especially appropriate to guide the balancing of the dosage against the diet desired."[1]

Most cases of diabetes go on for months, many for years, without being diagnosed. For example, in my series, out of 1135 cases which are available for statistics in this regard, at the most 286 cases, or 25 per cent, showed an acute onset of the disease. This shows the necessity for frequent urinary examinations.

It is inexcusable to neglect to examine the urine of any case coming for treatment. The wealthy parents of Case No. 1123, built a hospital for their community, but two doctors failed to examine the urine of their child and diabetes was diagnosed by a nurse. Similarly, the parents of Case No. 2568, took the precaution to send their children for medical inspection, prior to an European trip, but urinary examinations were omitted and the diagnosis of diabetes postponed for a year, to the sorrow and chagrin of the doctor.

I attach so much significance to this point that I believe if the physician is unable to secure the urine from the patient he should record this fact for his own self-protection. Practitioners in all branches of medicine should examine the urines of their patients or demand a recent urinary report. I except no specialist, whether he be surgeon, ophthalmologist, otologist, laryngologist, gynecologist, neurologist, orthopedist, or dentist. All would be incomparably rewarded if they made gratuitous examinations of the urine for albumin and sugar for all patients coming to them. The expense would be trifling, the good done would be enormous. Furthermore, such thoroughness would redound to the credit of those who adopted it. General practitioners should teach their patients, as a matter of routine, to have their own urines and those of their families examined each birthday. This is not fantastic. It is simply a part of the movement to have each member of the community undergo a physical examination each year.

(*a*) **Inexpensive Urinary Examinations.**—Examination of the urine should cost the patient little. Formerly I deprecated the routine examinations made in drug stores, but now I welcome them because

---

[1] Gray: Boston Med. and Surg. Jour., 1923, **188**, 168.

such examinations are so inexpensive. The mystery attached to a urinary analysis should be abolished. Recognized essentials alone should find place in an urinary report, which in turn should be expressed in the simplest terms and not be designed to impress the patients with awe. When I see two or even four full pages covered with a single urinary report and padded printed matter, yet showing on the face of it that modern analytical methods were not employed, I blush for the profession. When a urinary report was shown me for which a boy's father had paid $10, it was with considerable satisfaction that I taught the child to do the qualitative Benedict test for sugar, the materials for which can be purchased for 1 cent.

(*b*) **The Importance of a Physician's Laboratory.**—On the other hand, a physician's laboratory and his urinary examinations are often poor. It is not the rule for a physician to quantitate the sugar in the urine even by the fermentation test. The comparison between the outlay which the surgeon is willing to make for the conduct of his practice with that of the physician is most unfavorable to the latter. The surgeon almost invariably takes pride in his equipment, purchasing new apparatus and discarding old with a lavish hand. The physician seldom expends the fraction of this outlay in the development of a laboratory. This should be entirely different. The physician should take as much pride in a well-equipped and neat laboratory as the surgeon in his instrument case.

(*c*) **Causes which Lead to the Examination of the Urine of Diabetic Patients.**—(1) *Life Insurance Examinations.*—Life insurance examinations led to the detection of sugar in the urine of 14 per cent of 1698 male cases of my series.

TABLE 138.—DIABETES DISCOVERED AT EXAMINATION FOR LIFE INSURANCE.

Age at onset by decades, years.	Total No. of cases.	Sugar highest per cent, avg.	Per cent of total cases.			Range of duration.	
			Living.	Fatal.	Untraced.	Living, years.	Fatal, years.
11–20	6	0.95	83	0	17	1.5–11.3	
21–30	59	1.3	66	12	22	0.6–30.4	2.0–35.0
31–40	74	1.2	72	15	13	0.5–30.0	1.5–16.8
41–50	79	1.5	63	20	17	0.2–22.3	1.5–25.0
51–60	33	1.5	61	33	6	0.3–19.8	2.5–21.0
61–70	2	0	0	50	50	9.0	

The other causes which led to the examination of urine were those usually recorded in the symptomatology of diabetes, namely, polyuria, polydipsia, loss of weight, rapid gain in weight, weakness, pruritus, pains in the back or legs, but almost never polyphagia.

22

2. **The Volume of Urine in Twenty-four Hours.**—The quantity of urine frequently coincides with the quantity of sugar eliminated and von Noorden[1] gives a table to show this relation along with the co-existent specific gravities. (See Table 139.) The connection between volume, specific gravity and sugar percentage is by no means as close as his table would suggest. For comparison I have added to it figures based on 1127 successive cases of my own.

TABLE 139.—VOLUME OF URINE, SPECIFIC GRAVITY AND PERCENTAGE OF SUGAR COMPARED.

Volume of urine, cc.	Von Noorden. Specific gravity.	Sugar percentage.	Author.[2] Specific gravity.	Sugar percentage.
1,500– 2,500	1025–1030	2–3	1014–1038	2–8
2,500– 4,000	1030–1036	3–5	1010–1044	2–6
4,000– 6,000	1032–1040	4–7	1014–1036	2–8
6,000–10,000	1036–1046	6–9	1006–1036	.3–7

But the volume of urine may give little index to the severity of diabetes. Cases of diabetes decipiens are most common. Case No. 8 at onset of treatment showed 1030 cc of urine with 5 per cent of sugar, and twelve years later 1125 cc of urine with 2.4 per cent of sugar. Case No. 340 showed 5.8 per cent of sugar in 1860 cc of urine. Case No. 356 showed 5.8 per cent of sugar in 1035 cc of urine. In other words, the twenty-four-hour quantity of urine may be normal and yet contain a large amount of sugar. That a patient reports that he is voiding a normal quantity of urine, therefore, is no excuse for the neglect of a urinary examination. However, it is unusual for the urine to be normal in quantity unless the patient is sugar-free, just as it is unusual for a patient long under treatment to have a normal urinary volume. This is particularly true of severe cases who are upon low diets and consuming substitute foods such as broths with their liberal salt content and agar-agar jellies.

There are other exceptions to Table 139. Severe cases of diabetes passing through a period of restricted diet show a steady and daily diminution in the quantity of urine consistent with the restriction of carbohydrate, provided acidosis is absent. On the other hand, if acidosis appears, it is occasionally found that the volume of urine fails to decrease and may rise. The quantity of urine may be quite independent of the amount of sugar which is excreted. So far as I am aware the percentage of sugar as compared with urinary volume through the course of years has not been studied to determine its value in estimating changes in the renal efficiency of any given case.

[1] Von Noorden: Loc. cit., p. 325.
[2] Figures in each group based upon 10 successive cases.

A nearly normal quantity of urine, even with a large percentage of sugar, when patients first come for treatment is usually a favorable prognostic sign. On the other hand, a marked polyuria is by no means always an unfavorable omen. Case No. 585, Table 140, shows this very plainly. Onset of diabetes at forty-nine years of age, first seen at fifty-two years and eleven months on February 21, 1913. The first volume of urine collected from this woman was 6250 cc and the quantity of sugar excreted amounted to 500 grams, yet the patient despite various vicissitudes is alive over fourteen years after the onset of the disease; in other words, she has already lived within seven years of her normal life expectancy at the age the disease began. She is now sugar-free upon a diet of carbohydrate 76 grams, protein 45 grams, fat 130 grams. The blood-pressure is 250 mm. Hg systolic and 120 mm. Hg diastolic.

TABLE 140.—CHART OF CASE NO. 585. VOLUME OF URINE LARGE, YET COURSE OF CASE FAVORABLE.

Age at Onset in 1909, Forty-nine Years.   Greatest Weight, 190 lbs.

Date.	Vol. cc.	Specific gravity.	Diacetic acid.	Sugar, total gms.	Blood sugar, per cent.	Weight, lbs.
1913.						
Feb. 21	6250	1044	0	500	....	146
Mar. 9	2250	1039	0	126	....	146
23	2000	1033	0	68	....	
July 1	2115	1040	0	140	....	140
Aug. 4	2000	1025	0	2		
11	1500	1029	0	13		
18	1680	1027	0	2		
Nov. 4	2000	1036	sl +	27		
1914.						
Summer	Successfully shipwrecked off the coast of Ireland					
1916.						
Jan. 17	1900	1020	0	0[1]	....	146
1917.						
Jan. 2	2000	1029	0	56	....	146
1918.						
Mar. 5	....	....	....	60	0.27	137
Nov. 26	Nervous prostration					
1919.						
Apr. 29	1920	1009	s.p.t.	....	....	119d
May 5	....	....	....	....	0.10	
Oct. 28	1920	1010	0	....	....	128d
1920.						
May 15	2000	1006	0	....	....	137d
1921.						
Feb. 25	2000	1004	s.p.t.	....	0.21	138d
May 24	Fracture of neck of left femur. Successful recovery.					
1922.						
Mar. 15	....	....	....	....	0.18	
17	Twice successfully operated upon for cataract.					
Sept. 20	....	1004	0	0	0.18	
1923.						
Feb. 5	2500	1009	0	0	0.25	119d
Aug. 27	2000	1010	0	0	0.17	117

[1] Carbohydrate in diet, 40 grams.
d Dressed weights.

The greatest volume of urine in twenty-four hours in comparison to the weight of the patient was voided by Case No. 1151, who developed diabetes at the age of three years and came under my care at the age of ten years weighing 18.6 kilos in October, 1916. During the first sixteen hours at the hospital the volume of urine was 7200 cc and for the following twenty-four hours 7000 cc. If one should calculate on the same basis the total twenty-four-hour quantity of urine, it would amount to 10,800 cc, or 58 per cent of the body weight. Per minute he voided 7.5 cc and per hour per kilogram 24 cc.

The volume of urine should be expressed in cubic centimeters. This enables the percentage of the twenty-four-hour amount of sugar to be most readily calculated. An ounce of urine is actually 29.6 cc, but in clinical work one may reckon it as 30 cc, for the errors in collection of urine more than offset the trifling error in the equivalent. One quart of urine is equivalent to 946 cc. From experience with patients, I believe accurate enough figures are obtainable, except for scientific experiments, if we consider a quart of urine 1000 cc, and I am content with this rule because the error comes in reporting too little rather than too much urine. Naturally, such methods are absolutely barred when accurate work is being done. To avoid the necessity of measuring the urine, wide-mouthed, stoppered bottles graduated in cubic centimeter should be employed. The use of the metric system is essential both in recording the urine and in computing the quantity of sugar, and, indeed, for the diet as well. Most patients are glad to adopt it. The avoirdupois system involves too much labor. Few, if any, instances are recalled of a physician who was accustomed to record the volume of the urine and quantity of sugar by the avoirdupois system who knew the total amount of sugar voided by his patient in twenty-four hours. How could such a physician estimate the quantity of carbohydrate in the diet in grains to the ounce?

3. **The Specific Gravity.**—The specific gravity of the urine in diabetes is usually high, but Case No. 38 showed sugar in the urine when the specific gravity was 1.007. Case No. 1673 showed 0.34 per cent sugar in the urine with a specific gravity of 1.006, and Case No. 1151 showed 0.3 per cent sugar with a specific gravity of 1.004, and on two occasions traces of sugar not quantitatable by the Benedict test with a specific gravity of 1.002. A low specific gravity, therefore, is no more excuse for neglecting to examine the urine for sugar than is a normal quantity of urine. The specific gravity of the urine has taken on increased significance since it has been shown that variations in the specific gravity during the day indicate very satisfactorily the functional power of the kidney.

Perhaps no test of renal function is of so great value for the general practitioner or so simply performed.

The fixation of specific gravity is well illustrated in Table 141. The patient, Case No. 1086, was a man, aged sixty-nine years, with prostatic obstruction, and the following test was made ninety-six days subsequent to the removal of the prostate gland by Dr. A. L. Chute. It will be seen that during the whole twenty-four hours the specific gravity varied from 1.008 to 1.012. Along with the figures for the specific gravity are included those for salt and nitrogen. They do not, however, rise and fall with the specific gravity and their variation is much wider than that of the specific gravity. Consequently, they indicate greater renal efficiency. It is well to bear this in mind and not to become too despondent with the results of a two-hour renal test based upon specific gravities alone. Since the greatest excretion, as well as almost the highest percentage, of salt was with the lowest specific gravity, that evidence of functional power should be utilized in drawing conclusions.

TABLE 141.—THE FIXATION OF SPECIFIC GRAVITY. CASE NO. 1086.

Time. Oct. 31, 1916.	Volume, c.c.	Specific gravity.	Salt.		Nitrogen.	
			Per cent.	Grams.	Per cent.	Grams.
8 to 10 A.M.	130	1012	0.43	0.74	0.52	0.67
10 to 12 "	430	1008	0.53	2.0	0.32	1.3
12 to 2 P.M.	200	1012	0.4	1.2	0.54	1.1
2 to 4 "	155	1010	0.4	0.93	0.57	0.9
4 to 6 "	240	1010	0.42	1.4	0.43	1.16
6 to 8 "	270	1012	0.47	1.4	0.47	1.26
8 to 8 A.M.	1150	1012	0.57	4.4	0.47	5.4
Totals	2575			12.77		11.79

4. **The Sugars of Normal Urine.**—"The sugars of normal urine must consist of a considerable variety of reducing carbohydrate other than dextrose and fructose. A small portion may be derived from the sugar of milk. In the main they are derived from foreign, partly or wholly unusable, crabohydrate materials present in grains, vegetables, and fruits. Artificial decomposition products due to the heat used in cooking, canning, and baking probably contribute a considerable share. Pentoses and pentose compounds are doubtless represented, at least when fruit is eaten.

"The escape of such miscellaneous unusable carbohydrate material into the urine has no connection with the main carbohydrate metabolism, and therefore, none with the various problems of diabetes, except with reference to the correct interpretation of weak but positive tests for sugar in the urine. These foreign glycuresis products may sometimes be abundant enough to cause confusion or to give positive clinical tests for sugar. It is clear that one cannot expect to find any sugar reagent which will entirely discriminate between such foreign sugars and traces of real glucose. Excessively sensitive copper reagents, such as the copper-glycerol reagent described by Folin,[1] will show sugar in every urine."

"The sugars of normal urine cannot be entirely eliminated from the urine by abstaining from carbohydrate food, so that in addition to the precursors already referred to, one must also ascribe a part to the endogenous metabolism."[2]

5. **Tests for Glucose.**—(Dextrose, $C_6H_{12}O_6$).—It is the presence or absence of glucose in the urine which is important rather than the percentage of sugar, though a knowledge of the latter is essential for careful work. The quantity of sugar in the urine should be recorded in per cent and in grams for the twenty-four hours. The clinic upon diabetes given by Friedrich von Müller at the Boston City Hospital, in which he illustrated the total amount of sugar voided by the patient by exhibiting an equivalent amount of cane-sugar, was most impressive to patient and student. I constantly employ this method in teaching and there never fails some one in the audience who appears astonished at the pound of sugar, more or less, which has been excreted in twenty-four hours. The pound, not the per cent, leaves the desired indelible impression.

In most chronic diseases there is no criterion by which the success or failure of treatment can be readily estimated. Such is not the case in diabetes. One can tell when treatment is successful, for the patient should be free from sugar and acid and be happy and vigorous. While the twenty-four-hour quantity of sugar in the urine is not an absolute measure of diabetes, still in the vast majority of cases it is an accurate index. Taken alone the quantity of sugar eliminated is not of great significance, still less the percentage of a single specimen, but when compared with carbohydrate intake it is possible to determine quite definitely the condition of the patient. It would be deplorable if anyone, from the above statement, should lay undue stress upon this sign, because the strength, the weight, the mental attitude, the presence or absence of complications, and the acidosis are all important, but it remains true that this is the one feature of the disease which is of almost mathematical accuracy, though we often err in thinking of it alone.

The sugar in the urine of diabetic patients usually varies directly with the quantity of carbohydrate-forming material in the diet, to a lesser extent with the protein, still less with fat, save as that influences the total caloric intake. A change of diet is shown in

[1] Folin: Jour. Biol. Chem., 1915, **22**, 327.
[2] Folin and Berglund: Jour. Biol. Chem., 1922, **51**, 256.

the urine within a few hours and sugar may appear within a few minutes after food.

(*a*) **Qualitative Tests.**—Many of the qualitative tests for glucose are excellent, and nearly all have the advantage that although sugar is present in the urine of normal individuals, they fail to demonstrate its presence unless the sugar exists in a greater than normal amount. The Benedict test is the most generally useful. It requires a single solution, keeps indefinitely and the reaction offers less chance for error. Many false positive tests by this method, caused by concentrated urines, may be avoided by the use of slightly more Benedict's solution than originally directed.

(1) *Benedict's Test.*[1]—The technic of this test has been slightly modified from that first described by Benedict in order to aid in the performance of as many tests as possible at the same time and also to prevent chance, falsely positive tests. The method of heating the tubes in a water-bath rather than over a free flame, as directed by Benedict, was first suggested to me and used by B. H. Ragle. Later we found that Myers and Fine had previously suggested a similar procedure. The test is carried out as follows:

Seven cubic centimeters (an ordinary teaspoon holds about 5 cc) of Benedict's solution are placed in a test-tube. Eight (not more) drops of the urine to be examined are added, the tube is agitated to mix the urine and solution and then placed in water that is already boiling. After being in the boiling water for five minutes, the tube is removed and examined for evidence of reduction. In the presence of glucose the entire body of the solution will be filled with a precipitate, which may be greenish, yellow or red in tinge, according to whether the amount of sugar is slight or considerable. As used with urine the test is sufficiently delicate to detect quantities as small as 0.08 or 0.1 per cent sugar. A faint pea-green change in color represents about 0.08 to 0.1 per cent sugar. This pea-green color changes into a brownish tint when the urine contains about 0.5 per cent sugar. When the solution loses the greenish tint entirely and becomes brown, the urine contains from 0.5 to 0.8 per cent. Above this percentage the color of the solution gives very little aid in estimating the amount of sugar in the urine. The entire amount of copper in the 7 cc of solution is reduced (as determined by allowing the test to stand and observing a water clear supernatant fluid) by a urine of approximately 1.5 per cent glucose content. Frequently urines are tested which give a fluorescent appearance due to a very fine brick-red precipitation of the copper oxide. This seems to occur with severe diabetics who show sugar after eating certain fruits, are on low

---

[1] Benedict: Jour. Am. Med. Assn., 1911, **57**, 1193.

diets, and void large quantities of urine. Its appearance is related to the rapidity of reduction. It is so slight in amount that one is thrown off guard as to the amount of glucose present in the urine. On titration it is often found that there may be as much as 1 per cent sugar in a urine, which tested qualitatively might be estimated as 0.2 per cent.

The presence of a large amount of phosphate in the urine may produce a flocculent precipitate upon boiling with the copper reagent, but such a false positive test is very easily distinguished by that fact that it is not green but blue and also that it is coarsely flocculent and not in the fine suspension that the oxide of copper exhibits. Another source of falsely positive tests occurs when the urine is concentrated, amounting in twenty-four hours to less than 1000 cc. Under such circumstances creatinine is probably the disturbing factor. A false positive test of this character cannot be distinguished from a true test. The concentration of the urine therefore must be taken into account. Such an error can be excluded by a fermentation test. It should also be remembered that lactose will reduce Benedict's reagent, and positive tests during the latter months of pregnancy are not at all infrequent. Fermentation of such a urine will help to differentiate lactose from glucose. Traces of lactose are fermented by commercial yeast.

The chief points to be remembered in the use of the Benedict reagent are: (1) The addition of not more or less than 8 drops of urine, delivered from an unbroken medicine dropper; (2) the use of not less than 5 cc or more than 8 cc of Benedict's solution; (3) the transfer of the tube to water actually boiling where it should remain for five minutes; (4) the change in color and transparency of the solution is the criterion for a positive test for sugar.

The formula and directions for preparing the Benedict solution follow: They should be strictly adhered to in preparing the solution.

	Grams or cc.
Copper sulphate (pure crystallized)	17.3
Sodium or potassium citrate	173.0
Sodium carbonate[1] (anhydrous)	100.0
Distilled water to make	1000.0

The citrate and carbonate are dissolved together (with the aid of heat) in about 700 cc of water. The mixture is then poured (through a filter) if necessary, into a larger beaker or casserole. The copper sulphate (which should be dissolved separately in about 100 cc of water) is then poured slowly into the first solution, with constant stirring. The mixture is then cooled and diluted to 1 liter. This solution keeps indefinitely.

---

[1] The crystallized (10 molecules of water) Na_2CO_3 is more soluble; 270 grams of the crystals are equivalent to 100 grams of the anhydrous salt.

(*b*) **Multiple Qualitative Tests.**—The performance of a qualitative test for sugar in the urine requires scarcely three minutes, but when there are 10 to 20 urines to be examined the amount of time consumed is considerable. Time thus spent is wasted. With this in mind Myers and Fine examined simultaneously several urines qualitatively for sugar by utilizing a water-bath filled with saturated solution of calcium chloride.[1] (These writers also describe various practical methods for routine urinary examinations in hospitals.)[2] My former assistant, B. H. Ragle,[3] showed that a water-bath filled with water is quite satisfactory.

If Benedict's solution is used the directions are as follows: The water-bath, filled with 3 cm. water, is placed over a large flame. While the water is coming to a boil 5 cc of the reagent are introduced into the same number of test-tubes as there are urines to be examined. A very handy way is to have the tubes in a rack, and the solution can be siphoned into them from a bottle. Eight drops of urine are now put into each test-tube and the tubes immediately transferred to the actively boiling water-bath and left for five minutes. Within thirty seconds to one minute urines containing 0.5 per cent or more of sugar will have reduced the copper, and in five minutes any specimen with a pathological trace of dextrose will give a positive reaction.

The advantages of this method are that multiple qualitative tests for sugar may be made simultaneously with little labor, bumping is avoided, and test-tubes are less apt to be broken.

Dr. John A. Peterson, of Hingham, tells me that he has used this method for individual sugar tests, and I have adopted it as a routine method for patients to use at home. They call it the "teapot method," because a little teapot, reserved for the purpose, is so convenient for the test and the kitchen stove is far safer than to heat a test-tube over an alcohol lamp. A more refined method is to use an electric stove or point. A man can complete his test while shaving; it thus becomes a part of the day's routine.

(*c*) **Quantitative Tests.**—All quantitative tests for glucose in the urine are as unsatisfactory as the qualitative tests are satisfactory. It is one of the chief advantages of modern treatment that the need for these tests is nearly abolished. This field of chemistry has received the attention of chemists for years and still there remains debatable ground, although the last few years have clarified the situation considerably, and today we have relatively simple and accurate methods for the quantitative deter-

[1] Myers and Fine: Essentials of Pathological Chemistry, reprinted from the Post-Graduate, 1912–1913, New York, p. 127.

[2] Myers and Fine: New York Med. Jour., 1913, **97**, 1126.

[3] Ragle: Boston Med. and Surg. Jour., 1915, **163**, 746.

mination of glucose in urine. However, the more accurate of these methods, even though simple, necessitate the maintenance of a laboratory and can hardly be used by the general practitioner. Fortunately, with the modern treatment of diabetes these tests are not absolutely necessary, except as a matter of record, and some of the less accurate methods will answer the purpose very well. The simplification of the treatment of diabetes means everything to the practitioner and patient. The highest percentage of sugar found in the urines of my patients was with Case No. 2292. The onset of the disease was in June, 1920. The patient first came for treatment July 23, 1921 at the age of sixteen years and eleven months. The urine voided at this first visit at my office on July 23, 1921, was of specific gravity 1.045 and contained 14 per cent sugar. The quantitative analyses were checked twice by my assistant, Howard F. Root. The following twelve-hour specimen of urine voided during the night, after diet had been restricted, amounted to 1600 cc, with specific gravity of 1.042 and contained 8.5 per cent sugar. The patient was later treated with insulin, taking 20 units per day. With this he tolerated a diet of carbohydrate 66 grams, protein 72 grams, and fat 154 grams. He reports in May, 1923, that he is sugar-free most of the time and that his weight has increased 20 pounds. The best quantitative test for sugar for physicians who do not devote unusual attention to diabetes is the fermentation test.

(1) *Fermentation Test.*—To 100 cc of urine of known specific gravity, one-fourth of a fresh yeast cake, thoroughly broken up, is added and the whole is set away at a temperature of 85° to 95° F. Twenty-four hours later the urine is tested with Fehling's or Benedict's solutions. If a reduction is obtained it is set aside for further fermentation. Complete fermentation having been proved the specific gravity is taken after the urine has acquired its original (room) temperature. The difference in specific gravity multiplied by 0.23 gives the percentage. In the performance of the fermentation test for sugar a few crystals of tartaric acid should be added whenever the urine is alkaline. If the temperature of the urine is 76° F. (room) when the specific gravity is taken at the beginning and end of the test the result will be still more accurate. The physician who expends 3 cents of his own money for an yeast cake to perform this simple quantitative test for sugar usually knows far more about the treatment of diabetes than his brother practitioner who expends $10 of his patient's money for a laboratory report.

The test is most valuable in determining the presence or absence of traces of sugar. At the end of twenty-four hours, if the filtered urine which previously showed a doubtful test for sugar with

Fehling's or Benedict's solutions shows no reduction upon repetition of the test, it can be assumed that a fermentable substance, presumably glucose, was present. If further doubt exists, the use of the polariscope and the phenylhydrazin tests will help to settle the question.

(2) *Polariscopy.*—The determination of the percentage of sugar by means of the polariscope is the most convenient of all quantitative tests for glucose. The test is easily performed during the patient's visit and the result so obtained can be immediately utilized for treatment. The quantity of urine required for the test is small and quantitative solutions are not needed. It is not usually recognized that in the vast majority of cases simple filtration sufficiently clarifies the urine to allow of its examination. This saves a few minutes' time in one examination, but the aggregate of many hours in the course of a year. Should it be necessary to decolorize the urine, use infusorial earth. Magnus-Levy has pointed out that the employment of lead acetate introduces an error. Unfortunately in the presence of β-oxybutyric acid the polariscope gives too low a reading, for β-oxybutyric acid is levorotatory, whereas glucose (dextrose) is dextrorotatory. This error may be considerable, even amounting to as much as 57 grams sugar in twenty-four hours as in Case No. 235.

To obviate this the levorotatory power of the urine can be determined after fermentation, and this fraction of a percentage added to the percentage of sugar obtained before fermentation. But this calculation is not very satisfactory and, besides, requires a long time. Whenever, therefore, β-oxybutyric acid is present and accurate knowledge of the percentage of sugar in the urine is desired the Benedict test should be performed. In general the promptness with which the determinations with the polariscope can be made discounts this error in clinical work.

(3) *Benedict's Test.*[1]—"Like Fehling's quantitative process, the method is based on the fact that in alkaline solution a given quantity of glucose reduces a definite amount of copper, thus decolorizing a certain amount of copper solution. The copper is, however, precipitated as cuprous sulphocyanate, a snow-white compound, which is an aid to accurate observation of the disappearance of the last trace of color. The solution for quantitative work, which keeps indefinitely, has the following composition:

"Pure crystallized copper sulphate, 18 grams.

"Sodium carbonate, anhydrous, 100 grams or 270 grams of the crystalline salt.

"Sodium or potassium citrate, 200 grams.

[1] Benedict, S. R.: The Quantitative Estimation of Glucose in the Urine, Jour. Am. Med. Assn., 1911, **57**, 1193.

"Potassium sulphocyanide, 125 grams, or sodium sulphocyanide 100 grams.

"Five per cent potassium ferrocyanide solution, 10 cc.

"Distilled water to make a total volume of 1000 cc.

"With the aid of heat dissolve the carbonate, citrate, and sulphocyanide in approximately 600 cc of water and filter if necessary. Dissolve the copper sulphate separately in about 100 cc of water and pour quantitatively the solution into the other liquid, with constant stirring. Add the ferrocyanide solution, cool and dilute to exactly 1 liter. Of the various constituents the copper salt only need be weighed with exactness. Twenty-five cc of the reagent are reduced by 50 mg. (0.05 gram) of glucose."

The procedure for the estimation is as follows: "The urine, 10 cc of which should be diluted with water to 100 cc (unless the sugar content is believed to be low), is poured into a 50 cc burette up to the zero mark.

"Twenty-five cc of the reagent are measured with a pipette into a porcelain evaporating dish (10 to 15 cm. in diameter), 10 to 20 grams of crystallized sodium carbonate (or one-half the weight of the anhydrous salt) are added together with a small quantity of powdered pumice stone or talcum, and the mixture heated to boiling over a free flame until the carbonate has entirely dissolved. The diluted urine is now run in from the burette, rather rapidly, until a chalk-white precipitate forms and the blue color of the mixture begins to lessen perceptibly, after which the solution from the burette must be run in, a few drops at a time, until the disappearance of the last trace of blue color which marks the end-point. The solution must be kept vigorously boiling throughout the entire titration."

If the mixture becomes too concentrated during the process, water may be added from time to time to replace the volume lost by evaporation; however, too much emphasis cannot be placed upon the fact that the solution should never be diluted before or during the process to more than the original 25 cc. Moreover, it will be found that in titrating concentrated urines, or urines with small amounts of sugar, a muddy brown or greenish color appears and obscures the end-point entirely. Should this be the case the addition of about 10 grams of calcium carbonate does away with this difficulty. The calculation of the percentage of sugar in the original sample of urine is very simple. The 25 cc of copper solution are reduced by exactly 0.05 gram of glucose. Therefore the volume of diluted urine drawn out of the burette to effect the reduction contains 50 mg. of sugar.

When the urine is diluted 1 to 10, as in the usual titration of diabetic urines, the formula for calculating the percentage of sugar is the following:

$$\frac{0.05}{x} \times 1000 = \text{percentage in the original sample, wherein } x \text{ is}$$

the number of cubic centimeters of the diluted urine required to reduce 25 cc of the copper solution.

"In the use of this method chloroform must not be present during the titration. If used as a preservative in the urine it may be removed by boiling a sample for a few minutes, and then diluting to the original volume."

My laboratory assistant, Miss Evelyn Warren, suggested the use of white enamelware dishes instead of porcelain in the performance of the Benedict quantitative test. These serve the purpose admirably and the saving in expense is very considerable. The equipment of a diabetic nurse includes this apparatus.

(4) *Simplified Benedict's Test.*—The use of 25 cc of Benedict's solution is an appreciable expense item when one is performing 10 to 20 determinations a day and no less than the expense item is the time item for the reduction of 25 cc of the copper solution requires several minutes. Consequently, a modified Benedict's method sprang into use independently in several clinical laboratories making use of only 5 cc of the copper solution. Recently Millard Smith has shown that as used these modifications were not accurate. He, therefore, revised the test, made it still simpler

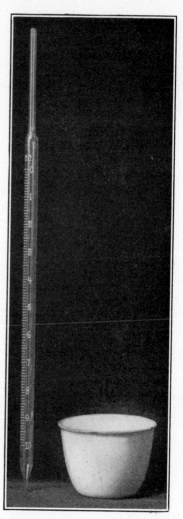

Fig. 15.—Apparatus required for a simplified quantitative Benedict test (p. 351).

and at the same time accurate. The new test, however, requires a slight change in the composition of Benedict's quantitative solution. The Benedict's quantitative solution, as modified by Smith for use exclusively with the 5 cc method, is as follows:

Pure crystallized copper sulphate	14.20 grams
Anhydrous sodium carbonate	100 "
Sodium citrate (5½H₂O)	200 "
Potassium sulphocyanide	125 "
Five per cent potassium ferrocyanide	10 cc.
Distilled water to make a total volume of	1000 cc.

"With the aid of heat dissolve the carbonate, citrate and potassium sulphocyanide in enough water to make about 800 cc of the mixture. Dissolve the copper sulphate (which has been accurately weighed) separately in about 100 cc of water and pour the solution into the other liquid with constant stirring. Add the ferrocyanide solution, cool and dilute to exactly 1 liter. Only the copper sulphate need be weighed with exactness." The sodium citrate should contain 5½ molecules of water and the sodium carbonate should be anhydrous. If it is necessary to use either with a different amount of water content, the weight should be corrected accordingly. The copper sulphate crystals should be pure blue and any white deposit of the anhydrous salt should be removed before weighing.

Five cc of this reagent are reduced by 10 mg. of glucose when used under the exact conditions to be described.

In buying the copper solution described in this modified method it should be emphasized to the druggist that this solution is different from the original Benedict quantitative copper solution. The reason that the original Benedict solution cannot be used with the modified method is explained by the fact that a reduction of copper solutions by glucose is a very delicately balanced reaction affected markedly by differences in acidity. The amount of copper which is reduced by a given amount of glucose is determined by the acidity, *i. e.*, with different acidities varying amounts of copper will be reduced by a given amount of glucose. Therefore, when the original method calls for the use of 25 cc of the copper solution, it is not permissible to add water to it to dilute it before titrating. By diluting 5 cc of Benedict's copper solution with 10 or 20 cc of water the acidity is markedly changed and a variable error of 20 to 30 per cent is encountered. To use such a modification it is necessary to standardize very carefully the amount of water added and the amount of copper and sodium carbonate used. This has been done in the above solution and with the following technic, used as directed, it is possible to obtain results identical with those by Benedict's original procedure.

Rules for Nurses in Performing the Simplified Quantitative Benedict Test.

Articles Required.

Ten cc Mohr pipette graduated in tenths of a cubic centimeter; small enamelware dish, 3 inches across and 2 inches deep; talcum powder; anhydrous sodium carbonate; water and flame.

The test can be performed by the aid of a kitchen gas burner or small alcohol stove. If the gas burner is not a small one and flares around the edges of the dish, put an asbestos plate or simply an iron cover over it.

The Determination.

1. Place 5 cc of the quantitative copper solution, accurately measured, in the dish.

2. Add 20 cc of water. Measure this with the Mohr pipette as the total dilution of copper solution should be quite accurate.

3. Add about half a thimble full of talcum powder.

4. Add 10 grams of anhydrous sodium carbonate. It is important to have this much carbonate. It may be weighed with sufficient accuracy by means of the food scales.

5. Dilute 1 part of urine with 9 parts of water unless the quantity of sugar is low. (A low percentage of sugar is shown by the qualitative Benedict test turning green instead of brown. With small quantities of sugar it is not necessary to dilute the urine.)

6. Bring the contents of the dish to boiling, maintain in this condition and then add, drop by drop, the urine from the graduated Mohr pipette until the blue color has entirely disappeared. Upon the first trial too much may be added, and therefore having noted the approximate quantity of urine required to reach the end-point, invariably repeat the test as a control. It is important that the total volume of the boiling solution should not decrease or increase (within reasonable limits *i. e.*, 5 to 8 cc) and this should be controlled by either vigorous boiling or the addition of water according as to which may be necessary.

Calculation.

Five cc of the copper solution are reduced by 0.01 grams of glucose. Consequently, the quantity of undiluted urine required to reduce the 5 cc of copper solution contains 0.01 grams of glucose.

$$\frac{0.01}{x} \times 100 = \text{per cent glucose in the urine.}$$

$x = $ cc of undiluted urine used in titration.

Example.—Fifteen hundred cc urine in twenty-four hours. Five cc used to reduce (decolorize) Benedict solution.

$$\frac{0.01}{5} \times 100 = 0.2 \text{ per cent.}$$

1500 × 0.002 (0.2 per cent) = 3 grams sugar in twenty-four hours.

Example.—If the urine had been diluted with 9 parts water, in other words, 10 times, the calculation would be:

$$\frac{0.01}{0.5} \times 100 = 2 \text{ per cent.}$$

1500 × 0.02 (2 per cent) = 30 grams sugar in twenty-four hours.

(5) *A Micro-modification of Benedict's Test.*—For this test Millard Smith[1] uses even less solution than the 5 cc modification and thus there is the advantage of using the original quantitative copper solution of Benedict unchanged. The test is performed in a minimum of time and the end-point is more distinct than in either the original method or the 5 cc modification. It is not necessary to calculate the final percentage of sugar for this can be read directly on the special pipette used for titrating.

Apparatus Needed.

A small ring stand with test tube clamp.
Micro-bunsen burner or small alcohol lamp.

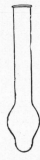

Titration tube as shown in Fig. 16. (A test tube of same size without the bulb may be used.)

One large bore Mohr pipette graduated to read directly in percentages of sugar.

One small bore Mohr pipette graduated to read directly in percentages of sugar.

The titration tubes and the pipettes may be obtained from Emil Greiner Co., 55 Fulton Street, New York City for a moderate sum.

One 1 cc Ostwald pipette.

Fig. 16. — Titration tube for micro-modification of Benedict test.

Determination.

"Accurately pipette 1 cc of Benedict's solution into the test-tube (held in the ring stand clamp) and then add 0.2 to 0.7 gram of anhydrous sodium carbonate. A small well dried pebble, or piece of quartz, or a pinch of talcum powder should also be added to prevent bumping.

[1] Smith: Jour. Lab. and Clin. Med., 1922, **7**, 3.

"Heat the mixture to boiling and add the urine from the Mohr pipette, until reduction is complete as evidenced by the disappearance of the blue color. For a urine expected to contain 1 per cent or less sugar, the large bore Mohr pipette is used, and for stronger urines or higher percentages the small bore pipette. The approximate strength of the urine, with a slight amount of experience, is easily estimated from the qualitative Benedict test. It has been found that with the use of the small bore Mohr pipette it is unnecessary before titration to dilute urines under 3 per cent in order to ensure sufficient accuracy. Urines over 3 per cent should be diluted to secure an accurate titration.

"For *rapid* reduction of the reagent vigorous boiling is essential, which may result in too rapid evaporation. This is avoided by allowing more time for reduction between additions of urine.

"The best results are obtained if the solution is kept *at* the boiling point by manipulation of the flame and the urine added slowly. A very small flame should be employed. *The tendency in this titration of sugar is to go past the end-point. This is because the reduction does not take place as rapidly as the ordinary titrations to which one is accustomed. When nearing the end-point the urine must be added slowly.* In urines of low sugar content the boiling should be rather vigorous at first in order to maintain a constant volume while the 1 to 2 cc of urine necessary to give complete reduction are being added. With a moderate amount of practice the regulation of the volume of the boiling solution becomes quite simple."

(6) *Colorimetric Method of Folin and Berglund[1] for Determination of Minimal Quantities of Sugar.*—This method is perhaps the simplest of the group of refined quantitative methods for sugar determination in urine. One should not be misled by thinking this method shows the percentage of glucose alone. (See p. 341.) It is so sensitive that the sugar content of normal urine may be readily determined and by proper dilution the concentration of sugar in diabetic urine may be determined with great accuracy. The method is based upon the procedure of Folin and Wu for blood-sugar determination and the interfering substances of the urine other than sugar are removed by shaking with Lloyd's alkaloidal reagent. The procedure is as follows:

If the urine shows a negative Benedict's test, it need not be diluted preliminary to treating with Lloyd's reagent, but for urines showing a positive test the following table will show appropriate preliminary dilutions for approximate percentages of sugar:

---

[1] Folin and Berglund: Jour. Biol. Chem., 1922, **51**, 209.

Approximate per cent sugar.

	Dilution.
0.08– 0.16	2 times
0.16– 0.30	4 "
0.30– 0.50	8 "
0.50– 0.80	10 "
0.80– 1.00	20 "
1.00– 2.00	50 "
2.00– 5.00	100 "
5.00–10.00	200 "
10.00–15.00	500 "

Five cc of undiluted urine which shows a negative Benedict's test or 5 cc of the diluted urine showing a positive test is placed in a flask together with 5 cc of tenth-normal sulphuric acid and 10 cc of distilled water. To the flask then add 1.5 grams of Lloyd's alkaloid reagent (this may be obtained from Parke, Davis & Co.) shake gently for two minutes and filter. The filtrate is then ready for the sugar determination after the method of Folin and Wu using 2 cc of the filtrate for a determination. The 0.2 and 0.4 mg. sugar standards used for the blood-sugar determination are also used. If the standard is set in the colorimeter at 20 mm. and the unknown moved, the calculation is as follows:

20 x 200 x strength of standard (0.2 or 0.4) x preliminary dilution, divided by reading of unknown = mg. sugar per 100 cc of urine.

Since urine sometimes contains polysaccharides as well as monosaccharides, it is possible to determine the total sugar by the same method after hydrolysis. Proceed as follows: "To 10 cc of the filtrate obtained after shaking with Lloyd's reagent add 1 cc of 10 per cent hydrochloric acid and heat in boiling water for seventy-five minutes. This heating should be done in test-tubes graduated at 20 cc for purposes of subsequent dilution. After hydrolysis, cool thoroughly and neutralize with normal sodium hydroxide. Phenolphthalein may be used as indicator, if desired, but is not necessary as the cloud produced from the material dissolved out of Lloyd's reagent furnishes an adequate indicator of the degree of neutrality required. Add the alkali until the cloud so formed does not disappear on shaking. Dilute the neutralized hydrolysate to the 20 cc mark. Then add a small pinch of Lloyd's reagent and invert half a dozen times. This is for the purpose of removing most of the coloring matter formed during the hydrolysis. Two cc of this more dilute filtrate are used for the determination. The standards used are the same and the calculation as given above is used, except that the final result is multiplied by 2."

(7) *Benedict's Colorimetric Method for Determination of Sugar in Urine.*—In 1918, Benedict and Osterberg[1] published a micro-

---

[1] Benedict and Osterberg: Jour. Biol. Chem., 1918, **34**, 195.

colorimetric method for the determination of sugar in normal urine. The method served its purpose very well except that it was quite laborious due to the necessary removal of certain nitrogenous products from the urine before the color reaction with picric acid could be applied. In a more recent paper[1] they have greatly simplified the method by the use of acetone at the time the color reaction is taking place, thereby eliminating the preliminary treatment of the urine with mercuric nitrate and sodium bicarbonate. They have found that this step was made necessary by the presence of creatinine and that acetone destroys the color which is formed by the interaction of picric acid and creatinine in alkaline solution, while at the same time it permits the color reaction between glucose and picric acid to go to completion.

The Method.—1. *Reagents.*—(*a*) Purified Bone-black. This is prepared from commercial bone-black (Benedict recommends that sold by Eimer and Amend). Animal charcoals should not be used. Two hundred and fifty grams of commercial bone-black are treated with about 1.5 liters of dilute hydrochloric acid (1 volume of concentrated acid diluted with 4 volumes of water) and the mixture is boiled for about thirty minutes. The bone-black is now filtered off on a large Buchner funnel and washed with water (preferably hot) until the washings are neutral to litmus. The product is then dried and powdered. The final product should be tested by shaking a portion (15 cc) of a glucose solution containing 1 mg. of the sugar in 2 cc of water with 1 gram of the bone-black and determining the sugar in the filtrate. There should be no detectable absorption of the sugar.

(*b*) Picric acid solution, 0.6 per cent.

(*c*) Sodium hydroxide solution, 5 per cent.

(*d*) Acetone solution, 50 per cent.

This should be prepared fresh every day or two by diluting some pure acetone with an equal volume of water.

(*e*) Glucose standard containing 1 mg. pure glucose in 3 cc of solution. Benedict states that this solution keeps "indefinitely" if preserved with a little toluene. Judging from past experience in the New England Deaconess Hospital Laboratory it does not keep as well in the average clinical laboratory. The danger may be avoided by preparing the standard with saturated benzoic acid solution according to the suggestion of Folin and Berglund. The latter method we have found to produce standards which keep without any detectable change after many months. The benzoic acid should not interfere in the determination.

2. *Procedure.*—"The urine should be diluted so that the specific gravity does not exceed 1.025 to 1.030. Fifteen cc of the urine

[1] Benedict and Osterberg: Jour. Biol. Chem., 1921, **48**, 51.

are then treated with about 1 gram of bone-black (smaller quantities of both may be used if desired) and the mixture shaken vigorously occasionally for a period of five to ten minutes. The mixture is then filtered through a small filter into a dry flask or beaker. The volume of the filtrate to be used in the determination depends upon its sugar content, but should never exceed 3 cc. Such a volume should be used as will contain about 1 mg. of sugar. Usually 1 to 2 cc is the right amount. The proper volume of the urine filtrate is measured into a large test-tube which is graduated at 25 cc, and if the volume used was less than 3 cc enough water is added to make the volume exactly 3 cc. Now add exactly 1 cc of 0.6 per cent picric acid solution and 0.5 cc of 5 per cent sodium hydroxide solution. Just before the tube is ready to be placed in boiling water add 5 drops of 50 per cent acetone taking care that the drops fall into the solution and not on the sides of the tube. Shake the tube gently to mix the contents, and place immediately in boiling water and leave for twelve to fifteen minutes. The standard solution should be simultaneously prepared by treating 3 cc of the standard glucose solution exactly as described for the unknown solution and heating simultaneously. After heating and cooling the tubes are made to 25 cc mark and the unknown read against the standard in a colorimeter."

The picric acid solution must be measured as accurately as the unknown or standard solutions. The alkali may be added with sufficient accuracy by measuring out about 10 drops from the same pipette into each tube. All tubes should receive the same number of drops. The acetone solution should be added last and the tubes placed in the boiling water within a minute afterward. The diluted acetone should not be over two days old. Each solution must be added so that it does not touch the sides of the tube but falls directly to the bottom. The standard and unknown must correspond in sugar content within reasonable limits. For the 1 mg. standard described above, the limits for the strength of the unknown are about 0.75 to 1.75 mg. of sugar. If less than 0.7 mg. of sugar are found in 3 cc of the unknown, a half strength standard solution should be employed, and the final colored solutions diluted to 12.5 cc instead of 25 cc. For clinical purposes the bone-black may be omitted if desired. Under such conditions figures will be obtained which are about 0.03 to 0.04 per cent too high. The method is also applicable to urines after they have been fermented with yeast.

6. **Tests for Other Sugars.**—Other sugars than glucose are occasionally found in the urine. It is rare that they cause confusion. It is not quite so easy to detect or to exclude them, as would appear from the description of the tests by which they

are said to be identified. Of these various sugars lactose is the one most commonly encountered.

(*a*) **Lactose** ($C_{12}H_{22}O_{11}$).—Lactose in the urine may give rise to confusion in the performance of Fehling's or Benedict's tests. Fortunately, the conditions in which it is liable to occur, pregnancy and the lactation period, are usually known to the physician, and it is then not considered of significance. It has also been found in the urines of nurslings. Lactose, like glucose, reduces copper, is dextrorotatory, but it yields a characteristic osazone with phenylhydrazin and does not ferment with pure yeast (saccharomyces-apiculatus). However, the osazone is very difficult to obtain from the urine and ordinary yeast is not to be depended upon for the fermentation test.

(1) *Rubner's Test.*—To 5 cc of urine in a test-tube, add 1 or 2 grams of lead acetate. Heat until bubbles appear and then add ammonium hydrate until the color changes. A deep yellow or brown color in the solution is distinctive of lactose, whereas in the presence of dextrose the color is a cherry-red.

(2) *Mucic Acid Test.*—This test does not distinguish between lactose and galactose, but the latter very rarely occurs. The test is, therefore, of considerable value in differentiating these two sugars from all other reducing sugars. It is performed as follows: To 100 cc of the urine add 20 cc of concentrated nitric acid and evaporate the mixture in a broad, shallow glass vessel, upon a boiling water-bath, until the volume of the solution is only 20 cc. At this point the fluid should be clear and a fine, white precipitate of mucic acid should separate. If the percentage of galactose present in the urine is low, it may be necessary to cool the solution and permit it to stand for some time before the precipitate will form. If the specific gravity of the urine is 1.020 or over, it is necessary to use 25 to 35 cc of nitric acid. Under these conditions the mixture should be evaporated until the remaining volume is approximately equivalent to that of the nitric acid added.

(*b*) **Pentose** ($C_5H_{10}O_5$).—Pentose is occasionally present in the urine, and probably will be encountered more frequently in the future now that attention has been called to it. It may be suspected when Fehling's test, performed in the ordinary way, fails to show reduction upon the second boiling, but later suddenly causes a partial reduction. Pentose neither ferments nor is it optically active.

(1) *Orcinol-hydrochloric Acid (Bial) Test.*—Bial's reagent is employed and is as follows:

Orcinol	15 grams
Fuming HCl	500 grams
Ferric chloride (10 per cent)	20 to 30 drops

To 5 cc of the reagent in a test-tube add 2 to 3 cc of urine and heat the mixture gently until the first bubbles rise to the surface. Immediately, or upon cooling, the solution becomes green and a flocculent precipitate of the same color may form. This test is more specific than the original orcinol test.

(c) **Levulose** ($C_6H_{12}O_6$).—Levulose is frequently present in the urine of severe diabetics. It is not easily identified. It is levorotatory, but so is β-oxybutyric acid, which is found under similar conditions. Levulose ferments with yeast, gives a positive Fehling and Benedict test, and yields the same osazone as does dextrose with phenylhydrazin. Levulose can, however, be differentiated by the Seliwanoff reaction, provided the following precautions are observed: (1) The concentration of the HCl must not be more than 12 per cent; (2) the reaction (red color) and the precipitate must be observed within twenty to thirty seconds of boiling; (3) glucose must not be present in amounts exceeding 2 per cent; and (4) the precipitate must be soluble in alcohol with a bright red color.

(1) *Seliwanoff's Test.*—Seliwanoff's reagent is prepared by dissolving 0.05 gram of resorcinol in 100 cc of dilute (1:2) HCl. To 5 cc of the reagent in a test-tube add a few drops of the urine under examination and heat the mixture to boiling. The presence of levulose is indicated by the production of a red color and the separation of a red precipitate. The latter may be dissolved in alcohol to which it will impart a striking red color.

A new method for the determination of levulose in the presence of dextrose is described by Loewe.[1]

(d) **Maltose** ($C_{12}H_{22}O_{11}$).—Maltose very rarely occurs in human urine, and has not been shown to be of clinical significance. Maltose is powerfully dextrorotatory, completely fermented by yeast, reduces copper slowly, and yields a characteristic osazone.

(e) **Glycuronic Acid** ($C_6H_{10}O_7$).—Glycuronic acid as such is not found in fresh urines, but conjugated glycuronic acids occurring in the urine spontaneously decompose and may cause confusion. Such conjugated glycuronic acids only appear after the ingestion of chloral hydrate, camphor, menthol, turpentine, or phenol in large enough quantities to be of significance. If this point is borne in mind confusion will not arise. Glycuronic acid reduces copper and bismuth, but does not ferment. It may be difficult to detect in the presence of pentose, although one can rely on the characteristic osazone of pentose if differentiation becomes necessary.

(f) **Substances Found in the Urine which give Rise to Confusion in Testing for Sugar.**—These may be divided into two groups;

---

[1] Loewe: Proc. Soc. Exp. Biol. and Med., 1916, **13**, 71.

those in normal urines and those in pathological urines. Of those met with in normal urine there are creatinin, especially if the urine is concentrated, earthy phosphates, uric acid, xanthin basis, peptone, glycuronic and glycosuric acids, mucus, indoxyl sulphates, and urates. These decolorize the blue solution, but do not give the red precipitate, which cannot be mistaken. In pathological urines albumin is the most troublesome, but this is easily counteracted by precipitating the albumin by the Esbach test and subsequently filtration. In doubtful cases, precipitation of uric acid, xanthin, hypoxanthin, creatins, and phosphates may be accomplished by adding 5 cc of 10 per cent solution of sodium acetate. The test is then applied to the filtrate.

7. **Methods for the Determination of the Urinary Acids.**—
(a) **Qualitative Tests.**—(1) *Diacetic Acid* (CH_3COCH_2COOH).—
The simplest method for the detection of acidosis by urinary examination is Gerhardt's ferric chloride reaction for diacetic acid. The test may be performed as follows: To about 10 cc of the fresh urine carefully add a few drops of an undiluted aqueous solution of ferric chloride, Liquor Ferri Chloridi, U. S. P. A precipitate of ferric phosphate first forms, but upon the addition of a few more drops is dissolved. The depth of the Burgundy-red color obtained is an index to the quantity of diacetic acid present. On account of the merely approximate value of the reaction I now record the intensity of the reaction as follows: $+$, $++$, $+++$ instead of in four degrees of intensity, Lüthje pointed out the fallacies of this method and Table 142 shows how unreliable Benedict and I have also found it to be.[1]

TABLE 142.—COMPARISON OF DIACETIC ACID AND β-OXYBUTYRIC ACID.

Diacetic acid, symbol.	β-oxybutyric acid, grams.
0	5.7 to 11.0
+	7.0 to 14.2
++	8.5 to 55.3
+++	13.3 to 51.0
++++	17.6 to 36.8

It should not be forgotten that if a patient is taking salicylates, antipyrin, cyanates, or acetates, the foregoing test will give a similar reaction, but one that cannot be mistaken if the solution is boiled for two minutes. Diacetic acid is unstable and the color disappears if due to it, but if due to the above substances the color is unchanged. Diabetic patients often take salicylates for pain of one kind or another, and therefore one must always be on the watch for this possibility. I have seen a patient on the verge of

[1] Benedict and Joslin: Carnegie Inst., Washington, Pub. 136, p. 25.

coma who was taking salicylates, and at the start confusion arose as to whether the ferric chloride reaction was due to diacetic acid or to salicyluric acid.   The vacation of another patient in Europe was abruptly terminated, so far as I can determine, by a falsely positive ferric chloride test due to the oil of wintergreen in an innocent official, compound rhubarb pill.

TABLE 143.—THE RELATION BETWEEN THE QUANTITY OF SODIUM BICARBONATE REQUIRED TO RENDER THE URINE ALKALINE AND THE ACID BODIES PRESENT.

NaHCO₃ required to render urine alkaline, grams.	Approximate acidosis in terms of β-oxybutyric acid, grams.
20	Under 15
30 to 40	20 to 30
40 +	30 to 40

With the test for diacetic acid the physician must be absolutely at home.   It is doubtful if 1 physician in 500 will employ any better test for acidosis, and only rarely is any other test necessary.

(2) *Acetone* (CH_3COCH_3).—The test for acetone was the first employed for the detection of acid poisoning, but the small rôle which Folin[1] has shown that acetone plays in the total acidosis led me to discard it, believing it better to concentrate time upon the quantitative estimation of the acidosis than to use several qualitative tests.   Folin demonstrated that most of the substance supposed to be acetone in the urine is really diacetic acid, and that Legal's test for acetone is really a very delicate test for both diacetic acid and acetone.   Weiland, quoted by L. Blum,[2] says that acetone may amount to 1.67 grams and yet the Gerhardt test for diacetic acid be negative, while at other times the presence of 0.1 gram of acetone in the twenty-four hours is sufficient to make the Gerhardt test positive.   The different tests for acetone are in reality tests for both acetone and diacetic acid.

The simplest and most reliable test for acetone plus diacetic acid is a modification of Rothera's test.   In a small test-tube (5 mm. x 50 mm.) or in a 15 cc centrifuge tube with tapered end, place enough crystals of ammonium sulphate to make the final mixture supersaturated.   Add 4 drops of the urine to be tested, 2 drops of a 5 per cent solution of sodium nitroprusside (this solution should be kept in the dark and preferably in an ice box; otherwise it spoils within a week) and 2 drops of concentrated ammonium hydroxide.   Agitate and thoroughly mix the contents of the tube by holding the open end of the tube in the fingers of one hand and quickly striking the bottom with the fingers of the other.   At the

[1] Folin: Jour. Biol. Chem., 1907, **3**, 177; Jour. Am. Med. Assn., 1907, **49, 128.**
[2] Blum: Ergebnisse der inneren Medizin und Kinderheilkunde, 1913, **2**, 454.

end of two or three minutes the maximum color will have appeared and the test may be read. Since the maximum color slowly turns into a muddy brown, one should read the test before this occurs. A little practise enables one to tell the point of maximum color formation. A positive test is evidenced by a range of color from a faint purplish-pink to a very dark purple. A faint pink may be called 1 plus and a dark purple which does not transmit light a 7 plus. One soon becomes accustomed to making the gradations between these two extremes. Usually the ferric chloride test becomes positive when the nitroprusside test is 5 plus. This is a valuable test in following the course of cases of pernicious vomiting. These are at times quite severe in degree at a stage when the ferric chloride test begins to be positive. It is also of value in watching the disappearance of the final traces of acidosis in treated cases of diabetes or in detecting early tendencies to returning acidosis. Again it should be remembered that salicylates give a strongly positive reaction with nitroprusside.

(3) *β-oxybutyric Acid* ($CH_3CH(OH),CH_2COOH$).—There is no simple qualitative test for β-oxybutyric acid.

(*b*) **Quantitative Tests.**—The determination of the extent of the acidosis is of prime importance in the treatment of any severe case of diabetes. I sympathize with any physician who must treat a severe case of diabetes without a knowledge of the degree of acid poisoning present. Fortunately, comparatively simple methods are at hand which are quite satisfactory in routine treatment; but even most of these simple methods are too complicated for a physician with a large practice who has only a few cases of diabetes in the course of a year.

(1) *Reaction of Urine.*—The most easily performed of the urinary tests are concerned with the reaction of the urine. Although the urines of normal individuals are frequently neutral or alkaline, this is seldom the case with urines of diabetics, for the protein-fat diet of the diabetic favors an acid reaction; despite the alkaline salts present in diabetic vegetables.

(*a*) *Total Titratable Acidity.*—The total titratable acidity of the urine is a very good index of the amount of acidosis and runs parallel with the ammonia excretion. The determination is made as follows: Transfer 20 cc of undiluted urine to a small beaker and add 15 grams of neutral potassium oxalate crystals. *Extreme care must be taken that the oxalate is neutral.* Add 3 or 4 drops of 1 per cent phenolphthalein in 95 per cent ethyl alcohol solution and titrate with $\frac{N}{10}$ NaOH to the first *faint* permanent tinge of red, using another beaker containing 20 cc of the urine as a guide. Calculate the total excretion of acid in terms of $\frac{N}{10}$ NaOH for the twenty-four hours. A normal individual excretes between 200 and

500 cc of $\frac{N}{10}$ acid bodies in twenty-four hours. Amounts considerably in excess of this quantity indicate acidosis.

It has been proposed to estimate the degree of acidosis by determining the quantity of alkali which it is necessary to give the patient to render the urine alkaline. I do not recommend this method, for I do not approve of giving alkalis to diabetic patients unnecessarily. It is mentioned to illustrate in a homely way the intensity of the diabetic acidosis. Ordinarily, 5 to 10 grams of sodium bicarbonate will render the normal urine alkaline, but in diabetic patients with an acidosis of moderate severity 20 to 30 grams are required, and in severe cases of acidosis 50 grams daily for a week or more make little impression, and even with doses of over 100 grams sodium bicarbonate in twenty-four hours the urines of patients in coma frequently remain acid. A table has been constructed by von Noorden showing approximately the quantity of acidosis which can be assumed to be present when various quantities of sodium bicarbonate are required to render the urine alkaline.

A more accurate method of determining the alkali tolerance has been described by Sellards,[1] and also by Palmer and Henderson.[2]

(2) *Ammonia.*—The quantity of ammonia in the urine is a measure of the reaction of the body to counteract the acidosis produced in it. To this extent its estimation gives a more accurate idea of the acid production of the body than any other of the urinary tests at our disposal, which simply show the quantity of acid leaving the body. The test, however, becomes of less value so soon as extraneous alkali is administered, because under such conditions the ingested alkali is used by the body in preference to ammonia. The normal amount of ammonia in the urine varies between 0.5 to 1 gram, and the ratio between the ammonia-nitrogen to the total nitrogen in the urine is fairly constant at 1 to 25 (4 per cent). In severe diabetes the ammonia may gradually increase, and in Case No. 344 it amounted to 8 grams in one day. The nitrogen upon this same day was 19.2 grams, giving an ammonia-nitrogen nitrogen ratio of 34.3 per cent. On another day this ratio reached 44.4 per cent, but the absolute quantity of ammonia was only 4.4 grams and the nitrogen 8.7. In fact, these high ammonia-nitrogen nitrogen ratios are ordinarily only obtained when the total quantity of nitrogen in the urine is small. The two tests which we have employed for the determination of ammonia follow:

(a) *Ammonia in Colorimetric Determination of Urine* (Folin and Bell[3]).—This method is based upon the power of permutit to

1 Sellards: Johns Hopkins Hosp. Bull., 1912, **23**, 289.
2 Palmer and Henderson: Arch. Int. Med., 1913, **12**, 153.
3 Folin and Bell: Jour. Biol. Chem., 1917, **29**, 329.

absorb the ammonia from interfering substances in the urine, the subsequent liberation of the ammonia from the permutit by treating with alkali and finally the Nesslerization of the liberated ammonia. This method in detail is as follows:

Transfer 2 grams of permutit[1] to a 200 cc volumetric flask. Add about 5 cc of water (no more) and with an Ostwald pipette introduce 1 or 2 cc of urine, or with a 5 cc pipette introduce 5 cc of previously diluted urine, corresponding to 1 or 2 cc of the original urine. With urines extraordinarily poor in ammonia it may be necessary to use 5 cc of urine, but in so far as it may be practicable, it is better not to use more than 2 cc and to employ a weaker standard (0.5 mg. of nitrogen) for the color comparison. Rinse down the added urine by means of 1 to 5 cc of water, and shake gently but continuously for five minutes. Now rinse the powder to the bottom of the flask by the addition of 25 to 40 cc of water and decant. Add water once more and decant, but if the urine is rich in bile, it is advisable to wash once or twice more. Add a little (5 cc) water to the powder, introduce 2 cc of 10 per cent sodium hydrate, mix, allow to stand about ten minutes and then add more water until the flask is about three-fourths full. Shake for a few seconds and then add 20 cc of Nessler's reagent prepared as described on p. 381. Mix, and let stand in the stoppered flask for ten minutes or as much longer as may be convenient. Fill up to the mark with water, mix and compare in the colorimeter with the standard. The standard should be made up from a stock solution containing 4.716 grams of ammonium sulphate of high purity plus 11.5 cc of concentrated HCl (specific gravity, 1.16) per 1000 cc. (This stock solution is used for making the standards for urine urea, urine total nitrogen, blood non-protein nitrogen and blood urea determinations.) One hundred cc of the stock solution are diluted to 1000 cc together with 11.5 cc of concentrated HCl. Ten cc of this dilute standard are placed in a 200 cc volumetric flask, 2 cc of 10 per cent NaOH added and the flask filled three-fourths full with water. It is Nesslerized at the same time as the unknown and with the same amount of Nessler's solution.

The unknown is compared in the colorimeter with the standard which is set at 20 mm., the unknown being moved. The calculation is then

$$\frac{20 \times 1 \times 100}{\text{reading of unknown}} = \text{mgs.}$$

[1] Permutit especially prepared for this determination must be used. It may be obtained from the Permutit Company, 30 East 42d Street, New York City by requesting permutit such as prepared for Professor Folin. Different specimens of permutit even from the same company may vary in their power to both take up ammonia and to liberate it in the presence of alkali. One should always test each new preparation of permutit purchased for these two properties in the presence of a known amount of ammonium sulphate which will represent the maximum amount of nitrogen that one is apt to encounter in a determination.

ammonia-nitrogen per 100 cc of urine, provided 1 cc of urine has been used for the determination. If 2 or more cc are used, the final result is divided by the number of cc of urine used.

(b) *Ronchese-Malfatti Method for the Determination of Ammonia.* —(a) To 25 cc of urine in a 200 cc Erlenmeyer flask, add about 25 cc of distilled water, about 10 grams (1 or 2 teaspoonfuls) of powdered potassium oxalate, and a few drops of indicator (phenolphthalein). Shake a few times to dissolve the oxalate, then titrate with tenth-normal sodium hydroxide until the first pink color is permanent.

(b) Take 5 cc of commercial formalin solution in a test-tube, add a few drops of phenolphthalein indicator, and then titrate with tenth-normal sodium hydroxide until a faint pink is obtained.

(c) Add this neutralized formalin to the urine, which has just been titrated, and titrate again with tenth-normal sodium hydroxide until the previous pink is again obtained.

(Calculation: The number of cc of tenth-normal alkali used in titration (c) multiplied by 0.0017 gives the number of grams of ammonia in 25 cc of urine.)

No account need be taken of the amount of sodium hydroxide used in titrations (a) and (b).

The method depends upon the fact that formalin combines with ammonium salts and forms hexamethylenetetramin with the liberation of an equivalent of acid which is titrated by means of standard NaOH.

$$4 \ NH_4Cl + 6 \ CH_2O = N_4(CH_2)_6 + 6 \ H_2O + 4 \ HCl$$

This method also gives the amino-acid nitrogen as well as the ammonia.

(3) *β-oxybutyric Acid.*—The tests for β-oxybutyric acid are all complicated, because they depend upon the extraction of the acid. Estimation of the β-oxybutyric acid based upon the difference between the quantity of sugar as determined by Fehling's fermentation and polarization tests are inaccurate. They simply suggest the presence of β-oxybutyric acid.

(a) *Black's Method.*—One hundred cc of urine are measured with a pipette into an evaporating dish and made distinctly alkaline by the addition of sodium bicarbonate. The urine is then evaporated to a thick syrupy liquid (4 or 5 cc) using the gentle heat of a water-bath or the low heat of an electric stove. After cooling the residue is made distinctly acid with strong hydrochloric acid, and is then formed into a thick paste, and later into a porous meal by the gradual addition of plaster of Paris. This porous meal is placed in an extraction apparatus (a Soxhlet or a modification of it) and extracted with about 60 cc of ether for three hours. The ether extract is then transferred to an evaporating dish, where the ether is allowed to evaporate spontaneously. The residue is treated with 5 cc of water and 0.4 gram of bone-black added to decolorize, then filtered, and washed until perfectly clear and made up to a known volume, usually 25 cc. The β-oxybutyric acid is determined with a polariscope, using the following formula:

$$\frac{\text{Angle observed} \times 100}{\text{Specific rotation of } \beta\text{-oxybutyric acid (24.12)} \times \text{length of polarizing tube in mm.}} = \text{grams of } \beta\text{-oxybutyric acid in 1 cc.}$$

(*b*) *Van Slyke-Fitz Methods for Determination of β-hydroxybutyric Acid, Diacetic Acid and Acetone in Urine*[1] *and Blood*.[2]—For the following simplified method for the determination of β-hydroxy-butyric acid, diacetic acid and acetone in the blood and urine I am greatly indebted to Drs. Van Slyke and Fitz of the Rockefeller Institute for Medical Research. The methods are based on a combination of Shaffer's principle of oxidizing hydroxybutyric acid to acetone, and of Denige's method for precipitating acetone as a basic mercuric sulphate compound. Oxidation and precipitation are carried out simultaneously in the same solution, so that the technic is simplied to boiling the mixture for an hour and a half under a reflux condenser, and weighing the precipitate which forms. Neither the size of sample nor mode of procedure have required variation for different urines; the same process yields accurate results for the smallest significant amounts of acetone bodies and likewise for the largest that are encountered. The precipitate is crystalline and beautifully adapted to drying and accurate weighing; but when facilities for weighing are absent the precipitate can be redissolved in 5 per cent hydrochloric acid and the mercury titrated by a suitable method, such as that of Personne.[3]

Solutions Required.

Twenty Per Cent Copper Sulphate. — Two hundred grams of $CuSO_4.5H_2O$ dissolved in water and made up to 1 liter.

Ten Per Cent Mercuric Sulphate.—Seventy-three grams of C. P. red mercuric oxide dissolved in 1 liter of H_2SO_4 of 4 normal concentration. The solution of the oxide is assisted by warming on a steam bath.

Fifty Volume Per Cent Sulphuric Acid.—Five hundred cc of sulphuric acid of 1.835 specific gravity, diluted to 1 liter with water. Concentration of H_2SO_4 should be 17 normal.

Ten Per Cent Calcium Hydrate Suspension.—Mix 100 grams of Merck's fine light "Reagent" $Ca(OH)_2$ with 1 liter of water.

[1] Van Slyke: Jour. Biol. Chem., 1917, **32**, 455.
[2] Van Slyke and Fitz: Ibid., **32**, 495.
[3] Personne: Sutton's Volumetric Analysis, 10th edition, p. 264.

Five Per Cent Potassium Dichromate.—Fifty grams $K_2Cr_2O_7$ dissolved in water and made up to 1 liter.

Removal of Glucose and Other Interfering Substances from Urine.—Place 25 cc of urine in a 250 cc measuring flask. Add 100 cc of water, 50 cc of copper sulphate solution and mix. Then add 50 cc of 10 per cent calcium hydrate, shake and test with litmus. If not alkaline, add more calcium hydrate. Dilute to mark and let stand at least one-half hour for glucose to precipitate. Filter through a dry folded filter. This procedure will remove up to 8 per cent of glucose. Urine containing more should be diluted enough to bring the glucose down to 8 per cent. The filtrate may be tested for glucose by boiling a little in the test-tube. A precipitate of yellow Cu_2O will be obtained if the removal has not been complete. White $CaCO_3$ precipitate means nothing.

Removal of Proteins from Blood and Plasma.—Ten cc of whole blood are measured into a 250 cc volumetric flask, half-full of water. Twenty cc of the mercuric sulphate solution are added, the flask filled to the mark, and shaken. The contents are filtered through a dry folded filter.

For plasma the procedure is the same except that only 8 cc are taken in a 200 cc flask with 15 cc of mercuric sulphate solution.

In the case of either whole blood or serum, 125 cc of filtrate, equivalent to 5 cc of the original sample, are taken for analysis.

Simultaneous Determination of Total Acetone Bodies (Acetone, Diacetic Acid and β-oxybutyric Acid) of Urine or Blood in One Operation.—Place in a 500 cc Erlenmeyer flask 25 cc of urine filtrate plus 100 cc of water or 125 cc of blood filtrate. Add 10 cc of 50 per cent sulphuric acid and 35 cc of the 10 per cent mercuric sulphate. Connect the flask with a reflux condenser having a straight condensing tube of 8 or 10 mm. diameter, and heat to boiling. *After* boiling has begun, add 5 cc of the 5 per cent dichromate through the condenser tube. Continue boiling gently one and one-half hours. The precipitate which forms consists of the mercury sulphate compound of the preformed acetone and of the acetone which has been formed by oxidation of the hydroxybutyric acid. It is collected in a Gooch or a medium density "alundum" crucible, washed with 200 cc of cold water, followed by a little 95 per cent alcohol, dried for an hour at 110° and weighed. Several precipitates may be collected, one above the other, without cleaning the crucible.

Acetone and Diacetic Acid.—These substances without the hydroxybutyric acid are determined exactly as the total acetone bodies, except that (1) no dichromate is added to oxidize the hydroxybutyric, and (2) the boiling must continue for not less than thirty-five nor more than forty-five minutes. Boiling for more than forty-five minutes splits off a little acetone from hydroxybutyric acid even without dichromate.

β-hydroxybutyric Acid in Urine.—The β-hydroxybutyric acid alone is determined exactly as total acetone bodies except that the preformed acetone and that from the diacetic acid are first boiled off. To do this the 25 cc of urine filtrate plus 125 cc of water are treated with 2 cc of 50 per cent sulphuric acid and boiled in the open flask for ten minutes. The volume of solution left in the flask is measured in a cylinder. The solution is returned to the flask, and the cylinder washed with enough water to replace part of that boiled off and bring the volume of the solution to 127 cc. Then 8 cc of the 50 per cent acid and 35 cc of the 10 per cent mercuric sulphate are added. The flask is connected under the condenser and the determination is continued as above.

β-hydroxybutyric Acid in Blood.—The following procedure enables one to determine separately in a single sample of blood both the acetone plus diacetic acid and the β-acid. The acetone and diacetic acid are precipitated as above described, and the filtrate poured as completely as possible through the Gooch or alundum crucible into a dry receiving flask. Of this filtrate 160 cc are measured into another Erlenmeyer flask and 10 cc of water are added. The mixture is heated to boiling under a reflux condenser, 5 cc of dichromate solution are added, and the determination continued as described for "total acetone bodies."

TABLE 144.—FACTORS BY WHICH MILLIGRAMS OF PRECIPITATE ARE MULTIPLIED IN ORDER TO GIVE RESULTS CALCULATED AS:

Determination.	β-hydroxybutyric acid.		Acetone.		Molecular equivalents.	
	Gms. per liter, urine.	Mg. per 100 c.c., blood.	Gms. per liter, urine.	Mg. per 100 c.c., blood.	C.c. $\frac{M}{10}$ acetone or β-acid per liter, urine.	Molecular concentration in blood or plasma.
Total acetone bodies[1]	0.0428	2.14	0.0238	1.19	4.11	0.000206
β-hydroxybutyric[2]	0.0460	2.30	0.0256	1.28	4.42	0.000221
		(2.44)		(1.37)		0.000235
Acetone and diacetic acid	0.0364	1.82	0.0203	1.015	3.50	0.000175

[1] The "total acetone body" factors are calculated on the assumption that the molecular ratio (acetone plus diacetic acid): (β-hydroxybutyric acid) is 1:2. Because the hydroxybutyric acid yields on oxidation only 0.79 molecule of acetone, the "total acetone body" factor is absolutely accurate only when the above ratio is 1:2. But with the range of mixtures encountered in acetonuria, when the ratio is usually between 1:2 and 1:3, with extreme limits of 1:1 and 1:4, the use of the above approximate factors for "total acetone bodies" will seldom involve a significant error. The actual errors in percentages of the amounts determined are as follows: ratio 1:1, error 3.7 per cent.; ratio 1:2, error zero; ratio 1:3, error 1.9 per cent.; ratio 1:4, error 3 per cent.

[2] The factors in parenthesis are the usual factors $\times \frac{170}{160}$, and are for use in determination of β-hydroxybutyric acid in blood when the acetone is precipitated and the β-acid determined in 160 c.c. of the filtrate.

In case only the β-acid is desired, or enough blood is taken for double portions, the slightly easier procedure used for urine may also be followed with blood.

Factors for Calculating Acetone Bodies in Urine when 25 cc of Filtrate, Equivalent to 2.5 cc of Urine, and in Blood when 125 cc of Filtrate, Equivalent to 5 cc of Blood are Used for Determination.— One mgm. of β-hydroxybutyric acid yields 8.7 mgm. of precipitate. One mgm. of acetone yields 19.7 mgm. of precipitate.

The amount of precipitate obtained from β-hydroxybutyric acid therefore corresponds to 79 per cent of the acetone that would be obtained if each molecule of hydroxybutyric yielded a molecule of acetone. The oxidation is complete in one and a half hours, and the conditions are so constant that duplicates usually check within 1 per cent.

8. Nitrogen.—The determination of the nitrogen in the urine is valuable because it furnishes an index to the quantity of protein which the patient is disintegrating. Incidentally, this is the easiest way to determine the quantity of protein in the diet. Since nitrogen constitutes 16 per cent of the protein molecule, we can multiply the quantity of nitrogen obtained in the urine by $6\frac{1}{4}$ to obtain the protein which it represents. We shall not be far wrong if to this we add 1 gram of nitrogen to offset the nitrogen of the feces, and consider this total quantity as representing the protein in the food. The determination of the nitrogen is also valuable because it is often useful to know the ammonia-nitrogen nitrogen ratio as well as the dextrose-nitrogen ratio.

Formerly large quantities of nitrogen were obtained in the urines of diabetic patients, but modern treatment with its restriction of protein makes these excessive quantities rare.

However, I have met with three such examples: Thus, Case No. 632 came to me upon a supposedly restricted diet, and the nitrogen in the urine amounted to 29.25 grams. The diminution of protein in the diet removed the sugar entirely from the urine, even though 12 grams of carbohydrate were added in the form of oatmeal. Case No. 616 was not sugar-free before her entrance to the hospital, but in the hospital easily became so. The urine upon March 18, 1913, amounted to 6615 cc, and contained 485 grams sugar and 67.9 grams nitrogen. She entered the hospital May 22, 1913, and the urine was free from sugar May 25. Five months subsequently the urine was examined and the quantity of nitrogen in the twenty-four hours amounted to 36 grams. Case No. 1196 is discussed in connection with the volume of the urine (see p. 468).

A daily analysis for nitrogen is expensive, but it is a simple matter to aliquot specimens of urine for a week and then obtain the average nitrogen excretion per day.

Two simple methods by which the nitrogen in the urine may be determined are here given. Each is based upon preliminary digestion of the urine with sulphuric acid-phosphoric acid-copper sulphate mixtures and final determinations of the ammonia content either by distillation and titration or by direct Nesslerization. Both methods have been devised by Prof. Folin and co-workers.

(*a*) **A Simplified Macro-Kjeldahl Method for Urine.**[1]—This method is a modification of the Kjeldahl method for the determination of nitrogen in urine which requires very little equipment and by which a urinary nitrogen determination can easily be finished in twenty to twenty-five minutes.

The hydrolyzing-oxidizing reagent is the same phosphoric-sulphuric acid mixture that is used in the micro method. To 50 cc of 5 to 6 per cent copper sulphate solution add 300 cc of 85 per cent phosphoric acid and 100 cc of concentrated sulphuric acid. Five cc of this mixture are used for the destructive digestion of 5 cc of undiluted urine. Ten per cent solution of ferric chloride is also required. The ferric chloride can scarcely be considered indispensable; but it hastens the digestion, and the iron hydroxide promotes even boiling during the subsequent distillation.

Transfer 5 cc of undiluted urine to a 300 cc Kjeldahl flask (Pyrex). Add 5 cc of the phosphoric-sulphuric acid mixture, also 2 cc of 10 per cent ferric chloride solution and 4 to 6 small pebbles (to prevent bumping). Boil in a hood over a micro-burner.[2]

Micro-burners are by far the best to use as a source of heat, because even inexperienced workers or students cannot go far astray with them; whereas, large Bunsen burners with their great variations in heating power are much more difficult to regulate. The micro-burner should give a good strong flame and the top of the burner should be not more than 1 cm. away from the bottom of the flask. Boil vigorously. In three to four minutes the foam which forms at first will entirely disappear and the flask becomes filled with dense white fumes. When this stage is reached (but no earlier), cover the mouth of the flask with a small watch-glass and continue the vigorous heating for two minutes. At the end of two minutes dilute urines will already be green or blue and concentrated urines will be a light straw-yellow, the black carbonaceous matter being completely destroyed. The flame should then be turned very low and the gentle boiling process should be con-

---

[1] Folin and Wright: Jour. Biol. Chem., 1919, **38**, 461.

[2] A very convenient clamp for holding the Kjeldahl flasks in position is the one listed as No. 24598 in Arthur H. Thomas Company's catalogue. The micro-burner which we use is listed under No. 1506 in Eimer and Amend's catalogue.

24

tinued for two minutes, making a total boiling period of four minutes, counting from the time the watch-glass was put in place. Remove the flame and let the flask cool for four to five minutes. At the end of four or not more than five minutes, add first 50 cc of water, then 15 cc of saturated sodium hydroxide (50 to 55 per cent) and connect the Kjeldahl flask promptly by means of a rubber stopper and ordinary glass tubing with a receiver containing from 35 to 75 cc of 0.1 N acid together with water enough to make a total volume of 150 cc, and a drop or two of alizarin red. Florence flasks, capacity 300 cc, of Pyrex glass make excellent receivers for this distillation. As soon as the connection is made with the receiver, apply the flame again at full force, but not directly under the center until the acid and alkali in the flask have had time to mix. The contents in the flask begin to boil almost at once and four to five minutes' boiling transfers the whole of the ammonia to the receiver. The contents in the receiver become heated of course, since no condenser is used, but under the conditions described the temperature reached is only 65° to 70° C.

The only precaution needed in connection with the titration of the distillate (without previous cooling) is that a faint red color shall be accepted as the end-point. The color will deepen on cooling, and when time permits it is more satisfactory to cool in running water before titrating.

While the operator is directed to make prompt connections with the receiver after the alkali has been added to the digestion mixture there is in point of fact very little danger of losing ammonia vapors by being unduly slow in closing the mouth of the flask. Similarly when the receiver contains too little acid and turns pink there is no need for extraordinary haste in adding more acid. The water, though warm, will hold considerable free ammonia.

It will be noted that the digestion period, thirty to forty minutes of ordinary Kjeldahl determinations, has here been cut down to four minutes and that the distillation period, twenty-five to forty minutes, has been cut down to five, and the only source of heat is an ordinary micro-burner. The delivery tubes are made from glass tubing, small enough to pass into the ready-made holes in rubber stoppers. For the sake of flexibility the delivery tube must consist of two parts connected with a short piece of rubber tubing. (See Fig. 17.) It may also be observed that the Kjeldahl flask need not be moved from the time the digestion is begun until the determination is finished, though this involves the continuous use of the hood. Where hood space is scarce the distillation can, of course, be conducted just as well at the desk.

One very satisfactory feature of this new process is that the preliminary steaming out of the condenser for an occasional nitrogen determination is replaced by a simple rinsing of the glass tube.

The simplified distillation process described above can also be used in other determinations involving the removal of ammonia; as, for example, in urea determinations. The elaborate metal condensers now found in every well equipped laboratory are practically superfluous.

The method described in this paper, as far as the destructive digestion is concerned, is primarily intended for urine only. It is not applicable to highly resistant materials, as for example milk, which cannot be completely destroyed within six minutes. Urines

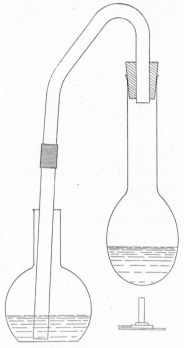

Fig. 17.—Apparatus for Folin and Wright's simplified Macro-Kjeldahl method.

containing much sugar belong in this class. If fuming sulphuric acid be substituted for ordinary sulphuric acid in the preparation of the hydrolyzing reagent, or if 2 cc of fuming sulphuric acid are used in addition to 5 cc of the regular reagent, sugar urines are readily destroyed within the required heating period of four to five minutes.

(b) **Micro-Kjeldahl Colorimetric Method.**[1]—Dilute 5, 10 or 20 cc of urine to 100 cc, mix and with an Ostwald pipette transfer 1 cc

[1] Folin: A Laboratory Manual of Biological Chemistry, 1919, New York, D. Appleton & Co.

of the diluted urine to a large hard glass test-tube. This pipette must be drained for fifteen seconds against the wall of the test-tube and then blown clean. With an ordinary pipette add 1 cc of phosphoric-sulphuric acid-copper sulphate mixture, together with a pebble or small piece of broken quartzware to prevent bumping.

The acid digestion mixture is made according to the directions given under the simplified Macro-Kjeldahl method.

Heat over a micro-burner, a hood being unnecessary, until water is driven off and fumes become abundant within the tube. This should take place in about two minutes. When filled with fumes close the mouth of the test-tube with a watch glass and continue the boiling at such a rate that the tube remains filled with fumes yet almost none escape. Within two minutes after closing the mouth of the test-tube the contents should become clear, and bluish or light green. Continue the gentle boiling for thirty to sixty seconds longer, provided, however, that the total boiling period, with test-tube closed, must not be less than two minutes. Remove the flame and let cool for a little less than two minutes, then add about 10 cc of water. Rinse the hot digestion mixture, sometimes turbid from silica, into a 200 cc volumetric flask, using for this purpose about 125 cc of water.

Transfer 10 cc of standard ammonium sulphate solution containing 1 mg. of nitrogen, the same standard as that used for urinary ammonia (see p. 363) into another 200 cc volumetric flask. Add 1 cc of the concentrated phosphoric-sulphuric acid mixture, to balance the acid in the unknown, and dilute to a volume of about 150 cc. When both flasks are thus ready give each flask a whirl and add 30 cc of Nessler's reagent (see p. 381). Shake a little more, dilute both flasks to the 200 cc mark and mix.

If the unknown Nesslerized digestion mixture is turbid, centrifuge a portion, giving a crystal clear fluid above a white sediment (silica). If the sediment is colored the Nesslerization was not successful, and the determination must be repeated. The standard is set in the colorimeter at 20 mm. and the unknown moved. The calculation is

$$\frac{20 \times 1 \times 2}{\text{reading of unknown}} = \text{grams.}$$

nitrogen per 100 cc of urine when 5 cc of the urine have been diluted to 100 cc and 1 cc of the diluted urine used for digestion.

9. **Albumin.**—The test for albumin in the urine should be performed at frequent intervals during the care of diabetic patients. Too often the diagnosis of diabetes leads to neglect of the general treatment of the case. As a rule when albumin appears, the percentage of sugar falls, even though the percentage of sugar in the blood remains high. Among 50 cases of diabetes of twenty years'

duration, 13 showed more than the slightest trace of albumin, whereas among the same number of cases under two years' duration, the number showing albumin was 2.

10. **Casts.**—From the time of Külz the irritation of the kidneys in the first stages of diabetic coma has been observed. Over and over again I have seen typical "showers" of casts at the beginning of diabetic coma. They may occur at times when the albumin in the urine amounts to the slightest possible trace. Casts in the urine, even though occurring in showers, do not necessitate the development of fatal coma, for these were found in the urine of Case No. 765 on December 6-7, 1915. (See Table 145.)

TABLE 145.—CASE NO. 765. SEVERE ACIDOSIS; "SHOWERS" OF CASTS WITHOUT COMA.

Date.	Vol., c.c.	Albumin.	Diacetic acid.	Ammonia, gms.	Sugar, urine, gms.	Carbohydrate balance, gms.	Soda administered.	Weight, lbs.	Alveolar air, CO_2 mm. Hg.
1915. Dec. 6-7	..	..	..	3.3[1]	3.6%	Showers	of granular	casts.	
7-8	1800	Slight trace	++	3.9	25	-20	0	88	26
8-9	1200	Slight trace	+++	2.6	7	-7	0	88	26
9-10	1200	Very slight trace	++	2.4	2	3	0	89	29
10-11	1600	Slightest possible trace	++	2.9	6	-1	0	89	32
11-12	1400	..	++	..	14	16	0	88	33
12-13	900	Slightest possible trace	++	1.5	9	-9	0	89	32
			Death	in coma,	Octob	er 26, 1	916.		

11. **Chlorides.**—The importance of a knowledge of the chlorides in the urine is due to the remarkable changes in weight of diabetic patients which are apparently related to the excretion and retention of sodium chloride. This subject is discussed under Influence of Sodium Chloride upon the Weight. (See p. 219.)

Folin's Simplified Method.[2]—Solutions required:

1. Standard silver nitrate: Dissolve 29.12 grams of silver nitrate in distilled water and dilute to 1 liter. One cc is equivalent to 10 mg. of NaCl.

---

[1] Ammonia in 14°.

[2] Folin Laboratory Manual of Biological Chemistry, 1922. D. Appleton & Co., New York.

2. Indicator: To 100 grams of ferric ammonium sulphate add 100 cc of water and 200 cc of concentrated nitric acid.

3. Standard ammonium sulphocyanate: Dissolve 20 grams of ammonium sulphocyanate in 1 liter of water and mix. Transfer 10 cc of the standard silver nitrate solution to a beaker, add 20 cc of water and 5 cc of indicator. Titrate with the sulphocyanate solution until the characteristic reddish end-point is reached. On the basis of the figure obtained, prepare 1 liter of ammonium sulphocyanate solution, which is equivalent to the standard silver nitrate solution.

With a pipette transfer 5 cc of urine to a beaker, add 20 cc of water, 5 cc of indicator and finally (with a pipette) 10 cc of silver nitrate solution. While stirring, titrate the surplus silver with the standard sulphocyanate solution until the first faint, but unmistakable, brown or reddish coloration is obtained. On standing or continued stirring the color may disappear, so the very first end-point must be taken.

Subtract the sulphocyanate used (in cc) from 10 and multiply by 10. This gives in mg., the amount of NaCl present in 5 cc of urine.

B. THE EXAMINATION OF THE BLOOD.

Since the last edition of this book was written the field of blood chemistry has received a remarkable stimulus due to the introduction of a System of Blood Analysis by Folin and Wu.[1] We are now able to take a comparatively small sample of blood and make a complete analysis of the blood for sugar, urea, non-protein nitrogen, uric acid, creatin, creatinin, and chlorides. Formerly each determination required as much and sometimes more blood than all of them together at present. A 10 cc sample of blood will permit of a complete chemical analysis. This does not include a gas analysis. For this the blood should be taken separately and either under oil or in a tube which is completely filled and tightly stoppered. Since all of these tests are seldom required on each sample of blood even less than 10 cc suffice. As a routine we precipitate 5 cc of blood and this requires that about 7 or 8 cc of blood be taken into the syringe. A 22-gauge needle and a 10 cc syringe may be used. For preventing the clotting of blood 2 mg. of potassium oxalate per 1 cc of blood should be placed in the bottle and the blood forced out of the syringe into the bottle with as little loss of time as possible. The bottle should be immediately corked and shaken vigorously for thirty seconds. Folin has introduced a new anticoagulant in a very convenient and effective form. This is a lithium oxalate impregnated cloth. It is made in the following manner.

[1] Folin and Wu: Jour. Biol. Chem., 1919, **38**, 81; 1920, **41**, 367.

Procure about 6 yards of 18-inch bird's-eye cloth, which comes under the trade name of Red Star Diaper Cloth, and cut it into 6-inch widths and 18-inch lengths. Determine the total weight of the strips of cloth. In a 2 liter beaker or flask dissolve 126.05 grams of oxalic acid crystals ($H_2C_2O_4.2H_2O$) in 1600 cc of distilled water. Add in small portions 74.06 grams of lithium carbonate and after shaking to get rid of the vigorous foaming, heat the solution to boiling. After the carbon dioxide has been driven off, pour the contents of the flask into a shallow dish and while still hot, draw the pieces of bird's eye through the solution, allowing them to drain a moment and then hanging them on a line to dry. Six yards of 18-inch bird's-eye cloth will take up nearly the whole of the above saturated solution. Proportionally smaller amounts may be made up if desired.

When the cloth is dry, weight again to determine the gain in weight and the percentage content of lithium oxalate. One then determines the weight of oxalate in a square inch and from this the size of the cloth to place in the blood bottle. The cloth takes up about 13 per cent lithium oxalate during the one treatment and it is best after drying to pass it through another lot of the lithium oxalate to bring it to 20 to 26 per cent concentration. One mg. of lithium oxalate will prevent 1 cc of blood from clotting.

The use of this cloth greatly facilitates the blood uric acid determination. It also affords a large surface area of oxalate which is exposed to the blood and consequently makes the oxalate more efficient as an anticoagulant.

Another helpful contribution has been made by Folin indirectly through a former pupil, Denis,[1] in solving the question of transportation of bloods for which a sugar determination is desired. Formerly a blood sugar demanded almost immediate attention due to the fact that the sugar content of the blood *in vitro* tended to decrease. They discovered that the addition of 1 drop of 40 per cent commercial formaldehyde to every 5 cc of blood would effectively destroy the enzyme which lowered the sugar content. Bloods treated thus have been kept as long as four days under ordinary laboratory conditions. This solves the laboratory problem for the general practitioner who cannot do his own blood-sugar test. He can draw the blood and send it at his convenience to the laboratory. All of the determinations may be made on blood thus treated excepting urea. Contrary to the statement of Denis and Aldrich we have been unable to make this determination accurately, due to the effect of the formaldehyde, even in such small quantities, on the Nessler reagent, which it precipitates.

[1] Denis and Aldrich: Jour. Biol. Chem., 1920, **44**, 203.

The different chemical determinations are made upon a water-clear filtrate obtained by removing the proteins from the blood. To obtain this filtrate the blood is diluted with 7 volumes of water and then treated with 1 volume of a tungstate solution and 1 volume of a sulphuric acid solution. This precipitates the blood protein which may then be filtered off.

1. **Precipitation of Blood Proteins.**—The solutions required are two, a two-thirds normal (0.667 N) solution of sulphuric acid, which it is best to carefully standardize, and a 10 per cent solution of sodium tungstate.

All brands of sodium tungstate are not equally good. At the present time the large chemical companies are not aware of this fact, and consequently, the reputation of the company or the apparent pure crystalline character of the tungstate is no indication that the tungstate will be suitable for blood work. Up to the present we have secured the best tungstate for blood work from Mr. H. J. Bean, Biochemical Laboratory, Harvard Medical School, Boston, Mass., or from the E. F. Mahady Co., 671 Boylston Street, Boston, Mass., who also have Mr. Bean's product. If this tungstate is used, we have not found it necessary to titrate the tungstate solution, but if other brands of tungstate are employed, they should be carefully titrated to determine if they have the proper degree of alkalinity. Ten cc of 10 per cent tungstate solution should require not over 0.4 cc of $\frac{N}{10}$ acid to neutralize it to phenolphthalein. Many tungstates are neutral or acid. It may be positively stated that these will not make effective blood protein precipitates.

In a flask or large tube are placed 7 volumes, usually 35 cc, of distilled water; 1 volume, 5 cc, of blood is then added, followed by 1 volume of the 10 per cent tungstate. After mixing, add slowly with shaking 1 volume of the two-thirds normal sulphuric acid. Allow to stand about five minutes or until the coagulum has turned a dull brown color and then filter. The filtrate should be water-clear, and alkaline to Congo red, but neutral or slightly acid to litmus. If formaldehyde has been added to the blood, previously, the filtrate will keep very well for two or three days, but if it has not been added, either 1 drop of formaldehyde for every 30 to 40 cc of filtrate or 2 or 3 drops of xylol should be added for preservation, in case the determinations are not to be made the same day.

2. **Blood-sugar Determinations. Solutions Required.** — (a) **Standard Sugar Solution.**—Dissolve 1 gram of pure anhydrous dextrose in saturated benzoic acid solution and dilute to a volume of 100 cc. Mix, and bottle. If pure dextrose is not available, a standard solution of invert sugar made from cane sugar is equally

useful. Transfer exactly 1 gram of cane sugar to a 100 cc volumetric flask; add 20 cc of normal hydrochloric acid and let the mixture stand over night at room temperature (or rotate the flask and contents continuously for ten minutes in a water-bath kept at 70° C.). Add 1.68 grams of sodium bicarbonate and about 0.2 grams of sodium acetate, to neutralize the hydrochloric acid. Shake a few minutes to remove most of the carbonic acid and fill to the 100 cc mark with saturated benzoic acid solution. Then add 5 cc more of benzoic acid solution (1 gram of cane sugar yields 1.05 grams of invert sugar) and mix. Transfer to a bottle; shake well, and stopper tightly. The stock solution made in either way keeps indefinitely. Two standard sugar solutions should be on hand: (1) A solution containing 1 mg. of sugar per 10 cc (5 cc of the stock solution diluted to 500 cc with a saturated benzoic acid solution); (2) a solution containing 2 mg. of sugar per 10 cc (5 cc of the stock solution diluted to 250 cc). The invert sugar solution has the advantage that it can be easily prepared from cane sugar, which is pure. The keeping quality of such solutions should be less good than those made from glucose, but we have encountered no trouble on that score. When good quality glucose is available, it is, of course, the one to use.

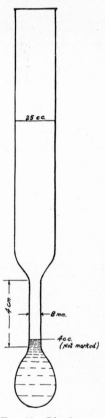

FIG. 18.—Blood-sugar tube.[1]

(*b*) **Alkaline Copper Solution.**—Dissolve 40 grams of anhydrous sodium carbonate in about 400 cc of water and transfer to a liter flask. Add 7.5 grams of tartaric acid and when the latter has dissolved add 4.5 grams of crystallized copper sulphate; mix, and make up to a volume of 1 liter. If the carbonate used is impure, a sediment may be formed in the course of a week or so. If this happens, decant the clear solution into another bottle.

(*c*) **Sugar Reagent.**—Transfer to a liter beaker 35 grams of molybdic acid (100 per cent) and 5 grams of sodium tungstate. Add 200 cc of 10 per cent sodium hydrate and 200 cc of water. Boil vigorously for twenty to forty minutes so as to remove nearly the

---

[1] Test-tubes of the sort, shown in Fig. 18 with and without graduation, are now made by The Emil Greiner Company, 55 Fulton Street, New York, and can also be obtained from Arthur H. Thomas Company, West Washington Square, Philadelphia.

whole of the ammonia present in the molybdic acid. Cool, dilute to about 350 cc, and add 125 cc of concentrated (85 per cent) phosphoric acid. Dilute to 500 cc.

(*d*) **Blood-sugar Tubes.**—See Fig. 18.

(*e*) **The Determination.**—Transfer 2 cc of the tungstic acid blood filtrate to a blood-sugar test-tube, and to two other similar test-tubes (graduated at 25 cc) add 2 cc of standard sugar solution containing respectively 0.2 and 0.4 mg. of dextrose. To each tube add 2 cc of the alkaline copper solution. The surface of the mixtures must now have reached the constricted part of the tube. If the bulb of the tube is too large for the volume (4 cc) a little, but not more than 0.5 cc of a diluted (1:1) alkaline copper solution may be added. If this does not suffice to bring the contents to the narrow part, the tube should be discarded. Test-tubes having so small a capacity that 4 cc fills them above the neck should also be discarded. Transfer the tubes to a boiling water-bath and heat for eight minutes. Then transfer them to a cold water-bath and let cool, without shaking, for two to three minutes. Add to each test-tube 2 cc of the sugar reagent. The cuprous oxide dissolves rather slowly if the amount is large, but the whole, up to the amount given by 0.8 mg. of dextrose, dissolves usually within two minutes. When the cuprous oxide is dissolved, dilute the resulting blue solutions to the 25 cc mark, insert a rubber stopper, and mix. It is essential that adequate attention be given to this mixing because the greater part of the blue color is formed in the bulb of the tube.

The two standards given representing 0.2 and 0.4 mg. of glucose are adequate for practically all cases. They cover the range from about 70 to nearly 400 mg. of glucose per 100 cc of blood.

It will be noted that in the process described we recommend cooling of the alkaline cuprous oxide suspension before adding the sugar reagent. This cooling is not essential and, in case of one or two determinations only, may be omitted. In a large series of determinations it is probably best to use it.

The standard nearest to the unknown in color is set at 20 mm. in the colorimeter and the unknown moved. The calculation is then:

$$\frac{20 \times 0.2 \times 500}{\text{reading of unknown.}} = \text{mg. glucose per 100 cc of blood when standard No. 1 is used.}$$

$$\frac{20 \times 0.4 \times 500}{\text{reading of unknown.}} = \text{mg. glucose per 100 cc of blood when standard No. 2 is used.}$$

Micro-chemical Methods for Analysis of Blood.—Hagedorn and Jensen have recently a new micro-chemical method for blood-sugar estimations by means of potassium ferricyanide.

3. **Non-protein Nitrogen.**—The remarkable efficiency of the kidneys of patients with diabetes has always impressed me, and the onset of renal disease in cases of diabetes of long duration has been far less frequent than most of us would anticipate. Proof of this is shown by the moderate changes of blood-pressure in cases of diabetes over long periods of time. (See p. 582.) On the other hand, in beginning coma renal involvement has always seemed to the author to be marked. Today the question arises as to whether this may not have been in part due to the alkaline treatment at such times, which forced an excessive quantity of acid through the kidneys. The increasing duration of life of patients with diabetes will show in a few years whether this is accompanied by a greater incidence of renal complications. Other evidence will be forthcoming upon the effect of high blood-sugar percentages over long periods of time upon the kidneys, as a result of insulin.

TABLE 146.—NON-PROTEIN NITROGEN IN DIABETES.

Non-protein nitrogen in 100 mgms. of blood, mg.	Number of analyses.	Age in years.		Phthalein tests.			Albumin present, per cent.	Blood-pressure.		Acidosis present, per cent.	Blood sugar.	
		Average.	Range.	Number.	Average.	Range.		Systolic average.	Diastolic average.		Average, per cent.	Range, per cent.
						1916[1]						
16–20	2	32	25–39	1	58	...	0	130	83	100	0.33	0.09–0.57
21–30	12	47	26–68	6	51	28–60	67	144	87	33	0.19	0.11–0.40
31–40	13	50	19–69	6	45	20–60	77	153	91	54	0.24	0.12–0.33
41 and over	9	50	22–69	4	34	5–56	89	152	80	40	0.20	0.10–0.50
						1922[2]						
16–20	4	31	16–51	1	42	...	0	146	77	0	0.21	0.17–0.29
21–30	43	40	9–69	17	51	26–80	7	130	78	21	0.19	0.05–0.45
31–40	55	41	7–73	30	55	22–90	2	129	79	18	0.21	0.06–0.39
41 and over	22	50	14–69	15	46	26–75	5	143	81	5	0.25	0.05–0.42

The non-protein nitrogen of the blood varies in normal individuals between 20 and 40 mg. per 100 cc blood. Table 146 shows a small number of analyses of non-protein nitrogen in two series of diabetics which were abnormal. Thus, of 36 analyses in 1916, there were but one-fourth (9) with 41 mg. non-protein nitrogen or over; of 124 analyses in 1922, but one-sixth (22). These figures confirm the impression of the tendency of the kidneys above mentioned. Both series of data show increasing non-protein nitrogen with advancing age. Acidosis appears to have exerted little influence. As to be expected there is a general tendency for the phenolphthalein excretion to decrease as the non-protein nitrogen increases. In the earlier series of data the blood-pressure also rises with the non-protein nitrogen. The fact that the greatest blood-pressure in the 1922 series (146 mm. Hg.) occurred when the non-protein

[1] 30 cases, 36 analyses. [2] 100 cases, 124 analyses.

nitrogen was between 16 and 20 mg. does not invalidate this statement because of the small number of determinations. The blood
sugar appears to have no relation whatsoever to the non-protein
nitrogen as shown by the average values and the ranges of the
blood sugars.

A premortal rise in non-protein nitrogen occurred in Case No.
3079, who entered the hospital on April 2, 1923, with gangrene
and septicemia due to streptococcus hemolyticus. The changes
in non-protein nitrogen, blood sugar, and glycosuria which occurred
in twenty-four hours are shown in Table 147. Death occurred one
hour after the last observation. The influence of "renal bloc"
upon the percentage of sugar in the blood has been noted by Fuller.[1]
It is certainly true that one often encounters falling percentages
of urinary sugar as coma advances. Fasting or inability to take
food may in part account for this phenomenon, but undoubtedly
"renal bloc" is one of the factors.

TABLE 147.—CASE NO. 3079. PREMORTAL RISE IN NON-PROTEIN NITROGEN.

Date.	Diacetic acid.	Sugar in urine, gms.	Diet in grams.				Non-protein nitrogen, mgs.	Blood sugar, per cent.	Blood CO_2 vols., per cent.	Insulin, units.
			C.	P.	F.	Cals.				
1922. Apr. 2	..	..	..	..	..	...	35.4	0.40	58	
	Amputation		left leg	half	way	between	knee	and ankle.		
2–3	0	21	60	17	2	326	....	....	..	5
3–4	0	46	62	37	38	738	....	....	..	10
4–5	0	45	74	42	44	860	....	....	..	20
5–6	0	0	..	..	..	...	75.0[2]	0.50		

(a) **Determination of Blood Non-protein Nitrogen.**—The tungstic
acid filtrate is used in this method which is part of "The System
of Blood Analysis of Folin and Wu." The filtrate is first digested
with a digestion mixture similar to that used in the urine Macro-
Kjeldahl method for nitrogen determination. The digested mixture
is then Nesslerized directly with a Nessler reagent specially modified by Folin and Wu. The solutions needed follow:

(1) *Digestion Mixture.*—Mix 300 cc of phosphoric acid syrup
(about 85 per cent H_3PO_4) with 100 cc of concentrated sulphuric
acid. Transfer to a tall cylinder, cover well to exclude the
absorption of ammonia, and set aside for sedimentation of calcium
sulphate. In the course of a week or so the top of the liquid may
be used. To 100 cc of the clear acid add 10 cc of 6 per cent copper

---

[1] Fuller: Jour. Metabl. Research, 1922.
[2] Blood specimen taken one hour before death.   Death occurred 4.30 P.M. April
5, due to streptococcus hemolyticus septicemia.   No coma.   Blood culture taken on
admission and before operation.

sulphate solution and 100 cc of water. The mixture may be prepared by diluting some of the digestion mixture used in the Micro-Kjeldahl method for the urine with an equal volume of water.

(2) *Nessler's Reagent (Modified).*—Transfer 150 grams of potassium iodide and 110 grams of iodine to a 500 cc Florence flask; add 100 cc of water and an excess of metallic mercury 140 to 150 grams. Shake the flask continuously and vigorously for seven to fifteen minutes or until the iodine has nearly dissolved. The solution becomes quite hot. When the red iodine solution has begun to become visibly pale, though still red, cool in running water and continue the shaking until the red color of the iodine has been replaced by the greenish color of the double iodide. This whole operation usually does not take more than fifteen minutes. Now separate the solution from the surplus mercury by decantation and washing with liberal quantities of distilled water. Dilute the solution and washings to a volume of 2 liters. If the cooling is begun in time, the resulting reagent is clear enough for immediate dilution with 10 per cent (2.5 normal) alkali and water, and the finished solution can at once be used for Nesslerizations.

The final Nessler solution is prepared from the above stock solution as follows. From completely saturated caustic soda solution containing about 55 grams of NaOH per 100 cc decant the clear supernatant liquid and dilute to a concentration of 10 per cent. (It is worth while to determine by titration that a 10 per cent solution has been obtained within an error of not over 5 per cent.) Introduce into a large bottle 3500 cc of 10 per cent sodium hydroxide solution, add 750 cc of the double iodide (stock Nessler's) solution and 750 cc of distilled water, giving 5 liters of Nessler's solution. This solution may be used for urine nitrogen, urine ammonia, urine urea, blood non-protein nitrogen and blood urea Nesslerizations.

(3) *Apparatus Needed.*—Blood non-protein nitrogen tubes (200 x 25 mm.) graduated at 35 cc and 50 cc. These may be obtained at any of the large chemicalware supply houses by asking for Folin non-protein nitrogen digestion tubes. A ring stand with test-tube clamp with which to hold the digestion tubes. Micro-bunsen burner.

The Determination.—Introduce 5 cc of the protein-free blood filtrate into a dry 75 cc test-tube graduated at 35 cc and at 50 cc. Add 1 cc of the digestion mixture. Add a dry quartz pebble or broken quartzware and boil vigorously over a micro-burner until the characteristic dense acid fumes begin to fill the test-tube. This is usually accomplished in from three to seven minutes. When the fumes are unmistakable, cut down the size of the flame so that the contents of the tube are just visibly boiling, and close the mouth of the test-tube with a watch-glass or a very small Erlenmeyer flask. Continue the heating very gently for two minutes from the time the fumes began to be unmistakable, even if the solution has become clear and colorless at the end of twenty to forty seconds. If the oxidations are not visibly finished at the end of two minutes the heating must be continued until the solution is nearly colorless. Such cases are very rare; the oxidation is almost invariably finished within the first minute. Allow the contents to cool for seventy to ninety seconds and then add 15 to 25 cc of water. Cool further, approximately to room temperature, and add water to the 35 cc mark. Add, preferably with a pipette, 15 cc of the Nessler solution described above. Insert a clean rubber stopper and mix. If the solution is turbid, centrifuge a portion before making the color comparison with the standard. The standard most commonly required is 0.3 mg. of N (10 cc of a solution prepared by diluting 30 cc of the stock ammonia-sulphate solution described under urine ammonia together with 11.5 cc concentrated HCl to 1000 cc) in a 100 cc flask. Add to it 2 cc of the sulphuric-phosphoric acid mixture, about 50 cc of water, and 30 cc of Nessler solution. Fill to the mark and mix. The unknown and the standard should be Nesslerized at approximately the same time. If the standard is set at 20 mm. for the color comparison, 20 divided by the reading and multiplied by 30 gives the non-protein nitrogen in mg. per 100 cc of blood.

4. **Chlorides.**—The determination of the chlorides in the blood gains importance from the fact that the water content of the body in diabetes varies so rapidly and to so great an extent. This is in addition to the value which such determinations have in the dietetic management of cases of nephritis and hypertension, complications not uncommon in diabetes.

This determination should be done upon plasma or serum taken under the same conditions as demanded for plasma CO_2 determination, i. e., without loss of CO_2. The tests devised by Whitehorn[1] may be made with tungstic acid filtrates, but in precipitating the plasma proteins half-strength sodium tungstate and sulphuric acid solutions are used. It depends upon direct titration with KCNS of the excess of a known amount of silver nitrate solution added to 10 cc of tungstic acid filtrate.

Reagents Required.
1. Silver nitrate solution (M/35.46).
2. Potassium sulphocyanate solution (M/35.46).
3. Powdered ferric ammonium sulphate (ferric alum).
4. Concentrated nitric acid (Specific gravity 1.42).

[1] Whitehorn: Jour. Biol. Chem., 1921, **45**, 449.

Preparation of Reagents.—Dissolve 4.791 grams of chemically pure silver nitrate in distilled water. Transfer to a liter volumetric flask and make up to the mark with distilled water. Mix thoroughly and preserve in a brown bottle. One cc equals 1 mg. Cl. (It is to be noted that the silver nitrate and nitric acid are not added to the protein-free filtrate simultaneously. To do so may result in the mechanical enclosure of silver nitrate solution within the curds, and a consequent error in the positive direction.)

Because sulphocyanates are hygroscopic, the standard solution should be prepared volumetrically. As an approximation about 3 grams of KCNS or 2.5 grams of NH_4CNS should be dissolved in a liter of water. By titration under the conditions specified under "Chloride Determination" and by proper dilution, prepare a standard such that 5 cc are equivalent to 5 cc of the silver nitrate solution.

The solid ferric alum is used rather than a solution, in order to insure a very high concentration in the mixture to be titrated. It is powdered in order to facilitate its solution.

(*a*) **Chloride Determination.**—Pipette 10 cc of the tungstic acid filtrate into a porcelain dish. Add with a pipette 5 cc of the standard silver nitrate solution and stir thoroughly. Add about 5 cc of concentrated nitric acid, mix, and let stand for five minutes, to permit the flocking out of the silver chloride. Then add with a spatula an abundant amount of ferric ammonium sulphate (about 0.3 grams) and titrate the excess of silver nitrate with the standard sulphocyanate solution until the definite salmon-red (not yellow) color of the ferric sulphocyanate persists in spite of stirring for at least fifteen seconds.

(*b*) **Calculation.**—5 minus titer (in cc) = mg. of Cl per cc of blood (or plasma).

Since each cc of thiocyanate solution used is equivalent to 1 cc of silver nitrate solution, the difference between the volume of silver nitrate solution taken and the excess determined by the titration, that is (5— titer), represents the volume which reacted with chloride at the ratio of 1 cc to 1 mg. of Cl. And the 10 cc of filtrate taken represents 1 cc of blood (or plasma).

To convert Cl figures into NaCl figures divide by 0.606. The same result may be more easily obtained by the following rule: To obtain mg. NaCl per 100 cc, divide mg. Cl per liter by 6, and subtract 0.001 of the result. Conversely, to obtain mg. Cl per liter, add to mg. NaCl per 100 cc 0.001 of itself and multiply by 6.

5. **Lipoids.**—The blood of diabetic patients can advantageously be examined for its content of lipoids. It is true, one seldom sees cases with 16.3 per cent of blood fat as Case No. 786, and in fact,

I have had no other among the 1062 analyses made in my laboratory. One reason for this may be that less fat is given now than formerly and another that the blood is examined for the lipoids before instead of after a meal. Notwithstanding these changed conditions, however, the lipoids have been almost invariably increased in diabetic patients. Of the cases examined, an increase was found in 26, a normal state in 2, and a decrease in none. The blood fat should be normal in all cases of diabetes and no case of diabetes should be considered cured otherwise. When carbohydrate and protein are unassimilated, they appear in the urine, but when fat fails of assimilation, it collects in the blood.

The normal variations of the lipoids in the blood and the changes which they undergo have been described on p. 192.

The method given below for the estimation of the blood lipoids is that now employed by Prof. Bloor, and kindly given me by him. It is a modification of this method published in 1914,[1] and of that in the first edition of this book.

"The method to be described depends on a new principle—the determination of the fat by precipitation in a water solution and comparison of the cloudy suspension so obtained with that of a similarly prepared standard fat solution by the use of the nephelometer. The determination may be completed in about three-quarters of an hour and may be carried out with from 0.5 cc to 5 cc of blood. Ordinarily about 2 cc are used. It has been found to be accurate to within 5 per cent of the total fat."

The material determined by the "total fat" method consists of total fatty acids and cholesterol.

The "total fatty acids" consists of fatty acids contained in combination in lecithin, cholesterol esters and fat of the blood. (In it would also be included any free fatty acids, soap or other compounds of fatty acids, not mentioned above, which may be present in blood—probably a negligible amount.)

The cholesterol is the total cholesterol—both that which is present in the free condition and that present in combination as cholesterol esters.

As found in normal human blood, the value "total fat" is made up approximately of 2 parts of "total fatty acids" to 1 part of cholesterol. The procedure is as follows:

"*Extraction.*—Two cc of freshly drawn and well-mixed blood are run in a slow stream of drops into a 50 cc graduated tube containing about 35 cc of a mixture of 3 parts alcohol and 1 part ether (both redistilled), which is kept in constant motion by rotating the tube. The solution is raised to boiling by immersion in a

---

[1] Bloor: Jour. Biol. Chem., 1914, **17**, 378.

water-bath (with frequent shaking to prevent superheating), cooled to room temperature, made up to volume with alcohol-ether, mixed and filtered. The extract if placed in tightly stoppered bottles in the dark will keep several months unchanged.

"*Determination.*—From 5 to 10 cc (ordinarily 10 cc) of the extract, containing about 2 mg. of 'fat,' are measured with a pipette into a tube graduated at 50 cc and saponified by evaporating just to dryness with 2 cc of $\frac{N}{1}$ sodium ethylate (made by dissolving cleaned metallic sodium in absolute alcohol). After evaporation is complete 5 cc of alcohol-ether are added and the mixture heated slowly to boiling. A similar solution of the standard is prepared by measuring 5 cc of the standard fat solution (see below) into a beaker and heating to boiling as above. The mixture is made to the 50 cc mark with distilled water. To standard and test solutions are added, as nearly simultaneously as possible, 10 cc portions of dilute (1 to 4) hydrochloric acid, the tube inverted once to insure mixing, and the solutions allowed to stand five minutes, after which they are transferred to the comparison tubes of the nephelometer."

If bubbles appear on the walls of the tubes they should be removed by inverting the tubes two or three times. The movable jacket on the standard tube is set at a convenient point, generally 20 mm. (Richard's nephelometer) and comparisons made by adjusting the jacket on the test solution until the images of the two solutions show equal illumination. Not less than five readings are taken, alternately from above and below, and the average taken as the correct reading.

"The standard solution used is an alcohol-ether solution of pure oleic acid of which 10 cc contain about 2 mg. of fat. The alcohol and ether used for the standard are freshly redistilled absolute alcohol and pure dry ether."

6. **Acetone in the Blood.**—It sometimes occurs that acidosis is present yet is not disclosed by the simple ferric chloride test for diacetic acid in the urine. Under such circumstances the test for acetone in the urine may be made, or better still, a qualitative test for acetone in the blood. The description of such a test follows.

(*a*) **Wishart Method for Detection of Acetone in the Blood.**—The blood is drawn into a syringe or tube containing a few crystals of potassium oxalate, then centrifuged for five minutes at medium speed. The test is made on the plasma with as little delay as possible, as there is liable to be some loss of acetone on standing.

To 4 drops of plasma add solid ammonium sulphate until plasma is thoroughly saturated and protein precipitated; then add 2 drops of a freshly made 5 per cent solution of sodium nitroprusside and 2 drops of concentrated ammonium hydrate. Thoroughly mix.

25

If the test is positive, in from one to ten minutes a color develops which runs all the way from a pale lavendar to that of a deep permanganate hue, in this way indicating whether much or little acetone is present. This is an adaptation to the plasma of the Rothera nitroprusside reaction as ordinarily used for urine. It is said to be sensitive to 1 part in 20,000.

(*b*) **Van Slyke-Fitz Methods for Determination of β-hydroxybutyric Acid and Acetone in Urine and Blood.** (See p. 365.)

7. Carbon Dioxide in Blood Plasma.—Whether in health or in disease, the reactions of the body remain nearly constant and the blood not only conforms to this general law but helps to enforce it. This end is accomplished in the presence of acidosis: (1) by removing the CO_2 from the blood by way of the lungs to make way for the stronger acid, the combining of the acid through the buffer; and (2) by saving of alkali through the excretion of acid phosphate through the kidneys. With the first of these measures we are concerned here and to a considerable extent a determination of the quantity of CO_2 in the blood is an index of the degree of acidosis. Van Slyke has devised a comparatively simple method by which the carbon dioxide combining capacity of the blood plasma can be determined, but before proceeding to a description of that, it may not be out of place to present certain of the factors which must be considered in order to estimate the significance of such a determination.

The blood plasma normally contains a certain amount of bicarbonate ($NaHCO_3$). An idea of the amount of bicarbonate can be obtained by measuring the quantity of CO_2 which is set free when a stronger acid, such as lactic acid, is added to the blood. The CO_2 thus obtained is expressed as volumes of CO_2 per 100 cc of blood (volumes per cent). Normal venous bloods contain between 48 and 58 volumes per cent of CO_2 and normal arterial bloods between 46 and 52 volumes per cent of CO_2. Despite the introduction of an acid, the blood preserves its normal degree of alkalinity to a certain point through the buffer action of the alkali (chiefly sodium bicarbonate) of the plasma and the proteins, especially hemoglobin. Just how much a reserve in alkalinity a given blood plasma may possess is comparatively easily learned by exposing the blood to an atmosphere of CO_2 until it has become saturated and then measuring the amount of CO_2 which has been taken up. This gives the alkali reserve capacity (combining power) of the blood for CO_2 of which the normal varies between 55 and 75 volumes per cent with an average of 65 volumes per cent. The actual CO_2 content in volumes per cent of the blood, or the alkali reserve of the blood for CO_2 expressed also in volumes per cent, are measures of its alkalinity. It is with this latter value in the routine of the clinic with which one usually deals, because the method of determination is simpler and because haste is unnecessary.

But, if one can take the time for actual determinations of the volume per cent of CO_2 in the blood, certain other values can be obtained which are of value in the interpretation of states of acidosis. For this purpose one makes use of the CO_2 diagram of Haggard and Henderson. This is a diagram in which ordinates express volume per cent and abscissæ express tension in mm. of mercury. Upon this diagram are recorded the volume per cent of CO_2 which the blood is found to contain when exposed to an atmosphere of CO_2 at three or more different tensions measured in mm. of mercury. By connecting these plotted points one obtains the *Dissociation Curve* for the volume per cent of CO_2 in the blood under these varying conditions. One can determine, then, by analysis the actual volume per cent of CO_2 in a portion of the sample of arterial blood and find its place on the dissociation curve. This point, known as the "A" point, projected downward will allow one to read on the abscissæ in terms of mm. of mercury the tension under which CO_2 must have existed in the arterial blood, which in turn is the same as that of the tension of the CO_2 in the alveolar air of the patient.

From facts thus obtained two other deductions can be drawn, namely, the hydrogen-ion concentration of the blood and the total amount of acid in the body. The former deduction is possible as shown by Henderson from the ratio $\dfrac{NaHCO_3}{H_2CO_3}$ with the use of a formula and its accuracy can be demonstrated by actual hydrogen-ion determinations. The latter deduction Bock, Field and Adair[1] have made.

TABLE 148.—CALCULATIONS OF BODY FLUID AND OF TOTAL ACID IN FOUR DIABETICS RECOVERING FROM COMA. (BOCK, FIELD AND ADAIR.)

Case.	Weight in kg.	Body fluid in liters.	Concentration of acid.	Total acid in gram mols.	Total acid in grams, diacetic acid.
No. 1	32	22.5	0.031	0.698	71.0
2	42	28.8	0.031	0.892	91.0
3	40	28.0	0.027	0.757	77.2
4	39	27.3	0.037	1.01	103.0

For the total quantity of acid in the body a specimen of normal blood was taken by them and known amounts of acetic acid were added to different portions and the CO_2 which the blood would take up at 40 mm. of mercury was determined. The data of the experiment were plotted and the curve thus obtained was used to find the amount of acid corresponding to the CO_2 bound at 40 mm.

[1] Bock, Field and Adair: Jour. Metab. Research. To be published.

in each of their patients. "We have assumed that the acid or acids in question are evenly distributed throughout the body fluids. The body fluids have been taken as 70 per cent of the body weight, and the concentration of acid has been multiplied by this volume. . . "

"It is convenient to have figures in grams as well as gram molecules, therefore the figures of column 4 have been multiplied by 103, the molecular weight of diacetic acid, which may be taken as a type of the foreign acids present."

For practicing physicians like myself the mysteries of blood-gas analysis are simplified by a letter I was fortunate enough to receive from Arlie Bock relating to his work at the Massachusetts General Hospital. For his letter with its accompanying diagrams and the privilege of inserting the same here, I am most grateful.

BOSTON, May 26, 1923.

"DEAR DR. JOSLIN: In the accompanying five figures I have attempted to reconstruct in a simple way the Haggard-Henderson CO_2 diagram as used in the study of our cases of diabetic coma.

"In the figures the volumes per cent of CO_2 are expressed by the ordinates, and the tensions of CO_2 by the abscissæ. The CO_2 dissociation curve is determined by exposing three or more samples of venous or arterial blood to different atmospheres of air and CO_2 in saturators in a water-bath at body temperature until equilibrium is reached. The amount of CO_2 taken up by the blood in each saturator is determined by means of a Van Slyke or other apparatus, the values obtained are plotted as in Fig. 19, and the best free-hand curve fitting the points is drawn through them. This curve represents the combination of CO_2 and blood over the range of changing tensions of CO_2 that may exist in the body, and since the amount of CO_2 carried by blood is chiefly concerned with the amount of alkali present in the blood, the level of the CO_2 curve is of interest in determining whether an acidosis, alkalosis, or a normal state exists at the time the observations are made. If the level of the curve falls below the zone (Fig. 20) now considered as normal for CO_2 curves, acidosis, as the term is now used, exists although the actual reaction of the blood may be kept normal down to quite low levels of the curve through the action of the lungs in blowing off CO_2 by means of increased ventilation. If a curve is obtained having a level above that of the normal zone an excess of alkali is present in the blood and the condition is known as alkalosis.

"In Fig. 21, the method of plotting the amount of CO_2 in arterial blood is shown. Arterial blood is obtained by puncture of the radial or brachial artery, the amount of CO_2 which it contains is

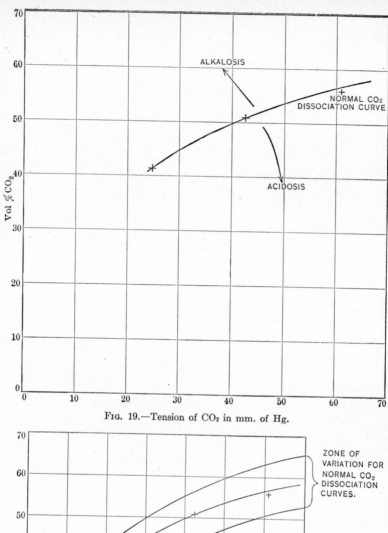

ALKALOSIS

NORMAL CO₂
DISSOCIATION CURVE

ACIDOSIS

FIG. 19.—Tension of CO₂ in mm. of Hg.

ZONE OF
VARIATION FOR
NORMAL CO₂
DISSOCIATION
CURVES.

FIG. 20.—Tension of CO₂ in mm. of Hg.

determined immediately, precautions being taken to exclude loss of CO_2 from the blood, and the value obtained is then placed on a CO_2 dissociation curve determined either from the same sample of arterial blood or on venous blood drawn simultaneously with the arterial sample. The point on the curve at which this value falls is known as the "A" point. In the case given in Fig. 21, the value is 47.8 volumes per cent. An ordinate drawn from this

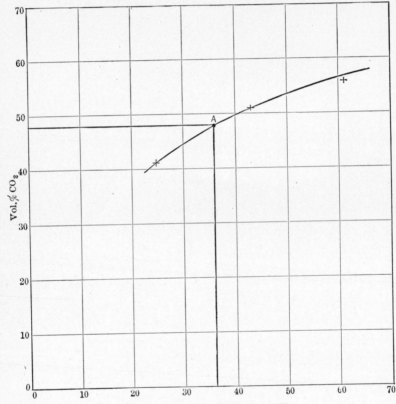

Fig. 21.—Tension of CO_2 in mm. of Hg.

point on the curve to the base line shows that the tension at which this amount of CO_2 in arterial blood existed in the body must have been about 36 mm. of mercury. In patients not subject to cardiac or pulmonary disease, the tension of CO_2 in arterial blood is the same as that of the CO_2 in the alveolar air, so that in the above case the tension of CO_2 in the alveolar air at the time the observation was made was 36 mm. of mercury.

"Now, it is of interest also to know the reaction of the blood,

expressed by the brief symbol pH. This can be easily obtained
with the data before us. We know from L. J. Henderson's original
observations that the reaction of the blood depends upon the ratio
of the free CO_2, or the CO_2 in solution in blood, to the combined
CO_2 in the form of sodium bicarbonate. Given the total CO_2
in arterial blood and the tension at which it exists, as in the above
case, we can determine the value of the ratio of free to combined

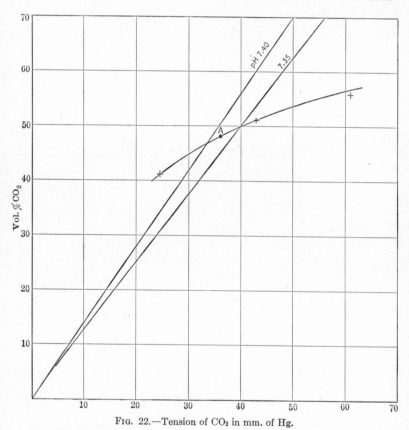

FIG. 22.—Tension of CO_2 in mm. of Hg.

CO_2 because the amount of free CO_2 is directly dependent upon
the tension or pressure at which it exists in the blood. Instead
of making this calculation for each determination we can calculate,
by means of the Hasselbalch formula, a series of pH values and
express them by the straight lines shown in Figs. 22 and 23. The
pH line passing through the A point on the curve thus gives the
reaction of the blood at the time of the observation.

"In Fig. 23, I have added two additional curves and several pH lines in order to show the general level of the CO_2 curve in diabetic coma, the low level to which the arterial CO_2 may fall in this condition, the change in pH from a normal of 7.37 to 7.20, and to indicate the response of the blood and body in general to insulin therapy. The rise in the level of the curve is due to the amount of alkali released from its combination with non-volatile acids such as those of the ketone group and thus made available for combination with CO_2. . . .

Sincerely yours,
A. V. Bock."

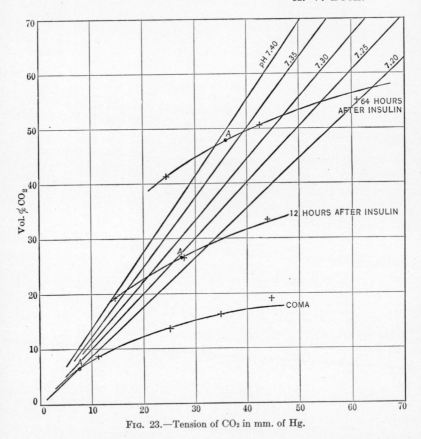

Fig. 23.—Tension of CO_2 in mm. of Hg.

(a) **Van Slyke's Method for Determination of Carbon Dioxide Capacity of Blood Plasma.**—The blood is drawn from a vein into the vessel containing potassium oxalate powder. Unless the blood is drawn under oil to prevent contact with air, it must not be submitted to any agitation except gentle inversion once or twice to mix the oxalate, and should be centrifugated at once, or two errors may occur. The chief error is due to escape from the plasma of carbonic acid, as a result of which approximately an equivalent of HCl diffuses from the corpuscles into the plasma. The net effect is that by internal aëration one can change as much as one-third of the plasma $NaHCO_3$ into NaCl. Unless the above precautions can be observed it is advisable to collect the blood in a syringe containing no gas space, or in a centrifuge tube under a layer of paraffin oil. In order to avoid the reverse, effect, viz., overaccumulation of CO_2 in the venous blood, it is advisable when ligature is used to release it as soon as the vein is entered, and to allow a short time for the stagnant blood to be washed out of the vein before the main sample is drawn. A second and lesser error, which appears to be significant only when the whole blood stands over an hour before centrifuging is due to apparent formation of organic acids by the corpuscle and results in lowering of the bicarbonate. The plasma once separated, however, may be kept for analysis at leisure, any loss of CO_2, by such reactions as $2NaHCO_3 = Na_2CO_3 + H_2CO_3$, being made good before the analysis by resaturating with CO_2 at alveolar tension as described below.

The clear plasma, being pipetted off, should, in case it is not convenient to determine its carbon dioxide capacity at once, be transferred to a paraffin-lined tube, where it will keep unchanged for a week if placed on ice.

In order to determine its alkaline reserve, the plasma is saturated with carbon dioxide at alveolar tension. For this purpose the plasma (about 3 cc if there is plenty of material), which should be at room temperature, is placed in a separatory funnel of about 300 cc capacity, and the funnel is filled with alveolar air from the lungs of the operator. The air is passed through a bottle full of glass beads before it enters the funnel, in order to bring the moisture content down to saturation at room temperature. If one blows directly into the separatory funnel, enough moisture condenses on the wall to appreciably dilute the plasma. The funnel is closed just before the stream of breath stops, and is shaken for one minute in such a manner that the plasma is distributed as completely as possible about the walls, forming a thin layer which quickly approaches equilibrium with the carbon dioxide in the air. After the shaking has lasted a minute, a fresh portion of the alveolar air or of 5.5 per cent carbon dioxide from a gas tank, is run into the funnel, and the shaking completed.

The determination of the carbon dioxide content of the saturated plasma is performed as follows: The carbon dioxide apparatus (Fig. 24) held in a strong clamp on a ringstand, is completely filled with mercury which should fill both capillaries above the upper stopcock. The mercury leveling bulb is placed about on a level with the lower cock. The cup at the top of the apparatus is washed out thoroughly with dilute ammonia followed by water, medicine droppers being convenient for this purpose. One cc of the saturated plasma is now introduced into the cup, and allowed to flow down into the upper stem of the apparatus. The cup is now washed with two portions of about 0.5 cc each of water, care being taken that no air enters the apparatus with the liquid. One small drop of redistilled caprylic alcohol, to prevent foaming, is now admitted into the capillary connecting the cup with the upper end of the apparatus, and about 1 cc of 5 per cent sulphuric acid is poured into the cup. Enough of the acid is now admitted into the apparatus carrying the caprylic alcohol along with it, so that the total volume of water in the apparatus is exactly 2.5 cc. A drop of mercury is now placed in the cup and allowed to flow down to the upper stop-cock in order to seal same, and make it capable of holding an absolute vacuum. The leveling bulb (the lower cock having remained open from the beginning of operations) is lowered to a point such that the surface of the mercury in it is about 800 mm. below the lower stop-cock, and the mercury in the apparatus is allowed to fall until the meniscus of the mercury has dropped to the 50 cc mark on the apparatus. As the latter is evacuated, bubbles of carbon dioxide are seen escaping from the water mixture in the vacuum.

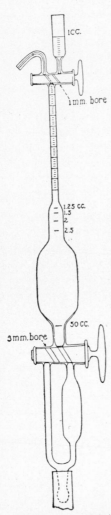

FIG. 24.—Van Slyke's pipette for determining the combining power of the blood for carbon dioxide.

In order to completely extract the carbon dioxide, the apparatus is removed from the clamp and shaken by turning it upside down about a dozen times. It is then replaced, the mercury leveling bulb still being at the low level, and the water solution is allowed to flow completely into the small bulb below the lower stop-cock. The water solution is drained out of the portion of the apparatus above the stop-cock as completely as possible, but without removing any of the gas. The mercury bulb is now raised in the left hand, and the lower stop-cock is turned with the right hand so that mercury is admitted to the apparatus through the left-hand entrance of the 3-way cock without readmitting the water solution. The leveling bulb is held beside the apparatus so that the mercury level in it is even with that in the apparatus, and the gas in the latter is under atmospheric pressure. A few hundredths of a cc of water will float on the mercury in the apparatus, but this may be disregarded in leveling. The volume of gas above the short column of water referred to is at once read off.

The calculation of the result into terms of volume percentage of carbon dioxide bound as bicarbonate by the plasma is quite complicated, and Van Slyke consequently computed a table which obviates the necessity of calculation. (Table 149.)

TABLE 149.—VAN SLYKE'S TABLE FOR CALCULATION OF CO_2 IN BLOOD.

Observed vol. gas $\times \dfrac{B}{760}$	C.c. of CO_2 chemically bound by 100 c.c. plasma.				Observed vol. gas $\times \dfrac{B}{760}$	C.c. of CO_2 chemically bound by 100 c.c. plasma.			
	15°	20°	25°	30°		15°	20°	25°	30°
0.20	9.1	9.9	10.7	11.8	0.60	47.7	48.1	48.5	48.6
1	10.1	10.9	11.7	12.6	1	48.7	49.0	49.4	49.5
2	11.0	11.8	12.6	13.5	2	49.7	50.0	50.4	50.4
3	12.0	12.8	13.6	14.3	3	50.7	50.9	51.3	51.4
4	13.0	13.7	14.5	15.2	4	51.6	51.9	52.2	52.3
5	13.9	14.7	15.5	16.1	5	52.6	52.8	53.2	53.2
6	14.9	15.7	16.4	17.0	6	53.6	53.8	54.1	54.1
7	15.9	16.6	17.4	18.0	7	54.5	54.8	55.1	55.1
8	16.8	17.6	18.3	18.9	8	55.5	55.7	56.0	56.0
9	17.8	18.5	19.2	19.8	9	56.5	56.7	57.0	56.9
0.30	18.8	19.5	20.2	20.8	0.70	57.4	57.6	57.9	57.9
1	19.7	20.4	21.1	21.7	1	58.4	58.6	58.9	58.8
2	20.7	21.4	22.1	22.6	2	59.4	59.5	59.8	59.7
3	21.7	22.3	23.0	23.5	3	60.3	60.5	60.7	60.6
4	22.6	23.3	24.0	24.5	4	61.3	61.4	61.7	61.6
5	23.6	24.2	24.9	25.4	5	62.3	62.4	62.6	62.5
6	24.6	25.2	25.8	26.3	6	63.2	63.3	63.5	63.4
7	25.5	26.2	26.8	27.3	7	64.2	64.3	64.6	64.3
8	26.5	27.1	27.7	28.2	8	65.2	65.3	65.5	65.3
9	27.5	28.1	28.7	29.1	9	66.1	66.2	66.4	66.2
0.40	28.4	29.0	29.6	30.0	0.80	67.1	67.2	67.3	67.1
1	29.4	30.0	30.5	31.0	1	68.1	68.1	68.3	68.0
2	30.3	30.9	31.5	31.9	2	69.0	69.1	69.2	69.0
3	31.3	31.9	32.8	32.8	3	70.0	70.0	70.2	69.9
4	32.3	32.8	33.4	33.8	4	71.0	71.0	71.1	70.8
5	33.2	33.8	34.3	34.7	5	71.9	71.9	72.1	71.8
6	34.2	34.7	35.3	35.6	6	72.9	72.9	73.0	72.7
7	35.2	35.7	36.2	36.5	7	73.9	73.9	74.0	73.6
8	36.1	36.6	37.2	37.4	8	74.8	74.8	74.9	74.5
9	37.1	37.6	38.1	38.4	9	75.8	75.8	75.8	75.4
0.50	38.1	38.5	39.0	39.3	0.90	76.7	76.7	76.8	76.4
1	39.1	39.5	40.0	40.3	1	77.8	77.7	77.7	77.3
2	40.0	40.4	40.9	41.2	2	78.7	78.6	78.7	78.2
3	41.0	41.4	41.9	42.1	3	79.7	79.7	79.6	79.2
4	42.0	42.4	42.8	43.0	4	80.7	80.5	80.6	80.1
5	42.9	43.3	43.8	43.9	5	81.6	81.5	81.5	81.0
6	43.9	44.3	44.7	44.9	6	82.6	82.5	82.4	82.0
7	44.9	45.3	45.7	45.8	7	83.6	83.4	83.4	82.9
8	45.8	46.2	46.6	46.7	8	84.5	84.5	84.3	83.8
9	46.8	47.1	47.5	47.6	9	85.5	85.3	85.2	84.8
0.60	47.7	48.1	48.5	48.6	1.00	86.5	86.2	86.2	85.7

Bar.	$\dfrac{Bar.}{760}$	Bar.	$\dfrac{Bar.}{760}$	Bar.	$\dfrac{Bar.}{760}$	Bar.	$\dfrac{Bar.}{760}$
		746	.981	762	1.003	780	1.027
730	.960	748	.984	764	1.006		
732	.962	750	.987	766	1.008		
734	.963	752	.989	768	1.011		
736	.966	754	.992	770	1.013		
738	.967	756	.995	772	1.016		
740	.971	758	.997	774	1.018		
742	.974	760	1.000	776	1.021		
744	.976	...	...	778	1.024		
	.979						

Plasmas of normal adults yield 0.65 to 0.90 cc of gas, indicating 53 to 77 volume per cent of carbon dioxide chemically bound by the plasma. Figures lower than 50 per cent in adults indicate acidosis. The normal figures for infants appear to be 40 to 55 per cent, much lower than for adults.

Caution in Setting up Apparatus.—The jaws of the clamp in which the apparatus is held should be lined with thick, soft rubber. The apparatus should be clamped very tightly because of the weight of the mercury.

In order to prevent the apparatus from slipping out of the clamp, an iron rod should be so arranged as to project under the lower stop-cock, so that it will support the apparatus from this point, in case it should at any time slip down from the clamp.

The temperature figures at the heads of columns represent the room temperatures at which the samples of plasma are saturated with carbon dioxide and analyzed. It is assumed that both operations are performed at the same temperature, which is also that of the solutions analyzed.

The figures have been so calculated that, regardless of the temperature at which the plasma is saturated, the table gives the volume (reduced to 0°, 760 mm.) of carbon dioxide that 100 cc of plasma are capable of binding at 20.°

If the figures in the table are multiplied by 0.94 they give, approximately (within 1 or 2 per cent), the volume per cent of carbon dioxide bound by plasma at 37.°

If the figures in the table are multiplied by 0.69 they give, usually within less than 5 mm., the alveolar carbon dioxide tension of the plasma donor as determined by the Fridericia apparatus.

If the figures in the table are multiplied by 0.01964, they give the milligrams of carbon dioxide bound by 1 cc of plasma.

The apparatus can be obtained from E. Greiner, 55 Fulton Street, New York.

8. **The Hydrogen-ion Concentration of the Blood.**—Human blood is slightly alkaline, having an hydrogen-ion concentration a little less than that of pure water. The hydrogen-ion concentration—pH— of oxalated normal blood is pH 7.35. In clinical acidosis the values for the oxalated blood may fall to pH 7.1, and Bock has found as low as pH 7.03 in diabetic coma. In artificially produced acidosis in dogs the pH may go as low as pH 6.9. A reaction of pH 7.6 or higher would be obtained only after the administration of alkalis. The buffer action of the carbonates of the plasma and the protein of the whole blood enables the blood to take up considerable amounts of acids or alkalis without appreciable change in hydrogen-ion concentration. Until practically all the plasma bicarbonate is taken up by acid, little or no change

occurs in the pH of the blood. After this point rapid changes in pH occur. It is at this stage that the buffer action of the protein is called upon to take up additional acids. The last resort of the patient in averting death from acidosis is thus the body proteins. A simple method for determining variations in the hydrogen-ion concentration of the blood has been devised by G. E. Cullen.[1]

C. EXAMINATION OF THE RESPIRATION.

1. **The Technic.**—Two types of apparatus are employed to learn the exchange of carbon dioxide and oxygen in man: The respiration calorimeter and the respiration chamber, which are the same in principle, and the respiration apparatus. In the closed chamber of the calorimeter and the respiration chamber, the oxygen admitted and the carbon dioxide withdrawn can be accurately determined in periods from one-half to one hour's duration, but it is better to take the average of the results obtained in three successive periods.

The respiration apparatus differs from the calorimeter and respiration chamber in that the patient is not in a closed chamber, but instead breathes through a nose- or mouth-piece. This is advantageous because the exchange of gases can be determined during short periods of fifteen minutes or less. It is disadvantageous however, because, the periods being so short, errors at the beginning and end of the periods are magnified, and further, because of the individual breathing through a nose-piece or mouth-piece an abnormal state is introduced. Unfortunately, in each form of mouth- or nose-breathing apparatus the error of a leak falls chiefly on the oxygen, because the patient and the apparatus constitute a closed circuit, and any diminution in gas in this circuit must be offset by the addition of oxygen. A more troublesome source of error and one difficult to avoid arises from the possibility of the patient exhaling carbon dioxide, which has previously accumulated in the body, at a more rapid rate than corresponds with the oxygen inhaled. The patient is said to "pump out" carbon dioxide. This error could only occur in the relatively short periods which are employed with the respiratory apparatus. There is also another error due to carbon dioxide which is lost by cutaneous respiration, and it has been calculated that this would lower the quotient 0.01 to 0.015. This also occurs only with the respiratory apparatus.

Many forms of apparatus have been invented to measure the basal metabolism of man and it is gratifying that the tendency is

---

[1] Cullen: Jour. Biol. Chem., 1922, **52**, 501.

all in the way of simplification. At present in the routine and investigative work at the New England Deaconess Hospital the Tissot is employed. Along with this the new student apparatus recently devised by Benedict is being introduced and it is possible that this will eventually be the apparatus for clinical work. As yet, it has not seemed justifiable to expend the money for a basal metabolism test of each diabetic. A single observation, with the necessary control tests on the same day, should not be given as much weight as the labor of securing the data would warrant. The variations in the metabolism of diabetics are far less than in the metabolism of patients of the thyroid.

Many pitfalls likewise lurk in the determination of the respiratory exchange of an individual. The carbon dioxide is the more easily estimated of the two gases, and in early experiments on metabolism investigators attempted to estimate this alone. The determination of oxygen is far more difficult. In dealing with the respiratory quotient, which depends on the relation of these two determinations to each other, the problem is still more complicated and all statements regarding the respiratory quotient of individuals must be accepted with caution. The general picture of the respiratory quotient in an individual is far more valuable as a guide to his true metabolism, if based on several experiments, than is the result of a single experiment. Similarly, it is probably safer to average the results of a series of cases than to attach great importance to figures obtained in an isolated experiment.

2. **The Respiratory Quotient.**—The relation which the volume of carbon dioxide exhaled bears to the volume of oxygen inhaled constitutes the respiratory quotient. The respiratory quotient has been discussed at length on page 254 to which the reader is referred. During the combustion of a food in the body a definite quantity of oxygen is consumed and carbon dioxide produced. The relation which the volumes of carbon dioxide and oxygen bear to one another constitutes the theoretical respiratory quotient of the substance. I will insert here examples showing how the respiratory quotient of alcohol and milk may be theoretically calculated, because the computations are based on different methods.

The oxidation of alcohol (C_2H_5OH) requires 3 molecules of oxygen 3 (O_2), for its complete combustion, as is indicated in the following equation:

$$C_2H_5OH = \begin{matrix} C_2 \\ H_4 \\ H\text{-}O\text{-}H \end{matrix} + 3(O_2) = 3(H_2O) + 2(CO_2). \qquad \frac{\text{Volume } 2(CO_2)}{\text{Volume } 3(O_2)} = 0.67, \text{ respiratory quotient of alcohol.}$$

The calculation of the theoretical respiratory quotient of milk is dependent upon the fact that milk is made up of known quantities

TABLE 150.—RESPIRATORY QUOTIENTS FOR PROTEIN, FATS, CARBOHYDRATES,[1] AND ALCOHOL.

Materials.	Oxygen required to oxidize 1 gram.		Produced in the oxidation of 1 gram.			Respiratory quotient $\frac{CO_2 \text{ c.c.}}{O_2 \text{ c.c.}}$	Heat.			
			Carbon dioxide.		Heat, cal.		Per gram of oxygen, cal.	Per liter of oxygen, cal.	Per gram of carbon dioxide, cal.	Per liter of carbon dioxide, cal.
	Weight, gms.	Volume, c.c.	Weight, gms.	Volume, c.c.						
Starch . .	1.185	829.3	1.629	829.3	4.20	1.000	3.54	5.06	2.58	5.06
Cane-sugar .	1.122	785.5	1.543	785.5	3.96	1.000	3.53	5.04	2.57	5.04
Milk-sugar[2] .	1.066	746.2	1.466	746.2	3.74	1.000	3.51	5.01	2.55	5.01
Animal fat .	2.876	2013.2	2.811	1431.1	9.50	0.711	3.30	4.72	3.38	6.64
Human fat .	2.844	1990.8	2.790	1420.4	9.54	0.713	3.35	4.79	3.42	6.72
Protein[3] .	1.367	956.9	1.520	773.8	4.40[4]	0.809	3.22	4.60	2.89	5.69
β-oxybutyric acid . .	1.368	968.0	1.286	860.0	4.69	0.889	3.40	4.85	2.78	5.46
Alcohol . .	2.085	1459.5	1.911	972.9	7.10	0.667	3.41	4.86	3.72	7.30

[1] Loc. cit., p. 223.

[2] These values apply likewise to dextrose and levulose.

[3] While this computation is based upon meat protein, the values will be essentially the same for all proteins. These values represent quantities found when burning protein not in a calorimetric bomb, but in the animal body.

[4] The heat of combustion of protein averages 5.65 calories per gram; deducting the unoxidized material in the urine, the heat per gram would be 4.40 calories. For discussion of this point, see Atwater and Bryant, Storrs (Connecticut) Agr. Exp. Sta. Rept., 1899, p. 73. Since this value has to deal with protein actually burned, it is not to be confused with the value 4.1 commonly used to calculate the calories from ingested protein of which a portion is assumed to be excreted undigested in the feces.

of milk-sugar, fat, and protein, and that the quantities of oxygen consumed and carbon dioxide given off in the combustion of each of these substances have been determined. These values, as well as some others, are shown in Table 150.

One liter of milk may be considered to contain 50 grams of carbohydrate, 40 grams of fat, and 33 grams protein.

$$
\begin{aligned}
&\text{C.} && (50 \text{ grams} \times 746.2) = 37,310.0 \text{ c.c. } CO_2 \\
&\text{F.} && (40 \text{ grams} \times 1431.1) = 57,244.0 \text{ c.c. } CO_2 \\
&\text{P.} && (33 \text{ grams} \times 773.8) = 25,535.4 \text{ c.c. } CO_2 \\
&&&\overline{\phantom{(50 \text{ grams} \times)} 120,089.4 \text{ c.c. } CO_2} \\
&\text{C.} && (50 \text{ grams} \times 746.2) = 37,310.0 \text{ c.c. } O_2 \\
&\text{F.} && (40 \text{ grams} \times 2013.2) = 80,528.0 \text{ c.c. } O_2 \\
&\text{P.} && (33 \text{ grams} \times 956.9) = 31,577.7 \text{ c.c. } O_2 \\
&&&\overline{\phantom{(50 \text{ grams} \times)} 149,415.7 \text{ c.c. } O_2}
\end{aligned}
$$

$$\frac{120,089.4 \text{ c.c. } CO_2}{149,415.7 \text{ c.c. } O_2} = 0.803, \text{ respiratory quotient of milk.}$$

The calculations to determine the respiratory quotient of an individual are still simpler, and are shown in an experiment discussed under the Total Metabolism in the following paragraph.

3. **The Total Metabolism.**—The total metabolism, with its variations in diabetic patients at different stages of the disease, has been discussed, beginning on page 200. The calculations by which the total metabolism of an individual can be determined when the oxygen consumed and the carbon dioxide exhaled are known are illustrated in the data of the following experiment (Table 151).

TABLE 151.—NORMAL INDIVIDUAL (E. P. J.). FASTING EXPERIMENT DECEMBER 23, 1914. WEIGHT, 65 KILOS. HEIGHT, 177.8 CM.

Period.	Duration, min.	sec.	CO_2 per min. cc.	O_2 per min. cc.	Respiratory quotient.	Calories per kilo per 24°.	Variation standard H. & B.	Variation from DuBois.
1	15	6	152	192	0.79	20.40		....
2	14	59	150	194	0.77	20.51	−14%	−20%
3	15	0	153	196	0.78	20.77		....

Average = 0.78
Total calories. per 24 hours = 1336.

First, the calculation of the respiratory quotient of this individual should be determined, and this is done as follows:

$$\frac{\text{Volume } CO_2}{\text{Volume } O_2} = \frac{152 \text{ cc}}{192 \text{ cc}} = 0.79, \text{ respiratory quotient.}$$

Since the body weight was 65 kilograms and 192 cc O_2 were inhaled for the whole body per minute, 2.95 cc (192 cc O_2 ÷ 65 kilos) were inhaled per kilo per minute, and as there are fourteen hundred and forty minutes in twenty-four hours 4284 cc or 4.284 liters oxygen (1440 × 2.95) were consumed per kilogram body weight per twenty-four hours. In order to express in terms of calories the heat which any consumption of oxygen represents, Williams, Riche and Lusk have constructed a useful table (see Table 152) showing the caloric value of a liter of oxygen for different non-protein respiratory quotients. The term "non-protein respiratory quotient" is explained in a later paragraph.

TABLE 152.—THE CALORIC VALUE OF ONE LITER OF OXYGEN FOR VARIOUS NON-PROTEIN RESPIRATORY QUOTIENTS AND THE PROPORTIONS OF THE ENERGY FROM CARBOHYDRATE AND FAT METABOLISM TO BE ASSIGNED TO CARBOHYDRATE AND FAT RESPECTIVELY. (WILLIAMS, RICHE AND LUSK.[1])

Respiratory quotient.	Calories for 1 liter O_2.		Carbohydrate, per cent.	Fat, per cent.
	Number.	Log.		
0.70	4.686	0.67080	0	100.0
0.71	4.690	0.67116	1.4	98.6
0.72	4.702	0.67231	4.8	95.2
0.73	4.714	0.67346	8.2	91.8
0.74	4.727	0.67460	11.6	88.4
0.75	4.739	0.67574	15.0	85.0
0.76	4.752	0.67688	18.4	81.6
0.77	4.764	0.67801	21.8	78.2
0.78	4.776	0.67913	25.2	74.8
0.79	4.789	0.68024	28.6	71.4
0.80	4.801	0.68136	32.0	68.0
0.81	4.813	0.68247	35.4	64.6
0.82	4.825	0.68358	38.8	61.2
0.83	4.838	0.68469	42.2	57.8
0.84	4.850	0.68578	45.6	54.4
0.85	4.863	0.68690	49.2	51.0
0.86	4.875	0.68800	52.0	47.6
0.87	4.887	0.68910	55.4	44.2
0.88	4.900	0.69019	59.8	40.8
0.89	4.912	0.69128	62.6	37.4
0.90	4.924	0.69230	66.0	34.0
0.91	4.936	0.69343	69.4	30.6
0.92	4.948	0.69450	72.8	27.2
0.93	4.960	0.69557	76.2	23.8
0.94	4.973	0.69664	79.6	20.4
0.95	4.985	0.69771	83.0	17.0
0.96	4.997	0.69878	86.4	13.6
0.97	5.010	0.69985	89.8	10.2
0.98	5.022	0.70092	93.2	6.8
0.99	5.034	0.70199	96.4	3.4
1.00	5.047	0.70307	100.0	0.0

Consulting this table of Williams, Riche and Lusk, it will be seen that the equivalent in calories for 1 liter of O_2 for a non-protein respiratory quotient of 0.79 is 4.789. (As a matter of fact, the respiratory quotient above obtained is not the exact non-protein

---

[1] Williams, Riche and Lusk: Jour. Biol. Chem., 1912, **12**, 357.

respiratory quotient, but this may be neglected unless the nitrogen excretion is distinctly abnormal.)[1] If we multiply 4.789 calories by the total number of liters of O_2 consumed per day, the number of calories per kilo per twenty-four hours is obtained, which would be in this case (4.789 × 4.284) 20.5 calories. It should be stated that this actually represents the metabolism for a period of fifteen minutes when the individual was under complete relaxation, and as quiet as possible. It by no means represents the average metabolism for the day. Even with this extreme basis of repose maintained during the experiment the weight of the oxygen inhaled was 550 grams and of the carbon dioxide exhaled 424 grams in the twenty-four hours.

4. **The Non-protein Respiratory Quotient.**—If the nitrogen in the urine is known, one can calculate the amount of oxygen employed by the body for the oxidation of the protein which it represents, and correspondingly, the amount of carbon dioxide simultaneously produced. If these computed figures are subtracted from the total oxygen and carbon dioxide obtained by direct experiment, the remainders represent the oxygen absorbed and carbon dioxide produced by the non-protein respiratory metabolism. The relation of these to one another constitutes the non-protein respiratory quotient. In the table of Williams, Riche and Lusk the proportions of the total energy from the katabolism of carbohydrate and fat assumed as produced from the two materials respectively for any known non-protein respiratory quotient between 0.70 and 1 given. Thus, a respiratory quotient of 0.70 shows that 100 per cent fat and no carbohydrate was oxidized, and a respiratory quotient of 1 shows exactly the reverse.

The calculations necessary for the determination of the non-protein respiratory quotient of an individual are given below. The example chosen for this purpose is that of a man undergoing a prolonged fast at the Nutrition Laboratory. (See p. 306 for the complete table.)

	Respiratory quotient.		Quantities oxidized.			Calories. per kilo. per 24 hrs.
Time.	Actual.	Non-protein.	Protein, gms.	Carb., gms.	Fat, gms.	
5th day of fast	0.73[2]	0.72	62	15	133	28

The values used for the computation of the above data were as follows:

CO_2 cc per min.	O_2 cc per min.	Nitrogen. grams per 24 hours
175	240	10.41

---

[1] It will be remembered that the respiratory quotient of protein is 0.81 which is nearly that here obtained for the total metabolism.

[2] Calculated for twenty-four hours.

10.41 grams nitrogen represents the nitrogen excreted per twenty-four hours or fourteen hundred and forty minutes, and $\left(\dfrac{10.41 \text{ gms.}}{1440 \text{ min.}}\right)$ 0.0072 gram is the excreted nitrogen per minute.

One gram of protein nitrogen, representing 6.0 grams body protein,[1] produces in its combustion 4750 cc CO_2, and consumes in its combustion 5910 cc O_2. Therefore (4750×0.0072) 34.20 cc CO_2 are produced per minute, and (5910×0.0072) 42.55 cc O_2 are consumed per minute, as a result of the protein metabolism.

In the experiments conducted that day, the total CO_2 eliminated per minute was estimated at 175 cc, and the total O_2 consumed per minute at 240 cc. These two amounts represented the total metabolism of protein, fat and carbohydrate for the day. If the oxygen and carbon dioxide per minute derived from nitrogen, which represents the protein metabolism, are subtracted from the total oxygen absorbed and carbon dioxide produced per minute, the remainders show the non-protein metabolism, or the metabolism which is based on the oxidation of fat and carbohydrate.

175 cc CO_2 per min.	=	total metabolism.	240 cc O_2 per min.	=	total metabolism.
34 " "	=	protein metabolism.	43 " "	=	protein metabolism.
141 " "	=	non-protein metabolism.	197 " "	=	non-protein metabolism.

$\dfrac{\text{Volume 141 cc } CO_2}{\text{Volume 197 cc } O_2}$ = 0.72, non-protein respiratory quotient. Consequently 4.8 per cent of the non-protein metabolism was due to carbohydrate and 95.2 per cent due to fat, according to Table 155.

5. Theoretical Respiratory Quotients as Calculated from the Diet.

—The theoretical respiratory quotient of a normal individual living upon protein and carbohydrate can be calculated as shown in the following table:

TABLE 153.—THEORETICAL RESPIRATORY QUOTIENTS.

Diet.[2]	Cal.	O_2.	CO_2.	Respiratory quotient.
Protein, 100 grams . .	414	95.69	77.38	
Carbohydrates, 563 grams	2365	466.73	466.73	
		562.42	544.11	0.967

The theoretical respiratory quotient of a diabetic individual in which the carbohydrate in the diet has been replaced by fat has

[1] In estimating the quantity of body protein burned from the nitrogen in the urine the equivalent 6 should be employed instead of 6.25.

[2] Magnus-Levy: Ztschr. f. klin. Med., 1905, **56**, 83.

been calculated by Magnus-Levy, and he has also inserted the deductions which must be made on account, (1) of 60 grams of dextrose, and (2) 20 grams of β-oxybutyric acid lost in the urine during the same period.

TABLE 154.—THEORETICAL RESPIRATORY QUOTIENTS.

Diet.[1]	Calories.	O_2 liters.	CO_2 liters.	Respiratory quotient.
Protein, 100 grams	414	89.2	72.0	
Fat, 250 grams	2365	504.9	356.8	
	2779	594.1	428.8	0.722
Dextrose, 60 grams	225.6	44.8	44.8	
	2554	549.3	384.0	0.699
β-oxybutyric, 20 grams	91	19.3	17.2	
	2463	530.0	366.8	0.692

Lusk[2] has calculated that when the dextrose-nitrogen ratio is 3.65 to 1, the quotient of protein is 0.632. The formation and excretion of acetone bodies also tend to lower the quotient, but such acid substances may react with sodium bicarbonate to set free carbon dioxide, so that the precise theoretical value of the quotient in diabetes cannot be determined. The actual observations in phlorizinized dogs and human patients with the 3.65 ratio are found to meet the theoretical expectations with quotients approximating 0.69.

6. **The Carbon Dioxide Tension of the Alveolar Air.**—The introduction of simple methods for the detection of acidosis by determination of the CO_2 in the alveolar air has been of inestimable value. In 1907, I spent a week in Naunyn's laboratory with Magnus-Levy in order to learn to study acidosis by familiarizing myself with the latter's method for the estimation of β-hydroxybutyric acid. The analysis was most time-consuming, as was also the quantitative test for ammonia by the Schlösing method, then commonly in use, which demanded an interval of three days even after the twenty-four-hour quantity of urine had been collected. The technic of Folin in 1912, and of others soon reduced this latter process to less than half an hour, but even then the result obtained respresented the average excretion for the preceding twenty-four hours, and in the presence of approaching coma the data were obtained too late. Therefore newer methods which enable the acidosis to be quantitatively estimated promptly have proved most

---

[1] The values used by Magnus-Levy for O_2 and CO_2 vary somewhat from those given in Table 153.

[2] Lusk: Arch Int. Med., 1915, **15**, 939.

helpful in treatment. At present three such methods are available for the detection of the CO_2 in the alveolar air, the Plesch-Higgins, the Fridericia and the Marriott. Probably the Plesch-Higgins is the most accurate, and those familiar with it in large hospitals prefer it. However, the other two methods are quite satisfactory, and the technic of either one can be learned by physician or nurse in a few minutes.

In the discussion of the carbon dioxide tension of the blood plasma, reference is made to the fact that the carbon dioxide of the blood diffuses so readily into the alveolar air of the lungs that the estimation of the latter in nearly all cases gives an index of the former. Because of the simplicity of the determination of the carbon dioxide in the alveolar air, it is today the best quantitative method which the physician has for the estimation of the acidosis of the patient.

Normally, the carbon dioxide tension of the alveolar air varies between 38 and 45 mm. mercury, 5.3 to 6.3 per cent. If abnormal acids are present in the blood, these displace a proportionate amount of carbon dioxide, and as the carbon dioxide tension in the alveolar air bears a direct relation to that in the blood, it is evident that the carbon dioxide in the alveolar air will vary likewise. A low carbon dioxide tension of the alveolar air therefore indicates an acidosis. If the carbon dioxide tension lies between 38 and 32 mm. mercury a slight acidosis is present, between 32 and 28 a moderate acidosis, and if it falls below 25 mm. Hg. the acidosis is extreme. The lowest value with recovery in my group of cases has been 11 and the lowest obtained in the series was 9, and that occurred in a patient in coma.

Hornor[1] found in an analysis of 300 observations of the alveolar CO_2 tension of my cases that when the carbon dioxide tension of the alveolar air was less than 25 mm. mercury the ammonia was 3 grams or more, when the carbon dioxide tension varied between 25 and 33 mercury the urinary ammonia varied between 3.7 grams and 1.15 grams, and when the carbon dioxide tension was 33 mm. mercury or over the ammonia was less than 2 grams. He also studied the carbohydrate balance in these cases, and learned that it was invariably negative when patients showed a tension of less than 25 mm. mercury, and in three-quarters of the cases was negative when the tension was between 25 and 33 mm. mercury, but that at a higher tension the carbohydrate balance was usually positive and invariably so when the carbon dioxide tension was above 36 mm. mercury. The ferric chloride reaction was also observed, and was found to vary from negative to strongly positive, not only

---

[1] Hornor: Boston Med. and Surg. Jour., 1916, **175**, 148.

when the carbon dioxide tension of the alveolar air was at 36 mm., but also at 23 mm.

Case No. 1120, a child with onset of diabetes at the age of six years, entered the hospital eight months later as he was recovering from definite diabetic coma. Under treatment he thoroughly recovered from acidosis, but upon repeated trials increase of food led to the return of both sugar and acidosis. In one of these attempts to build up his nutrition severe acidosis occurred on a diet containing no carbohydrate, 42 grams protein and 70 grams fat. Typical hyperpnea without cyanosis developed and repeated observations showed the CO_2 tension of the alveolar air to be 15 mm. Hg. By fasting and without the use of alkalis the patient promptly came out of this state, but he later died from inanition without a trace of acidosis, representing the third mortality from inanition which I had had at that time.

(*a*) **Fridericia**[1] **Method.**—This method possesses the advantages of being simple and involving the use of apparatus which may be easily transported to the bedside. One hundred cc of alveolar air are collected in a closed chamber and then cooled from the temperature of the body to that of the room. The carbon dioxide in this air is then absorbed with a 20 per cent aqueous solution of potassium hydrate, thereby creating a partial vacuum which in turn is equalized with water. This water is then subjected to atmospheric pressure, when the amount of carbon dioxide replaced by water can be read in percentage of atmospheric air by reading the height in cm. to which the column of water has risen in the closed 100 cc chamber. This percentage may be changed to mm. of mercury pressure by multiplying by the difference between barometric pressure at the time of the test, and this varies in Boston between 770 mm., and 750 mm., and the tension of aqueous vapor at 37.5° C., which is 48 mm. mercury. This will make a factor which lies between 722 and 702. As the reading of 760 is much the more common at sea level, for clinical purposes the factor 715 ± may be used satisfactorily. The patient should be in the same position and quiet for ten minutes prior to the performance of the test.

After a normal inspiration the end *A* of the apparatus is inserted between the lips and the patient is instructed to expire forcibly through the apparatus with cocks *C* and *D* open, so that there is a free passage from *A* to *B*. The tube remains in the mouth throughout the entire expiration, and the cock *C* is then closed, thus retaining between cocks *C* and *D* the last 100 cc of expired air. (As the exchange of air in the upper respiratory passage is

---

[1] Fridericia: Berliner klin. Wchnschr., 1914, **51**, part 2, 1268.

200 cc, and the exchange of air from the alveoli is 800 cc, it is plain
that with any care at all a sample of alveolar and not upper respiratory air will be obtained.)   The apparatus is now immersed in
a glass tank of water at room temperature and allowed to remain
there five minutes.   At the end of five minutes about 10 cc of 20

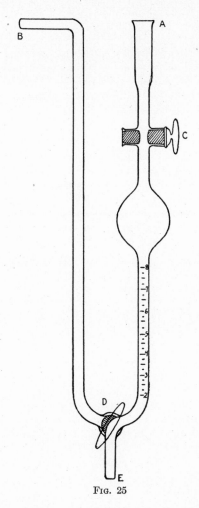

Fig. 25

per cent aqueous solution of potassium hydrate are poured into the
apparatus through orifice *B*. A little of this potassium hydrate
will leak through the hole in cock *D* to chamber *C–D*. Now cock
D is turned to the left so that chamber *C–D* is closed and chamber
B–D is also closed. The small amount of potassium hydrate in

chamber $C–D$ is shaken in the chamber for a moment. Then with apparatus in upright position cock D is turned so that there is a continuous passage from C and B, and the amount of potassium hydrate which will run into the chamber $C–D$ is allowed to do so. Now cock D is turned to the left until $B–D–E$ is a continuous passage, and in this way potassium hydrate is allowed to escape into the water tank. Chamber $C–D$ still contains 2 or 3 cc of potassium hydrate solution, and should be thoroughly washed with this solution. Every point in the surface of chamber $C–D$ must be touched by the alkaline solution. This is accomplished by shaking very thoroughly the potassium hydrate in chamber $C–D$. The apparatus is again immersed in the tank of water, cock D is turned to the left until water rises into $C–D$ through $E–D–C$, and the apparatus left in the water five minutes. At the end of this time the apparatus is raised until the bottom of the meniscus of the water in chamber $C–D$ is level with the top of the water in the tank. Now cock D is turned to the right until water runs through $E–D–B$ to the level of water in chamber $C–D$, which is now closed. Then cock D is turned farther to the right until $C–D–B$ is a continuous chamber. The apparatus is then again immersed to the bottom of the glass tank and the water in the arm $B–D$ of the apparatus should be at the same level with the water in the chamber $C–D$ and continuous with it. If this is not so, then the amount of water in $B–D$ should be changed until it reaches the height of the column of water in $C–D$. The reading is now taken in cm. of the height to which the column of water stands in $C–D$, and this is so graduated as to represent the percentage of CO_2 which was absorbed by alkali and replaced by water. This completes the test.

The apparatus is prepared for the next test by opening cock C so that A to B is a continuous passage. The fluid in the apparatus is allowed to escape. Orifice B is put under the faucet and cold water allowed to run through the apparatus, taking care to shake sufficiently at the time, so that water touches all of the inside of the apparatus. Repeat. Then pour through orifice B about 10 cc of 4 per cent solution of boric acid. Rinse the apparatus very thoroughly with this acid so that there shall be no alkali remaining adherent to its sides. Wash again with cold water. Leave the apparatus so that the cocks to A and B are open, thereby allowing any water in the apparatus to drain out.

From the above it will be seen that the apparatus necessary is, first, the Fridericia appliance,[1] a glass tank, whose depth is equal to the length of the Fridericia apparatus, a wash bottle containing 20 per cent solution of potassium hydrate and another wash bottle

---

[1] Apparatus may be purchased from Emil Greiner, 55 Fulton Street, New York.

containing 4 per cent solution of boric acid. It is convenient to add an indicator, such as alizarin or litmus, to the alkaline and acid fluids.

(*b*) **Marriott's Method.**[1]—A very simple method has been devised by Marriott for the determination of the CO_2 in the alveolar air. The apparatus is portable and the test requires but a few moments for execution. Two procedures are involved: The collection of the alveolar air and the analysis of the sample.

"*Principle of the Method of Analysis.*—The method depends on the fact that if a current of air containing carbon dioxide is passed through a solution of sodium carbonate or bicarbonate until the solution is saturated, the final solution will contain sodium bicarbonate and dissolved carbon dioxide. The reaction of such a solution will depend on the relative amounts of the alkaline bicarbonate and the acid carbon dioxide present. This, in turn, will depend on the tension of carbon dioxide in the air with which the mixture has been saturated and *will be independent of the volume of air blown through, provided saturation has once been attained.* High tensions of carbon dioxide change the reaction of the solution toward the acid side. Low tensions have the reverse effect; hence the reaction of such a solution is a measure of the tension of carbon dioxide in the air with which it has been saturated.

"The reaction of such a solution may be determined by adding to it an indicator such as phenolsulphonephthalein which shows over a considerable range of reaction definite color changes. A certain color indicates a certain reaction.

"Solutions of a given reaction may be prepared by mixing acid and alkaline phosphates in definite proportions. Such solutions may be kept unaltered for long periods of time and can be used as standards for comparison.

"*Collection of the Alveolar Air.*—With an ordinary atomizer bulb, which will deliver approximately 50 cc of air, force approximately 600 cc of air into the rubber bag and clamp the outlet tube with the pinch-cock. While the subject is at rest and breathing naturally and at the end of a *normal* expiration, place the tube in the subject's mouth and close his nose, allowing him to breathe from and into the bag four times in twenty seconds, emptying the bag with each inspiration; the observer should indicate when breathing should be in or out. More frequent breathing will not greatly alter the results. After breathing twenty seconds, at the end of an expiration and while the bag is inflated, clamp the tubing with the pinch-cock and use the air contained in the bag for analysis. The analysis should be made within three minutes, as carbon dioxide rapidly escapes through rubber.

[1] Marriott: Jour. Am. Med. Assn., 1916, **66**, 1594.

"In the case of comatose patients, the rubber bag should be inflated with approximately 1000 cc of air. The comatose patient should be allowed to breathe out of and into the bag for at least thirty seconds, since it is feasible to have him completely empty the bag of air, at each inspiration. It is necessary to use some form of mask.

"A mask is also necessary for collecting alveolar air from infants as well as from comatose patients. This may be improvised, as suggested by Marriott, by means of a nipple of a wide-mouth (Hygeia) nursing bottle and a piece of thin rubber tissue (dental dam).

"*Technic of Analysis.*—Fill the test-tube one-fourth full with standard bicarbonate indicator solution. Then place the capillary nozzle tube in the outlet tube of the bag and, by releasing the pinch-cock, allow the alveolar air from the bag to pass rapidly through the solution in the test-tube for about one minute or until no further color changes occur. The tube is then stoppered and the color immediately compared with that of the standard solutions, by placing it in the center section of the comparison box and the standard solutions most nearly approaching its color on either side. Examination should be made, if possible, at temperatures from 20 to 25° C; if the room temperature is above or below this, the specimen should be immersed in water at about 25° C. while being saturated with the gas being examined.

"*Results.*—If the simple conditions described above for the collection and analysis of air samples are complied with, duplicate determinations usually agree within 2 mm. More than one determination should be made in every instance, especially in confirmation of a low tension, since errors in the technic of collection of the sample lead to too low rather than to too high results. In the case of failure of successive determinations to agree, the fault is much more likely to lie in the collection than in the analysis of the sample."

In normal adults at rest, the carbon dioxide tension in the alveolar air, determined as described above, varies from 40 to 45 mm. Tensions between 30 and 35 mm. are indicative of a mild degree of acidosis. When the tension is as low as 20 mm., the individual may be considered in imminent danger. In coma, associated with acidosis, the tension may be as low as 8 or 10 mm. In infants, the tension of carbon dioxide is from 3 to 5 mm. lower than in adults.

"Alveolar" air collected as described above, is essentially air which has come in equilibrium with the venous blood in the pulmonary capillaries. The tension of carbon dioxide is approximately that in the venous blood. "Alveolar" air collected by the Haldane or Fridericia methods is air which has come in approximate equilibrium with the arterial blood, and hence is of a carbon dioxide tension from 10 to 20 per cent lower.

SECTION V.

THE DIET IN HEALTH AND IN DIABETES.

A. THE DIET OF NORMAL INDIVIDUALS.

1. **Caloric Needs of the Body.**—The metabolism of normal individuals varies greatly, as Lavoisier, 1743–1794, was the first to prove by experiments in respiratory metabolism. A normal ration for a man weighing 70 kilograms (154 pounds) when at moderate work would contain approximately 2800 calories, but if he weighed 60 kilograms (132 pounds), 2400 calories, or 40 calories per kilogram body weight. Individuals with sedentary occupations require far less and I agree with Chittenden, about 2100 calories, or 30 calories per kilogram body weight. By a calorie is understood the amount of heat necessary to raise the temperature of 1 kilogram of water 1° C., or what is approximately the equivalent, 1 pound of water 4° F.[1] The heat liberated by 1 gram of various foodstuffs during this combustion in the body is shown in the following table. In clinical diabetic computations the decimals may be omitted:

TABLE 155.—CALORIC VALUES OF FOODS.

1 gram.	Calories.		Calories.
Carbohydrate	4	actually	4.1
Protein	4	"	4.1
Fat	9	"	9.3
Alcohol	7	"	7.1

The caloric needs of the body vary not only from day to day and hour to hour, but from moment to moment. It is convenient to remember that 1 calorie per kilogram body weight per hour represented the metabolism of a group of normal individuals at the Nutrition Laboratory while at rest in a horizontal position and 1.2 calories per kilogram per hour while sitting in a chair.

---

[1] This is a large calorie, often written with a capital C; a small calorie deals with 1 gram instead of 1 kilogram.

In other words, 20 per cent more energy was required by these individuals to sit in a chair than to lie on a couch. If the subject is asleep lying down and awake sitting up, the difference may be 35 to 40 per cent. On the other hand, if the greatest possible care is taken to be as quiet when erect as when horizontal, the difference may be only 8 per cent. If the individual is in a comfortable steamer chair or propped up in a semi-reclining position with a back-rest, the metabolism is 3 per cent less than when lying flat in bed.[1] At the Nutrition Laboratory 89 normal men at rest eliminated on the average 25.5 calories per kilo body weight per twenty-four hours, the total output per twenty-four hours being 1609 calories, and 68 normal women eliminated on the average 24.9 calories, calculated per kilogram of body weight per twenty-four hours, a total output of 1355 calories for the twenty-four hours of the day. Too often in dietetic computations it is assumed that the caloric needs of the body can be accurately estimated. As a matter of fact, the error in such computations is considerable, and it is absurd to expect to compute the needs of the individual when up and about, whether normal or diabetic, more closely than within 10 to 20 per cent of the real value. The reason for this is apparent if one observes the attitudes and motions of individuals in a street car. The one is quiet, the other restless, the one avoids exertion, the other is all activity. In disease these differences of habit and disposition are accentuated. One patient with 40 calories per kilogram body weight will gain pounds, the other will barely hold her own weight. A diabetic patient, Case No. 1541, confined to her bed with hemiplegia for a year remained sugar-free, held her weight constant and the diet, accurately weighed by a trained nurse for the entire period, amounted to 20 calories per kilogram body weight for twenty-four hours.

As an illustration of the amount of work which can be performed by 1 calorie of energy, I learn from my friend, Prof. Benedict, that the expenditure of 1 calorie of heat is required to rise from a sitting position in front of a door, turn the key in the door, and sit down. A single 16-candle-power carbon lamp gives off in heat the equivalent of about 45 calories per hour, which represents a little less than the basal metabolism of an adult weighing 50 kilograms.

Standards of basal metabolism for age, sex and height have been created in the last few years. The two most commonly employed are those of Harris and Benedict of the Nutrition Laboratory and of DuBois of the Cornell Laboratory. A description of the manner in which these standards were made and of the method by which

---

[1] Sonderstrom, Meyer and DuBois: Arch. Int. Med., 1916, **17**, 872.

the metabolism of an individual can be determined or predicted is described on pp. 203 and 400.

It is desirable for us all to visualize calories and to that end various concrete examples of what calories derived from food will enable an individual to do are given on p. 414.

To walk one hour on a level road at the rate of 2.7 miles an hour requires 160 calories above that of the resting metabolism (Lusk). The amount of energy expended in walking on a level road can be calculated with more accuracy as follows: If the individual weighs 60 kilograms and walks 1000 meters (3281 feet) he is said to have travelled (60 × 1000) 60,000 horizontal kilogram-meters. For each horizontal kilogram-meter 0.0005 calories are required. This would represent an expenditure of (60,000 × 0.0005) 30 calories, which should be added to the resting metabolism of the individual during the time required to walk the given distance. A man weighing 60 kilograms who walks 4 miles an hour would expend [60 (kilograms) × 4 (miles) × 1609.3 (meters in 1 mile) × 0.0005 (calories per horizontal kilogram-meter)] 193 calories. To this figure should be added 60 calories, on the basis of 1 calorie per kilogram body weight per hour, which would have been expended by the individual at rest if one desires to obtain the total expenditure of heat. The basis for calculations of this type is direct measurement. It should be remembered that the weight—60 kilograms —represents the naked weight of the individual plus the weight of his clothes. If a pack weighing 5 kilograms is carried, then the calculations must be on the basis of 65 kilograms.

If the individual ascends a height, the calculations are somewhat different. The unit is the vertical kilogram-meter. The weight of an individual in kilograms multiplied by the height ascended in meters gives the vertical kilogram-meters. The heat equivalent of the mechanical work evolved in 426.5 vertical-meters is 1 calorie. Thus, if an individual of 60 kilograms body weight walks up 10 flights of stairs each 3 meters high, he would expend $\frac{(60 \times 10 \times 3)}{426.5}$ 4.2 calories. As the mechanical efficiency of the body is only about 20 per cent, it is necessary to multiply this figure by 5 in order to determine the actual energy expended (4.2 × 5) namely, 21 calories. Here we are dealing with figures based on estimate and not on direct experimentation. To this figure must be added the calories necessary for horizontal progression, as well as the calories required during the same period of resting metabolism. Two calories might, therefore, be added for the forward progression, and 3 calories more for the three minutes of time of resting metabolism. In other words, a man of 60 kilograms walking up 10 flights of stairs each 3 meters (10 feet) high, in three minutes would expend the heat equivalent of 26 calories or about 3 calories per flight. This would in effect double his basal metabolism.

The metabolism of a group of men standing was 12 per cent more than when in the horizontal position, according to Smith.[1] He also found that walking at 2 miles an hour nearly doubled the standing requirement and at 4 miles an hour increased it threefold.

The basal metabolism of a fasting individual weighing 60 kilograms (132 pounds) has been determined by Benedict (see pp. 306 and 307) and found to vary between 1845 and 1318 calories during the thirty-one days of the fast. Not only did the total calories decrease as the fast progressed, but the calories per kilogram decreased as well. How important a rôle undernutrition plays in the metabolism has already been discussed at length, (See pp. 247 to 254).

It has been estimated that an individual weighing 70 kilograms (154 pounds) requires, under the varying conditions set forth in Table 156, the given number of calories.

TABLE 156.—CALORIES REQUIRED DURING TWENTY-FOUR HOURS BY AN ADULT WEIGHING 70 KILOGRAMS (154 POUNDS).

Condition.	Calories per kilogram body weight.	Calories per pound body weight.	Total calories.
At rest	25–30	11–14	1750–2100
Light work	35–40	16–18	2450–2800
Moderate work	40–45	18–20	2800–3150
Hard work	45–60	20–27	3150–4200

Farmers in various parts of the United States have been shown to consume on an average 3500 calories. One is apt to conclude that an individual doing heavy work requires additional calories for the entire twenty-four hours. This is by no means true. With the cessation of work the metabolism falls abruptly. Furthermore, the actual period of heavy work is short and represented by minutes rather than hours. If of a pessimistic nature one has only to watch street laborers to be convinced, though a far more enjoyable and as scientific a proof is furnished by the minutes spent in actual play by the teams of football. In an entire game, the minutes in which the ball was in play numbered 11, according to the stop watch observations of the late Prof. Harold C. Ernst and Mr. Robert Fisher tells me that in the Boston College—Holy Cross game of 1922 the ball was in play 11 minutes and 23 seconds. Carpenter[2] found 30 calories per hour additional were required by a typist when writing at the rate of 50 words a minute compared with sitting still and reading.

[1] Smith, H. M.: Gaseous Exchange and Physiological Requirements for Level and Grade Walking, Carnegie Inst., Washington, D. C., Pub. No. 309.
[2] Carpenter: Jour. Biol. Chem., 1911, **9**, 231.

Normal boys twelve or thirteen years of age have been shown by DuBois[1] to produce 25 per cent more heat than adults when compared according to his linear formula of body surface. Gephart[2] in a study of the dietary at St. Paul's School came to the conclusion that the boys whose average ages fell between thirteen years and six months and sixteen years and one month ate approximately 5000 calories daily. For these same boys, the calculated basal metabolism would amount to about 1700 calories. It is therefore evident that children require proportionately more food per kilogram or pound body weight. The metabolism of girls has been found to differ from that of boys or women. Standard tables for the estimation of the metabolism of infants, boys and girls are still unsatisfactory. This is especially true for girls and is set forth in the discussion of the basal metabolism of diabetic girls in Carnegie Monograph, No. 323, p. 90.

2. **Composition of the Diet.**—The ordinary diet for a man at moderate work would contain about 400 grams of carbohydrate, 100 grams of protein (equivalent to 16 grams of nitrogen, approximately eliminated as 14 grams in the urine and 2 in the feces) and 100 grams of fat. This would amount to 2900 calories in the twenty-four hours, or about 40 calories per kilogram for an individual weighing 70 kilograms. These figures would be proportionately reduced both for those of lower body weight and for those with lighter occupations, who would require nearer 30 calories per kilogram. As age advances the metabolism requirements are lessened, thus if 1677 calories are required for basal metabolic needs at thirty years, 1542 are required at fifty and 1407 at seventy years of age. The Harris and Benedict data for these figures are shown in Table 157.

TABLE 157.—DECREASING METABOLIC NEEDS WITH ADVANCING YEARS. HARRIS AND BENEDICT PREDICTION TABLES.[3]

Male, age in years	30	50	70
Height 170 cm.	648	513	378
Weight 70 kg.	1029	1029	1029
Calories in twenty-four hours	1677	1542	1407

TABLE 158.—THE PROPORTION OF CARBOHYDRATE, PROTEIN AND FAT IN THE NORMAL DIET.

Food.	Quantity, grams.	Calories, per gram.	Total calories.
Carbohydrate	400	4	1600
Protein	100	4	400
Fat	100	9	900

[1] DuBois: Arch. Int. Med., 1916, **17**, 887.
[2] Gephart: Boston Med. and Surg. Jour., 1917, **176**, 17.
[3] For the simple method of calculating the metabolism by the Harris and Benedict standard, see p. 735; also consult Boothby's and Wilder's charts pp. 460 and 461, for DuBois methods as well as p. 754.

The figures given above are very different from the old Voit standard in which the carbohydrate was placed at 500 grams, the protein at 125 grams and the fat at 55 grams. The more I observe the diets of non-diabetic patients, the more I have come to believe that adults eat less than has generally been supposed. The figures given above are high rather than low. Students in one University which I visited evidently ate below their requirements, and the reason was possibly attributable to the cafeteria system. At boarding houses they would have been more free to take liberal portions. The war, here as elsewhere, rendered less necessary the teachings of Chittenden[1] upon the dangers of over-nutrition. The inhabitants care more for their money than for surplus food.

3. **Carbohydrate.**—From the preceding statements it will be seen that 55 per cent of the energy of the diet of the normal individual consists of carbohydrate. These figures are only approximate, but they leave no doubt as to how large a place sugar and starch occupy in the daily ration. (See p. 415.) What percentage of carbohydrate is furnished by sugar is problematical. We do know, however, that the average individual was supposed to consume 84 pounds of cane sugar during the year 1921. This would amount to 105 grams, or 0.2 pounds, per day, which would amount to about one-fourth of the carbohydrate calories.

The proportion of carbohydrate in the normal diet varies in different countries, reaching its maximum in the tropics and its minimum in the arctic zones. The people in India take 484 grams carbohydrate daily, while the Eskimos get along very comfortably upon 52 grams. Table 159 is arranged by modifying somewhat a similar table of Lusk's.[2]

It shows well the adaptability of different races to different diets. That the Eskimos live upon 52 grams of carbohydrate daily should greatly encourage diabetic patients. All who treat diabetics should be very thankful that there is a race of Eskimos through which proof is afforded that it is perfectly possible to maintain life on a diet in which carbohydrate is largely replaced by fat.[3]

The composition of the diet also varies in the same race from time to time and this has been interestingly described by Mendel.[4]

[1] Chittenden: Physiological Economy in Nutrition, New York, 1904, p. 474.

[2] Lusk: The Fundamental Basis of Nutrition, New Haven, Yale University Press, 1914, p. 31.

[3] It must be acknowledged, however, that today the Danish Government supplies the Eskimo with more than this quantity of carbohydrate. Krogh: A Study of the Diet and Metabolism of Eskimos, Copenhagen, 1913.

[4] Mendel: Changes of the Food Supply and Their Relation to Nutrition, New Haven, Yale University Press, 1916.

Attention has already been called to the increase in the consumption of sugar in the United States during the last century. Rübner noted that the consumption of meat per capita in Germany had risen three and one-half times during a hundred years prior to the war. The effects of undernutrition during the war were manifest generally in Europe and America, but the total dietary restriction obscures the results of qualitative changes. (See p. 115.)

TABLE 159.—VARIATIONS IN DIET ACCORDING TO RACE.

Race.	Weight, kilos.	Protein, gm.	Carbohydrate, gm.	Fat, gm.	Total calories.
Eskimo . . .	65	282	52	141	2604
Bengali . . .	50	52	484	27	2390
European . . .	70	118	512	65	3055
American[1] . . .	70	100	400	100	2900

4. **Protein.**—The protein burned in the metabolism of a healthy individual from day to day depends chiefly on the protein supplied by the diet. Muscular exercise has little effect upon it, since that is dependent upon carbohydrate or fat, with a preference for the former. Even in the early days of fasting the protein metabolism changes but little from that in health. With a diet rich in carbohydrate and fat and low in protein the protein metabolism is easily brought to less than 50 grams per day, but with an excess of protein in the diet it may rise to 150 or 200 grams. A liver well stored with glycogen protects the body protein of a fasting man for a day just as carbohydrate in the diet, but on a second day fails because the glycogen is nearly exhausted.

TABLE 160.—THE EFFECT OF FASTING UPON THE PROTEIN METABOLISM OF A LEAN AND A FAT DOG.

Falck's lean dog.		Falck's fat dog.	
Fasting days.	Grams protein catabolized per day.	Fasting days.	Grams protein catabolized per day.
1– 4	26.1	1– 6	29.9
5– 8	24.6	7–12	26.7
9–12	33.9	13–18	26.1
13–16	38.0	19–24	22.3
17–20	31.9	25–29	20.0
21–24	3.9	30–34	16.8
		35–38	15.7
		40–44	13.0
On the twenty-fifth day the dog died.		45–50	13.6
		55–60	12.2
		Dog still healthy after sixty days.	

"The influence of the available supply of body fat upon the protein metabolism of fasting," as cited by Sherman,[2] "is shown

---

[1] Added by E. P. J.

[2] Sherman: Chemistry of Food and Nutrition, the Macmillan Company, 1919, p. 205.

27

by the following observations of Falck, on the protein metabolism of two fasting dogs—the one lean, the other fat." (See Table 160.) The fat dog was healthy thirty-five days after the lean dog died.

The quantity of protein in the normal diet is somewhat below 100 grams. Presumably patients visiting a physician and consequently not in perfect health would be living upon a somewhat restricted diet. Even allowing for this, the values, 8 to 14 grams, which represent the usual urinary nitrogen excretion of my non-diabetic adults, is lower than might be expected from older writers.

Prof. Cannon writes me that he has "reports from 46 different students who have lived carefully and made thorough reports of their conditions during four days, on the last of which unusual exercise was taken. The average excretion of nitrogen for these 46 students, on the four days in succession, was 12, 12.16, 12.38 and 12.29 grams." If we raise the nitrogen by allowing the difference for that eliminated in the feces, the total elimination of nitrogen would be 14 grams, and this would represent the equivalent of 88 grams protein ($14 \times 6.25 \times 88$) as the normal metabolism of these students. A group of 12 students in the International Young Men's Christian Association College, at Springfield, Massachusetts, excreted 13 to 14 grams nitrogen in the urine daily while upon an unrestricted diet. It will be found of great advantage to accustom oneself to estimate the protein content of the diet of patients in terms of nitrogen as well as in protein, and to control one's calculations by determining the nitrogen in the urine. Such controls, however, will not be of value if the patient is undergoing rapid changes of diet or weight.

When Prof. Chittenden's[1] epoch-making studies appeared, many felt that he went to extremes, but today his statements appear very moderate. He wrote "Food requirements must with necessity vary with changing conditions. . . all the results so far obtained in this investigation with a great variety of persons point to the conclusion that the real demands of the body for protein food do not exceed 50 per cent of the amount generally consumed. Half of the 118 grams of protein food called for daily in ordinary dietary standards is quite sufficient to meet all the real physiological needs of the body. . . "

Low protein diets are perfectly compatible with life and the more the supply of carbohydrate and fat and the more frequent the protein meals the lower they can be reduced. The fact that Karl Thomas could reduce his protein metabolism to between 2 and 3 grams daily is not proof that it is desirable to do so. Two-

---

[1] Chittenden: Loc. cit., p. 416.

thirds of a gram of protein per kilogram body weight appears to be a safe minimum. It is not a wise minimum when allowance must be made for growth, repair of injuries, convalescence from disease and heavy muscular work. The possibility of maintenance of nitrogenous equilibrium upon a very low protein intake has been demonstrated for diabetics by Newburgh and Marsh. (See p. 525, and Petrén, see p. 529.)

The term protein is a broad one, and until recent years in dietary programs comparatively little account has been taken of its components. The old formula for hemoglobin, $C_{758}H_{1203}O_{228}N_{195}FeS_3+P$, though by no means accurate, gives some idea of its complexity. The individual nitrogenous substances (amino-acids) which are found in protein are seventeen in number, and the different proteins vary in the percentages of each of these present. The complete proteins—namely, those which are essential for constructing the different parts of the body—contain the same amino-acids and such proteins are represented by milk, meat, fish and egg proteins. In gelatin and some vegetable foods, important amino-acids are lacking and it is, therefore, important that such incomplete proteins shall not be furnished diabetic patients, particularly children, when on a low diet. Osborne and Mendel[1] have carefully studied the value which various proteins exercised upon growth and have shown that whereas upon milk or a mixed diet young rats grew normally, if a single incomplete protein— gliadin—was given, they appeared well, but remained dwarfs, and resumed normal growth only when returned to milk or mixed diet.

The quantity of protein necessary to keep in nitrogenous equilibrium has been found by Thomas[2] to vary according to the source.

TABLE 161.—RELATIVE QUANTITIES OF PROTEIN REQUIRED TO MAINTAIN NITROGENOUS EQUILIBRIUM.

Protein.	Gm.
Meat	38
Milk	31
Rice	34
Indian corn	102
Potato	38
Bean	54
Bread	76

Furthermore, a possibility exists that protein may be formed in the body from the addition of nitrogen to the decomposition products of sugar (methyl-glyoxal, lactic acid, pyruvic acid) in the form of alanin.

5. **Fat.**—The quantity of fat in the normal diet varies, partly from choice and partly from economic reasons. In general, in

[1] Osborne and Mendel: Jour. Biol. Chem., 1913, **15**, 311; 1915, **23**, 439; 1916, **24**, 37; 1916, **25**, 1; 1916, **26**, 1 and 293.
[2] Cited by Lusk: Loc. cit., p. 416.

those cases where the carbohydrate in the diet is high, the fat is low, and *vice versa*.   The Voit standard placed the fat at 55 grams, but a series of 1300 dietary studies of families, carried out among different races and in different countries, showed that the average quantity of fat eaten was about 135 grams (4.5 ounces) per person per day, the variation recorded being from 45 to 390 grams per person per day.[1]

The more agreeable varieties of fat, such as butter, cream and oil, are expensive foods, counterbalanced to some extent, it is true, by their not being wasted.   Fat is also concentrated food, not only because it has twice the caloric value of either carbohydrate or protein, but because it occurs more frequently in pure form. Oil, butter, and lard contain little water, whereas, except for pure sugar and starch, most carbohydrates and proteins are diluted five to ten times with water.

The chief source of error in calculating the total caloric value of the diet and especially of the diabetic diet is in the estimation of fat.   Thus for many years I have considered that, on an average, lean meat and fish contained 10 per cent fat and have taught patients to reckon 3 grams of fat to each ounce of meat or fish. This figure is unquestionably correct for poultry and very lean meat, and is very high for most varieties of fish, such varieties as cod, haddock and flounder containing only 1 per cent, but an analysis of a mixture of ten portions of cooked meat exactly identical with similar portions about to be served patients at the New England Deaconess Hospital was made at the Nutrition Laboratory, and showed 14.4 per cent fat.   It is, therefore, better to reckon 5 grams of fat to the ounce of meat when the patient is taking several varieties.

Bacon is variously estimated, but I have adopted 50 per cent as an average value for the fat in cooked bacon.   Analyses from different sources show the fat of cooked bacon varies from 37 to 79 per cent.   Portions of bacon lose varying quantities of weight in the cooking, as shown in the following table:

TABLE 162.—LOSS OF WEIGHT OF BACON DURING COOKING.

Uncooked, grams.	Cooked, grams.	Loss.	
		Grams.	Per cent.
80	46	34	43
200	100 .	100	50
50	17	33	66
60	23	37	62
30	10	20	67
110	30	81	73
160	—	—	—
240	41	199	83

[1] Holmes and Lang: Fats and Their Economical Use in the Home, U. S. Dept. Agriculture, 1916, Bull. No. 469,

Through the courtesy of Miss Katherine Blunt, I am able to insert an extensive series of analyses of bacon. These make it very evident that our caloric values for bacon must be very crude unless all the fat in the frying pan is utilized. The protein appears to vary even more than the fat in the cooked bacon. Figures like these upset our preconceived ideas about dietary values and show the necessity of carefully arranged dietary studies upon diabetic patients.

TABLE 163.—COMPOSITION OF VERY FAT BACON COOKED (KATHERINE BLUNT).

	Fat, per cent.	Protein, per cent.	Ash, per cent.	Water, per cent.	Loss by cooking, per cent.
Much cooked	61.9	30.3	7.7	0.3	82
	64.5	28.1	6.2	0.3	79
Lightly cooked	71.4	21.8	2.7	1.9	65
	75.2	18.5	...	2.6	69
	80.3	12.0	2.1	2.8	58

Eggs in some cities by law must weigh a pound and a half a dozen, and average 60 grams (2 ounces) apiece. Such eggs contain approximately 6 grams of protein and 6 grams of fat. The German tables generally figure the fat at 5 or 5½ grams. How gross our caloric reckonings are is obvious if a collection of eggs is weighed and the minimum and maximum weights noted. The weight of the heaviest egg was 72 per cent more than that of the lightest. (See Table 164.)

TABLE 164.—VARIATIONS IN WEIGHTS OF EGGS WITH THE SHELLS.

Number eggs weighed.	Minimum, grams.	Maximum, grams.	Variation, per cent.
9	52	63	21
12	40	62	55
11	56	63	12
12	51	69	35
12	48	66	38

The weight of egg shells is usually about 7 grams.

These examples will serve to show that doctors, nurses and patients should not take their dietetic calculations of calories too seriously, and that carbohydrate, protein, fat and calories should be recorded in whole numbers and not in decimals.

6. **Caloric Values which Every Doctor Should Know by Heart.**— The quantity of carbohydrate, protein and fat found in an ordinary diet must be known by a physician if he wishes to treat a case of diabetes successfully. If he cannot calculate the diet he will lose the respect of his patient. The value of the different foods in the diet can be calculated easily from the diet Table 165. This is

purposely simple, because a diet chart, to be useful, must be easily remembered. With these food values as a basis it is possible to give a rough estimate of the value and composition of almost any food. Various foods are also classified according to the content of carbohydrate (see p. 436) in 5, 10, 15 and 20 per cent groups, and the lists are so arranged that those first in each group contain the least, those at the end the most. This is a practical and sufficiently accurate arrangement, because except in the most exact experiments the errors in the preparation of the food are too great to warrant closer reckoning. It is practically impossible, except when accurate analyses of the diet are made, to reckon the carbohydrate for the twenty-four hours closer than within 5 to 10 grams, and we had best acknowledge that fact. It is really surprising, however, how reliable the figures are if we do not push the matter to extremes. For example, the protein was analyzed in 10 portions of cooked lean meat, similar to 10 other portions served the same day at the New England Deaconess Hospital. In these analyses it was found that the protein content was 30 per cent.

TABLE 165.—FOOD VALUES IMPORTANT IN THE TREATMENT OF DIABETES.

30 grams (1 oz.) Contain approximately.	Carbohydrates, grams.	Protein, grams.	Fat, grams.	Calories.
Oatmeal, dry weight . . .	20	5	2	118
Shredded wheat	23	3	0	104
Uneeda biscuits, two . . .	10	1	1	53
Cream, 40%	1	1	12	116
Cream, 20%	1	1	6	62
Milk	1.5	1	1	19
Brazil nuts	2	5	20	208
Oysters, six	4	6	1	49
Meat (cooked, lean) . . .	0	8	5	77
Chicken (cooked, lean) . . .	0	8	3	59
Bacon	0	5	15	155
Cheese	0	8	11	131
Egg (one)	0	6	6	78
Vegetables 5% group (mixture)	1	0.5	0	6
Vegetables 10% group (mixture)	2	0.5	0	10
Potato	6	1	0	28
Bread	18	3	0	84
Butter	0	0	25	225
Oil	0	0	30	270
Fish, cod, haddock (cooked) .	0	6	0	24
Broth	0	0.7		3

7. **Household Measures.**—Repeatedly physicians have requested me to arrange the above table in terms of household measures. To a considerable extent this is impracticable because the diabetic diet deals with so small a quantity of carbohydrate. An earnest attempt to do this has been made, using the sensible table arranged

for general food values by F. W. White,[1] and the 100-calorie portions so much in vogue and described in the excellent book of Rose,[2] but without success. The only safe way for diabetic patients at the commencement of their training is to weigh their food. After

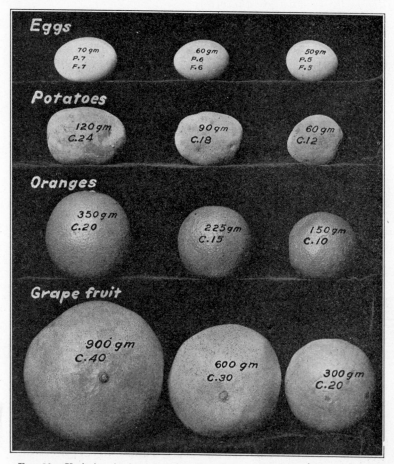

Fig. 26.—Variations in the sizes of common foods. $C.$ = carbohydrate; $P.$ = protein; $F.$ = fat. The food values recorded are for gross weights and only approximate.

a few days of weighing, patients can select utensils which conform to the size of the portions of their own special diets and use these exclusively. As a matter of fact practically all of my patients use

[1] White: Food Values in Household Measures, F. H. Thomas Co., Boston.
[2] Rose: Feeding the Family, The Macmillan Co., 1916, p. 13.

scales at one time or another in the course of treatment. The variety which has served me best is the 500 gram scale manufactured by John Chatillon and Sons, 85 Cliff Street, New York City. These scales have been of great service to diabetics.

In order to illustrate the errors which easily rise from general statements about foods, the accompanying illustration, Fig. 26 is inserted.

B. THE DIET OF DIABETIC INDIVIDUALS.

1. **Caloric Needs of the Diabetic.**—The diet of the diabetic patient should contain, except for brief intervals, the minimum number of calories which the normal individual would require under similar conditions. I am convinced that many normal individuals must live upon less than 30 calories per kilogram, and repeatedly one sees diabetic patients over fifty years of age who live upon less for long periods of time. Table 166, shows the wide variation in calories per kilogram body weight of those of my diabetic cases whose metabolism was tested between 1908 and 1917. In Table 167, the variation in basal metabolism is shown before and after treatment with insulin.

TABLE 166.—POSTABSORPTIVE METABOLISM OF ADULT DIABETICS ARRANGED ACCORDING TO CALORIES PER KILOGRAM BODY WEIGHT.

Calories per kilogram body weight per 24 hours.	Average calories per kilogram body weight per 24 hours.	Number of observation days.	Number of cases.	Average basal metabolism. By days, per cent.	By cases, per cent.
15 to 20	19	33	18	−16	−13
21 to 25	23	175	61	−11	− 9
26 to 30	28	122	45	0	+ 1
31 to 35	32	51	25	+15	+14
36 to 40	38	16	5	+14	+18
41	41	1	1	+22	+22

The average calories per kilogram body weight per twenty-four hours for all days and all cases was 26 calories.

If the physician allows his patient to go untreated and excrete sugar and β-oxybutyric acid in the urine instead of burning these substances in the body, he must add for each gram of sugar so lost 4 calories (actually 4.1) and for each gram of β-oxybutyric acid 5 calories (actually 4.693). I use the figure 5 calories for 1 gram β-oxybutyric acid because, along with this acid, a certain amount of acetone and diacetic acid also escape so that the allowance of 5 calories for all three is undoubtedly too low rather than too high. Case No. 344, p. 362, shows the importance of the loss of acid bodies as well as of sugar.

Fig. 26, p. 423, shows: 1. How readily errors may occur in estimating the food values of the diet unless definite quantities of foodstuffs are prescribed.

TABLE 167.—BASAL METABOLISM AND RESPIRATORY QUOTIENT OF DIABETIC PATIENTS BEFORE AND AFTER TREATMENT WITH INSULIN.

Case No.	Date before treatment, 1922.	No. of days treated.	Age, yrs.	Height (net), cm.	Weight (net), kg.	Gain in weight.		Calories per 24 hours.		Gain in calories.		Respiratory quotient.		Blood sugar.	
						Actual kg.	Per cent.	Before.	After.	Actual cals.	Per cent.	Before.	After.	Before, per cent.	After, per cent.
632	Dec. 1	18	41	177	49.6	0.3	0.6	1115	1186	71	6.4	0.76	0.79	0.14	0.13
866	Oct. 14	101	39	186	39.9	3.1	7.8	854	977	123	14.4	0.80	0.81	0.12	0.17
1542	Oct. 4	111	42	164	33.6	2.6	7.7	903	1033	130	14.4	0.78	0.76	0.31	0.26
1889	Nov. 13	68	17	156	28.4	2.9	10.2	849	1031	182	21.4	0.86	0.83	0.16	0.20
1970	Dec. 4	51	52	156	51.7	0.5	1.0	1198	1204	6	0.5	0.83	0.78	0.24	0.20
2256	Nov. 9	98	18	165	23.1	3.4	14.7	821	887	66	8.0	0.76	0.78	0.31	0.19
2448	Oct. 20	52	19	172	43.5	6.3	14.5	1355	1341	−14	−1.0	0.76	0.82	0.28	0.14
2687	Dec. 11	37	25	164	43.2	−0.1	−0.2	1119	1303	184	16.4	0.75	0.83	0.24	0.27
2729	Nov. 7	35	22	181	48.2	0.8	1.7	954	1012	58	6.1	0.78	0.81	0.22	0.14
2801	Oct. 19	88	15	161	38.0	1.5	4.0	1090	1352	262	24.0	0.76	0.79	0.35	0.39
2972	Dec. 21	34	67	151	33.7	2.1	6.2	931	921	−10	−1.1	0.79	0.75	0.25	0.22

TABLE 168.—ESTIMATED DIET OF CASE NO. 1147 PRIOR TO TREATMENT.

Food grams.	Carbohydrate, grams.	Protein, grams.	Fat, grams.
Eggs, 12	0	72	72
5 per cent. vegetables, 450 . . .	15	8	0
Milk, 2000	96	64	64
40 per cent. cream, 240	8	8	96
Butter, 90	0	0	75
Meat, 120	0	32	20
Bread, 100	60	10	0
Totals	179	194	327
	4	4	9
Total calories	716	776	2943

Total calories 4435 ÷ 72 (kilograms) = approximately 60 calories per kilogram body weight.

2. The absurdity of reckoning food values to the fraction of a gram unless actual analyses of each food as served are made.[1]

Errors in eggs may compensate themselves, because the eggs average about 60 grams (and must so average in some communities); errors in potatoes, oranges and grapefruit must necessarily be very great. The largest of the three potatoes is actually a small potato; the potato weighing 60 grams is about the size of an egg; the oranges from left to right are sold under the trade names of 126, 170 and 250 (to the box) and the grapefruit under the trade names of 28, 64 and 96 (to the box).

It is partly on account of the ease with which large errors in the carbohydrate content of food may occur that it is desirable to give to patients with a low carbohydrate tolerance their carbohydrate in the form of 5 per cent vegetables exclusively, for an error in weighing, reaching 120 grams (4 ounces), would amount to but a few grams of carbohydrate.

And this is not all, for when acidosis is extreme, Benedict and I have shown that the metabolism is increased about 15 per cent, and consequently more calories are required to meet this demand. It is seldom one can obtain definite knowledge of a patient's diet before treatment is begun, but with Case No. 1147, the figures appeared reliable, though they show an attempt to lower the carbohydrate in the food. A lady, aged thirty-five years, with diabetes of two and a half years' duration lost in a little more than this interval 66 pounds. On October 6, 1916, the volume of urine was estimated at 6000 cc, and the sugar was found to be 5 per cent or 300 grams—the equivalent of a loss of 1200 calories in

---

[1] Ladd and Palmer illustrate this point well in Table III of an article in Am. Jour. Med. Sci.; 1923, **166**, 157.

twenty-four hours. She reported her daily diet to have been as shown in Table 168, on p. 426.

After a two weeks' stay in the hospital she felt more content with a diet of 1600 calories than she did upon her diet at entrance, and her weight was constant during the last four days. It is obvious that the saving of food entailed hereby would be considerable. It is the diet of the untreated diabetic which is expensive.

2. **Carbohydrate.**—The total carbohydrate in the diet of diabetic patients is almost invariably restricted, and even with insulin the quantity prescribed seldom exceeds 100 grams. This is a decrease to approximately 25 per cent of the normal carbohydrate ration, and so radically changes the composition of the normal diet as to make it self-evident that rapid changes from a normal to a diabetic diet containing even 100 grams carbohydrate might easily cause indigestion in normal as well as in diabetic individuals. One of the advantages of fasting and undernutrition is the avoidance of indigestion at the beginning of treatment.

The character of the carbohydrate has comparatively little effect upon its assimilability. It is true that levulose behaves under certain conditions in a manner peculiar to itself, but as a rule its effect is not noticeably distinguishable, perhaps because not sufficiently investigated. For a discussion of the behavior of levulose in diabetes see pp. 289 and 539. Various methods have been employed to test the assimilation of the different carbohydrates and the evidence is presented in the following paragraphs. The results of oral tests have been described already. (See p. 167.)

(*a*) **The Assimilability of Starch and the Various Sugars.**—The assimilability of sugar can be tested by the oral, subcutaneous, and intravenous methods of administration, and Allen[1] has pointed out in detail the striking differences which result. The oral method is convenient, but inaccurate on account of variation in the rate of absorption. The intravenous method merely gives the saturation limit of the blood and tissues for sugar which can take place without sugar overflowing the kidneys, and hence is affected by slight variations in renal permeability. The subcutaneous test is the best test of all of the power of the body to utilize sugar. By it errors in absorption are minimized, the liver avoided, and the actual efficiency of the tissues in storing or burning the sugar is determined.

The relations of the tests are brought out interestingly by the case of levulose. "The oral tolerance of levulose is not much less than that of dextrose, because the liver stops nearly all levulose. The intravenous tolerance of levulose is approximately the same

---

[1] Allen: Glycosuria and Diabetes, Harvard University Press, 1913.

as that of dextrose, for the value represents a more immediate saturation limit. The subcutaneous tolerance of levulose is a very small fraction of that of dextrose, because this method tests the power of the general tissue to utilize levulose, and this power is easily exceeded." In other words, the intravenous method shows the saturation limit, the oral method furnishes a test for the hepatic function, and the subcutaneous method shows the utilization by the tissues.

Blumenthal found that the amount of sugar injected into a rabbit sufficient to cause glycosuria varied between 1.8 and 2.8 grams per rabbit (about 0.8 gram per kilo) in injections lasting from one to two minutes, and he records that the saturation limits of dextrose and levulose are almost equal. For galactose it is much less; for saccharose and lactose it is very small. Comessatti found the tolerance to be between 2 and 2.5 grams of dextrose; by having rabbits run in a treadmill the tolerance was raised about 20 per cent. Glucose is so frequently given today by the intravenous route that excellent opportunities are afforded for studying its effect. So far as glycosuria is concerned, one hears nothing; emphasis is rather placed on the danger of reactions if the glucose is not freshly prepared within six days.

The rate of injection is an important factor. Woodyatt, Sansum and Wilder[1] have urged very strongly the importance of time in determining sugar tolerance. Tolerance must be measured and expressed in grams of glucose or other sugar per kilogram of body weight per hour of time. They point out that sugars administered by the stomach take varying lengths of time to be absorbed, according to the motor power of the stomach and intestines, and even if sugars are given subcutaneously or by any other route, which demands absorption as a prelude to their entering the blood, the rates at which they enter the blood will depend upon the rates at which they are absorbed. They have devised a method by which solutions of the various sugars can be easily and painlessly injected into animals or man for hours at a time. By the use of these methods, they found that a man can utilize 0.85 gram of glucose per kilogram of body weight per hour for from six to twelve hours without producing any glycosuria, or even diuresis. In other words, a man weighing 70 kilograms when resting comfortably in bed may and did receive and utilize 60 grams of glucose by vein per hour without glycosuria. This would amount to 252 calories per hour. This apparently is the normal tolerance limit for glucose. In cases of exophthalmic goiter, the intravenous tolerance was found to be as low as 0.65 gram per kilogram per hour. For lactose it was nearly zero. If twice the normal tolerance

[1] Woodyatt, Sansum and Wilder: Jour. Am. Med. Assn., 1915, **65**, 2067.

limit for glucose—that is 1.7 grams per kilogram per hour—are given about 10 per cent of the same is lost in the urine, but if glucose is given at a rate faster than 2 grams per kilogram per hour, 50 per cent of all the glucose injected appears in the urine when constant conditions have been secured.

In a normal individual, the greatest rate of glycosuria which can be produced by feeding any quantity of glucose by mouth is limited, and at most approximates that which is produced by an intravenous injection at the rate of 1.8 kilogram per hour. Hence it would be reasonable to believe that when sugar is given by mouth in health, it is never absorbed faster than at this rate.

The above investigators also found that when glucose was given at rates exceeding 0.85 gram per kilogram per hour and the glucose begins to accumulate in the tissues and pass out into the urine, it carries water with it. When the sugar is given at the rate of 5.4 grams per kilogram per hour marked diuresis results—thus, in a dog the urine output rises rapidly to the vicinity of 350 cc per hour. If each hour the dog received enough water to make good the loss, this rate of diuresis or a higher one could be maintained for long periods of time. If enough water is not given to counterbalance the urinary loss, the volume of urine decreases, the dog suffers from thirst and death may ensue. On the other hand, if too much water is given with the hourly injections of glucose of 5.4 grams per kilogram per hour, there is danger of stopping the heart mechanically. In giving intravenous injections of glucose there are then two things to avoid: Too great dehydration on the one hand, and heart failure, from imposing too much mechanical work, on the other. These can both be avoided by knowing the number of grams of glucose which enter the body hourly, and what volume of water is removed by such a rate of sugar injection.

(1) *Glucose.*—The tolerance for glucose is apparently unaffected by season or sex, and there is no constant difference for the various races. It is interesting that children are supposed to have a far higher tolerance than adults, but Allen's experiments with young animals were to the contrary. The increased tolerance in children might be explained by their increased activity. In general, the tolerance for glucose, like that of other carbohydrates, varies inversely with the rapidity of its absorption. Its assimilation is increased in fever. The occasional appearance of glycosuria in fever is considered by Allen not to invalidate this statement, because that is a toxic glycosuria. Actual increased temperature favors tolerance, possibly by rendering the kidneys less permeable, but chiefly by increasing utilization in the tissues. The influence of muscular work in increasing the tolerance for dextrose has been proved by experiments upon animals and is analogous to the effect of work

upon the assimilation of carbohydrates in general. Glycosuria may be produced experimentally by intravenous, subcutaneous, and intraperitoneal administration of sugar, though not by oral administration even when as much as 200 grams are taken, according to Folin and Berglund. It is not produced by rectal injections.

Various methods have been employed to test the presence of diabetes by the administration of glucose. Naunyn's[1] is as follows: The patient has a breakfast of 80 to 100 grams of bread and a cup of coffee with milk. Two hours later he is given 100 grams of dextrose. If glycosuria occurs to a degree which can be determined quantitatively, the diminished power of assimilation for dextrose is demonstrated. Mere traces in the urine are disregarded. The term "alimentary glycosuria" in connection with such tests should be dropped. (See p. 166.) In Bright's disease the test may be obscured, and in diabetes, complicated by Bright's disease, the effect may not show itself.

Higgins[2] has studied the time at which the various sugars begin to be burned in the body by the change in the gaseous exchange and especially in the respiratory quotient. He found that glucose and maltose were not utilized as food as soon as the other sugars —sucrose, lactose and levulose—for the former begin to be burned in twenty to thirty minutes, but the latter within ten minutes. He further observed a distinct difference in men between the metabolism of glucose and of levulose and galactose.

We often erroneously think of an excess of sugar in the blood as being removed by the kidneys. As a matter of fact, this is not the case, for the kidneys remove only a trifle of the excess of the sugar. They by no means regulate the percentage of sugar in the blood. By far the greater portion of the sugar is removed from the blood by the tissues as Meltzer and Kleiner[3] have so beautifully demonstrated and Woodyatt, Sansum and Wilder have confirmed.

(2) *Saccharose.*—LeGoff[4] found that saccharosuria and glycosuria resulted in 100 per cent of the cases after 100 grams cane sugar were administered orally. This probably explains why glucose instead of saccharose is employed in making carbohydrate tolerance tests. Caution must be exercised in the interpretation of such tests in the light of the recent work of Folin and Berglund.

Saccharose has little place in the diet of primitive races, and Allen has pointed out a possible connection between the increased use of saccharose and the increased incidence of diabetes. (See p. 145.) Until the increased incidence of diabetes is thoroughly proved one must be slow to consider this relation established.

[1] Naunyn: Loc. cit., p. 102.
[2] Higgins: Jour. Phys., 1916, **41**, 258.   [3] See p. 34.
[4] Cit. by Allen: Compt. rend. de l'Acad. des Sc., 1911, **157**, 1785.

(3) *Lactose.*—The poor assimilation of lactose is remarkable because it is the one distinctly normal sugar. This lack of assimilation holds in diabetes as well as in health. It is perhaps due to the fact that lactose is broken up into galactose and dextrose before it is absorbed. Folin and Berglund[1] write instructively as follows: "Almost all authorities assign a much higher limit of assimilation for milk-sugar than for galactose, 100 to 150 grams for the former, against 20 to 40 grams for the latter. It is certainly true that much more sugar is excreted from 100 grams of galactose than from 200 grams of lactose, but with respect to the assimilation limits based on quantitative sugar determinations and glycuresis there is scarcely any difference between the two. Ten grams of milk-sugar, corresponding approximately to the amount taken with a single glass of milk, is sufficient to produce a temporary, but unmistakable increase in the sugar of the urine.

"The interesting fact about the sugar excretion after lactose ingestion is that *lactose* (as well as galactose) is present in the urine unless the amount taken is very small—less than 30 grams. This is instructive, for *it indicates that there is no mechanism in the digestive tract for preventing the absorption of soluble but incompletely digested carbohydrate materials. If such are not absorbed it is only because the activity of the endocellular enzymes is capable of accomplishing the hydrolysis during the transit of soluble carbohydrates through the mucous membrane of the intestine.* In the case of lactose the endocellular hydrolytic activity is easily exceeded, and this disaccharide is absorbed. Lactose, as such, is supposed to be unusable, and it is customary to refer to the occasional occurrence of milk-sugar in the urine of pregnant women as proof of how completely unassimilable milk-sugar really is.

"We do not think that the question of the assimilability of milk-sugar can yet be considered as definitely settled. The old experiments based on the injection of known quantities of milk-sugar into the blood and finding the whole of it in the urine can no longer be considered conclusive, because under such conditions the sugar in the urine would be increased by virtue of superimposed glycosuria. Our own experiments have not furnished conclusive evidence, but the fact that the excretion of milk-sugar comes to a definite end in the course of a few hours suggests that a part of the absorbed lactose may be utilized. The question of whether or not some lactose is utilized seemed to us unimportant in comparison with the problem of why milk-sugar taken by mouth results in less total sugar excretion than is obtained from the galactose corresponding to the same quantity of milk-sugar. One hundred grams

[1] Folin and Berglund: Jour. Biol. Chem., 1922, **51,** 251.

of galactose will give twice as much sugar in the urine as 200 grams of lactose.   Our attempts to solve this problem have yielded extraordinarily interesting results, but our investigation is not yet completed, and the statements and interpretations here given we explicitly consider only as a preliminary communication.   When the hydrolysis of the milk-sugar during absorption from the intestinal tract is quantitative, as it presumably is in normal infants, then the giving of milk-sugar is the same as the giving of equal quantities of galactose and glucose.   The difference between the adult and the nursing infant with reference to the power of splitting lactose can be eliminated by giving pure glucose and pure galactose— equal amounts of each.   This was done, the subject taking 100 grams of galactose plus 100 grams of glucose and the sugar excretion was less than one-fifth as great from the mixture of the two sugars as from the milk-sugar and is less than one-tenth as great as the excretion obtained from 100 grams of galactose when taken alone. The figures are 0.37, 2.8 and 5.7 grams, respectively.

"The results given show that the extent to which galactose is retained and utilized by the human organism depends on the quantity of available glucose."

(4) *Galactose.*—All agree that galactose is poorly assimilated, and yet it is fermented with more difficulty than either dextrose or levulose.   It is on a par with glucose or levulose as a glycogen former.   It scarcely increases the percentage of blood sugar, but 100 grams of galactose may yield as much as 10 grams of sugar in the urine, whereas 200 grams of glucose will not yield a trace.

(5) *Maltose.*—Maltose to the amount of 200 grams has extremely little effect on the level of the blood sugar of normals and no effect upon the sugar in the urine.   It is commonly agreed that maltose is tolerated less well by diabetics than any other form of sugar.

(6) *Levulose.*—(See also p. 289.)   Levulose does not cause an increase in the percentage of blood sugar (whole blood) even when 200 grams are taken.   Folin and Berglund found a slight increase in the plasma, from 0.102 per cent to 0.110 per cent.   Frequently, glycuresis was observed lasting for several hours, but this was proved *not* to be due to levulose.   Later experiments made probable that this glycuresis was caused by decomposition products of the levulose to which Folin and Berglund ascribe the nausea and diarrhea and indeed the laxative effects of various sugars—maple sugar, molasses, and certain candies.   Although levulose was not demonstrated in the urine, it was found in the blood at the height of its absorption from the digestive tract and the above authors conclude that the slight rise of sugar in the plasma from 0.098 per cent before to 0.112 per cent, twenty minutes after its ingestion, is made up one-third by levulose.   The assimilation limits for levulose are so high that they can scarcely be exceeded.

Folin's and Berglund's interpretation of the fate of absorbed fructose is as follows: "The liver retains fructose as well as every other usable sugar to a greater extent in proportion to its weight than do the general tissues such as the muscles. But such retentions by the liver are never even approximately quantitative, and a large fraction of absorbed sugar, possibly the greater part, gets by this organ. Other tissues, such as the muscles, take up sugar from the plasma of arterial blood, and it is this general absorption which prevents excessive accumulations of sugar in the blood. But tissue sugar like blood sugar is normally and predominantly glucose, partly because the major part of our carbohydrate food is made up of glucose, partly because all other usable sugars are gradually converted into this essential sugar. The tissues being relatively well stored with glucose and empty of other sugars, such as fructose, may well be able to absorb these other sugars from the blood so nearly completely that the venous blood used for our analyses shows only traces. The glycogen formation may or may not begin immediately, and at all events need not be the immediate cause for the rapid disappearance of levulose from the blood."

(7) *Dextrin.*—Dextrin given in large doses produced no increase in the level of the blood sugar and no increase in the level of the preformed sugar of the urine but the urine did contain an abundance of the dextrin. The elimination of dextrin was at its height the morning of the day following the ingestion of dextrin and continued for four days. Evidently dextrin or a dextrin-like product had been absorbed from the digestive tract and only slowly found its way into the urine. Since it was not found in the blood, presumably it was absorbed by the tissues and was gradually released and eliminated later.[1]

(8) *Inulin.*—Inulin is a polysaccharide of levulose and in this respect comparable with starch, which is a polysaccharid of dextrose. It occurs in the roots of many composites such as the tubers of dahlia and artichoke. No enzymes in the alimentary tract are known to convert it into sugar, but the normal acidity of the gastric juice may effect a partial hydrolysis of inulin to levulose. The bulk of the inulin is decomposed in the gastro-intestinal tract into non-carbohydrate products.[2] Following the feeding of inulin to phloridzinized animals Lewis and Frankel[3] found no increase in glycosuria which one would expect if any of the inulin had been converted to levulose. Consequently, there appears to be no reason for the employment of inulin in the diabetic diet except to

---

[1] Folin and Berglund: Loc. cit., p. 431.
[2] Editorial, Jour. Am. Med. Assn., 1914, **63**, 326.
[3] Lewis and Frankel: Jour. Biol. Chem., 1914, **17**, 365.

afford bulk. Sandmeyer[1] reported that inulin was absorbed only up to about 43.5 per cent of that ingested. "Inulin has been suggested as a possible carbohydrate for the diabetic because it yields levulose on splitting and there is some indication that levulose can be better tolerated than glucose. The higher animals have no enzyme capable of splitting inulin, and therefore its conversion into levulose in the body is dependent on the acid of the gastric juice. Lewis[2] has shown that inulin is poorly utilized by man. Intestinal fermentation attends its use, and the value of inulin in the diet is questionable."[3]

The use of inulin in the diabetic diet I am sure should be restudied. Our tests with artichokes at the New England Deaconess Hospital have been encouraging and will be continued.

(9) *Algæ.*—The nutritive value of the carbohydrate in lichens and algæ was investigated by Mary Swartz. Lichens and algæ have been used as food by man from the earliest times, being resorted to particularly when there is scarcity of cereal crops or in famine. Tons of marine algæ are eaten annually in various parts of the world particularly in Japan. Irish moss is the most common food of this type in the American dietary, being employed in the making of blanc mange. Dulse is particularly used in Scotland and is quite abundant in New England where it is dried and eaten as a relish.

Of the 10 species of marine algæ studied by Swartz the hemicelluloses which they contained were made up chiefly of pentosans and galactans. When these hemicelluloses are injected into an animal subcutaneously or intraperitoneally, they are excreted through the kidneys and can be recovered unaltered in the urine. The pentosan of dulse is completely eliminated in four or five days, and the carbohydrates of Irish moss, salep and sinistrin, in one to three days. Feeding experiments show that these hemicelluloses most readily attacked by bacteria disappear most completely from the alimentary tract. The average coefficient of digestibility for man is, in the case of the pentosan of dulse and the mannan of salep, 99 per cent notwithstanding their apparent resistance to amylolytic enzymes and the hydrolyzing influence of the gastric juice; their disappearance seems, therefore, directly attributable to bacterial activity, and the possibility of sugar formation by this agency having been demonstrated, it remains to be shown by means of respiration experiments to what extent materials so hydrolyzed can serve as true nutrients for the organism.

In striking contrast to the above hemicelluloses stand the

[1] Sandmeyer: Ztschr. Biol., 1895, **31**, 32.
[2] Lewis: Jour. Am. Med. Assn., 1912, **58**, 1176.
[3] Wardall, Ruth A.: Jour. Am. Med. Assn., 1917, **69**, 1859.

galactans, (of which agar agar is an example), with their high degree of resistance to bacterial decomposition; they show in man, an average digestibility of approximately 25 per cent, in dogs of 45 per cent. It is manifestly impossible to treat of the digestibility of hemicelluloses as a class, in view of such diversity in the groups. Not only must each type receive special consideration, but distinction must be drawn between soluble and insoluble forms, as is illustrated by the pentosans, the ratio of the digestibility coefficient of the former to the latter being approximately 100 to 50 in man, and 75 to 25 in dogs.[1] In general their disappearance from the alimentary tract appears to be proportional to their decomposition by microörganisms, and thus there is little justification for any especial claim as a source of energy and nutrition. Their bulk makes them of value in constipation and they also serve as a source of inorganic salts.

(10) *Mushrooms.*—"The value of the mushroom is in its flavor, for it is seen to have no extractable carbohydrate, and Mendel[2] has shown that its nitrogen does not occur as protein, but in an unavailable form."[3]

(*b*) **The Estimation of the Carbohydrate in the Diabetic Diet.**— The quantity of carbohydrate in the various foods is easily calculated and far more simply than is usually thought. This is not true if one desires scientific accuracy, for in that event analyses of the food given the patient must be made. In any estimation of carbohydrate in the diabetic diet one must not overlook the possibility of 58 grams of carbohydrate being formed out of 100 grams of protein and 10 grams out of the glycerol of 100 grams of fat. The "total glucose" value of the three foodstuffs would be, therefore, 100 grams C. × 100 per cent + 100 grams P. × 58 per cent + 100 grams F. × 10 per cent.

(*c*) **Carbohydrate in Vegetables.**—*Loss in Cooking.*—It would appear perplexing to determine the amount of carbohydrate in the various vegetables which the patient eats in twenty-four hours. Diabetic patients have too much to do in their daily work to be encumbered with unnecessary details of arithmetic. An attempt to force accuracy to the extent of a gram may result in loss of accuracy to the extent of an ounce by the patients' giving up weighing entirely.

For convenience I have classified the vegetables and fruits which enter into the diabetic diet under four headings—those containing approximately 5 per cent, 10 per cent, 15 per cent, and 20 per cent carbohydrate. (See Table 169.)

---

[1] Swartz, Mary D.: Trans. Conn. Acad. Arts and Sciences, 1911, **16**, 247.
[2] Mendel: Am. Jour. Phys., 1898, vol. **1**.
[3] Wardall, Ruth A.: Jour. Am. Med. Assn., 1917, **69**, 1859.

TABLE 169.—FOODS ARRANGED APPROXIMATELY ACCORDING TO CONTENT OF
CARBOHYDRATES.[1]

VEGETABLES[2]

1 per cent to 3 per cent	5 per cent. 3 per cent to 5 per cent.	10 per cent.	15 per cent.	20 per cent.
Lettuce	Tomatoes	String beans	Green peas	Potatoes
Cucumbers	Brussels	Turnip	Artichokes	Shell beans
Spinach	sprouts	Kohl-rabi	Parsnips	Baked beans
Asparagus	Water cress	Squash	Lima beans	Green corn
Rhubarb	Sea kale	Beets	(canned)	Boiled rice
Endive	Okra	Carrots		Boiled macaroni
Marrow	Cauliflower	Onions		
Sorrel	Egg plant	Green peas		
Sauerkraut	Cabbage	(very young)		
Beet greens	Radishes			
Dandelion	Leeks			
greens	String beans			
Swiss chard	(canned)			
Celery	Broccoli			
Mushrooms	Pumpkin			

FRUITS.				
Grapefruit				
Ripe olives (20 per cent fat)		Watermelon	Currants	Plums
		Strawberries	Apricots	Bananas
		Lemons	Pears	Prunes
		Cranberries	Apples	
		Peaches	Huckleberries	
		Pineapple	Blueberries	
		Blackberries	Cherries	
		Gooseberries		
		Oranges		
		Raspberries		

It is true that there is considerable variation in each group, but the average content is not far from that represented, the error being on the lower side. This does not hold for string beans, for often trouble occurs from the beans having developed into maturity, thus greatly increasing their content in carbohydrate. Canned string beans usually contain smaller beans than fresh string beans and for this reason are placed in the 5 per cent group. So with many of the other vegetables, the more advanced the stage of development, the more carbohydrate. Many an unexplained trace of sugar in the urine has undoubtedly occurred in this way. The carbohydrate content of peas is also most variable.

A deduction should be made in the percentage of carbohydrate in the vegetables of the 5 and 10 per cent groups because a part

[1] Percentage values for foods in this table will be found included in the comprehensive Table 247, p. 703.

[2] Reckon average carbohydrate in 5 per cent vegetables as 3 per cent and 10 per cent vegetables as 6 per cent.

of the carbohydrate is in the form of cellulose, and this is not assimilable. Then too, there are pentosans and, though these through bacterial decomposition in the intestinal tract may yield calories, they do not act as carbohydrate. For this reason 3 per cent and 6 per cent represent more accurately the content of available carbohydrate in the 5 per cent and 10 per cent vegetables. This being the case, it is convenient and fairly accurate to consider 30 grams, or 1 ounce of 5 per cent vegetables, to contain 1 gram carbohydrate and the same quantity of 10 per cent vegetables 2 grams of carbohydrate. The vegetables in the 15 per cent and 20 per cent groups should be reckoned at their full value.

Many of the vegetables under the 5 per cent group contain very little carbohydrate; for instance, lettuce contains 2.9 per cent, spinach 3.2 per cent. The vegetables are arranged in each group in sequence according to their content of carbohydrate.

Indeed, one will not be very wrong if he considers the total carbohydrate of the 5 per cent vegetables which a diabetic patient will eat as 10 to 20 grams in the twenty-four hours. As an actual fact, 300 grams of a mixture of 5 and 10 per cent vegetables served to a diabetic patient at the New England Deaconess Hospital were found by analyses at the Nutrition Laboratory to contain 10 grams carbohydrate.

(1) *Thrice-cooked Vegetables.*—Vegetables lose carbohydrate in the cooking, and this loss is favored (1) by changing the water in which they are prepared two or three times, and (2) by preparing the vegetables in finely divided form so that the water can have easy access to the whole mass. Von Noorden[1] pointed out that 100 grams of raw spinach contained 2.97 grams carbohydrate, but cooked spinach only 0.85 gram. Similarly, 100 grams of ripe peaches contained 9.5 grams carbohydrate, but when boiled and the water changed, only 1.8 grams. Allen[2] has utilized this method of removing carbohydrate from vegetables and thus allows patients to have bulk in their diet. He terms vegetables so prepared "thrice-cooked vegetables." "Under these conditions the vegetables may be boiled through three waters, throwing away all the water. Nearly all starch is thus removed. The most severe cases generally take these thrice-cooked vegetables gladly and without glycosuria." Patients often say that it makes little difference to them whether the vegetables are thrice washed or not. It is easy and useful to add a little salt, and if desired the vegetables can be flavored with meat juices or meat extracts.

The carbohydrate content of "thrice-cooked" or "washed"

---

[1] Von Noorden: Loc. cit., p. 122.
[2] Allen: Boston Med. and Surg. Jour., 1915, **173**, 241.

vegetables has been studied by Wardall.[1] The extractions were made by starting the vegetables in cold water and bringing this to the boiling-point and maintaining it at this temperature for one minute. Hot water was added for each of the other extractions, and all were boiled one minute. If the first extraction is kept at 150° F., as has sometimes been recommended, the second extraction leads the list in the power of reduction and in fermentation, the first extraction ranking after the third or fourth. With the exception of canned asparagus, the four or five extractions necessary to remove all reducing substances left the vegetable still attractive in flavor and appearance. For practical purposes three extractions will probably be found sufficient.

(2) *Lettuce and Cabbage.*—Lettuce and cabbage are the most useful 5 per cent vegetables. Bulletin No. 28, Office of Experiment Stations, U. S. Department of Agriculature, gives 2.9 per cent as the average percentage of carbohydrate in the former and 5.6 per cent for the latter. By its bulk lettuce satisfies the appetite and is far more agreeable than the insipid washed vegetables. In fact it has replaced these entirely at the New England Deaconess Hospital. When large quantities, as the above for lettuce, of a single vegetable are employed, one must not depend on the group analysis. Cabbage is the poor man's 5 per cent vegetable. It can be eaten daily for months, raw and cooked, without repugnance. Its composition is so constant that the amount tolerated can readily be determined. Case No. 866 was sugar-free at the hospital with difficulty and in the course of eight months the lowest blood sugar was 0.13 per cent. When he went to sea on a lumber schooner and lived almost exclusively on cabbage for his vegetable, he returned after one month not only without glycosuria but with a blood sugar of 0.1 per cent. In the spring of 1922, he went to sea again, returning to the hospital in October without glycosuria and with a blood sugar of 0.12 per cent. Whether there is any peculiar virtue in cabbage other than the above I am unaware, but a physician in New York extols the useful effects of cabbage water in diabetes. Could there be glukokinin in it?

(3) *Potatoes.*—The variation in the percentage of carbohydrate in potatoes before and after cooking is negligible, save with potato chips, in which it more than doubles. The loss of protein is slight, but if soaked in cold water before boiling the loss of protein is 25 per cent and of mineral matter 38 per cent. If the potatoes are not soaked, but dropped at once into boiling water the loss is much decreased and if the potatoes are boiled with the skins on the loss is very slight. Emphasis should be laid upon the comparatively

[1] Wardall: Jour. Am. Med. Assoc., 1917, **69**, 1859.

small amount of carbohydrate in potato in comparison with its bulk and in comparison with the percentage of carbohydrate in bread. A considerable number of my milder cases of diabetes, by giving up bread and bread preparations entirely, have been able to eat potatoes freely. In prescribing potatoes for diabetic patients it is desirable to designate baked potatoes, for these can be eaten with the skins if pains are taken to have them carefully cleaned with a scrubbing brush in the kitchen. This is advantageous in two ways: The skins are quite an addition to the meager diet of the diabetic, and, furthermore, they counteract constipation.

(4) *Nuts.*—Nuts containing 15 and 20 per cent carbohydrate are probably far less objectionable than most other foods with a similar carbohydrate content. This is due to the fact that in such nuts as almonds a larger part of the carbohydrate is in the form of pentosan, galactan, or other hemicelluloses some of which probably do not readily form glucose. (See p. 435.)

The usefulness of nuts in the diabetic dietary would furnish an interesting problem for investigation. The danger of nuts to the diabetic rests not in the content of carbohydrate, but rather in their high percentage of protein and fat. Ignorant diabetics often eat nuts as freely as they would 5 per cent vegetables and wonder why they develop glycosuria and acidosis. Case No. 1930, quite mild when her treatment was inaugurated, went home, ate nuts about as freely as some 5 per cent vegetables, escaped diabetic coma, but only through severe undernutrition from which a special nurse and insulin are rescuing her. The downward course of her case followed the excessive use of nuts.

The protein of nuts is valuable and Morgan and Heinz[1] found the protein of almond meal to have a biological value superior to that of wheat gluten.

Sherman cites the digestion experiments of Jaffe upon California fruitarians whose diet consists of fruits and nuts and concludes that "apparently the fruits and nut diet was as readily and almost as completely digested as would be expected of ordinary mixed diet." Sherman further states that fruitarians, both adults and children, maintain a well-nourished condition on diets of fruits and nuts which are moderate in total food value and low in protein content, and considers this strong evidence that the nutrients are well digested and efficiently utilized in metabolism.

It is well known of course, through the work of Osborne, that the vegetable proteins are not all equally efficient in supplying the nitrogen requirement of normal growth and development for the reason that some lack essential amino-acids. Probably this

[1] Morgan and Heinz: Jour. Am. Med. Assn., 1919, **72**, 730.

is true of nut proteins but these have not been so extensively studied. The protein of the Brazil nut has been demonstrated to be completely adequate for normal growth and development of young animals. The vegetable and animal fats are supposed to be equally well digested, but they differ in their vitamins which are more conspicuous in fats of animal origin.

(5) *Fruit.*—Fruit is most desirable for a diabetic patient if his tolerance will allow him to take it. The taste is agreeable, it serves instead of a dessert, and so relieves the patient of the embarrassment of sitting idly at the table when others are eating. The best varieties of fruit for diabetic patients are grapefruit (5 per cent), strawberries (7.4 per cent), and oranges (11.6 per cent). These fruits are safer than apples (14.2 per cent) for the patient, because they contain 5 to 10 per cent less carbohydrate and are more satisfying. Furthermore, it is less easy thoughtlessly to eat an orange than an apple and thus break dietetic restrictions. To a diabetic an apple is devoid of skin, seeds and core. A small apple contains 1 tablespoonful of sugar, a moderate-sized apple 2 tablespoonfuls and a large apple 3 tablespoonfuls. Even the 20 per cent carbohydrate fruit, banana, contains scarcely more carbohydrate than a small apple, because it weighs only about 100 grams. A small apple weighs 120 grams. Unfortunately, steaming an apple removes little of the carbohydrate which it contains.

Equivalent weights of various fruits which contain approximately 10 grams of carbohydrate are given in Table 170.

TABLE 170.—EQUIVALENTS OF 10 GRAMS CARBOHYDRATE IN VARIOUS FRUITS.

Orange pulp	100
Grapefruit pulp	200
Strawberries	150
Blackberries	100
Raspberries	75
Peaches	75
Blueberries	65
Banana	50

(6) *Grapefruit, Oranges, Lemons.*—The quantity of carbohydrate in a very small orange is not far from 10 grams. My children counted for me the number of compartments in 48 oranges, and found these to vary between nine and eleven in 43 instances, but in 3 there were 12 and in 2 were 13 compartments. Consequently, one will not be far wrong to consider that 1 compartment of a small orange contains 1 gram carbohydrate.[1] The same statement

[1] According to a recent authority there were 16 oranges with 10 sections, 9 oranges with 11, and 1 orange with 12. Two lemons counted contained 10 sections each, and 1 grapefruit, 11 sections. Irving Bailey, aged eight years.

will likewise apply to a small-sized grapefruit. It is interesting to note how constantly inconsistent the variations are in the amount of edible portions in small, medium, and large oranges as prepared for patients by a nurse. Grapefruit vary more, but it is not difficult to select one of moderate size or to take less of a large one. Table 171, shows these variations. Gross appearance and the weight of the edible portion do not correspond.

TABLE 171.—Weights of Grapefruit, Oranges and Bananas Compared with Edible Portions as Determined by a Nurse.

Grapefruit.				Orange.				Banana.		
	Whole, grams.	Edible portion, grams.	%		Whole, grams.	Edible portion, grams.	%	Whole, grams.	Edible portion grams.	%
Small	347	145	42	Medium	260	118	46	149	92	62
Large	677	320	47	Large	275	116	42	149	91	61
				Small	252	113	45	121	74	61
Florida				Medium	253	101	40	125	79	63
				Large	308	141	46	136	84	62
				Small	260	108	42	119	74	62
California				Medium	278	121	44	160	96	60
				Large	282	129	46	119	73	61
						—		145	89	61
					Average		44	167	101	61
								158	97	61
								153	94	61
					Average			141	87	61

The observations recorded in Table 171, prompted me to pursue the matter further, for it was evident that inaccuracies must creep into the dietetic calculations in this way. In Tables 172 and 173 are shown analyses made for me by Edward M. Frankel, Ph.D., on aqueous extracts of oranges and grapefruit after cautions were taken to remove the bulk of the protein and cellulose with lead acetate. The results, therefore, represent the amounts of water-soluble carbohydrate calculated as glucose after hydrolysis. No account is taken of the insoluble material on the assumption that such carbohydrate not soluble in water is of the hemicellulose type, which has been shown not to be utilized by the human body.

Frankel has added data on the acidity of the fruit calculated as citric acid, because it has been pointed out by Greenwald[1] that this substance is converted quantitatively by the diabetic organism into glucose.

The quantity of levulose in oranges is discussed on p. 298.

The edible portion of a grapefruit or orange as prepared by a nurse is about 45 per cent of the total weight, as shown in Table 171, but upon more accurate analysis about 77 per cent, as shown in Table 172. Trust the diabetic, if left to himself, to extract

[1] Greenwald: Jour. Biol. Chem., 1914, **17**, 115.

all the edible portion from all fruits. Half a grapefruit would contain from 12 to 23 grams of carbohydrate and half an orange from 5 to 10 grams.

TABLE 172.—ANALYSES OF ORANGES.

Made by Edward M. Frankel, Ph.D., New Haven, Conn.

Sold as	Size.	Gross weight, grams.	Edible portion, grams.	%	Grams of sugar as glucose.	Percentage of edible portion.	Total acidity as citric acid, grams.	Percentage of edible portion.
Florida	Small	188	152	81	12.0	7.9	1.5	1.0
"	Small	169	143	85	12.3	8.6	...	...
"	Medium	214	172	80	12.4	7.2	1.2	0.7
"	Medium	215	179	83	15.7	8.8	...	...
"	Large	290	222	80	19.6	8.4	1.3	0.6
"	Large	357	282	79	19.7	7.0	...	...
"	Large	310	243	78	20.4	8.4	...	...
California	Small	189	149	79	10.9	7.3	...	...
"	Small	178	149	84	10.9	7.3	...	...
"	Medium	250	188	75	17.5	9.3	2.2	1.2
"	Medium	236	170	72	16.2	9.5	1.6	0.9
"	Medium	270	203	75	17.2	8.5	...	...
"	Medium	264	193	73	15.4	8.0	...	...
"	Large	287	220	77	16.5	7.5	1.4	0.6
"	Large	322	219	68	19.3	8.8	1.3	0.6

TABLE 173.—ANALYSES OF GRAPEFRUIT.

Made by Edward M. Frankel, Ph.D., New Haven, Conn.

Sold as	Size.	Gross weight, grams.	Edible portion, grams.	%	Grams of sugar as glucose.	Percentage of edible portion.	Total acidity as citric acid, grams.	Percentage of edible portion.
Porto Rico	Small	401	301	75	24.0	8.0	2.4	0.8
"	Small	428	318	74	26.7	8.4	2.3	0.7
California	Medium	581	449	77	31.8	7.1	6.5	1.4
"	Medium	550	394	72	23.8	6.0	6.4	1.6
"	Large	676	515	76	34.8	6.8	5.6	1.1
"	Large	773	606	78	46.6	7.7	6.7	1.1
Florida	Small	538	409	76	25.0	6.1	4.2	1.0
"	Medium	712	539	76	34.2	6.3	5.0	0.9
"	Medium	724	585	81	44.8	7.7	6.2	1.1
"	Large[1]	834	624	75	40.3	6.5	5.4	0.9

Similar analyses for lemons are shown in Table 174.

TABLE 174.—ANALYSES OF LEMONS.

Sold as	Gross weight, grams.	Edible portion, grams.	%	Grams of sugar as glucose.	Percentage of edible portion.	Total acidity as citric acid, grams.	Percentage of edible portion.
California . .	92	50	54	0.576	1.15	3.10	6.20
California . .	90	42	47	0.518	1.20	2.83	6.75
Messina . . .	87	60	69	0.459	0.77	3.82	6.35

[1] Greener than the others.

(7) *Bananas.*—Bananas were seldom prescribed for diabetic patients because the content of carbohydrate is so high, being equivalent to that in potato. In recent years, however, I have recommended them more and more because of their comparative uniformity in size. It is infinitely safer for a patient to be told that he can have a banana of moderate size than an ounce of bread, though each would contain the same amount of carbohydrate. For the same reason they are safer than potatoes. Anything which introduces a moderate degree of definiteness into the diabetic diet is advantageous. In general the riper a banana, and for that matter any vegetable or fruit, the more the starch in it has changed to sugar, and also the more carbohydrate it contains. Since unripened fruits with their lower carbohydrate content can be made palatable by cooking, a way is afforded for diabetic patients to use them.

(8) *Ripe Olives.*—Ripe olives make a pleasing change in the diet. They contain 4 per cent carbohydrate in contrast to green olives, which contain 1.8 per cent. Furthermore, ripe olives are more easily digested. Five ripe or 10 green olives contain 1 gram carbohydrate and a ripe olive contains a gram and a green olive half a gram of fat. The quantity of protein in 10 olives is about 1 gram.

(9) *Distilled Vinegar.*—Distilled vinegar contains no protein, fat, or sugar because it is made from a dilute alcoholic distillate. Cider, wine, malt and sugar vinegars are made of fermented juices, infusions or solutions, *not distilled,* and may contain small amounts of sugar, etc. For analyses of vinegar, see p. 714.

(10) *Milk.*—The carbohydrate in milk is in the form of lactose and can be reckoned at 5 per cent or 1.5 grams per 30 cc, or 1 ounce. It is the same in skimmed milk and whey; but cream and koumyss contain about 3 per cent, or 1 gram carbohydrate to the ounce. Buttermilk contains essentially the same quantity of carbohydrate and protein as milk, but only a trifling amount of fat. Fermented milk may contain 3 per cent sugar. I could not understand for years why doctors so frequently gave it to their patients but the reason is plain. It represents undernutrition and the physician who prescribed skimmed milk or buttermilk for his mild diabetic patient was employing a modern therapeutic agent.

One quart of milk contains about 600 calories, of skimmed milk[1] 300 calories, of cream with 20 per cent butter fat 2000 calories, and of 40 per cent cream 3700 calories. Milk contains so many desirable food elements that it is always desirable to insert some of it as milk or cream into the diet.

---

[1] So-called "skimmed milk" upon one occasion by analysis contained 4 per cent butter fat.

(11) *Oatmeal.*—Oatmeal is two-thirds carbohydrate. In calculations one should always be guided by the dry weight, because the different preparations vary greatly in bulk and weight when cooked. It would be of great advantage to diabetics if uncooked oatmeal could be bought in 1 ounce packages, so that the diabetic could secure constant portions. It is by far the most desirable cereal for the diabetic. (See Table 200, p. 537.) The subject of oatmeal treatment of diabetes is discussed at length on p. 532.

(12) *Bread.*—The carbohydrate in white wheat bread amounts to about 53 per cent. If the bread is toasted, enough water is lost to raise the percentage of carbohydrate in the toast to about 60 per cent. If the bread is made without sugar and with water instead of milk the carbohydrate content is lowered and may amount to only 45 per cent. Coarse breads if made without sweetening or milk would contain slightly less carbohydrate. It is undesirable to give bread to diabetic patients unless their tolerance is very high, because they can take so little without causing glycosuria that the bread is simply an aggravation. An error in weight of 1 ounce of a 5 per cent vegetable amounts to 1 gram carbohydrate, of potato to 6 grams, but of bread to 18 grams. Crackers and zwieback contain still less water than toast, and in consequence the percentage of carbohydrate is raised to the neighborhood of 70 per cent.

Diabetic breads are discussed on p. 728.

So much do I fear to give bread to a diabetic for dread he will overstep the limits that I am apt to prescribe a standard biscuit or cracker like an Uneeda biscuit, two of which contain about 10 grams carbohydrate, 1 gram of protein and 1 gram of fat, or a Shredded Wheat biscuit, 23 grams carbohydrate, 3 grams protein, the equivalent of which is three Triscuits.

Bread is a great temptation. Total abstinence in respect to bread for the diabetic is as desirable as total abstinence in respect to alcohol is for human kind.

3. **Protein.**—The quantity of protein required by diabetic patients varies with the age, weight, and activity of the case as well as with the condition of the kidneys. It is a safe rule at the beginning of treatment to attempt to increase the protein gradually up to the same quantity as that required by a normal individual.

Until the Chittenden low protein diet is proved to be entirely satisfactory for healthy individuals over a long period of years it is best not to have recourse to it for long periods in the treatment of diabetes. Temporarily small quantities may be given, but safety lies not far from 1 gram protein for each kilogram body weight for adults, but for children considerably more is required. In the arrangement of the diets of severe diabetics the protein must be restricted to less than 1 gram per kilogram body weight in order to increase carbohydrate and fat. With low protein intake the ketogenic-antiketogenic ratio can be lowered. (See p. 525.) Protein stimulates the metabolism more than any other kind of food, favors acidosis and, as has already been said, can lead to the formation of 58 grams of glucose for every 100 grams protein metabolized. Reference has already been made to the excessive quantities of protein ingested by diabetic patients when living upon an unprescribed diet (see p. 236) and will be made to the similarly large quantities of protein metabolized both by patients in the course of acid intoxication (see p. 632) and rarely during the course of fasting when inanition is extreme (Case No. 1011, p. 238).

It has been claimed that vegetable proteins give rise to less carbohydrate in the diabetic organism than do animal proteins. As a matter of fact, carbohydrate may be formed out of any protein.

Janney[1] has studied the formation of glucose from protein in diabetes by feeding pure proteins to fasting, phloridzinized dogs. He found that no difference existed in the sugar-producing capacity between animal and vegetable proteins because of their respective origins, but that the glucose yielded in metabolism could be demonstrated to vary directly with the amount of glucogenetic amino-acids contained in each individual protein. Thus the wheat protein gliadin which contains 43.7 per cent of the highly glucogenetic glutamic acid yields 80 per cent of glucose in metabolism. Indeed gliadin yields the largest amount of glucose of all proteins hitherto examined and casein and ovalbumin the least. The quantity of glucose yielded by various proteins is shown in Table 175.

TABLE 175.—GLUCOSE YIELDS OF INGESTED PROTEINS (JANNEY).

Casein, per cent.	Ovalbumin, per cent.	Serum, per cent.	Gelatin, per cent.	Fibrin, per cent.	Edestin (hemp protein), per cent.	Gliadin (wheat protein), per cent.	Zein (corn protein), per cent.
48	54	55	65	53	65	80	53

The amount of sugar formed from protein, therefore, is dependent upon the glucose-yielding amino-acids of protein and not upon the carbohydrate content of protein, which is negligible. Janney's experiments showed that no great variation existed in the amount of glucose produced from muscle obtained from various species of animal, including man, and that the percentage obtainable was 58, corresponding to a glucose-nitrogen ratio of 3.4 to 1. (See p. 245.)

It is evident that closer attention should be paid to this glucose formation from protein, and that the carbohydrate derived from

[1] Janney: Arch. Int. Med., 1916, **18**, 584.

protein should be added to the carbohydrate given as such in the diet in estimating the diabetic's power to burn carbohydrate.

Diabetic breads and also patent diabetic foods may contain a small quantity of carbohydrate, yet the protein in them is high and capable of furnishing a large amount of glucose. The result is that such commercial products may actually produce as much glucose in a diabetic as does ordinary bread. However, one must not be wholly governed by analytical conditions, as Janney has pointed out, for although vegetable and animal protein yield glucose according to their content of amino-acids, it is quite possible that the vegetable proteins will be less well digested owing to the form in which they are eaten, and thus less protein is assimilated, and in consequence less glucose formed.

The restricted allowance of carbohydrate with an unrestricted allowance of protein and fat must be held responsible for many untimely diabetic deaths. For the more the doctor curtailed the carbohydrate, the more he yielded to the appetite of his patient by increasing protein and fat and then both physician and patient wondered why glycosuria persisted. Indeed, it was not until von Mering and Minkowski with their depancreatized dogs and Lusk with his phloridzinized dogs showed the constancy of the dextrose-nitrogen ratio in total diabetes that the profession fully appreciated the carbohydrate-forming qualities of protein.

(*a*) **Meat and Fish.**—The chemical composition of meat and fish is simplified by the fact that except in liver and shell-fish, carbohydrate is absent. Even in liver the quantity of carbohydrate is almost negligible when we consider the amount and frequency with which this article of food is eaten. The glucose-forming power of meat is quite constant for different animals and in clinical dietetic calculations can be reckoned at 60 per cent.

The chief difficulty in computations of the nutritive value of meat and fish is due to the varying content of fat. Thus, the edible portion of chicken may contain on the average only 2.5 per cent of fat, whereas lean ham may contain 14 per cent of fat, fat ham as much as 50 per cent, and smoked bacon 65 per cent, though lean smoked bacon 42 per cent. It is obvious, therefore, that without accurate analyses of the fat in meat, only an approximate idea can be had of its caloric value. For these reasons I have little sympathy with those who record the protein and fat contents of their diets in decimals, but much sympathy with the poor patients who labor for an obviously false accuracy.

Fish differs from meat chiefly in the small quantity of fat. Even salmon, which contains more fat than most other fish, showed in its analysis only 12.8 per cent fat, shad 9.5 per cent, and herring and mackerel 7.1 per cent. In general, other kinds of fish show

6 per cent or less of fat. Halibut steak, for example, contains 5.2 per cent, and cod 0.4 per cent. Preserved fish, however, is quite rich in fat; thus sardines contain 19.7 per cent. In substituting fish for meat, my patients are taught to add from $\frac{1}{2}$ to 1 teaspoonful of olive oil to the diet for each 30 grams of fish.

The quantity of protein in meat also varies considerably and usually falls as the percentage of fat rises. Tripe is an exception. In 100 grams the protein amounts to 17 per cent and the fat is but 9 per cent. A value of 20 per cent for protein in uncooked lean meat represents about the average, and this is increased to 25 per cent or more when the meat is cooked. The quantity of protein in fish is very slightly less than that in meat. Shell-fish make agreeable additions to the diet: (1) They are desirable because they are palatable; (2) they are bulky foods and so are satisfying; (3) they furnish a separate course at a meal. Half a dozen oysters or clams are quite sufficient. The edible portion of a medium-sized oyster on the shell weighs on the average half an ounce, and half a dozen oysters would amount to 90 to 100 grams. The six would contain about 6 grams protein, 1 gram fat, and 4 grams carbohydrate—the equivalent of 50 calories. Half a dozen clams on the shell (edible portion) weigh 35 grams and contain 0.7 gram carbohydrate, 3 grams protein, and a negligible quantity of fat.

(*b*) **Broths.**—Broths are so extensively used upon fasting days in the treatment of diabetes that their composition deserves notice. In the Composition of American Food Materials, Bull. 28, U. S. Dept. of Agriculture, the average of three analyses of bouillon shows it to contain protein 2.2 per cent, fat 0.1 per cent, carbohydrate 0.2 per cent. This is based on the supposition that all the nitrogen is present in the form of protein, which all understand is not actually the case. It is apparent that patients taking 1 quart of bouillon or broth in a day must get considerable nitrogenous material. Frequently bouillon cubes[1] are used by patients. These consist chiefly of common salt; the amount of meat extract present ranges from 8 to 28 per cent; and the third important ingredient is plant or vegetable extract, which constitutes from 3 to 30 per cent.

In a research with Riche upon the metabolism of amino-acids, Lusk[2] had occasion to investigate the nutritive value of Liebig's Extract of Beef. As a result of his metabolism experiments upon fasting dogs in the calorimeter, he reached the conclusion that "Liebig's Extract is without influence upon the metabolism in spite of the glandular activity it is known to induce."

Reference is made on p. 469 to the large quantity of salt in the

---

[1] Bouillon Cubes, Bulletin No. 27, U. S. Dept. of Agriculture, November 5, 1913.
[2] Lusk and Riche: Jour. Biol. Chem., 1912, **13**, 155.

broth prepared at the New England Deaconess Hospital, and the full analysis of the broth is there given. Believing the matter of still greater importance, I enlisted the help of Prof. Mendel, and through him analyses of various broths in use in small and large hospitals in Boston have been made by Mr. A. H. Smith, of New Haven, Conn. These are given in Table 176, and to these other analyses of various broths examined at the Connecticut Agricultural Experiment Station have been added.

The table shows that the quantity of salt in the broths is quite considerable and that it varies markedly in the different broths. One quart of broth at one hospital, for example, would contain 20 grams of salt, while at another less than 1 gram.

It is satisfactory to record that all broths agree in being free from carbohydrate. It becomes evident, therefore, why edema is so apt to occur during the course of modern diabetic treatment. The quantity of salt in broths should certainly not exceed 0.5 per cent and if there is any tendency to edema, all salt should be eliminated.

The percentage of fat in the broth as shown by the ether extract is almost invariably slight. The broth C–1, in which the percentage was so considerable, was a sample sent from the hospital kitchen to the diet kitchen; it did not represent the actual form in which the broth was served the patients.

The variation of the total nitrogen in the broths is marked and is the most important feature brought out by these analyses. Here again it should be remembered that the higher analyses represent broths submitted for examination to Mr. Smith, and that if the sediment of the broths as well as the fat were removed the values for nitrogen would not only be less but also more uniform. It will be seen that in broth D–2 over 10 grams of nitrogen were present to the liter, and that the protein-nitrogen in this broth amounted to 61 per cent of the total. In general, it is a safe statement to make that nearly three-quarters of the total nitrogen in broths is made up of protein- and amino-nitrogen. Such a large quantity of protein demands cognizance and must be allowed for in any dietetic computations. It is notable that the broths with high values for nitrogen were broths from private hospitals and were the broths usually given all the hospital patients rather than to diabetic patients. It is obvious, therefore, that broths for diabetic patients should be prepared in a different manner than the rich broths for other patients who are often overfed with design.

In general, therefore, thin, clear meat broths, agreeably seasoned, lightly salted, can be considered desirable for diabetic patients. If the broths are concentrated, form a jelly when cold, are served without complete removal of the fat and the sediment, they are

TABLE 176.—ANALYSES OF BROTHS. MR. A. H. SMITH, NEW HAVEN, CONN.

Hospital.	Total solids, per cent.	Ash, per cent.	Chlorine as NaCl, per cent.	Ether extract, per cent.	Carbohydrates.	Total nitrogen, per cent.	Protein nitrogen, per cent. of total.	Extractive nitrogen, per cent. of total.	Amino nitrogen, per cent. of total.	Remarks.
A-1	2.45	0.42	0.07	0.26	No reduction test	0.26	39.3	45.7	15.0	A beef broth, unsalted; very turbid, but settling quickly to a water-clear broth; some fat; with salt this would be very palatable.
B-1	4.39	2.38	2.02	0.27	No reduction test	0.25	34.1	38.1	27.8	A light yellow, slightly turbid chicken broth; salted and very palatable.
C-1	9.85	0.10	0.03	4.53	No reduction test	0.12	12.7	52.0	35.2	A light yellow clear broth, considerable yellow fat; it tasted flat and a trifle bitter; was much too fat and it lacked flavor.
C-2	8.76	0.38	....	0.63	No reduction test	0.54	84.3	14.9¹	....	This was a thick, white, jelly; there was no salt in it, but it was palatable; very characteristic taste of mutton; small amount of fat.
C-3	1.49	0.41	0.22	0.07	No reduction test	0.16	43.9	35.7	18.8	This was a clear, light yellow broth, palatable though unsalted; had no definite taste.
D-1	7.54	0.99	0.77	0.12	No reduction test	0.86	83.7	9.1	7.2	When cold this broth was a brown jelly; flavored with spices and onion; very little salt; carried a small amount of fat well; tasted fairly good.
D-2	12.53	3.14	1.73	0.12	No reduction test	1.09	61.0	23.5	15.5	When cold this broth was a dark brown jelly with small amount of fat; it was salted and was very palatable; was very concentrated.
D-3	7.73	1.24	1.10	0.13	No reduction test	0.91	88.0	6.9	5.6	When cold this broth was a light brown, thin jelly with sediment in it; it seemed to contain vegetable extracts; unsalted or slightly salted and most palatable.
Station No.										
13342	2.10	0.28	0.05	0.04	None	0.23	....	....	....	Mutton bone.
13343	1.42	0.36	0.03	0.04	None	0.23	....	....	....	Veal bone.
13344	1.32	0.30	0.05	0.04	None	0.20	....	....	....	Beef bone.
13345	0.92	0.32	0.03	0.03	None	0.15	....	....	....	Beef bone.
13346	0.90	0.18	0.03	0.04	None	0.16	....	....	....	Mutton bone.
13347	1.85	0.30	0.05	0.02	None	0.28	....	....	....	Veal bone.
13348	0.69	0.19	0.03	0.04	None	0.10	....	....	....	Chicken.
13349	1.60	0.48	0.06	0.03	None	0.24	....	....	....	Clams chopped.
13391	1.93	0.30	0.07	0.04	None	0.20	....	....	....	Clams unchopped.

¹ The sum of extractive and amino-nitrogen.

29

unsuitable and, unless account is taken of their nutritive value, will seriously impair the value of dietetic calculations. Undoubtedly such broths have repeatedly prolonged the periods required to make patients sugar-free.

Protein for diabetics should be given in the form of Class A proteins according to Banting, Campbell and Fletcher.[1] These Class A proteins—meat, eggs, fish, milk—are desirable instead of broths which contain amino-acids and thus use up insulin without, at the same time, serving for tissue replacement.

(*c*) **Increased Utilization of Carbohydrate in Absence of Protein.**— The effect of a low protein diet upon the assimilation of carbohydrate was first strikingly brought out by Klemperer,[2] who showed that even dextrose would be assimilated to a considerable degree by a severe diabetic patient provided the protein in the diet was low. Clinicians of the older school beginning with Cantani, appreciated the importance of restricting the quantity of protein, though Bouchardat, and still earlier Prout, Watt and Rollo saw the dangers of overfeeding. But it is only within the last few years, when the necessity of avoiding acidosis by balancing the glucose-forming material in the diet against fat-forming factors, that the profession appreciated why glycosuria could increase by feeding protein. It is a credit to the older investigators that they sensed the truth even though they knew nothing of amino-acids.

Far less protein is given the diabetic today than ever before. This may be possible with the help of insulin allowing more calories, but we should not forget that such masters of diabetic treatment as Cantani and Naunyn fed much more.

Naunyn, for example, frequently mentions 125 grams protein (20 grams nitrogen) (500 grams cooked = 625 grams uncooked meat) in the dietaries of his patients, though I am inclined to believe he usually employed a somewhat smaller amount. The tolerance of the diabetic for protein, should be determined just the same as is the tolerance for carbohydrate; it should be determined in the presence of carbohydrate and fat as well. Protein is indispensable to a diabetic, and his tolerance for carbohydrate and fat, must be subservient to it. Eventually a protein may be found in which the amino-acids containing an uneven number of carbon atoms, which are the ones giving rise to sugar, are especially low, just as a fat, intarvin, with an uneven number of carbon atoms has been constructed which does not give rise to the formation of β-oxybutyric acid. Unfortunately, if we avoid the amino-acids with uneven numbers of carbon atoms and give those with an

---

[1] Banting, Campbell and Fletcher: Jour. Metab. Research, 1922, **2**, 547.
[2] Klemperer: Die Therap. der Gegenwart, 1911, **52**, 447.

even number of carbon atoms, we are offering our patient good material for the formation of β-oxybutyric acid.

(*d*) **Dextrose-nitrogen Ratio.**—The quantity of dextrose which can be formed from the protein molecule has already been discussed on p. 243. In dietetic computations I think it safest to consider the maximum quantity of sugar in the urine which can be attributed to the protein in the diet is 58.4 per cent, which is Lusk's dextrose-nitrogen ratio. (3.65 grams dextrose: 1 gram nitrogen, equivalent to 6.25 grams protein.) For convenience in clinical computations the value 60 per cent may be employed. Lusk points out that the quantities of sugar in the urine in excess of the ratio of 3.65 grams dextrose for 1 gram nitrogen, are an indication that the patient is taking carbohydrate and so far all my data support this view. The theoretical maximum of carbohydrate which can be formed from protein is 83 per cent.

Lusk also found the same D : N ratio in the case of a severe diabetic, and he has termed a D : N ratio of 3.65 : 1 the fatal diabetic ratio, but further study of this ratio showed him that it is not necessarily of fatal omen.[1] Minkowski found that 2.65 grams of dextrose appeared in the urines of his depancreatized dogs for each gram of nitrogen, thus giving a D : N ratio of 2.65 : 1.

(*e*) **The Carbohydrate Balance.**—The carbohydrate balance represents the difference between the total quantity of carbohydrate as such ingested in the diet and the sugar excreted in the urine during the same period. When the quantity of carbohydrate in the diet is greater than the quantity of sugar in the urine the patient is said to have a positive carbohydrate balance. When the carbohydrate in the diet is less than the quantity of sugar in the urine the carbohydrate balance is said to be minus or negative. Under the latter circumstances it is evident that the sugar in the urine is derived either from sugar stored in the body or is being formed out of protein, or fat. If it simply represents stored-up sugar, within a few days the negative carbohydrate balance will promptly change to zero and perhaps eventually to a positive balance. Case No. 8, in Table 177, will illustrate this, but Case No. 2095, shows it in more modern form. (See Table 178).

This moderate case of diabetes, Case No. 8, first came under observation June 28, 1899, and for the first twenty-four hours during which the urine was collected the intake of carbohydrate was not known. Upon the following day no carbohydrate at all was administered, but sugar had existed for so considerable a period in the body that time was necessary for its excretion. The minus carbohydrate balance of 65 grams, therefore, was simply due to retained sugar

---

[1] Lusk: Arch. Int. Med., 1909, **3**, 1.

in the body. This is plainly shown because upon the following day, when 10 grams carbohydrate were allowed, the sugar in the urine decreased to 13 grams, constituting a minus carbohydrate balance of 3 grams; but a day later upon the same diet the urinary sugar completely disappeared and the carbohydrate balance was plus 10 grams. Six months later the tolerance for carbohydrate

TABLE 177.—THE CHANGE IN THE CARBOHYDRATE BALANCE FROM NEGATIVE TO POSITIVE. CASE NO. 8. AGE AT ONSET, SIXTY YEARS. NORMAL EXPECTATION OF LIFE, FOURTEEN YEARS AND TEN MONTHS. THE PATIENT LIVED FOURTEEN YEARS. TREATMENT ACCORDING TO NAUNYN.

Date, 1899.	Diacetic acid, grams.	Sugar in urine, grams.	Carbo-hydrate intake.	Carbo-hydrate balance.	Weight, pounds.	Remarks.
June 28 . .	0	61	?	?	161	Diabetes discovered.
30 . .	0	65	0	−65		
July 1 . .	0	13	10	− 3		
2 . .	0	0	10	+10		
1900						
Jan. 1		4	45	+41	174	
1909						
Oct. 12 . . ++		19	54	+35	..	Carbuncle.
17 . . +		0	76	+76		
21 . . 0		0	70	+70	146	
1911						
May 18 . .	0	42	65	+23	..	Pneumonia.
1912						
Sept. 11 . .	0	10	30	+20	143	
1913						
April 20		21	?	..	140[1]	Hemiplegia.
June 17		2.4%	?	..	..	Pneumonia; died.

TABLE 178.—CHANGES IN CARBOHYDRATE AND GLUCOSE BALANCES. CASE NO. 2095. AGE AT ONSET, TWENTY-SEVEN YEARS, DEC. 1920.

Date.	Urinary sugar.		Diet in grams.			Carbo-hydrate balance.	Glu-cose balance.	Weight, lbs.	Blood sugar.	Insu-lin, units.	Remarks.
	%	gm.	C.	P.	F.						
1921											
Feb. 21	9.0	54	53	25	0	−1	+14	131			
22[2]	3.7	37	99	57	0	+62	+95	132	0.20		
25	0	0	16	6	4	+16	+20	131			
28	0	0	61	33	9	+61	+81	132	0.08		
Mar. 7	0	0	131	67	22	+131	+172	131			
14	0	0	205	74	52	+205	+253	130	0.08		
1922											
Feb. 7	0	0	175	74	85	+175	+227	132	0.11		
Apr. 26	0.5	8	88	37	43	+ 80	+113	115	0.17	..	Temperature 102°, jaundice in March
May 19	0	0	140	60	68	+140	+182	115	0.11		
Sept. 13	0	0	175	75	85	+175	+227	122	0.18		
1923											
Mar. 14	0	0	148	64	72	+148	+194	124	0.12	2	
21	0	0	147	73	121	+147	+209	126	0.18	2	
28	0	0	171	77	133	+171	+230	124	..	3	
Apr. 2	0	0	171	77	133	+171	+230	125	0.08	3	
6	0	0	171	77	141	+171	+231	126	..	3	

[1] March 23.
[1] Acidosis present (slightly +) on this day only.

had risen to 41 grams. It rose somewhat during the subsequent years, persisted during a carbuncle, fell with an attack of pneumonia, then again fell, and in 1913, the patient died of a second attack of pneumonia three months after a cerebral hemorrhage in the fourteenth year of the disease. I do not believe this patient could have tolerated for fourteen years as low a carbohydrate intake as that advocated by Newburgh and Marsh, namely 40 grams, but I do believe that she would have been better off if her protein had been restricted.

Case No. 2095, a minister, married three years, aged twenty-seven years, developed symptoms of diabetes in December, 1920, and came for treatment February 21, 1921, seven weeks later. He followed the scheduled regimen at that time employed, the negative carbohydrate balance changed to positive and with a high-carbohydrate, low-fat diet remained sugar-free and held his weight one year. He then returned to see if insulin would put him back in the pulpit. I tell him that is probable, but at any rate it has put him into mine, for his case preaches that (1) 9 per cent of sugar is consistent with a mild diabetes, if (2) treatment based upon a high-carbohydrate, moderate-protein and low-fat diet is begun early; and that (3) tolerance can be maintained when the diet is always faithfully followed, as Allen and Sherrill have claimed; (4) with preservation of weight; (5) absence of glycosuria; (6) a normal percentage of blood sugar; (7) a recuperative power with three units of insulin which allows a gain in strength, mental vigor and weight; (8) raises the question as to whether a similar amount of insulin nearer onset might have brought the patient closer to a state of complete recovery. Compare Case Nos. 2962, 3078, pp. 47 and 74.

On the other hand, a minus carbohydrate balance which is persistent is indicative of severe diabetes with the formation of sugar from protein. The severity of the diabetes in such a case is also shown by the fact that when a minus carbohydrate balance is permanently present, acidosis is extreme. (See Case No. 344, p. 574.) It will be seen that the carbohydrate balance was minus on June 28, and July 4, 6, 10 and later remained at quite a uniform figure, although the carbohydrate intake was varied to a considerable degree, but increased along with the severity of the diabetes. During the year represented by these days, the quantity of nitrogen was not very far from 16 grams, and with allowance for fecal nitrogen might be taken as 18 grams, representing the metabolism of approximately 112 grams protein. From this enough sugar could be formed to account for the minus carbohydrate balance if 60 grams of sugar are derived from 100 grams protein in accordance with Lusk's D : N ratio of 3.65 : 1. Unlike the temporary minus balance in

Case No. 8, it will be seen that the minus carbohydrate balance in Case No. 344, was persistent and in consequence the acidosis was extreme. The remarkable change in the carbohydrate balance toward the end of life took place after the patient had developed diffuse tuberculosis and was about to die. Attention is called especially to the disappearance of acidosis at this time. It is referred to in the discussion of Allen's theories of diabetes, under Treatment, and again in the Section upon Tuberculosis.

The cases above cited are illustrations of changes in the carbohydrate balance over considerable periods of time. They indicate at a glance that, when the diet is being rapidly altered, the carbohydrate balance is not a true index of the carbohydrate utilized and should not be regarded as such. A true carbohydrate balance demands a constant diet with the patient in nitrogen equilibrium as well.

(*f*) **The Glucose Balance.**—The term "glucose balance" is employed frequently instead of "carbohydrate balance," including under glucose the carbohydrate of the diet, 58 per cent of the protein and 10 per cent of the fat. It is not wholly satisfactory, because it implies that all the protein and fat consumed are immediately oxidized and the carbohydrate which can be formed out of them at once has entered into the metabolism. Shaffer and Wilder are correct in utilizing the urinary nitrogen as a guide to the actual amount of protein entering into the metabolism. It is quite a question, however, whether this will suffice and, for one, I am skeptical whether the carbohydrate, fat and protein of the diet, even basing the latter on nitrogen excretion, accurately represent the actual metabolism of these three substances. If an exact knowledge of the carbohydrate, protein, and fat burned is desired, recourse must be had to the respiratory metabolism aided by the nitrogen excretion and even here it is only the uninitiated who will pin all their faith on the respiratory quotient as the crucial factor in such determinations.

The glucose balance is shown in Table 178, along with the carbohydrate balance. I inserted a column for the words "Glucose Balance" on my hospital charts, but I confess in practice I seldom refer to the data. The tolerance of a hospital diabetic changes so rapidly from day to day that its worth is vitiated. Woodyatt's[1] classic example follows. For a friendly, but searching criticism of Woodyatt's position, see an article by Allen.[2]

To the total glucose and the glucose balance of the diet Woodyatt attaches great weight. In his opinion it matters little whether the glucose comes from carbohydrate yielding 100 per cent glucose, protein yielding 58 per cent glucose, or from fat yielding 10 per cent

[1] Woodyatt: Arch. Int. Med., 1921, **28**, 125.
[2] Allen: Jour. Metab. Research, 1923, **3**, 61,

glucose, or whether the glucose has its source in food consumed or body tissue burned. He has described in detail his experience with a severe diabetic, and to his article the reader is referred. Four days of severe undernutrition failed to render the urine sugar-free at entrance to the hospital, but this was accomplished later with intermittent fasting, first for two days, and subsequently after an interval of feeding, with one day. By period V the tolerance of the patient had improved so that with carbohydrate 92 grams, protein 103 grams, and fat 70 grams, total glucose 159 grams, he excreted but 50 grams sugar thus making a glucose balance of 109 grams. He was then placed upon two radically different diets; the first, with low-protein and high-fat, consisting of carbohydrate 84 grams, protein 11.5 grams, and fat 162 grams, total glucose 116 grams and the second, carbohydrate 28 grams, protein 118 grams, and fat 160 grams, and with these latter two diets having a glucose value of 116 grams and 112 grams, respectively he remained sugar-free.

In conclusion, therefore, when dealing with either the carbohydrate or glucose balance, let us remember that neither expresses what is taking place in the body unless the patient is on a constant diet for a week or more and in caloric, even if not in nitrogenous, equilibrium and that these terms, even at their best, hint merely at what is taking place in the body, but are by no means representative of the potential carbohydrate and glucose balances which may be growing from day to day while the recorded figures stand still.

4. **Fat.**—(*a*) **The Value of Fat to the Diabetic.**—Fat forms the bulk of the diabetic patient's diet. Even with the most modern ideas on treatment the statement holds. Whereas in the normal diet it furnishes less than one-third of the total calories, that diabetic diet is exceptional which is not made up one-half of fat, and there are few diabetic diets in which fat does not represent two-thirds, and frequently it comprises three-fourths and occasionally eight-ninths of the total.

It is surprising how readily in the past double and even treble the quantity of fat ingested by normal individuals was borne by the stomach of the diabetic patient. It is, however, unwise to push the administration of fat too energetically for fear of causing a dislike for it or even indigestion. I once prevented a diabetic boy from enjoying and deriving benefit from sardines, with their accompanying oil, by allowing him to eat the first time as many as he liked. He promptly ate a boxful and the disgust Case No. 4 then acquired for sardines was never overcome. Perhaps this is one reason why I still avoid high ketogenic-antiketogenic ratios. Frequently I see patients who have taken large quantities of fat with obvious benefit for long periods. Case No. 8 (p. 104) must have taken 150 grams of fat daily for fourteen years and died at the age of seventy-three. The quantity of carbohydrate in her diet for the greater part of the time was below 75 grams. The fat could hardly be said to have done injury in this case, for the patient out-lived most of her family. Case No. 564, Table 179, age at onset sixteen years, eats 170 grams daily—too much, I acknowledge. His case is interesting because four years ago he was three and a half months in getting sugar-free, and for a large part of the time showed acidosis. After four years of diabetes, he passed his pre-liminary examination for Harvard. A brief abstract of his case is given below to show that, even formerly, patients sometimes did surprisingly well.

TABLE 179.—CASE No. 564. THE COURSE OF SEVERE DIABETES IN A BOY OF SIXTEEN YEARS. TREATMENT BEGUN IN DECEMBER, 1912.

Date.	Urine.				Carbo-hydrate in diet, grams.	Sodium bicarbo-nate, grams.	Naked weight, pounds.
	Volume, c.c.	Diacetic acid.	Total NH₃, grams.	Total sugar (polar.), grams.			
1912							
Dec. 17–18	5430	+++	...	230	160	16	99
18–19	5100	sl. +	5.2	130	160	16	99
19–20	4710	++	...	180	135	16	100
20–21	4710	++	...	190	125	16	99
21–22	4050	++++	...	115	125	16	100
22–23	3840	++	...	119	115	16	100
23–24	4020	+++	...	137	75	16	99
1913							
Jan. 1– 2	4140	++	...	89	50	20	101
2– 3	4440	+++	...	115	50	20	100
3– 4	3420	+++	...	75	50	20	101
4– 5	3120	++	...	37	15	20	103
5– 6	4200	+	...	143	165	20	104
6– 7	2100	++++	...	13	15	..	106
9–10	2700	++++	3.8	49	40	..	102
Mar. 31							
April 1	945	....	1.1	0			
7– 8	1240	sl. +	...	0	...	..	113
1914							
Jan. 5	2000	0	...	0			
1915							
April 26	1800	0	1.0	0	50	..	134 (dressed)
1916							
Sept. 23 [1]	700	..	0.7	0	...	..	129 (dressed)
Oct. 18–19	1600	+	...	6			
Dec. 20–21	800	0	...	0	...	..	134 (dressed)
1917							
Jan. 25–26	1000	+	1.0	0	45		
1920							
May 11[2]	2600	0	...	0	55	..	104
1922							
Nov. 16	Died. Perforation.		Gastric ulcer.		Autopsy.		

[1] May 1, 1915, blood sugar, 0.13 per cent; Sept. 23, 1916, blood sugar, 0.13 per cent.
[2] May 11, 1920, blood sugar, 0.1 per cent.

Case No. 564, came under observation November 30, 1912, at the age of sixteen, three weeks after his onset, which occurred without previous symptoms after an important football game. Volume of urine 8 quarts during the day. The marked acidosis at that time led me to make very gradual changes in the diet and the sugar in the urine decreased from presumably more than 500 grams a day before entrance to the hospital to 230 grams on the first day after entrance, December 17–18, 1912. The patient was discharged, with 42 grams of sugar in the urine on February 13–14, 1913. Under the close care of his physician and a trained diabetic nurse he became sugar-free March 31, 1913, and remained sugar-free, with the rarest exceptions, until his death by perforation of a gastric ulcer on Nov. 16, 1922. It was not by accident he lived so long, because his physicians were F. G. Brigham, B. H. Ragle and Bertnard Smith.

The Eskimos live largely upon fat. Their duration of life can hardly be known with accuracy, and many of the men die as a result of their hazardous seafaring occupations. The duration of life of the Eskimo women should furnish an interesting study.

How much fat should a diabetic patient eat? Plainly, from what has been and will be recorded in the next section, this does not depend upon the capacity of his digestion. The safest answer would be as little as possible above the normal ration of 50 to 100 grams. Unquestionably the quantity will vary from time to time, and it may increase with years without detriment to the patient. Nevertheless, I am always glad to see a diet with a carbohydrate-fat ratio under 1 : 2, and dread to see one with a ratio above 1 : 3.

Fat is most agreeably taken as cream, and cream which contains 20 per cent butter fat is usually better borne than a richer cream. It is seldom advisable to allow more than half a pint (240 cc) of cream, although patients prefer to increase the quantity of cream at the expense of other forms of fat in the diet. Rather than increase the quantity of cream increase its richness in fat. There is no other form of food from which a diabetic patient can derive more pleasure for its caloric value and yet with less harm to himself than from cream. Half a pint of 20 per cent cream contains approximately 50 grams of fat, and yet the quantity of carbohydrate in cream of this richness is but little over 8 grams, and may be estimated in clinical work as 8 grams or 1 gram to the ounce. Occasionally, patients bear butter better than cream, and, as a rule, fresh unsalted butter is preferred. Thirty grams of butter contain 25 grams of fat, and this is a welcome addition to the diet. Intarvin is of about the same strength, 85 per cent fat, but actually less, because it is a higher fatty acid. Oleo or butterine contains no sugar and has about the same percentage of fat as butter and the cost is approximately one-half that of first-class butter. Lard, being nearly 100 per cent fat can be used to advantage more than it now is in the diabetic's diet. Crisco, also nearly 100 per cent fat, is often more welcome than lard, because of its lack of flavor. Oil is an ideal diabetic food, because it is a pure fat. Oil is so desirable for a diabetic that I hesitate to have a patient take more than 15 grams (1 tablespoonful) lest he weary of it. If oil is disliked upon vegetables it can be taken in small quantities after meals as a medicine.

Italian patients naturally bear olive oil unusually well. An Italian diabetic patient under my care at the Boston City Hospital with typhoid fever not only passed through the disease uneventfully upon oatmeal gruel and olive oil, but incidentally became sugar-free and developed no acidosis. Olive oil forms an excellent lunch for diabetic patients, and is useful upon retiring to combat insomnia. It is the diabetic patient's cough medicine; it relieves the symptoms of his hyperacid stomach. Peanut, corn or cotton-seed oil may be substituted if expense is a factor. Cod-liver oil is very readily taken by children and of much value.

(b) **The Danger of Fat to the Diabetic.**—Fat is the chief source of the dreaded acidosis, though to this in lesser degree the amino-acids of the protein molecule with even numbers of carbon atoms contribute as well. Fat, therefore, at one time may save the life of the diabetic, but at another period may destroy it.

One of the most potent agencies in the prevention of acidosis is the withdrawal of fat from the diet. The absence of acidosis in totally depancreatized animals and in a human case of pancreatic insufficiency like that of Spriggs and Leigh[1] is to be explained by the non-absorption of the fat given.

One cannot treat diabetes successfully without increasing the quantity of fat and to what extent depends somewhat upon the attitude of the clinician. Fortunately, however, there are certain definite criteria. On the one hand it is unreasonable to give less than in health, and on the other more than the patient can take without developing acidosis, or more than enough to bring his weight up to 10 per cent below normal.

Allen has again made us all his debtors by a series of experiments upon diabetic dogs which show the insidious way in which fat is harmful in the manner in which it has been customarily employed in the treatment of diabetes. "Fat unbalanced by adequate quantities of other foods is a poison."[2] And Shaffer, Woodyatt, Newburgh and Marsh, Petrén, Wilder, Campbell, Strouse, Ladd and Palmer all contributed formulæ to show the adequate quanti-

[1] Spriggs and Leigh: Jour. Am. Med. Assn., 1915, **65**, 1952.
[2] Allen: Am. Jour. Med. Sci., 1917, **153**, 313.

ties of other foods. Newburgh and Marsh and Petrén courageously demonstrated that patients did not die in the hospital while living upon a high-fat, but low-carbohydrate and very low-protein diet, even before the explanation therefor was perfectly plain. Shaffer[1] has assiduously studied the ketogenic and antiketogenic properties of foods and shown that two molecules of aceto-acetic acid, representing two molecules of a higher fatty acid, are offset by one molecule of glucose and to this Wilder[2] agrees and that acidosis occurs when this ratio is exceeded. Woodyatt[3] places the ratio as 1 molecule fatty acid to 1 molecule of glucose, which ratio Hubbard and Wright[4] adopt. This is based on the supposition earlier adopted by Shaffer that 1 molecule of a higher fatty acid is offset by 1 molecule of glucose.

Various formulas have been devised by which to calculate the maximum amount of fat which a diabetic patient can take with a given tolerance for carbohydrate. All agree that the protein should be kept low, certainly not over 1 gram per kilogram body weight and permanently not below 0.66 gram per kilogram. Shaffer and Wilder each base the quantity of protein in their formulæ upon the nitrogenous metabolism as determined by the urinary nitrogen excretion. Likewise all would concede that the patient should be in nitrogenous as well as in caloric equilibrium.

Shaffer's formula is as follows:

$$\frac{(\text{Calories of Basal Metab.} \times 120\,\%) - (\text{Grams Urinary Nitrogen} \times 100)}{50} = G \times 2.$$

Given: basal metabolism 1000 calories : urinary nitrogen 8 grams. Thus, if the basal metabolism is 1000 calories and 200 calories are added for hospital activity, we have 1200 calories from which must be subtracted the 8 grams of urinary nitrogen $\times$ 100 = 800, leaving 400 to be divided by 50, or 8, a quotient representing the lowest quantity of glucose in grams which could burn the amount of ketone molecules represented in the protein and fat of the equation. Since the glucose must be burned continuously and in all parts of the body, Shaffer multiplies the result by 2, for a safe margin, making 16 grams glucose.

The glucose calories would be, therefore, carbohydrate	16 grams $\times$ 4 =	64
The protein calories would be 8 $\times$ 6.25 = protein	50 grams $\times$ 4 =	200
The fat calories would be $\frac{1260 - 264}{9}$ = fat	104 grams $\times$ 9 =	939
		1200

Wilder uses two formulæ:

$$C = 0.024\ M - 0.41\ P \qquad \text{Formula 1}$$
$$F = 4\ C + 1.4\ P \qquad \text{Formula 2}$$

[1] Shaffer: Jour. Biol. Chem., 1922, **50**, 26.
[2] Wilder: Jour. Am. Med. Assn., 1922, **78**, 1878.
[3] Woodyatt: Arch. Int. Med., 1921, **28**, 125.
[4] Hubbard and Wright: Jour. Biol. Chem., 1922, **50**, 361. Hubbard and Nicholson: Ibid., 1922, **53**, 209.

"In these formulæ, F is the number of grams of fat, C the number of grams of carbohydrate, P the number of grams of protein allowable, and M the total caloric requirement. The calculation is further simplified by the nomographic chart." (See Fig. 28, p. 461).

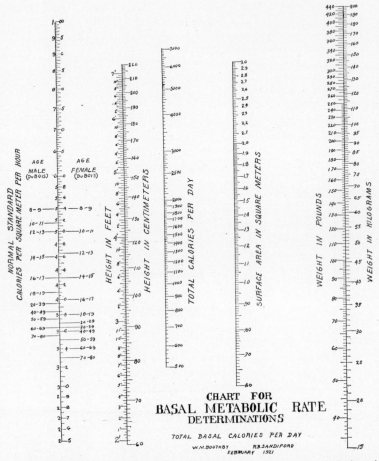

Fig. 27.—Boothby and Sandiford's chart for quick and accurate calculation of normal basal food calory requirement. The weight is located on the weight scale and the height on the height scale with pins (needles set in wooden handles). A straight edge connecting these two points crosses the surface area scale at the patient's surface area. The normal standard is located on the left hand scale. The line connecting this point with the surface area crosses the calory scale at the basal twenty-four-hour calory requirement.

The protein can be taken at 0.66 gram per kilogram body weight and, as the diabetic metabolism is so much below standard, a standard metabolism will allow enough calories for moderate activity. Charts for rapid calculations of basal metabolism and optimal diets

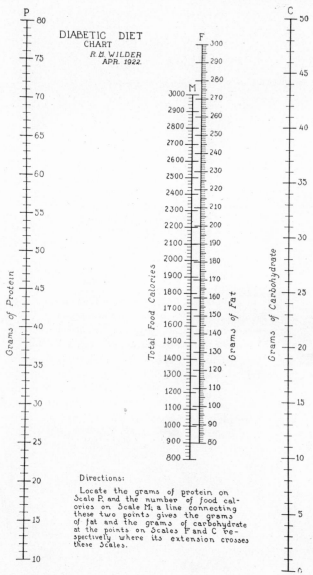

Fig. 28.—Diabetic diet chart: The grams of protein are located on Scale P, and the number of food calories on Scale M; a line connecting these two points gives the grams of fat and the grams of carbohydrate at the points on Scale F and C, respectively, where its extension crosses these scales.

have been devised at the Mayo Clinic and these appear on pp. 460 and 461. These are described in Wilder's article previously cited.

Woodyatt, assuming a ratio of 1.5 grams fatty acid to 1 gram glucose, gives three formulæ for the estimation of the fat for the quantity of glucose tolerated. The glucose in the diet is estimated by formula (1):

$$(1), \ G \ = \ C \ + \ 0.58 \ P \ + \ 0.1 \ F$$

The fatty acids are estimated by formula (2):

$$(2), \ FA \ = \ 0.46 \ P \ + \ 0.9 \ F.$$

Assuming that when the ratio $\frac{FA}{G}$ exceeds 1.5 ketonuria develops, the maximum quantity of fat is shown in formula (3):

$$\frac{C \ + \ 0.58 \ P \ + \ 0.1 \ F}{0.46 \ P \ + \ 0.9 \ F} \ = \ 1.5 \ = \ F \ = \ 2 \ C \ + \ 0.54 \ P \text{ or simply}$$

$$(3), \ F \ = \ 2 \ C \ + \ \frac{P}{2}$$

Conclusions Regarding Fat—Carbohydrate Ratios and Formulæ.— (1) It is rarely necessary to give the maximum quantity of fat, which the carbohydrate allows without acidosis, to any diabetic and for practical purposes one can say wholly unnecessary with either insulin or, apparently, intarvin at our disposal. (2) If the urine is sugar-free, one need not worry about acidosis if the fat is twice the carbohydrate, or even thrice the carbohydrate provided the protein is but 1 gram per kilogram of the patient's body weight, and if the protein is reduced to 0.66 gram per kilogram and the calories not over 30 per kilogram the fat can be four times and probably five times the carbohydrate with safety. A still lower protein would allow a still higher fat-carbohydrate proportion, but this is best avoided. If a doctor wishes to give more than 3 grams fat for 1 gram carbohydrate, he had best use insulin to raise the carbohydrate tolerance or intarvin to avoid the formation of ketone bodies.

Fat in any form is absorbed by the diabetic patient quite as well as by normal individuals, except in those rare cases of pancreatic diabetes. One such case (No. 670) was seen by me a few days before coma. In this instance diabetes occurred after partial loss of the gland from acute pancreatitis. The case is reported in detail by Jurist.[1]

Fat, however, is not well absorbed by the dog made diabetic by the removal of the pancreas. This fact explains one of the diffi-

[1] Jurist: Am. Jour. Med. Sci., 1909, **138**, 180.

culties experienced in producing acidosis in dogs. When Allen succeeded in making a dog with severe diabetes gain or even hold his weight by forced feeding of fat, increasing acidosis occurred.[1]

(*c*) **The Increased Assimilability of Carbohydrate in Absence of Fat.**[2] —Notwithstanding that sugar is not formed from fat, the addition of fat to a diet upon which a severe diabetic patient is sugar-free can easily be followed by the appearance of sugar in the urine, and the converse is equally true. It would seem as if the fat molecules displaced the sugar molecules from their attachments in the body and set them free for excretion. Allen[3] with insulin and Leclercq[4] without insulin have demonstrated this clearly. The increase of sugar following the addition of fat to the diet is well shown in Case No. 513, Table No. 225, p. 632, for the period extending between August 12–13 to August 19–20. The preceding sentence represents my original interpretation. Today I should ascribe the increased glycosuria partly to loss of tolerance, caused by the infection (carbuncles) and in part caused by acidosis brought on by the complete exclusion of carbohydrate from the diet with simultaneous administration of fat. I question if the man could have recovered today without insulin, but I believe if he had been placed upon the test diets, T. D., 1, 2, 3, 4, 5 and then worked up to $C_4 PF_7$ or $C_5 PF_9$, he would have had a better chance.

The remarkable power by which the individual can gradually become accustomed to a fat-protein diet is well shown by many diabetic patients. Thus, Case No. 344 took 372 grams of fat on an oatmeal day September 15–16, 1910. The acidosis on this day was extreme, as shown by the excretion of 27.6 grams β-oxybutyric acid. Formerly many diabetic patients took 100 grams fat in the form of cream in addition to that in bacon, butter, eggs and fat meat. Von Noorden's oatmeal cure called for 200 to 300 grams butter and one is led to ask if the simultaneous ingestion of the large quantity of carbohydrate did not save the patient's life?

Very recently Weeks, Renner, Allen and Wishart[5] in studies upon fasting and diets in epilepsy observed a remarkable hyperglycemia which developed in every case on a high-fat diet, but not with any of the other diets.

(*d*) **Synthetic Fat, Odd Carbon Atom Fat, Intarvin.**—From fat the diabetic develops acidosis and dies, but not from all kinds of fat, thanks to Max Kahn and Ralph H. McKee of Columbia University. The harmful fat is that with the even number of carbon atoms, but as the common edible fats in the animal and vegetable

---

[1] Allen: Am. Jour. Med. Sci., 1917, **153**, 313.

[2] Work in progress in other clinics will necessitate the revision of various sentences upon this page. October 8, 1923.

[3] Allen: Loc. cit., p. 196. [4] Leclercq: Loc. cit., p. 467.

[5] Weeks, Renner, Allen and Wishart: Jour. Metab. Research, 1923, **3**, 317.

kingdoms, such as stearic acid ($C_{18}H_{36}O_2$), palmitic acid ($C_{16}H_{32}O_2$), and oleic acid ($C_{18}H_{34}O_2$), are all even number carbon atom fats and as the diabetic must have fat he has had no recourse, but to live upon them and take his chances. The story of the discovery of an odd number carbon-atom fat follows:

Knoop[1] demonstrated that fatty acids in the course of their oxidation in the body lost two carbon atoms at a time from the fat acid chain. Dakin[2] confirmed and added to the Knoop theory by showing that in the catabolism of fats under normal conditions there is a rapid oxidation of the fat acid radical, such as $C_{18}H_{36}O_2$, to butyric acid, $C_4H_8O_2$, and that this is in turn also rapidly oxidized to CO_2 and H_2O provided there is simultaneous oxidation of a sufficient amount of carbohydrate. In diabetics the mechanism is different. As usual the fats are broken down to the butyric acid stage but here, instead of continued oxidation, the butyric acid $C_4H_8O_2$ is decomposed first into β-oxybutyric acid ($CH_3CHOH.CH_2COOH$) and then to diacetic acid (CH_3COCH_2COOH). This final transformation is what led to Rosenfeld's oft quoted remark that fats burn only in the fire of carbohydrate.

Embden clarified the situation when he found that only those fat acids of even number of carbon atoms yield diacetic acid when transfused through the liver of a dog. Presumably this earlier work led Ringer[3] to conceive the idea that since oxybutyric acid was derived from only those fatty acids with an even number of carbon atoms one should seek for a fat with an uneven number of carbon atoms which a diabetic could assimilate without danger of acid poisoning. He argued that if such fats could be made to burn in the body, acidosis might be avoided because the β-oxybutyric acid could not be formed. Ringer, however, was unsuccessful in his attempts to prepare the odd number carbon atom fat. Janeway and Mosenthal also saw similar possibilities, but it was left to Max Kahn to carry to completion the manufacture of such a fat.

The fat used for the manufacture of intarvin, this new fat, was stearic acid and out of this was produced magaric acid $C_{16}H_{33}COOH$. This is easily purified, then united with glycerol to form a neutral fat. The substance is of a white creamy color, odorless and tasteless, melting at 38° C, neutral in reaction. When cold and granulated it is quite palatable.

By means of this fat Max Kahn has been able to bring about the disappearance of acidosis with a group of diabetics. In one case 150 grams of fat were given daily. Also in a normal individual in whom acidosis was artificially produced by fasting, its disappearance was accomplished by the use of this synthetic fat.

[1] Knoop: Hofmeister Beiträge, 1905, **6**, 150.
[2] Dakin: Jour. Biol. Chem., 1909, **6**, 203.
[3] Ringer: Jour. Biol. Chem., 1913, **14**, 48.

The fat does not cause nausea nor is it disagreeable. Ninety-five per cent of the ingested fat was utilized according to analyses of the feces.

Through the courtesy of Professor McKee, I have been able to use this synthetic fat at the New England Deaconess Hospital. I can confirm the statements above quoted that it is not disagreeable and is readily eaten. Its efficacy in preventing acidosis has not been as yet sufficiently tested by me. It would appear to be ideal in the instance of acidosis in the presence of an infection and it is particularly with such cases that I wish to employ it.

Furthermore, it can logically be recommended to those cases with whom the fat carbohydrate ratio is above 3 : 1. Indeed that might appear to be an arbitrary rule for its employment and perhaps in the course of time one may change this rule to the use of intarvin whenever the patient's fat-carbohydrate ratio must be raised above an even lower ratio in order to maintain nutrition.

5. **Alcohol.**—In no disease is the employment of alcohol more useful or more justifiable, but it cannot be taken with impunity, for neuritis rather easily develops in undernourished patients. Alcohol furnishes an agreeable form of food in a diet which is often disagreeable, and the quantity of nutriment which it contains is by no means negligible. Alcohol is the only food material which is free from the special characteristics of carbohydrate, protein and fat and as it is of nutritive value might be of special advantage to diabetics. Alcohol is not convertable directly into either glucose or fatty acids, *i. e.*, neither ketogenic or antiketogenic. There is no evidence that alcohol is etiologically harmful save from the production of obesity. With but one patient have I a record that he gave up alcohol, increased sweets and developed diabetes. As to its action in protecting protein Mosenthal and Harrop[1] conclude that "the addition of an equal number of calories of protein, fat or alcohol to a low caloric carbohydrate-free diet in cases of diabetes mellitus results in the assimilation of considerable amounts of nitrogen when the protein is used, a favorable nitrogen balance in only occasional instances with fat, and no change in the nitrogen equilibrium when alcohol is given." Higgins, Peabody and Fitz[2] from tests upon themselves when upon a carbohydrate-free diet found that alcohol did not stop the progress of the acidosis or show any antiketogenic action. Coincidental with its administration there was further increase in the oxygen consumption and in the disagreeable subjective symptoms.

Few of my cases have taken alcohol and still fewer take it now than in years gone by. In former days with our crude notions

---

[1] Mosenthal and Harrop: Arch. Int. Med., 1918, **22**, 750.

[2] Higgins, Peabody and Fitz: Jour. Med. Research, 1916, **34**, 263.

30

about diet 15 to 30 cc of alcohol were often useful, when the patients were given excessive quantities of fat. Though Allen originally suggested its use in fasting at the beginning of treatment, he discarded it so soon that I doubt if a dozen of my patients received it under such circumstances. They preferred to go without it, requesting that it be discontinued on account of the nausea which it produced. Diabetic patients require no alcohol and as yet I have not found it necessary or desirable to have a license to prescribe it, and this statement applies to my assistants as well. Thirty cc of alcohol are to be found in approximately 60 cc of whisky, brandy, rum, or gin, or 300 cc of most of the sugar-free wines. Thirty cc of alcohol are equivalent to (30×7) 210 calories. Few of my patients ever took as much alcohol as this, but half the quantity will replace about 5 per cent of the total diet, and allows the omission of $\dfrac{(105)}{9}$ 12 grams of fat. This does not appear of great moment, but it would amount to 2100 calories in twenty days. Alcohol may be administered in various forms which are free from sugar. These are specified in the diet tables on p. 716.

The effect of alcohol must be more thoroughly studied with the calorimeter. Allen and DuBois[1] found its ingestion was occasionally followed by respiratory quotients higher than would theoretically be expected.

Allen and Wishart's[2] studies of the effect of alcohol upon two diabetics "support the prevailing belief that ethyl alcohol is not converted into sugar in the body. At the same time, they are interpreted as signifying that the addition of calories in the form of alcohol in excess of the patient's caloric tolerance produces a return of glycosuria and other diabetic symptoms.

"The experiments also corroborate the prevailing view that alcohol is not converted into acetone in the body. No antiketogenic action was demonstrable; on the contrary a slight production of acetone seemed to be caused when alcohol was given in considerable quantities. Luxus diets formed by the addition of alcohol or a mixture of fat and alcohol to a standard diet gave rise to very much less acidosis both chemically and clinically than similarly excessive diets built up by the addition of fat alone. The former therapeutic use of alcohol is thus justified, with respect to the lessened danger of acidosis when part of the fat of a high caloric diet is substituted by alcohol. The experiments do not establish such a fact for undernutrition diets, or warrant attempts to prevent combustion of fat by administration of alcohol. On the contrary, the conversion of an undernutrition diet into a luxus

[1] Allen and DuBois: Arch. Int. Med., 1916, **17**, 1010.
[2] Allen and Wishart: Jour. Metab. Research, 1922, **1**, 304.

diet by addition of alcohol may result in an actual increase of acetone. . . .

"The experiments with alcohol, if fully confirmed, are of crucial importance in supporting the undernutrition treatment They add to the existing evidence that the assimilative power of the diabetic organism is limited not only in respect to carbohydrate (preformed or potential) but also in respect to total calories as such. . . . In confirmation of the view that the harmfulness of excessive fat in diabetes does not consist merely in its possible conversion into either sugar or acetone but preëminently in the overload of the total metabolism, it is found that alcohol, which is clearly recognized as not convertable into sugar or acetone in the body, produces a return of glycosuria and other symptoms when added to the diabetic diet in quantities exceeding the caloric tolerance."

Leclercq[1] likewise demonstrated on two patients with severe diabetes the production of hyperglycemia in consequence of adding excessive calories to the diet in the form of either fat or alcohol. It is readily conceivable that replacing a certain amount of fat might lower glycosuria and acidosis, and Fuller[2] found this true in most cases of mild and moderate diabetes. "This effect is most pronounced when the alcohol is substituted for the caloric equivalent of fat, but is also frequently manifest, when the alcohol is given as an addition to the previous diet. These effects are usually lacking in diabetic cases of great severity."

6. **Liquids.**—It is rarely necessary to restrict the liquids at the beginning of treatment in diabetes. The diminution of the carbohydrate in the diet usually leads to a corresponding diminution in the thirst and quantity of urine. I hesitate to restrict liquids in severe diabetes for fear too little liquid will be available for the body with which to eliminate the acids that may have been formed. On the other hand in the course of treatment, if the patient is upon an undernutrition diet, he may take liquids too freely in the form of broths, cocoa, tea and coffee to make up for food.

The metabolism increases 3 per cent according to Benedict and Carpenter[3] when large quantities of liquids are drunk. The increase has amounted to 16 per cent. Liquids also impose a demand upon the metabolism if they are taken cold. The quantity of heat required of the body to raise the temperature of a glass of ice-water to body temperature is not negligible. Patients on the verge of coma often upset the digestion by drinking large quantities of liquids rapidly. This is avoided by allowing only half a glass of

[1] Leclercq: Jour. Metab. Research, 1922, **1**, 308.
[2] Fuller: Jour. Metab. Research, 1922, **1**, 609.
[3] Benedict and Carpenter: Carnegie Inst., Washington, Pub. No. 261, p. 247.

liquid at a time, though the patient is instructed to take that every half hour. Case No. 1196, continually voided large quantities of urine, but usually I could find a cause such as the ingestion of 20 or more grams of salt, bouillon cubes in variable number or 21 half-grain saccharin tablets a day. Ice-water should be discouraged.

The free administration of liquids at the approach of coma is, next to insulin, the most important factor in rescuing the patient. At such a time the liquids should be introduced by mouth, by rectum, and as a rule subcutaneously.

Graphic charts of the liquids ingested and excreted are often seen on hospital rounds. These are very crude affairs. In recording the intake, even if everything that flows is regarded as intake, there are amusing inconsistancies. While an egg, in an egg-nog is liquid, it escapes being recorded if boiled to the point of coagulation, cream is liquid, ice cream solid, vegetables and fruits are solid, though they contain 85 per cent more or less of water, potatoes are 75.5 per cent water and meat 77 per cent. The retained water of an enema is forgotten. Errors also creep into the estimation of the quantity of liquids excreted. The water in the feces is seldom estimated, the excretion of water by the skin is most variable, depending largely on the amount of exercise, the excretion by the lungs is entirely neglected and this amounts to about 300 cc, Dr. Carpenter tells me. Finally, as DuBois pointed out to members of the Interurban Club, in the combustion of each 60 grams of sugar there are 5 cc of water formed, of 100 grams of protein 41 cc of water, of 100 grams of beef fat, 107 cc of water.

7. Sodium Chloride.—Salt is of great service to the diabetic patient. If it is withdrawn from the diet the weight falls, due to excretion of water, and the skin and tissues of the patient become obviously dry. In the early days of the fasting treatment patients often lost much weight because water alone was allowed. For example, I learned of one case who lost 13 pounds in four days in this manner. Conversely, when broths are freely given during fasting it is not uncommon, particularly in the presence of acidosis, to see a patient gain weight, and invariably such patients feel better than those who lose.

Butter may contain a large amount of salt. Analyses of 695 samples of butter reported in Bulletin 149, Bureau of Animal Industry U. S. Department of Agriculture, show an average of 2.51 per cent salt in finished butter.

Salt is very freely used by diabetic patients. I do not remember to have ever seen a diabetic patient who took too little salt. One of my fasting cases was accustomed to shake it into his hand to eat. Patients will often salt their broths, although they contain considerable salt. An analysis of the duplicate portion of the broth which Case No. 765 drank in three days is recorded in Table 180.

TABLE 180.—BROTH TAKEN BY CASE NO. 765 IN THREE DAYS AT THE NEW ENGLAND DEACONESS HOSPITAL.

Volume of broth ingested in three days, 1220 c.c.

	Total grams.	Per cent.	Total calories per 100 c.c.
Salt	10.7	0.88	0.0
Nitrogen	2.57	0.21	5.2
Fat	0.6	0.05	0.5

The same patient used 26 grams of salt from the salt-celler during the week which included two fasting days and five other days upon which she took 300 grams washed vegetables and from 150 to 225 grams fish or lean meat. To avoid such excessive use of salt, nurses are advised to serve no salt with broths.

Case No. 982, a young man with onset of diabetes at the age of twenty, excreted 40.3 grams of sodium chloride on February 15, 1916, and a few days later the aliquoted urine of two days contained 89.6 grams. Upon inquiry I learned from his nurse that in addition to the ordinary amount of salt in the food as it was prepared the young man filled a salt-cellar each morning and emptied it before night. Table 181.

TABLE 181.—EXCESSIVE INTAKE OF SODIUM CHLORIDE BY A DIABETIC BOY.

Date.	Vol., c.c.	NaCl, grams.	Diacetic acid.	Nitrogen, grams.	Sugar, grams.	Carbo-hydrate, grams.	Protein, grams.	Fat, grams.	Calor-ies.
1916									
Feb. 14–15	1920	40.3	0	10.9	0	61	72	106	1486
18–19	2880	44.8	0	12.4	0	101	103	143	2103
20–21	1800	44.8	0	12.4	0	101	103	143	2103
			SALT	IN DIET	RESTRICTED.				
22–23	2010	15.0	..	11.8	0	122	107	143	2199
23–24	1290	15.0	..	11.8	0	131	97	144	2208
24–25	1050	15.0	..	11.8	0	119	95	144	2152

The quantity of sodium chloride in 30 grams of cooked bacon at one hospital amounted to 3.3 grams and at another hospital to 7.3 grams.

An oatmeal cure is accompanied by the use of much salt. In the preparation of the standard 240 grams dry oatmeal a cook would employ about 10 grams salt. This may be of importance in the explanation of the edema which often accompanies the oatmeal cure.

Vegetable foods are rich in potassium and, as any farmer's child who salts the cattle Sunday mornings knows, deficient in sodium. It is not strange, with our free use of vegetables, that diabetic patients, like cattle, crave salt. But there is still another reason, because when an excess of potassium is eaten, it is quickly discharged and along with the potassium goes sodium as well. A meat diet requires little salt.

Attention may be called to the low excretion of salt in coma. In one case (No. 1053) two days before death the quantity of salt was 1.28 grams, and in the twenty-four hours preceding death amounted to but 0.44 gram. Magnus-Levy's[1] series of cases of severe acidosis showed a low salt excretion particularly in those which were fatal. It is possible that under such conditions renal insufficiency may enter in.

[1] Magnus-Levy: Die Oxy-Buttersäure, Leipzig, F. C. W. Vogel, 1899.

SECTION VI.

TREATMENT.

A. PREVENTION.[1]

THERE are entirely too many diabetic patients in the country. Statistics for the last thirty years show so great an increase in the number that, unless this were in part explained by a better recognition of the disease, the outlook for the future would be startling. In 1900, the death-rate from diabetes in the registration area of the United States was 10 per 100,000 and in 1920, 16 per 100,000. In the same period in Boston, it rose from 14 to 23 on the same basis. There are probably 1,000,000 diabetics in the United States. Therefore, it is proper at the present time to devote attention not alone to treatment, but still more, as in the campaign against typhoid fever, to prevention. The results may not be quite so striking or so immediate, but they are sure to come and to be important.

The prophylactic and etiological treatment of diabetes will surely play an important rôle in the future, and it is already plain that progress will be along two lines: (1) Toward the early detection of the disease; and (2) toward the prevention of the development of the disease in those susceptible to it. The whole trend of Naunyn's teaching favors the energetic treatment of the slightest evidence of diabetes. Only by following this plan are regrets avoided. The importance of the treatment of incipient pulmonary tuberculosis is not greater than that of the treatment of incipient diabetes. The tendency to diabetes frequently remains latent for a long time, and this is well illustrated by the appearance of diabetes in the children before it occurs in the parent. In many instances the disease breaks out temporarily before the glycosuria becomes permanent. Case No. 129 showed sugar in the urine in 1901, at the age of three years "at a time when she appeared out of condition. Examining frequently after that I failed to find it

---

[1] On pages 471 to 473, there are sentences and occasionally paragraphs which are taken from a paper by the writer in the Jour. Am. Med. Assn., 1921, **76**, 79.

and did not look for it again until in February, 1905, when she appeared like a full-fledged case of diabetes." Death occurred in coma in July, 1907.

Case No. 235 showed 1.3 per cent of sugar in the urine January 3, 1901, at the age of twenty-six years, one month after an attack of severe catarrhal jaundice. The glycosuria disappeared at once on restriction of diet and did not return after resumption of a liberal diet containing sugar. December, 1904, right pyelonephritis, urine sugar-free; January 3, 1905, sugar appeared with a moderate amount of acetone, but no diacetic acid, and the patient became sugar-free with a strict diet and, until July, 1906, was able to eat freely of toast, oatmeal, potato, rice or oranges without glycosuria. Death in coma May 4, 1910.

Case No. 1008, showed sugar in the urine on repeated occasions at the age of forty years, was carefully treated for sixty days and later no sugar was found, but it reappeared when the patient was fifty-one, and he came under my observation three years later, with severe diabetes.

1. **Early Diagnosis.**—The only way in which an early diagnosis of diabetes will ever be made is to search for it. It is possible that tests of the blood may soon give us still earlier hints of the presence of the disease, but at present the only practical method is to make frequent examinations of the twenty-four-hour quantity of urine or single specimens one hour after meals.

(*a*) **A Plea for Early Diagnosis.**—"Diabetes does not develop over night."[1] It is well known that diabetic patients come too late for treatment. If the disease is detected early it is far more susceptible to diet. It is easier to diagnose than tuberculosis. Funck deplored the scant attention paid to the discovery of a trace of sugar in the urine, which was often more a harbinger of death than an apical tuberculosis. How considerable was the interval between the date of the onset and the beginning of treatment can be inferred by the loss of weight that occurred during this period in 600 of my cases. The reduction below the maximum weight amounted on the average to 30 pounds. One of the reasons for this delay in diagnosis is the neglect of frequent or routine urinary examinations. Thus, in 77 successive cases of diabetes, in which the patients were especially questioned with this in view, it was found that in 30 instances there had been no urinary examination before the disease was discovered, and in 18 instances the interval since the previous examination was three or more years. Therefore, it is necessary to establish the custom of urinary examinations being made more frequently and more universally. Every

---

[1] John: Ohio State Med. Jour., 1921, **17**, 826.

one should have the urine examined on his or her birthday. Start the custom with the children and it will persist to old age. How easily new cases of diabetes can be brought to light, the subjoined incident will disclose:

March 30, 1920, there came to my office a woman with diabetes. She was given the usual examination with suggestions for treatment, and as it was impracticable for her to enter the hospital, she was taught on the spot to examine her urine. She went home and shortly after contracted pneumonia and died. But in the intervening days amid her household cares she found time and took enough interest to examine the urines of ten others in her boarding house, and in so doing discovered the presence of diabetes in a boy. She gave him sound advice and sent him to his own physician, who also subsequently died and eventually the boy came to me, telling this story. On the day she learned the Benedict test and made these ten urinary examinations for her friends, Louisa Drumm, Case No. 1796, was seventy-nine years and four months old.

The physician should take pride in the prevention of diabetes in his practice. Obese patients should be frankly told that they are candidates for diabetes. The physician should consider it as important to prevent his patients acquiring diabetes as he feels it incumbent on himself to vaccinate them against smallpox or typhoid fever, or to protect them from exposure to tuberculosis.

The results of life insurance examinations (see p. 122) show how useful such examinations are, and it is a hopeful sign that the insurance companies are offering to examine gratis at frequent intervals the urines of their policy holders. No physician should see a patient without examining the urine at least every six months, and no physician should discharge a patient after a contagious disease without examining the urine. The urine should be tested before departure from a hospital as well as at entrance. But the responsibility for urinary examinations rests not alone upon the family physician. It is the duty of all specialists either to examine the urines of their patients or to assure themselves that such examinations have been recently made, and the time is not far distant when this course will be adopted by progressive dentists as well. One of the greatest aids to this policy has been the establishment of laboratories where patients and physicians can secure examinations of urine at trifling cost. Such institutions have come to stay.

A routine fasting blood sugar estimation for every patient is insisted upon by John[1] just as the Wassermann test is routinely applied.

Recognizing the hereditary and familial tendency, relatives of

---

[1] John: Texas State Jour. Med., February, 1923.

a diabetic patient should always be kept under supervision, and urinary examinations should be made at more frequent intervals than in other individuals. Particularly should the urines of such individuals be carefully examined when conditions arise which would favor the development of diabetes. A family physician should treat not only the patient he is called in to see but should take an active interest in the other members of the family as well. One should also endeavor to prevent the outbreak of diabetes by instructing individuals hereditarily burdened (1) to control the total quantity of food eaten by their body weight; and (2) to take carbohydrate almost exclusively in the form of starch rather than sugar, and never to indulge in unusual quantities of carbohydrate, such as candy, maple sugar, or sweet fruits. (3) It would be a great mistake to consider the diet alone of importance. Mental relaxation and physical exercise should be promoted. If we are to bring about a decrease of diabetes in the community it will be with measures such as these. Every agency which promotes health and physical development tends to prevent an outbreak of the diabetic tendency. "It is easier to keep well than to get well." (Greeley.)

It would be most unfortunate for two individuals each hereditarily burdened with diabetes to wed, though by care in environmental conditions the consequences of heredity might be averted and the tendency decrease in the third generation.[1]

Who would say that the onset of diabetes in George M., Case No. 2151, aged twenty years could not have been prevented? His grandfather and father had diabetes. His weight was 29 per cent above standard for his age, and he reports eating two whole pies a day and a whole bottle of cream on his pudding on Sunday. Now, he has cataract though the diabetes is mild.

2. **Prevention.**—Real headway against the ravages of a disease begins with its prevention rather than with its treatment. Prevention implies a knowledge of the predisposing agency.

(a) **Obesity.**—Overweight predisposes to diabetes. The individual overweight, is at least twice, and at some ages forty times, as liable to the disease. For the prevention of more than half of the cases of diabetes in this country, no radical undernutrition is necessary; the individual is simply asked to maintain the weight of his average fellow man. (See Table 255, p. 761.) Obesity affords a splendid opportunity for the physician in which to practice preventive medicine. The individual who allows himself or herself to become fat may easily develop diabetes. It is desirable to spread the information that those live longest who above the age of thirty-

---

[1] Pribram: Ztschr. f. klin. Med., 1914, **81**, 120.

five years are 5 to 10 per cent below the average normal weight and that so little an excess of weight as 5 per cent is fraught with danger. Patients should be cautioned against gaining weight at any period, but particularly after infectious diseases, pregnancy, the climacteric, and following changes from an active to a sedentary mode of life. Since obese patients are prone to diabetes, they should have frequent examinations of the urine made. Although emphasis is usually laid upon the appearance of sugar in the urine with a patient losing weight, it cannot be too strongly emphasized that it is a common occurrence for sugar to appear in the urine when a patient is gaining weight. The first hint of diabetes occurred in Case No. 1207 when she weighed 142 pounds in 1895, but the disease did not become established in full force until 1912, when her weight was 248 pounds. In 1917, her weight was 200 pounds, and in 1921, she was "in the very best of health."

Diabetics who had never been obese according to medico-actuarial weight standards were found to have been 10 per cent over weight when compared with Dreyer's standard. These data are obtained by Root and Miles[1] in a study of 133 diabetic men and women from my clinic. The greater the previous obesity the greater the duration in these cases.

(b) **Infectious Diseases.**—In the presence of a wasting disease, diabetes is almost unknown. With the advent of tuberculosis and cancer, it may almost disappear. This is the foundation for the modern treatment suggested by Dr. Allen, who substituted for these wasting diseases the symptom, emaciation, without the disease. If the principle of low nutrition is effective in treatment, how much more will it be effective in prevention? And this the statistics of these 1,000 cases prove.

The development of diabetes following infectious diseases is less common than I anticipated before a careful search of my own cases was made. (See p. 148.) Cases of diabetes following infectious disease, however, are so startling when they do occur and at times, though by no means always (see the case of Schmitz, p. 130), are apt to be so severe that the physician should always examine the urines of patients during an infectious disease, during convalescence and without fail before discharging the patient. This is doubly important because a nephritis might be disclosed even though diabetes were not. The usefulness of urinary examinations will become increasingly apparent just as soon as busy physicians get the habit of testing the urine for albumin and sugar in the patient's home with as little formality as they make a test of the blood-pressure.

---

[1] Root and Miles: Jour. Metab. Research, 1922, **2**, 173.

(c) **Pregnancy.**—During pregnancy sugar is apt to occur in the urine. The subject will be discussed more in detail later on under the Treatment of Diabetes in Pregnancy. It is mentioned here simply to emphasize the point that mild cases of glycosuria, which go untreated in pregnancy, may later on in the same or in subsequent pregnancies become aggravated cases of diabetes. Perhaps some, and I suspect many, of the cases of diabetes in pregnancy may be really renal glycosuria. With blood-sugar examinations this point can probably be cleared up within a few years. At any rate it is perhaps unnecessary to exclude absolutely the last trace of sugar from the urine in pregnancy when the sugar amounts to only 0.2 or 0.3 per cent on a diet which contains as much as 100 grams of carbohydrate or more, particularly if the percentage of sugar in the blood is normal. It is essential that the percentage of sugar should be kept as low as this, and upon the first indication of an increase routine diabetic treatment should be instituted. Blood sugar tests have taken away much of the anxiety which a trace of sugar during pregnancy formerly elicited. Observation of such cases over many years may also cast light upon the problem as to whether a renal glycosuric in the course of time becomes a true diabetic.

(d) **Gall Stones.**—Whereas cirrhosis of the liver appeared but 8 times in 1993 fatal cases as a cause of death, diseases of the gall-bladder, as revealed by the presence of gall stones, are often associated with diabetes. The gall-bladder and the ducts of the liver are so near the pancreas that it is not unreasonable to suppose that frequently the pancreatitis which may lead to the destruction of the islands of Langerhans may actually originate in the gall-bladder region. If this premise is correct, one should hope to prevent diabetes by taking especial pains to cure promptly any diseases of the gall-bladder which can be diagnosed. Of 36 cases of so-called alimentary glycosuria seen by Eustis,[1] 15 showed definite gall stone disease. Six of these later presented symptoms of definite diabetes.

The influence of gall stones in the development of diabetes was strikingly shown in Case No. 954, described in the section upon the Etiology of Diabetes, p. 146.

The mildness of the character of the diabetes which occurs in association with gall stones is notable. Some of the most favorable cases occuring in my practice have been of this type. Several cases of diabetes associated with gall stones have done remarkably well when the inflammation about the gall stones has subsided. They suggest that surgical intervention might be advantageously

---

[1] Eustis: New Orleans Med. and Surg. Jour., 1923, **75**, 449.

employed in other selected cases. Case No. 18, age at onset of diabetes thirty-five years, first seen by me in August, 1900, at the age of thirty-nine years, showed no symptoms of diabetes for the following years; previously she had symptoms of gall stones. These symptoms disappeared, though the roentgen-ray demonstrated in 1916 the presence of calculi, and three years later, in 1919, despite a blood-pressure of 200/110, attacks of biliary colic occurred and the patient was operated upon and gall stones found. The patient finally died of chronic nephritis in 1922.

Case No. 309, went through a period of involuntary fasting and loss of weight because of digestive symptoms, sugar disappeared, tolerance trebled and roentgen-ray showed gall stones.

One of the most remarkable cases is that of Case No. 845. She noticed polyuria, sent her urine to a chemist for examination, who reported 6.58 per cent sugar. Her history showed previous attacks of inflammation in the gall-bladder region and in 1913, she was operated upon and gall stones found. There has been no recurrence of the gall-bladder trouble. Her diabetes has remained so mild that she goes for months without more than a trace of sugar in the urine and usually with none and is in better health today, 1923, than at any time since coming to me for treatment in March, 1915.

Still another case, Case No. 310, is striking. This patient developed diabetes at the age of seventeen years, gall stones were definitely diagnosed at the age of twenty-one years, and the duration of her diabetes was twenty-one years. Unfortunately, as described on p. 318, she died at sea.

Dr. Allen has quoted a whole series of interesting cases relating to diseases of the pancreas and liver in which sugar disappeared.

The favorable course of diabetes with 73 patients in the presence of gall stones is shown in Table 182. The average age at the diagnosis of gall stones in this series of cases was forty-five years, and the average age at the onset of diabetes was forty-seven years. It would seem clear that the gall stones preceded the diabetes rather than that the diabetes preceded the gall stones, despite numerous, seeming inconsistencies with this statement in the table. Twenty-two of these patients were males, 51 females and 69 of the total number, 73, were married. The average age at operation for gall stones in 26 cases was forty-five years. In 4 of these cases the average age at death was fifty-three years, showing a duration after operation of two and seven-tenths years, and in 20 others who are still alive the average is already fifty-two years, showing a duration since the operation of seven and two-tenths years. Two cases who had operations are untraced.

TABLE 182.—DIABETES IN ASSOCIATION WITH GALL STONES. TOTAL, 73. FEMALES, 51; MALES, 22.

Case No. and sex.	Age at: Diagnosis of gall stones, years.	Age at: Onset of diabetes, years.	Duration of diabetes, years. Living, Jan., 1923.	Duration of diabetes, years. Fatal.	Age at operation.
8 F.		60		14	58
18 F.		35		25	
177 M.	25	46	22		
200 M.	54	61		5	66
228 F.		55		11	47
268 F.	47	35	13		
273 M.	56	56		9	
309 F.	20	35	25		
310 F.	21	17		21	
422 F.	45	52	12		43
457 F.	43	55		7	
469 F.	52	55	11		
488 M.	40	59		5	48
560 M.	40	66	Untr.		
568 F.	48	57	14		55
639 F.	55	55	13		
697 M.	54	49	23	2	57
727 F.	52	52	8		49
799 F.	35	44		7	
839 M.	55	55	23		52
845 M.	57	59	8		28
954 F.	49	50	11		
981 F.	27	28	Untr.	5	
992 F.	52	42	31	2	
1061 F.	28	47	Untr.		
1062 F.	43	43	10		43
1170 M.	35	40	7		
1182 F.		38	6		
1210 F.	39	28	11		
1244 F.	43	43	8		44
1245 F.	49	44	6		27
1289 F.		58	8	5	28
1331 F.	44	44	6		
1389 F.	27	25	6		
1390 F.	28	31	6	5	
1391 F.	60	57	10		
1462 F.	48	40			
1531 F.	52	52	4		
1592 F.	28	28	6		28
1594 M.		36		::	
1672 M.	23	43	3	15	
1674 M.	60	63	7		60
1708 F.	43	46	5	::	
1741 M.	50	56	Untr.		
1785 M.	59	59	3		
1807 F.	51	37	8		
1815 F.	39	39	6		39
1900 F.	52	53	11	::	52
1987 F.	49	56	5	::	49
1994 M.	36	46	9	::	36 and 46
2071 F.	41	53	2		
2102 F.		42	2		
2115 M.	70	73	2		
2116 F.	60	60		6	
2139 F.	56	50	8		
2148 M.	41	40		13	
2164 M.	49	51	11		31
2190 M.	31	27	8		35
2200 M.	35	35	9		
2219 M.	64	61	2		
2283 M.	58	62	2		
2308 F.		43	1		
2373 F.	53	53	1		53
2386 F.	37	45	2		
2398 M.	24	46	Untr.		
2416 F.		25	3		
2491 F.	41	46	10		52
2493 F.		45	2		
2605 F.	47	47	1		47
2659 F.	68	69	2		
2688 F.	45	45	7		44
2763 F.	44	47	1		44
2766 F.	39	38	2		
Average	46	48	5	11	44

The favorable duration of life of diabetic patients with gall stones is remarkable, whether they have been operated upon or not. Thus, of the 17 fatal cases the duration of the disease was ten years and in the living up to January 1, 1923, is already eight years. It would appear that if one is to have diabetes the gall stone variety is to be preferred.

My advice to non-diabetic patients with gall stones is to be operated upon not only because of the danger of repeated attacks of gall stones and of the danger of a subsequent carcinoma, but also because of the danger of the development of diabetes. In diabetic patients my advice is to have the gall stones removed when the conditions of time, place, surgeon, and physician are all propitious.

(e) **Hygiene.**—(1) *Physical Hygiene.*—Any agency which promotes physical or mental hygiene is a step toward the prevention of diabetes in the predisposed, and the abatement of its severity when it has appeared. It should be recorded to the credit of Dr. A. J. Hodgson[1] that for years in dealing with his patients he has urged that they "should be kept mentally indolent and physically active." A good many young men may have escaped diabetes by going to war. (See p. 120.) I have never forgotten the remark of Dr. Sabine, of Brookline, that in the course of his long practice he had observed that those of his patients who had taken active camping trips in the woods bore the stress of modern life best. By this means exercise was combined with mental relaxation. That the good effects of each last for months is not hard to believe. It is only natural to conclude that if the muscles, in which is stored one-half of the carbohydrate of the body, are kept in good condition by training, a favorable effect must be exercised upon the general metabolism of carbohydrate. The man who, in middle life, gives up hard physical work and is promoted to an office chair with increased mental worry is exposed to diabetes.

Finally, it is astonishing how much exercise a diabetic in training can take. One of my severe cases living on a strict diet several years ago walked between 20 and 30 miles in one day. H. H., Case No. 1889, while taking insulin walked 10 miles a day and occasionally thereby accelerated an hypoglycemic reaction. Since taking insulin Case No. 632 has raised his standard of muscular efficiency from 71 per cent up to 89 per cent according to measurements of R. Fitz.

Mental Hygiene.—The change in the mental attitude of patients during the course of treatment is a gratifying encouragement to the physician. Untreated diabetics after a moderate number of years

[1] Hodgson: Jour. Am. Med. Assn., 1911, **57**, 1187.

usually show mental depression, and with women this often becomes pronounced. In the first ten years of my experience with diabetes I was much impressed with the tendency of such patients to cry, but even then, with the methods in vogue, it was interesting to see how depression disappeared with the decrease or disappearance of sugar in the urine. This could not be explained by the mental encouragement which a patient derived from his knowledge of the decrease in sugar excretion. Even when patients became free from sugar but developed acidosis mental symptoms often improved, and to so great an extent that one could say that with treatment, even though it did end in coma, the patient enjoyed life far more thoroughly than when untreated, his life ended with debility or tuberculosis. Greeley explained to my patients how diabetes has largely been robbed of its terrors. He urged the simple life as a great aid in treatment and told them not to try to be first in the Iberian village and be ill, but rather to be second in Rome and keep well. He told them to have a hobby, and not to make it a labor; to be cheerful and to keep their minds occupied, and as far as possible to continue the previous currents of their lives.

Heavy responsibilities should be avoided as well as nervous upsets and emotional excitements. It is almost as dangerous for a diabetic to get angry as for a man with angina pectoris. Case No. 1157 had been sugar-free for five days, but it came back when he had an important conference with one of his superintendents.

Psychological tests were applied by Miles and Root[1] to 40 diabetic patients prior to the introduction of insulin, and an average decrement of 15 per cent was found at the beginning of treatment in their performance of memory and attention tasks. With treatment the patients improved rapidly in psychological status but did not quite reach normal.

In accuracy and quickness of movements 5 treated diabetics of long duration were 20 per cent below normal.

(*f*) **Effect of Exercise.**—The effect of exercise upon the utilization of carbohydrate has excited interest for many years. Von Noorden, referring to this subject, writes: "Wide individual differences exist with regard to this matter. It is found that some patients can tolerate much more carbohydrate when taking plenty of exercise; with others this is not the case, muscular work doing them more harm than good."[2] At the Nutrition Laboratory a small series of experiments were conducted by Benedict and myself and published in 1910.[3] Allen and DuBois[4] have also recorded a

---

[1] Miles and Root: Arch. Int. Med., 1922, **30**, 757.

[2] Von Noorden: Diabetes Mellitus, E. B. Treat Company, 1905, p. 177.

[3] Benedict and Joslin: Metabolism in Diabetes Mellitus, Carnegie Inst. Pub. 136, p. 217.

[4] Loc. cit., p. 466.

slight rise in the respiratory quotient of a severely diabetic patient undergoing mild exercises during two respiration experiments. The evidence collected in the two laboratories was not enough to warrant general conclusions, but in so far as it went, it tended to show that during exercise there was a slightly increased combustion of carbohydrate, as shown by a rise in the respiratory quotient and also a rise in the total metabolism. Nehring and Schmoll[1] concluded that muscular activity in diabetics was also at the expense of glycogen from the fact that it was possible in many instances to reduce the sugar excretion by controlling the muscular activity. This is also fully in accord with the experiments made by Mohr[2] in which he found with a diabetic dog that there was a noticeable increase in the respiratory quotient during walking, and therefore he concluded that diabetics can burn but little glycogen until there is the most urgent need for it.

The blood sugar is lowered according to Sakaguchi[3] by exercise and this would seem probable from the development of an insulin reaction in Case No. 1889, when he took a walk of 10 miles, but not otherwise.

The following clinical observations are of interest: Case No. 112, a doctor, and a good observer, noticed that the quantity of sugar in the urine always decreased while on hard camping trips in Maine, although the diet contained the same, or probably more, carbohydrate than when he was at home. Case No. 22, a Harvard professor, said to me in 1901 that "mental work makes sugar, manual work burns it up." Case No. 511, shows sugar when hard at work in the city, but when quite as occupied with mental work in the country, but with more exercise and a similar diet, shows no sugar. Since my attention has been directed to this question by Allen's experimental work, I recall instances of diabetics who were able to carry on severe muscular labor, although the diabetes was of extreme severity. One striking case of this type was a railroad inspector, who traversed several times a day alone in a handcar many miles of railway, and yet maintained fair health, much to the astonishment of his physician and myself. I was always impressed in former days of treatment by the better results frequently obtained by ambulatory as compared with the hospital treatment at that time, provided the same degree of attention was given to the details of the diet and hygiene of the patient. According to the result of recent work it would seem now as if this was in part due to the individual maintaining his ordinary vocation, and thus undergoing considerable muscular work.

[1] Nehring and Schmoll: Ztschr. f. klin. Med., 1907, **31**, 59.
[2] Mohr: Ztsch. f. exper. Path. u Therap., 1907, **4**, 939.
[3] Sakaguchi: Mitt. d. Med. Fakultät d. Kais. Universität zu Tokyo, 1918, **29**, 471.

31

Finally, upon investigation of 29 cases of diabetes of fifteen or more years' duration, it is apparent that in many of these considerable activity was maintained throughout life.

Allen[1] has found that diabetic dogs with a known constant limit for tolerance of carbohydrate or protein upon vigorous exercise in a treadmill showed a marked increase in tolerance, as demonstrated both by the sugar in the urine and in the blood. He further says that dogs which have for months regularly shown glycosuria whenever they were given 100 grams of bread, on exercise became able to take 200 grams of bread as a regular daily ration without glycosuria. With patients, he has observed results sufficiently favorable to warrant recommending exercise as an addition to treatment, and he goes on to say that in a patient free from glycosuria with a persistent hyperglycemia, one fast day with exercise may reduce the blood sugar as much as several fast days without exercise.

(*g*) **Syphilis** is discussed on p. 605.

B. CLASSIFICATION FOR TREATMENT.

1. **Classification for Treatment.**—A classification of diabetic cases based upon the assimilation of carbohydrate will always be found helpful in their treatment. It is customary to divide cases of diabetes into three types; mild, moderately severe and severe. Such a classification, however, can never be arbitrary, because cases which at first appear to belong to the severest type of the disease may run a favorable course and cases showing at the outset only a small quantity of sugar may prove to be quite intractable. For this reason Naunyn did not pretend to be able to distinguish accurately between types. Furthermore, up to the present time it has nearly always been considered that diabetes was a progressive disease, and that each patient, if he lived long enough, was destined to pass through the three stages. Time alone will decide whether this unfortunate conception of the malady may be given up. In illustration of the above, Case No. 344 belonged to the type of mild diabetes for nearly four years, but gradually the character of the disease changed, and ultimately reached its greatest severity in this patient; tuberculosis then intervened, acidosis disappeared, and he died, four years after the onset, of tuberculosis rather than of coma. The diabetes had resumed its mild character. Case No. 8 responded so well to treatment as to justify being classed as mild in type, and even at the end of fourteen years was only moderately severe, death ensuing without acidosis but as a result of arteriosclerotic complications.

---

[1] Allen: Boston Med, and Surg. Jour., 1915, **173**, 743.

Case No. 552 appeared to belong to the severe type of diabetes, but after prolonged treatment improved so much as to reach the border-line of the moderately severe group. Diabetes in children is usually looked upon as severe, but a distinct fraction of these cases prove to be mild. The mere presence of 9 per cent of sugar in the urine when the patient is upon an unrestricted diet is no proof of severity. (See Case No. 2962, p. 55.) Of the last 100 cases seen in 1915, 12 were considered as severe cases, 52 moderate and the remaining 36 cases mild, but the last 100 cases prior to March 1, 1917, the statistics were 8 severe, 47 moderately severe, and 45 mild. In 1923, of 100 consecutive cases recently seen 2 were considered severe, 21 moderately severe, and 77 mild.

Most diabetics are mild and the percentage of mild cases to the total number of diabetics has been constantly increasing.

In this book the classification of diabetes is based upon the supposition that severe cases of diabetes have a tolerance from 0 to 10 grams carbohydrate, moderately severe cases have a tolerance from 10 to 50 grams of carbohydrate, and that the remaining cases are mild. I have not yet brought myself to the point of determining the severity in terms of glucose tolerance. Units of insulin will undoubtedly soon be in vogue for purposes of classification, perhaps with the patient upon 1 gram of carbohydrate, 1 gram of protein and 2 grams of fat per kilogram body weight. If no insulin is needed the case can be regarded as mild, if less than 30 units are required to prevent glycosuria, the case can be called moderate, and cases requiring 30 or more units can be called severe. By this standard about 5 per cent of my cases taking insulin would be classified as severe.

The presence, absence or intensity of acidosis affords an unsatisfactory basis for classification. Even the mildest case of diabetes by restriction of carbohydrate and increase in the amount of fat can be made to develop an acidosis which will be mild, moderate, or severe in degree.

The respiratory quotient in the series of 113 cases by Benedict and myself proved to be 0.73 for the severe and 0.77 for the moderately severe as well as the mild. But the respiratory quotient depends in such large measure on the diet as to render it an undesirable method by which to differentiate cases of diabetes even if it were practicable. Then, too, the rise in the quotient which has been observed with fasting diabetics confuses the picture.

Any of the above classifications of diabetes denotes the state of the disease at the moment, but gives no information concerning the response of the patient to treatment. Consequently a working classification with this in mind has been adopted at the New England Deaconess Hospital. For the purpose of treatment it is not of so much interest to be told that a patient is a severe or a mild diabetic as it is to be informed whether he is doing very well (A), fairly well (B), not very well (C), or is in a dangerous condition (D). To arrive at such a decision is not difficult with a knowledge at hand of the urine (sugar, diacetic acid, albumin), the diet (carbohydrate, protein, fat) the weight, pulse and blood-pressure. For convenience, upon the slip which gives these data the letters A, B, C, D are printed. Somehow when you yourself deliberately or someone else deliberately scores your patient (D) it makes more of an impression upon the mind than simply to gather from the accumulated reports that he is not doing well. This working classification has proved very helpful. It should save some lives.

2. **Classification for Prognosis.**—It is still more difficult to classify cases of diabetes for prognosis. The past is not a guide. Hitherto a case of diabetes occurring in an individual under the age of thirty years would usually be set down as severe, even though he readily became sugar-free; exceptions occurred now and then when the quantity of sugar was a mere trace and the patient obese. Diabetes beginning at sixty years of age should not shorten the duration of life, provided there is adherence to dietetic rules. Cases often appear severe when first seen, but upon further acquaintance it is found that this is due to some alleviable circumstance, such as the presence of an infection, or, more commonly, the sudden institution of a fat-protein diet with its attendant acidosis. One cannot too strongly emphasize the mild character of most cases of diabetes.

The presence of obesity, a favorable heredity, an early diagnosis, or the history of benign diabetes of several years' duration with gain rather than loss in tolerance, the retention of body weight, are good prognostic signs, but a placid, cheerful, brave and honest disposition, inherent or acquired, is fully as important.

C. DIETETIC TREATMENT.

1. **General Discussion.**—The dietetic treatment of diabetes is extraordinarily simple and yet so engrossing that unless the physician takes care he will fall into schematic ways and forget that it is the patient who comes for treatment and not the diabetes. Each case is to itself. The etiology of the disease in each instance should be carefully investigated and faulty habits corrected. It will often be found that the symptoms which annoy the patient bear little relation to diabetes, and these should be appropriately treated. This is particularly true in the diabetes of middle life and old age, which is so often accompanied by complications. This broad view of the case should be maintained throughout the course of treatment, and whenever unsatisfactory results are ob-

tained the whole situation should be investigated anew to determine whether some radical change in the plan of treatment should be adopted. A surgeon often overlooks grave medical complications in his cases simply because his attention is absorbed by the surgical aspect of his patient. More than once I have discovered in my own practice, as well as in that of others, the existence of advanced tuberculosis which had previously escaped attention.

Patients with diabetes often come to the physician in a state which is endurable. It is the function of the physician to improve upon this state. Only too frequently treatment in the past has done the patient more harm than good, but the fault lies not in the principles of treatment, but rather in their application. The physician who undertakes to treat the patient with diabetes whose condition is comfortable resembles the surgeon who, operating for an interval appendix, assumes a responsibility far greater than when acute symptoms make such an operation imperative.

In illustration of this point I would cite the following instance:

Case No. 473, aged forty-eight years, buried a child of diabetes at the age of fifteen years. During November, 1911, she began to lose weight, and though two quarts of urine were voided, no sugar was found in two *morning* specimens of urine either early in November or December. On December 5, 1911, a little sugar was discovered. January 24, 1912, she consulted a "specialist." The quantity of urine was then 6 quarts, the percentage of sugar 7 per cent, making the total quantity of sugar for the day nearly a pound.

The "specialist" *radically restricted the carbohydrate in the diet* and three days later, in consultation with her family physician, I found her in coma. This is one of the cases which led me to consider the first year following the detection of the disease to be the diabetic's danger zone. It is one of the cases which formerly would have gone down in the literature as "acute diabetes." How needless a death!

The responsibility for the management of the diet of a diabetic patient should always rest upon one individual. As a rule that individual is the patient, but at times another member of the household. Children who are above the age of ten years should be taught to plan their own diet. They readily learn to do this and in so doing make their elders blush. In fact it is more important for diabetic children to learn what and how much to eat than all the knowledge which their schools afford, for upon this information their life depends. A child at five years should be familiar with the Benedict test and what a positive test means for him. Perhaps it is because this personal responsibility is so deeply felt in the management of little children that the treatment of diabetes in them proceeds so uniformly and always produces results so much better than are expected. Conversely, the failure of diabetic patients to do well in the open wards of large hospitals has been due not so much to the alleged dishonesty of the patient as to the division of responsibility among several nurses. Errors in the diet or in the collection of the urine must be promptly traced to their source.

The treatment of a patient with diabetes lasts through life. Treatment must therefore be adjusted to this condition and should be so arranged that it can be continued for years without harm. The more concrete one's directions to a diabetic the more likely they are to be followed; likewise the easier it is for the doctor to discover the severity of the case, and later to see why this diet has worked well and that diet worked poorly. It is well nigh impossible to correct the diet unless the patient is following some definite plan, eating a certain daily total of carbohydrate, protein, and fat. It is impossible for the patient to play his part and to follow the plan unless we make it simple. This is the reason why card after card of directions for patients has been tried. This also explains why whole numbers instead of decimals have been employed in computing the food values of the diet.

The reasons for the treatment prescribed should be made real to the patient from the very start. It should be visibly demonstrated to him that the quantity of sugar which he is excreting amounts to a pound, more or less, in twenty-four hours, and as his diet is curtailed he should be shown that the sugar in the urine decreases. The quantity of sugar and starch in the common foods which he is to eat or not eat, but will see constantly before him, should be impressed upon him. He should learn that a large apple weighs 300 grams (10 ounces) and contains 3 tablespoonfuls of sugar, that a moderate-sized apple contains 2 tablespoonfuls, and that a small apple weighs about 100 grams, almost a quarter of a pound, and contains 1 tablespoonful of sugar, the same amount as in a medium-sized orange. It is worth while to set forth the dangers of bread by comparing the 18 grams carbohydrate in 30 grams (1 ounce), with the same amount which is contained in 540 grams (18 ounces) of 5 per cent vegetables, or even 900 grams of lettuce. It takes but a moment to point out that in a Uneeda biscuit are 5 grams of carbohydrate, in a Triscuit 8 grams, and in one Shredded Wheat biscuit 23 grams, that an egg has 6 grams of protein and 6 grams of fat. The patient may not learn all the food values, but he must be taught what kind of food he is to eat, what it weighs, or its size. If he does not know but one 5 per cent vegetable, let him live upon that until he learns another. In hospitals there should be daily lessons. The patient is at school to learn how to save his life. Time should be taken at the beginning of treatment to describe thoroughly to the patient the plan of procedure and the necessity of his being under close observation until the urine is sugar-free and until he understands how to keep it so. The diabetic patient should be made to realize that he has a lesson to learn, and the earlier he learns it, the sooner he can be discharged.

Office visits are sufficient for the treatment and education of the patient, but they are time consuming. The urine should be examined at the visit, preferably a twenty-four-hour specimen, because precise directions must be given at once, otherwise the patient may continue an improper diet needlessly. Orders should be written down in the patient's notebook just as carefully as they are in the hospital's order book. At each visit a specimen of the twenty-four-hour quantity of urine should be brought, or better sent, in advance, together with a written list of the character and weighed quantities of the food eaten during the same period. So soon as carelessness in this regard is condoned, indifference to other advice follows. The advantages of having the patient bring a written diet list are twofold: (1) It is more accurate, and (2) it saves an enormous amount of the physician's time. (See p. 682.) The changes in weight of the patient should be recorded. The specimen of urine should be that of the twenty-four hours immediately preceding the visit, but if it is not, do not neglect to immediately secure and test a specimen while the patient is at the office. In diabetes one cannot be in too close touch with the actual condition of the patient at the moment.

Urinary tests were not taught formerly, because doctors could not keep the urines sugar-free. Today the situation is altered and any modern patient knows that without urinary examinations a diabetic cannot secure the best results. Patients weary of testing the urine, but only under very exceptional circumstances should they be allowed to omit making the test. A daily negative Benedict reaction gives confidence and, on the other hand, in the presence of danger, it is never wise to follow the habits of the ostrich.

In what follows, treatment is based primarily on urinary examinations, and secondarily on the estimation of the blood sugar. Since Gray's studies and the advent of insulin the usefulness of the examination of several single specimens of urine in a single day has become apparent. The study of the blood lipoids is in its infancy and it is seldom as yet therapeutically useful in the individual case. Even examinations of the blood sugar are not yet sufficiently simple to be available to most physicians, and furthermore, not enough experience has been gained to indicate arbitrarily how one should proceed when the urine has become sugar-free and the blood sugar is persistently high. Nevertheless, the ratio of blood tests to urine tests is constantly increasing and I expect will continue to increase in my practice. Probably the fact that so few patients can secure blood tests after leaving the hospital makes me depend so much on urinary examinations.

Undernutrition widened the horizon for the diabetic, but insulin has given him back his old world of work and joy. Without undernutrition a large share of the wonders attributed to insulin would not have been forthcoming. One can well stand aghast at the thought of the deaths which would result from the greatly increased insulin diets had not the prevention and treatment of coma become matters of routine. The simplicity of undernutrition shows its worth and the increasing duration of life of diabetics since its introduction, is largely, though by no means wholly, to be explained by it. But it must not be forgotten that the first year of diabetes following the discovery of the disease is the diabetic's danger zone. Yet diabetes is an out-and-out chronic disease, and the greatest mortality from it should occur not in the first year following its discovery but in later years. It is my firm belief that the first year of a diabetic's life should be his safest, and that the reason that this has not been the case is best explained by the method of treatment to which he has been subjected rather than to a lack of treatment.

Formerly two-thirds of all the fatal cases of diabetes I had seen died in diabetic coma. In all but 20 of the fatal cases in children death has been due to coma. My records show that of all those diabetic patients who have succumbed to the disease during the first year of its course, coma claimed 77 per cent. If the first year of the disease is the patient's danger zone, it can be as truly said that the danger and almost the only danger is coma, and brushing aside all technicalities, coma must be considered from the practitioner's standpoint as synonymous with acid poisoning. Therefore, in the plan of treatment which follows it will be seen that from beginning to end the prevention and treatment of acid poisoning is constantly kept in mind. If acidosis exists when the patient comes for treatment, he must be in daily communication with his physician.

Diabetic Creed.—Never before has the plan of campaign for the treatment of diabetes appeared so clearly defined. Never before this year of 1923, thanks to insulin, has it been possible to look to treatment with so much hopefulness. For my own practical guidance I have adopted a diabetic creed but, like the best of the creeds, alterations in it are to be anticipated.

I believe (1) that *diabetes mellitus* should be considered so probable in any person who has 0.1 per cent or more of sugar in the urine by any of the common tests that such a person should be watched for life.

2. That *normal weight,* or less, should be insisted upon in each diabetic, suspected diabetic, or relative of a diabetic, since over-nutrition is the most common antecedent of diabetes.

3. That *mildness* of the diabetes should be assumed and the patient treated accordingly until the contrary is proved. Hence, the nearer the proportions of carbohydrate, protein, and fat in the diabetic diet conform to those of the normal diet, always avoiding glycosuria, the better it is for the patient, even at the sacrifice of weight, though not of strength.

4. That *reversal of the diet,* namely high fat and low carbohydrate, assumes the contrary, severity of the diabetes, and is dangerous both in principle and in practice and unless accompanied by a minimum protein intake, frequently ends in coma by directly causing acidosis.

5. That *undernutrition* (*a*) prevents diabetes and (*b*) is the foundation stone of diabetic treatment. Undernutrition resembles in its action our best drugs, morphine and digitalis. These frequently give surprisingly good results, even when they are carelessly employed, but they often do harm, and their true worth is only disclosed when they are prescribed with intelligence. If hunger can be avoided, a smaller number of patients will yield to temptation, break treatment, and in consequence die of coma.

6. That *extreme inanition* with loss of body protein is not worth while *simply to render the blood sugar normal,* since this procedure may change a mild or a moderate case into a severe case, usually resulting in (*a*) abandonment of diet with resulting temporary benefit from the extra food but followed by early death, or (*b*) fatal inanition after a somewhat longer life. In either case life is shorter and less comfortable than when treatment is less rigorous.

7. That *acidosis,* the chief cause of death in diabetes, is more easily prevented in 99 cases than treated in 1 and therefore diabetics when ill from any cause should (1) go to bed, (2) keep warm, (3) take a glass of hot water, tea, broth, orange juice, or oatmeal watergruel every hour, (4) empty the bowels with an enema, (5) call a doctor who, if he finds acidosis, probably will give them insulin, digitalis and caffeine, may wash out their stomachs, and inject a subcutaneous solution.

That *gangrene,* the other diabetic enemy, should be avoided by extreme cleanliness, care and exercise of the feet by all diabetics over 50 years of age.

8. That the *immediate aim* of practice should be to simplify treatment and to encourage physicians to develop in their *own* communities, homes and boarding houses, clinics, or departments in

hospitals to which they may take or refer their patients for a diabetic education.

9. That any patient with a tolerance of less than 100 grams of carbohydrate should (a) test his own urine for sugar, (b) keep sugar-free, and (c) take home food scales and use them until he can keep sugar-free without them.

10. That *firm persistence* in a strict diabetic diet (a) finds ample justification in the many patients kept alive by it to profit by insulin with its assurance of gain in weight, strength, and mental vigor; and (b) is essential to safety and success in the use of insulin. Insulin utilizes rather than replaces the advances in diabetic treatment hitherto achieved.

Technic of Dietetic Treatment.—To render the urine of the diabetic patient sugar-free at the beginning of treatment is one of the simplest tasks which confronts the physician. Formerly this was considered to be an achievement, but now it is considered simply a matter of routine. But it is not without its danger. Formerly, and by that I mean scarcely a decade ago, when carbohydrate was the only food element carefully regulated for the diabetic this was alone curtailed, and to make up for its loss the patient was urged to devour, not merely eat, protein and fat *ad libitum*. Thereby the ketogenic-antiketogenic balance was upset, acidosis appeared, the patient was then set down as a severe case, the carbohydrate in consequence still more curtailed and as a result the really severe case either died suddenly soon after entrance to the hospital or just barely escaped with his life. The moderately severe diabetics automatically were transformed into severe and many even of the mild type progressed into the moderate group. The doctor, who treated his diabetics the most, had the severest cases for patients and thought his practice unique. I was then almost afraid to send a patient into the hospital believing it safer to allow the patient to eat his accustomed diet at home, gradually reducing the carbohydrate to a moderate degree. In this way the severe cases escaped immediate death and the moderately severe and the mild lived with comparative comfort. Considering all the fat and protein the patients were urged to eat it is a wonder so many survived. There were so many cases of "acute diabetes" that the average duration of life for all diabetics was about three years.

Undernutrition then entered upon the stage, introduced by Guelpa and Allen, though earlier recognized by Weintraud, Naunyn and in this country intuitively perceived by Hodgson. The results were remarkable. Patients became sugar-free who were never sugar-free before, hospital stay was shortened and the number of severe cases was materially reduced, coma was far less frequent and the average length of life of my diabetics rose to four and eight-tenths years. However, diabetic accidents still occasionally occurred and unstable diabetics, the old, the long-standing, the very fat and the diabetics with high metabolism such as those suffering from goiter or from dietary excesses did not react well to abrupt fasting. The ketogenic-antiketogenic balance was here upset by endogenous rather than by exogenous factors and the exceptional case developed coma. Notwithstanding its presence, coma was encountered with undernutrition far less than with the previous overnutrition. It was at this stage that the old practice of gradually changing the diet proved of service and I found safety in omitting fats, thereby somewhat securing the advantage of undernutrition and at the same stroke lessening the formation of ketone bodies, and also by diminishing the carbohydrate and protein until the results of undernutrition so much improved the tolerance that enough of the carbohydrate was burned to prevent acidosis. With this regimen hospital deaths from coma during treatment were abolished and the entrance of new patients into the hospital was not a cause for alarm. Forced by lack of assistants before entering the army, a series of test diets was instituted by which to make the patient sugar-free. Of these there were five. Fat was absent from all with the design to reduce the source of acid bodies to the minimum, protein was gradually reduced and the carbohydrate curtailed in steps from 200 grams to 15 in five days. These diets were a great time saver, gave the nurses a definite program and worked so well that the statement is warranted that I have heard of or experienced but two cases of diabetic coma when they were employed with patients not already in the clutches of coma. A few years later a series of Maintenance Diets was added and though these cannot be employed as schematically, they have helped the writer much. These diets tended toward deficiency in calories; they thus avoided coma but promoted inanition. Before describing these diets further or the alterations made in them the next element in the improvement of diabetic treatment which took place will be described.

The practical importance of endogenous metabolism for the diabetic as well as for Benedict's fasting normal man was the note then sounded by Newburgh and Marsh, and explained in detail by Woodyatt. Utilizing a diet of undernutrition, which perhaps they scarcely appreciated at first, and a protein ration far below bodily requirements Newburgh and Marsh demonstrated that with 15 grams of carbohydrate, 10 grams of protein and 89 grams of fat, acidosis did not develop. They pointed out that it was no more harmful to furnish the diabetic exogenous fat for consumption than to compel him to subsist upon his own. Other advantages

and disadvantages of their program will be discussed later. (See
p. 525.) It will suffice for present needs to say that as a result of
their teachings I returned into my Test and Maintenance Diets a
portion of the fat taken away. This was all the more readily done
because the result of the metabolism tests at the Carnegie Laboratory
upon normals and diabetics in undernutrition had vividly shown
that the value of a pound of body weight was equivalent to 1500
calories. With slight additions it was easy to insert into the series
of diets even more calories without the diets losing their function
of undernutrition. Likewise a lower protein ration was utilized,
about 1 gram per kilogram body weight, though not as low as
that of Newburgh and Marsh or of Petrén, of which more anon.
(See p. 529.)

The need of balanced diets began to be gradually recognized.
Shaffer and Woodyatt started the current in this direction, and
Woodyatt's formula by which the ketone forming elements of the
diet could be estimated and balanced against the antiketone elements
was the first to gain general adoption. In a word, his formula
$\left(F = 2C + \dfrac{P}{2} \right)$ indicated that the fat in the diet should not be
more than twice the carbohydrate plus half the protein. (See p.
462.) Woodyatt emphasized the necessity of estimating the
total glucose in the diet, counting for each gram of carbohydrate
1 gram of glucose, for each gram of protein 0.58 gram glucose
(which for convenience one may safely reckon at 0.6), and for each
gram of fat 0.1 gram glucose. From the total glucose of the diet
thus computed the sugar in the urine can be subtracted to get the
glucose balance. For the other formulæ of Woodyatt and Shaffer,
see pp. 459 to 462.

The dietetic treatment of diabetes today thus rests upon a
surer foundation than ever before. There are still different systems,
but undernutrition is utilized in one stage or another in all, and
all diets are planned to be adjusted so properly that the ketone-
forming elements shall be so related to the antiketone-forming
elements that acidosis shall not result. As a rule so much carbohydrate can be burned by the patient that this question eventually
does not arise. Indeed, this will rarely, if ever, take place if the
protein in the diet is held at 1 gram per kilogram body weight
and the grams of fat at not more than three times the grams of
carbohydrate. If the patient is not sugar-free upon this schedule,
the protein should be reduced to $\frac{2}{3}$ of 1 gram per kilogram
body weight. The grams of fat can then be raised with a fair
degree of safety to four times the grams of utilized carbohydrate.
Should the patient not remain sugar-free with this combination,
until dietetic theories were revolutionized by insulin, undernutri-

tion was the only recourse. Yet with insulin the best results are obtainable only when the tenets of the above program are followed to the letter.

The dietetic treatment of the average diabetic is extraordinarily simple. Upon entrance to the hospital if the patient is placed upon Test Diet 1 and at the end of each twenty-four hours progresses to the diet of the following day, that patient will be a rare exception who will not become sugar-free before the four Test Diets are completed and the first Maintenance Diet is reached, as outlined in Table 183. Even should a trace or a few tenths per cent of sugar remain in the urine, this usually disappears during the days of under-nutrition of the early Maintenance Diets. So striking have been the results obtained with these diets that I have been impressed as never before with the inherent mildness of diabetes, even in the presence of high percentages of sugar. Indeed, the early untreated case who shows 9 per cent of sugar is about the most amenable to treatment. The refractory cases are the long-standing ones with low percentages of sugar upon moderate diets.

TABLE 183.—TEST AND MAINTENANCE DIETS.

	Diets.	Total diet.				Carbohydrate (C)						Protein and fat (PF)					
		Carbohydrate.	Protein.	Fat.	Calories.	5 per cent vegetables.	Orange.	Oatmeal.	Shredded wheat.	Uneeda.	Potato.	Egg.	Cream 20 per cent fat.	Bacon.	Butter.	Meat.	
TEST	T.D.1	181	46	44	1304	300	300	....	3	4	240	3	120	..	..	....	1
	T.D.2	101	35	43	931	300	300	....	1	2	120	3	120	..	..	....	2
	T.D.3	66	24	37	693	300	300	....	½	2	...	2	120	..	..	....	3
	T.D.4	34	15	30	466	300	200	....	...	1		1	120	..	..	....	4
MAINTENANCE	C1+PF1	14	15	30	386	300	...	....	..	..	...	1	120	..	..	....	1
	C2+PF2	22	19	37	497	300	100	....	..	..	...	2	60	..	15	....	2
	C3+PF3	32	24	37	557	600	100	....	..	..	...	2	60	..	15	....	3
	C4+PF4	42	29	52	752	600	200	....	..	..	...	2	60	30	15	....	4
	C5+PF5	52	32	66	930	600	200	15	..	..	...	2	60	30	30	....	5
	C6+PF6	64	44	83	1179	600	200	30	..	..	...	2	120	30	30	....	6
	C7+PF7	74	52	88	1296	600	300	30	..	..	...	2	120	30	30	30	7
	C8+PF8	84	61	94	1426	600	300	30	..	2	...	2	120	30	30	60	8
	C9+PF9	98	65	106	1606	600	300	30	½	2	...	2	180	30	30	90	9
	C10+PF10	109	66	119	1771	600	300	30	1	2	...	2	180	30	45	90	10
	C11+PF11	135	80	135	2075	600	300	30	1	2	120	2	240	30	45	120	11
	C12+PF12	159	84	135	2187	600	300	30	1	2	240	2	240	30	45	120	12

The diet of the patient for the first day he begins treatment is not a matter of indifference. Decision rests upon his previous diet or the quantity of sugar which he is known to void in the twenty-four hours. I rarely give the patient an opportunity to continue his former diet for a few days at the beginning of treatment to serve as a baseline, because experience shows that he will not do this, but actually modifies it according to his own ideas as to what he thinks best for himself to eat. As a rule he radically restricts his diet in carbohydrate and frequently as a result will develop acidosis. Consequently in practice it will be found wiser to err on the safe side by giving the patient on the first day too much rather than too little carbohydrate, and the quantity selected, —181 grams, Test Diet 1, represents about half the carbohydrate which the healthy individual consumes. Likewise the protein and fat are correspondingly reduced so that the patient weighing 60 kilograms or 132 pounds actually receives upon the first day of treatment not far from half the food he was accustomed to take and the proportions of the different elements of the food in the diet to one another are preserved. The diet, therefore, for the first day simply represents about half the food the patient was eating, and hence indicates what undernutrition will accomplish alone. If this diet was continued, it is quite probable that many patients upon it would eventually become sugar-free and thus maintain a high tolerance.

The second day's diet, Test Diet 2, far more resembles a standard diabetic diet. The carbohydrate amounts to 101 grams, one-third to one-fourth that of the normal individual. The protein is not far from the minimum required, $\frac{2}{3}$ gram per kilogram body weight for the diabetic of 60 kilograms, and while the fat of the first day's diet remains unchanged, the relative proportion of fat to carbohydrate as compared with the first day's diet is about doubled. The total calories upon this diet are the same as those in the standard diet of Newburgh and Marsh. Not uncommonly the urine of a patient will become sugar-free upon this diet, illustrating the mildness of the disease. Having proved his innocence he escapes condemnation and life sentence and punishment with a diet of carbohydrate far below that which his disease deserved. If sugar-free upon Test Diet 2 it is a simple matter to trade the patient to a Maintenance Diet of a corresponding quantity of carbohydrate which will at the same time contain more liberal amounts of protein and fat. This is accomplished by the use of C_9PF_9, the carbohydrate (C) and the protein and fat (PF) for the ninth day of the Maintenance Diets. It is quite possible that the details of the protein and fat for these days may need to be altered. Both on account of the higher total glucose value in C_9PF_9 and the increased calories the patient upon this diet may show glycosuria and therefore will need to drop to C_8; on the other hand, he may be able to proceed to C_{10}. Above a diet represented by C_{10} one should seldom go unless very confident that the patient has an adequate tolerance for carbohydrate. The reason for this is that when one reaches 100 grams of carbohydrate in the diet, additions in carbohydrate must consist of foods containing high percentages of carbohydrate, and errors, innocently and easily, may creep into the patient's dietetic regimen. Thus a patient cannot readily eat more than 100 grams of carbohydrate in the form of 5, 10 and 15 per cent vegetables, oatmeal, grapefruit, strawberries, and orange. Above this level his carbohydrate must begin to be taken in the form of a banana, which to be sure is very useful, because a single banana contains about 20 grams of carbohydrate, in potato which is far less easily measured, or in bread which is almost invariably dangerous and therefore does not appear in the diet schedule at all.

The third day's diet utilizes undernutrition still more, and by lowering the carbohydrate to 66 grams gives still more relief to the islands of Langerhans. As a result carbohydrate oxidation is favored, constituting a protection against acidosis, which is helped still further by the reduction of protein and fat to so low a figure that the body is forced to supply these elements from its own stores and metabolism is thereby reduced. Money earned is far less apt to be squandered than money given. I cannot escape the conviction that the diabetic who is forced to draw upon his own body tissues for protein and fat will involuntarily reduce his demands upon these to a lower figure than when they are furnished in food. Ladd and Palmer recently have stated that in their studies endogenous fat was less likely to give rise to acidosis than exogenous fat.

The fourth day's diet progresses along the lines already outlined above but undernutrition is invoked still more vigorously while at the same time the proportion of fat to carbohydrate is increased so that for each gram of carbohydrate the patient received approximately 1 gram of fat instead of taking from 4 to 6 grams of carbohydrate to 1 gram of fat as in health.

In the first type of Test Diets a fifth Test Diet day was introduced. This has been found to be unnecessary, partly because protein metabolism has been lessened through the introduction of calories in the form of fat, but more especially because of insulin. So many patients became sugar-free before Test Diet 5, that it became superfluous and was therefore combined with the first Maintenance Diet, which originally contained carbohydrate 10, protein 11, and fat 6 grams, but now contains carbohydrate 14, protein 15, and fat 30 grams.

The endeavor to develop to the fullest extent the diabetic's power to utilize carbohydrate is the principle underlying the gradation of the Maintenance Diets. In practice it has been found that if undernutrition was maintained to a greater or lesser extent for a few days the quantity of carbohydrate which could be utilized was found to steadily increase. Consequently the carbohydrate in the Maintenance Diets has been increased about 10 grams for each day and the protein and fat less rapidly advanced. Diabetics are not so bad as painted. They have far more tolerance for carbohydrate than is often supposed. One must give them a chance to demonstrate what they can do, and unless some such scheme is adopted, it is difficult to find out. To follow the schedule of Test and Maintenance Diets in every case would be absurd because of variations in age, weight and occupation of the patient. It is a very simple matter, however, to modify these. It may be found that the carbohydrate tolerated is for the sixth day (C_6) but that the protein and fat requirements are for quite a different day, and the patient may be discharged on C_6PF_8. Even such a modification might be inadequate, because the patient may need more calories, and these are introduced very simply, either by the addition of cream to the diet or by changing the cream from the 20 per cent to the 40 per cent variety or by adding butter or oil. The only aim of the schedule is to simplify orders for the nurse in the hospital, treatment for the doctor in his practice and at the same time to enable patients to become sugar-free, and to acquire the allotment of carbohydrate which their disease deserves with protein and fat sufficient for maintenance.

Weighing the food is almost easier than approximating it in the treatment of a diabetic and demands almost less intelligence on the patient's part. However, occasionally it is desirable to use food equivalents. Those necessary for the utilization of the Test and Maintenance Diets are given below.

Food	Weight in grams.	Approximate equivalent.
5 per cent vegetables . . .	300	Three moderate portions
Orange	300	One and one-half large size
Oatmeal, dry weight . . .	30	One large saucerful
Potato	240	Two medium-sized potatoes
Cream	30	Two tablespoonfuls
Bacon	30	Four crisp strips
Butter	30	Three medium portions
Meat	90	One moderate portion

Every once in a while I see a patient who has been in the Outpatient Department of the Massachusetts General Hospital and have been impressed by the excellence of the scheme there adopted in the treatment of poor diabetics. The method which they employ with many patients is not based upon weights but largely upon portions, tablespoonfuls, and with it they secure excellent results.

Reappearance of Glycosuria.—Glycosuria frequently disappears while the diet is being increased. For this reason it is often well to disregard a few tenths of sugar in the urine when the patient is upon a low maintenance diet, because this will very likely vanish as the diet progresses. This is readily explained first because the increased diet is still one of undernutrition and second because the patient is regaining tolerance for carbohydrate.

Elderly patients with arteriosclerosis, particularly those with gangrene, often show this feature in a striking fashion. With the elderly the reaction to a change in diet takes place far more slowly than with the young. Perhaps this is a protective mechanism,

TABLE 184.—THE SIMPLICITY OF THE TREATMENT OF DIABETES WITH TEST AND MAINTENANCE DIETS.

CASE NO. 2851, BOY, AGED TWELVE AND EIGHT-TENTHS YEARS, DURATION TEN MONTHS. URINARY SUGAR 8.2 PER CENT, BLOOD SUGAR 0.4 PER CENT AT OFFICE VISIT OCTOBER 21, 1922. ENTERED N. E. D. HOSPITAL, OCTOBER 29.

Day.	Wgt., lbs., net.	Urine.		Blood sugar, per cent.	Diet.				Diet orders.	Insulin, units.
		Di-ace-tic.	Sugar, per cent.		C., gr.	P., gr.	F., gr.	Cal., gr.		
1	87	0	0	....	64	30	18	538	T.D. 2	0
2	87	0	0	0.12	42	29	39	635	C 4 PF4	0
3	88	0	0	....	52	30	53	805	C 5 PF5	0
4	87	0	0	....	63	43	65	1009	C 6 PF6	0
5	87	0	0	....	73	51	70	1126	C 7 PF7	0
6	87	0	0	....	84	54	70	1129	C 8 PF7	0
7	88	0	0	0.07	95	54	71	1235	C 9 PF7	0
8	87	0	0	....	106	53	71	1275	C10 PF7	0
9	87	0	0	....	118	55	71	1331	C10½ PF7	0
10	87	0	Trace	....	130	57	71	1387	C11 PF7	0
11	87	0	0	0.10	130	57	71	1387	C11 PF7	0
12	88	0	0	....	130	57	71	1387	C11 PF7	0
13	88	0	0	0.08	130	57	71	1387	C11 PF7	0
14										

CASE NO. 2959.—WOMAN, AGED FIFTY YEARS, DURATION FOUR MONTHS.

1	163.5	0	5.1	....	1	7	14	158	T.D. 2	0
2	.....	0	2.9	0.27	66	24	37	693	T.D. 3	0
3	.....	0	1.1	....	34	15	30	466	T.D. 4	0
4	.....	+	0.4	....	14	15	30	386	T.D. 5	0
5	.....	0	0.2	....	22	13	18	302	C 2 PF2	0
6	.....	0	0.1	....	28	25	17	365	C 3 PF3	0
7	.....	0	0.1	....	43	38	63	891	C 4 PF6	0
8	.....	0	0	....	54	50	75	1091	C 5 PF7	0
9	.....	0	0	....	63	59	87	1271	C 6 PF8	0
10	.....	0	0	....	74	60	93	1373	C 7 PF9	0
11	.....	0	0	....	89	62	95	1459	C 8 PF9	0
12	.....	0	0	....	96	63	94	1482	C 9 PF9	0
13	.....	0	0	....	107	62	92	1504	C10 PF9	0
14	.....	0	0	....	141	67	95	1687	C11 PF9	0
15	163.0	0	0	0.11	152	68	95	1735	C12 PF9	0

because when the sugar is readily reduced in an elderly person serious symptoms may occur such, for example, as the hypoglycemia reported with Case No. 2716 on p. 178.

The second alternative, namely, an increase in tolerance during treatment, is most important and especially important with cases who are receiving insulin. Case No. 2962 gained tolerance after discharge and an insulin reaction thereupon developed.

TABLE 184.—THE SIMPLICITY OF THE TREATMENT OF DIABETES WITH TEST AND MAINTENANCE DIETS.—(*Continued.*)

CASE NO. 3040, GIRL, AGED ELEVEN YEARS, DURATION NINE MONTHS.

Day.	Wgt., lbs., net.	Urine.		Blood sugar, per cent.	Diet.				Diet orders.	Insulin, units.
		Di-ace-tic.	Sugar, per cent.		C., gr.	P., gr.	F., gr.	Cal.		
1	73	0	3.0	....	67	25	29	629	T.D. 2	1-0-2
2	72	0	0.2	....	66	24	37	693	T.D. 3	3-4-5
3	75	++	0.3	0.16	52	32	53	813	C 5 PF5	5-0-5
4	75	Sl+	0	....	54	41	64	956	C 5 PF6	5-0-5
5	76	0	0	....	63	51	70	1086	C 6 PF7	5-0-5
6	74	0	0	....	74	52	76	1188	C 7 PF7 20% Cr. 120	5-0-5
7	73	0	0	....	84	53	77	1241	C 8 PF7 20% Cr. 120	5-0-5
8	74	0	0	....	96	54	77	1293	C9 PF7 20% Cr. 120	5-0-5
9	74	0	0	....	107	56	77	1345	C10 PF7 20% Cr. 120	5-0-5
10	75	0	0	....	131	60	77	1457	C11 PF7 20% Cr. 120	5-0-5
11	74	0	0	0.08[1]	156	61	78	1570	C12 PF7 20% Cr. 120	5-0-5

CASE NO. 3078, AGED THIRTEEN AND FIVE-TENTHS YEARS, DURATION SIX MONTHS.

Day.	Wgt., lbs., net.	Di-ace-tic.	Sugar, per cent.	Blood sugar, per cent.	C., gr.	P., gr.	F., gr.	Cal.	Diet orders.	Insulin, units.
1	81	Sl+	4.0	....	23	13	15	279	T.D. 2	2-0-0
2	81	0	0.6	0.29	66	24	37	683	T.D. 3	4-0-0
3	83	0	0.2	....	52	32	53	813	C 5 PF5	4-4-4
4	83	0	0	....	64	42	70	1054	C 6 PF6 20% Cr. 120	5-0-5
5	83	0	0	....	75	45	77	1173	C 7 PF6 20% Cr. 150	5-0-5
6	84	0	0	....	86	50	92	1372	C 8 PF6 20% Cr. 180	5-0-5
7	83	0	0	....	99	50	86	1390	C 9 PF6 20% Cr. 210	5-0-5
8	84	0	0	0.12	111	52	102	1570	C10 PF6 20% Cr. 240	5-0-5
1923 5/3	..	0	0	....	135	55	96	1624		

[1] Blood sugar taken one day later.

TABLE 184.—THE SIMPLICITY OF THE TREATMENT OF DIABETES WITH TEST AND MAINTENANCE DIETS.—(*Continued.*)

CASE NO. 3323, WOMAN, AGED FIFTY-TWO AND ONE-TENTH YEARS, DURATION FOUR AND SEVEN-TENTHS YEARS.

| Day. | Wgt. lbs. net. | Urine. | | Blood sugar per cent. | Diet. | | | | Diet. orders. | Insulin units. |
		Diacetic.	Sugar per cent.		C. gr.	P. gr.	F. gr.	Cal.		
1	117½	+++	9.1	....	33	13	15	319	T.D. 2	0 0-1
2	118¼	++	4.0	0.30	101	35	43	931	T.D. 2	2-4-5
3	118	0	0.2	....	66	24	37	693	T.D. 3	5-6-7
4	119½	0	0.3	....	44	39	81	1061	C 4 PF6 20% Cr. 120	8-9-10
5	120	0	0	....	48	43	105	1309	C 4 PF6 20% Cr. 240	10-10-10
6	120	0	0	....	58	54	124	1564	C 5 PF7– P 4145 20% Cr. 240	10-10-10
7	120	0	0	0.23	58	54	137	1681	ditto	10-10-10
8	119¾	0	0	....	58	54	137	1681	ditto	10-10-10
9	120¾	0	0	....	58	54	137	1681	ditto	10-10-10
10	121½	0	0	....	58	51	98	1381	ditto	10-10-10
11	121½	0	0	....	58	53	136	1668	ditto	15-0-10

CASE NO. 3324, BOY, AGED TWELVE AND SIX-TENTHS YEARS, DURATION THREE WEEKS.

Day.	Wgt. lbs. net.	Diacetic.	Sugar per cent.	Blood sugar per cent.	C. gr.	P. gr.	F. gr.	Cal.	Diet. orders.	Insulin units.
1	76¼	++	9.0	....	63	23	31	623	T.D. 2	0-1-2
2	75¾	+	2.0	0.21	66	24	37	693	T.D. 3	3-4-5
3	76¾	0	0.1	....	64	46	82	1178	C 6 PF6	5-5-5
4	78¼	0	0.1	....	73	44	83	1219	C 7 PF6	5-5-5
5	79	0	0	....	84	45	84	1272	C 8 PF6	8-0-7
6	79½	0	0	0.10	96	47	84	1328	C 9 PF6	8-0-7
7	79½	0	0	....	106	47	84	1368	C10 PF6	8-0-7
8	80½	0	0	....	107	54	89	1445	C10 PF7	8-0-7
9	80¾	0	0	....	119	55	89	1497	C10½ PF7	8-0-7
10	81¼	0	0	....	131	60	89	1565	C11 PF7	8-0-7
11	79½	0	0	....	131	58	89	1557	C11 PF7	8-0-7
12	80¾	0	0	....	131	58	89	1557	C11 PF7	8-0-7

The return of glycosuria in the course of treatment demands action. If the patient is upon Maintenance Diets, the simplest plan is to recede by a day when the restriction of carbohydrate and of calories may immediately clear the urine. If this is not successful still further recession may be tried. However, since the introduction of single specimen days, that is, the testing of each specimen of urine throughout the twenty-four hours, it frequently comes to light that the reason for the appearance of the sugar was simply due to the unbalanced diet. Correcting this by shifting the carbohydrate from the offending meal to another often solves the difficulty. The adjustment is made as indicated when insulin is employed along with the diet as shown in Table 2.

The return of sugar demands fasting whenever there is the slightest suspicion that the diet has been broken by design. This was the rule when treatment by fasting was first adopted. It is a pity now that it is not as strictly enforced. In hospitals it simplifies the treatment enormously. So soon as it is understood that the reappearance of sugar means a fast until glycosuria disappears from the twenty-four-hour quantity of urine, there is little tendency to break over the diet. Furthermore, most patients are thrifty enough to see the disadvantage of paying their board with no return. The rule must be rigidly enforced with children, because with them disobedience means death.

Determination of Tolerance for Protein.—Protein to the extent of 1 gram per kilogram body weight is borne by nearly all patients and I am very loathe to allow the protein to remain permanently below this figure save in the elderly and those with impaired kidneys. By further restricting the carbohydrate either temporarily or permanently this can usually be avoided. It is always necessary to bear in mind that one food which the diabetic patient cannot do without is protein and to it everything else must be subordinate. Body protein must be spared. Newburgh and Marsh emphasized the importance of fat in this regard. (See p. 525.)

The Caloric Needs of the Patient.—The total number of calories which a diabetic requires varies not only with each case, but varies with each case each day. Schematic rules do not hold. This will be seen in Table 166, in which the great variation in the basal metabolism of diabetics is shown. There it will be found that the average caloric needs were essentially the same as for a large group of normal men and women, about 25 calories per kilogram body weight reckoned per twenty-four hours.[1] Great variations in caloric requirements are also shown in this table since they vary from 19 calories to 41 calories per kilogram body weight. If this variation exists while at rest, how much more it must exist during the various activities of different individuals! Furthermore, one must remember that the number of calories consumed per hour varies enormously. During sleep, Benedict's fasting man burned 1 calorie per kilogram body weight per hour the day before the beginning of the experiment, while during the daytime and awake although still at rest, the number of calories rose to 1.05. During the fast while asleep the metabolism on the same basis dropped to 0.85 calorie, and when awake to 0.95 calorie. In the previous section it has been pointed out

[1] The error should not be made of concluding that an energy loss of 25 calories per kilogram body weight in the fasting state can be replaced by a diet with the corresponding number of calories. In reality a considerably greater number of calories would be required, due to the specific dynamic action of the food ingested.

that an individual weighing 60 kilos walking at the rate of 2 miles per hour would require twice and at 4 miles an hour thrice the calories of the standing metabolism which in turn is 12 per cent more than in the horizontal position. Habits of individuals vary widely. Some are quiet and some are active. All these considerations should be clearly borne in mind by doctors and patients in order not to allow themselves to be held too rigidly by any caloric fetish. Patients coming for treatment with severe acidosis consume from 10 to 20 per cent more calories per kilogram body weight than patients after they have become sugar- and acid-free. How low the caloric requirements go is well illustrated by Case No. 1085 (see p. 175) and by Case No. 866 (see p. 97).

The caloric requirements of patients over long periods of time were determined with unusual accuracy in 2 cases. The first was Mrs. P., Case No. 1541, who had suffered a hemiplegia. She was constantly under the strict supervision of one of my nurses trained in diabetes. Obviously, in this patient exercise was greatly curtailed and during one year she maintained her weight while living on a diet computed to be 20 calories per kilogram body weight.

TABLE 185.—TABULATION OF DIABETIC. DIET OF A MAN, AGED FIFTY-TWO YEARS, FOR FIFTEEN MONTHS (CASE No. 2207). (See p. 502.)

Date.	Carbohydrate.	Protein.	Fat.	Calories.	Remarks.
Oct. 14, 1921	126.45	95.69	124.99	2,015	Living in country; some golf.
Nov. 15, 1921	155.90†	86.73	115.55	2,010	Living in country; some golf.
Dec. 14, 1921	121.01	66.59	137.50	1,988	Living in country; some exercise.
Jan. 18, 1922	135.03	75.16	118.50	1,908	Living in country; some exercise.
Feb. 19, 1922	119.78	107.36	116.16	1,953	Living in country; some exercise.
Mar. 14, 1922	109.81	68.47	87.83	1,502*	At Atlantic City; some exercise.
April 16, 1922	104.16	90.16	125.33	1,907	Living in country; some golf.
May 15, 1922	125.20	100.03	123.83	2,015	Living in country; some golf daily.
June 16, 1922	116.54	61.45*	121.49	1,805	Living at seashore cottage; no golf.
July 24, 1922	98.28	101.61	138.33	2,044	Living in country; golf daily.
Aug. 15, 1922	143.50	114.33†	144.00†	2,327†	Motoring and playing some golf.
Sept. 16, 1922	113.48	110.66	133.00	2,091	Living in country; golf daily.
Oct. 15, 1922	106.80	109.30	106.16	1,819	Living in country; some golf.
Nov. 14, 1922	76.08*	73.66	113.83	1,623	Living in N. Y. City; no golf; very little exercise.
Dec. 14, 1922	103.58	86.33	93.99*	1,569	Living in N. Y. City; no golf; very little exercise.
Totals	1755.70	1357.53	1810.49	28,576	
Averages	117.00	90.00	120.00	1,905	
Maximum†	155.70	114.33	144.00	2,327	
Minimum*	76.08	61.45	93.99	1,502	

* Sugar-free throughout whole period. Weight from 155 to 160 pounds, naked.
† January 29, 1923. The above checked and corrected. I have vouchers for all the above entries. Signed, Case No. 2207.

Another patient, Case No. 2207, aged fifty-two years, submitted to me Table 185 on page 501. The weight of this patient varied from 155 to 160 pounds, 70 to 73 kilograms. His average daily diet amounted to 27 calories per kilogram body weight, the maximum being 32 calories per kilogram body weight and the minimum 21 calories per kilogram body weight.

A comparison of the calories received by a series of patients just before discharge from the hospital with their theoretical needs was made by Dr. J. H. Townsend unbeknown to me. These are recorded in Table 186. The lower number of calories of Case No. 1469 was due to recent glycosuria overlooked through a faulty Benedict solution. This girl with diabetes of six years' duration has gained $16\frac{1}{4}$ pounds since she began insulin.

TABLE 186.—CALORIES PRESCRIBED IN HOSPITAL COMPARED WITH THEORETICAL NEEDS.

No.	Age.	Sex.	Height.	Weight.	Surface area.	Cal. for quiet in hosp.	+ 20 per cent cal. for mod. activ.	Dis-charge diet.	Cals. per kilo.	Insulin units, daily.
3315	69	F.	5, $5\frac{3}{4}$	63.6	1.73	1380	1660	1568	24.7	0[1]
3309	61	F.	5, 4	75.0	1.81	1460	1750	1789	23.9	0
1469	16	F.	5, $8\frac{1}{2}$	44.8	1.51	1440	1730	1386	30.9	30
2448	20	M.	5, 8	51.4	1.59	1580	1880	1795	35.0	50
2776	11	F.	4, $9\frac{1}{2}$	27.7	1.09	1150	1380	1382	50.0	15
3317	51	M.	6, $2\frac{1}{2}$	78.1	2.04	1840	2210	2027	26.0	8
3270	17	M.	5, 8	50.8	1.59	1620	1940	2084	41.0	4
685	53	F.	5, 3	57.7	1.60	1330	1600	1634	28.3	6
585	62	F.	5, $5\frac{1}{2}$	53.0	1.59	1280	1540	1654	31.2	0
3321	26	F.	4, $11\frac{1}{2}$	40.6	1.32	1160	1390	1500	36.9	18
992	53	F.	4, $11\frac{1}{2}$	50.4	1.45	1210	1450	1557	30.9	15
3322	50	M.	5, $6\frac{1}{4}$	71.0	1.80	1630	1960	2137	30.1	0
3325	38	F.	5, 11	60.4	1.78	1540	1850	1962	32.5	15

2. **The Management of Mild Cases of Diabetes.**—The mild case of diabetes is the case which demands the most energetic treatment, but hitherto has received the least. These cases are analogous to the cases of incipient tuberculosis. As in tuber-culosis, a "cure" may not be effected, but the disease is held in check. Emphasis should be placed on freedom from glycosuria. Naunyn's dictum that "many a severe case was originally mild, but neglected," should not be forgotten.

These patients should be taught to take long vacations, secure an abundance of sleep, avoid excess in mental and physical labor, shun obesity, and provide for daily exercise. It is best to be frank with such patients, and warn them of the danger of neglecting treatment.

The diet of such patients is not a great hardship though often

[1] Never had any.

it is resented more than a closely limited diet by the severe diabetic. With these individuals it is hard to have patience.

Formerly the reduction of carbohydrate to 100 grams would often suffice to stop the glycosuria. In our enthusiasm for new methods it should not be forgotten that even in the past good results were obtained with the majority of diabetics, and that gradual restriction of carbohydrate was the means employed. Incidentally, this is good proof that most diabetics are not severe. The simple omission of butter, cream, or both for a time, will lead to a great reduction in the sugar excreted, which will be accentuated if the protein is limited to between 1 gram and $1\frac{1}{2}$ grams per kilogram body weight. Combined with the above the exclusion of actual sugar from the dietary and the substitution of potato (20 per cent carbohydrate) for bread (60 per cent carbohydrate) will frequently secure a sugar-free urine. It is onerous for a patient to eat 100 grams of starch in the form of potato, but enjoyable to consume it as bread. This method of treatment is very successful with my good-natured and usually obedient, fat doctor-patients.

The milder cases of diabetes in a few weeks attain a tolerance of more than 100 grams carbohydrate. Such cases should limit the quantity of carbohydrate in their diet for years, even though no signs of sugar appear. It is interesting to note that many of these patients like Case No. 1287, feel better and have less digestive trouble if the quantity of carbohydrate is held at about 125 grams to 150 grams even though they tolerate more. Such individuals live apparently in perfect health, and there is always satisfaction in the belief, and I think justification for it, that treatment has prevented the progress of the disease. Mention of these cases is is made in the discussion of the Cases of Twenty or More Years' Duration, p. 678.

The Management of Severe Cases of Diabetes.—It would be wrong to give the impression that the treatment of diabetes is entirely free from anxiety. It is true that it is much simpler and causes infinitely less worry to the physician than heretofore, but these patients are in most unstable equilibrium and a little upset of trivial character may lead to much danger. The physician who treats severe diabetes successfully must constantly be in close touch with his patient. Insulin has lessened the responsibility for the care of the severe but intelligent diabetic, but increased the responsibility for the welfare of the others.

3. **The Dietetic Treatment of the Severe Diabetic.**—Diabetics of the severe type do not become sugar-free without the interpolation of a fast day. I have not had experience enough with the diets of Petrén, Newburgh and Marsh either to confirm or disagree with their theory that the diabetic can be made sugar-

free upon a diet such as the latter which consists of carbohydrate 14 grams, protein 15 grams, and fat 89 grams. In practice the interpolation of one fast day usually rids the patient of sugar, and as many as four consecutive days of fasting have not been employed for at least one year prior to the introduction of insulin. For my patients a day without food accomplished at that time what nothing hitherto did, and for this weapon I am most grateful, though fortunately now it is rendered unnecessary, thanks to insulin. The introduction of fasting, or a "half-day," in the routine of dietetic treatment has been of inestimable value in prolonging the lives of several children so that they have preserved for years the spark of life which now insulin kindles to a full flame. The children who were fed for comfort died. The children who were kept sugar-free with painstaking adherence to the principles of undernutrition are here today. I do not want to forget the advantages which have accrued to the severest of my patients as a result of an occasional day without food.

The stimulus of a little carbohydrate to the utilization of a larger quantity of carbohydrate in a subsequent meal is definite. A number of patients with a carbohydrate tolerance of 10 to 15 grams in the twenty-four hours have reached this only by this means. Their method has been to take about 1 or 2 grams of carbohydrate in the form of lettuce or of grapefruit one hour before each of the three chief meals. The possibility of good effects from these "activating" carbohydrate meals came to my attention through the work of Benedict and Osterberg.[1] H. Gray[2] proved its efficacy with several of my patients. Case No. 1542, relied upon such expedients to hold out during the nine months before insulin arrived. Prof. MacLeod called my attention to the fact that experimentally carbohydrate was activating in this manner only when it was given by mouth and not by the intravenous route. It would appear that a little carbohydrate stimulated the islands of Langerhans to increased secretion. This is important and confirms me in the desirability of giving diabetics the carbohydrate which they can utilize rather than arbitrarily condemning them for life to a carbohydrate which is far, far below their original capacity to burn. Is it not possible that if the carbohydrate is radically restricted for weeks, months, or years to a point below what can be burned, the ability to burn carbohydrate will also fall? The usefulness of activating carbohydrate meals may be of a more general importance than in the immediate effects produced. A six meal schedule is arranged as follows: 1. Intervals between meals should be two and a half hours, except that the

[1] Benedict and Osterberg: Jour. Biol. Chem., 1918, **34**, 217.
[2] Gray: Boston Med. and Surg. Jour., 1922, **186**, 763.

first extra meal may be taken any time between one and two and a half hours before the regular breakfast. Illustration:

A.M.		Noon.		Night.	
1st extra:	5.30–7.00	2d extra:	10.00	3d extra:	3.30
Breakfast:	8.00	Lunch:	1.00	Supper:	6.00

2. Calorie Value of Meal.—The first extra is to be the smallest meal of the day, the breakfast which follows is to be the smallest of the three main meals, and the smaller it is, the better.

3. Composition of Meal.—The extra meals are to be mainly carbohydrate, usually in the form of lettuce or fruit because these are the most convenient and the former furnishes bulk. Breakfast is the meal at which carbohydrate is least well tolerated. It is often desirable to precede it with an extra activating meal even if it is not required to prevent glycosuria.

The carbohydrate ration of severe diabetics is therefore what he can tolerate, but the protein ration can be more definitely predicated. It should not fall below $\frac{2}{3}$ of a gram per kilogram body weight, or should it rise above 1 gram per kilogram body weight. Only by restricting the protein to this minimum is it possible to supply the diabetic with the maximum calories in the form of fat without the production of acidosis. We cannot be too grateful to the laboratory workers who have made so much more definite the proportions of carbohydrate, protein, and fat which diabetics can safely take. If the severe diabetic cannot be sugar-free with maintenance calories distributed between carbohydrate, protein, and fat, the only recourse for him is to undergo undernutrition to such an extent that his metabolism is reduced to such a level that a smaller quantity of carbohydrate, protein and fat will hold him in equilibrium.

The actual quantity of carbohydrate, protein, and fat which the diabetic metabolizes each day is very different from the actual quantity of carbohydrate, protein, and fat which he consumes or is prescribed for him to consume. The work of DuBois and Richardson shows this, and emphasis has been put upon it by Woodyatt, Shaffer, Newburgh and Marsh, and many others, yet we constantly forget it. Therefore, when a diet of undernutrition is prescribed for a diabetic, he should lead the life of undernutrition and stay abed. If he is up and about, the increased metabolism produced may counterbalance the good effects of the low diet prescribed. If he is allowed to live as formerly, he will supply from his own body tissues the calories of protein and fat for his daily needs which his diet lacks. It is true that he may not be as great a spendthrift of his own tissues as he would of food, but since his own resources are chiefly protein and fat, the amount of ketones formed can be deleterious. By keeping quiet the stimulus to carbohydrate utilization which exercise affords is sacrificed, but it is safer to forego this asset temporarily than to run the danger of the incomplete oxidation of large quantities of body fat. Until the diet contains at least two-thirds of a maintenance diet, the diabetic is safer abed.

Severe cases of diabetes cause the most worry at the beginning of treatment. A gastro-intestinal upset, a careless alteration of diet, anxiety, excitement, overexertion, a mild intercurrent disease or an infection may favor the outbreak of coma.

For these severe cases a trained diabetic nurse permanently in charge of the patient is of the greatest assistance to the patient and family. Certain of my severest cases have had nurses for long periods. Any diabetic who can afford the luxury of a diabetic nurse is fortunate. It is the best insurance he can take out for his life. If patients fully realized the advantages of a nurse, these would be in even greater demand than now. Several of my diabetic cases consult me but twice a year because they depend upon their nurse. If a nurse is not available, success in treatment depends upon the thorough education of the patient. The wise live long; the ignorant succumb early. Once having thoroughly mastered the essentials of treatment, these patients need little supervision. They manage themselves quite well and frequently give useful suggestions for their own treatment and that of others.

Case No. 632 has faithfully carried out treatment for ten years and his course is an encouragement to all. In fact most of the first severe cases treated with insulin both in this and other clinics, have been "pedigreed" diabetics, who by their own tenacity have kept life in the body. I have never seen a diabetic patient do well who had wholly given up diet, and I confess that I have had considerable opportunity to observe such cases. The family, the friends, the patient, and the doctor will all get along more comfortably if the diet throughout the whole course of the disease is kept at a point where sugar remains absent from the urine. The attitude of the patients themselves under the two conditions is very different. In the former, is the weak, complaining, melancholic, tearful patient, with complications of the nerves, eyes, or skin almost invariably present. In the latter group there is far more freedom from despondency and though pathetic to see, hope remains. With insulin both types are vanishing.

D. Summaries of the Treatment Employed in Four Successive Groups of Cases.

The treatment of diabetes is changing so rapidly that it is difficult to grasp its essential features from a study of individual cases. Consequently, in the following tables are summarized the treatment of four groups of cases of diabetes, each consisting of 30 cases, seen in chronological periods between 1915 and 1923. The composition of the diet during the first and last weeks of hospital stay is given and for comparison is calculated per kilogram body weight. The duration of the disease to death or of the living cases to January 1, 1923, shows the results obtained. Finally, the preliminary method of treatment is indicated, namely, whether it commenced with fasting or with preparatory treatment, that is, diminution of fat and protein prior to the fast, though often by this plan the patients became sugar-free and actual fasting was not used at all, or with the use of test diets.

In the last three columns the question of acidosis is considered. In the early cases but few showed its absence throughout, either developing it in the hospital or entering with it. A gratifying decrease in the number of cases who developed acidosis is evident. In the fourth group a record of acidosis has not been included because it dropped almost immediately with insulin.

The criteria for the selection of cases in the table were: (1) That the patients should have been over fifteen years of age; and (2) should have remained at least two weeks in the hospital. All cases recorded in these tables left the hospital alive except Case No. 904, who died with a carbuncle. It is hoped that the introduction of this method of presenting results of treatment will prove a valuable innovation in our management of diabetes. Undertaken with little conception as to what the average results would be, it shows quite clearly the errors in the past and indicates where the weak places in modern diabetic treatment lie.

1. **Body Weight.**—Weight was lost by all groups save the fourth which was treated with insulin. In the first and second groups the losses amounted to 3.07 and 2.87 kilograms respectively, but it will be noticed in the third group the loss was but 1.6 kilograms per patient. With the fourth or insulin group the steadily decreasing loss was changed to a slight gain of 0.5 kilogram.

During the stay of the first group of patients treated, the loss of weight per day per patient was approximately 100 grams, in the second group 125 grams, and in the third group 57 grams per day per patient. If this loss of weight should arbitrarily be reckoned in caloric equivalent as described on page 222, namely, allowing 3300 calories for each kilogram lost—it would be equivalent to 10131, 9471 and 5280 calories respectively. Since the average weight of the patients was 60, 59 and 56 kilograms, this would represent the equivalent of 5.1, 7.5 and 3.3 calories per kilogram body weight per day. Add these endogenous calories to the exogenous ingested and the calories in the four groups are almost identical.

Table 187.—The Treatment of Thirty Cases of Diabetes between April 6, 1915 and March 18, 1916.

Case No.	Age at onset, yrs.	Days in hospital	Weight in kilograms Entrance	Weight in kilograms Exit	First week Carbo-hydrate	First week Protein	First week Fat	First week Alcohol	First week Calories Total	First week Calories Per kilo	Last week Carbo-hydrate	Last week Protein	Last week Fat	Last week Alcohol	Last week Calories Total	Last week Calories Per kilo	Duration in years to Jan. 1, 1923, or to death.	Fasting.	Treatment begun with exclusion of fat, preparatory treatment.	Acidosis Present Developed after entrance.	Acidosis Present Decreased after entrance.	Acidosis Present. Developed after entrance.	Absent during hospital stay.
263	34	17	62	59	6	16	16	12	326	5.0	9	28	49	5	762	12	13.8	+	:	+	:	:	+
877	50	25	77	?	31	48	80	0	1037	13.0	53	51	89	0	1217	?	11.0	:	+	:	+++	:	
902	36	23	59	57	16	43	3	0	0	0.0	9	35	45	0	420	7	4.1	:	+	:	:	:	++
908	20	20	43	45	12	7	7	5	66	2.0	36	41	69	0	725	15	2.7	:	+	:	:	:	
181[1]	44	63	50	49	12	0	0	0	8	0.2	2	46	38	10	591	12	26.0	:	+	:	:+	:	
912	40	15	60	57	35	22	18	3	389	6.0	43	49	49	0	778	14	22.0	:	+	:	+++	:	
919	47	25	53	50	28	5	8	13	164	3.0	25	44	59	2	722	14	4.8	:	+	:	:	:	
552[1]	29	34	43	39	5	4	2	0	193	4.0	17	52	61	0	740	19	3.7	+	+	+	:	+	+
935	46	27	53	48	12	16	4	0	148	3.0	67	27	38	0	516	11	10.2	:	+	:	:	:	
955	47	19	84	76	21	30	23	0	409	5.0	27	76	93	0	1384	20	7.0	:	+	:	++	:	
953	18	21	74	76	10	20	9	0	188	3.0	28	67	60	0	973	13	7.2	:	:	:	:	:	
958	30	48	44	43	7	11	5	0	105	2.0	17	55	58	0	857	20	18.0	+	+	:	:	+	+
960	51	36	90	68	19	27	9	0	251	3.0	43	49	115	0	1191	18	10.4	+	:	:	:	:	
965	46	24	53	85	6	14	7	0	161	2.0	5	96	115	2	1592	19	1.0	:	:	:	+ :	:	+
966[1]	39	23	52	55	28	1	0	0	112	2.0	20	54	79	0	971	18	8.2	:	+	:	:	:	
969	42	34	75	55	15	30	18	0	338	7.0	43	57	80	0	1026	19	0.6	+++	:	:	++	:	
560[1]	66	30	44	69	19	31	11	1	264	4.0	19	67	98	0	1317	19	10.6	:	:	:	:+++	:	
684[1]	55	16	40	45	6	6	2	11	148	3.0	0	28	31	0	467	10	2.3	:	:	:+	:	+	+
765[1]	22	25	92	37	13	9	3	0	118	3.0	41	45	69	0	795	22	7.1	+	:	:	:	:	
970	59	36	90	89	14	28	14	0	281	3.0	40	75	107	0	1322	15	7.1	:	+	:	:	:	
983	55	27	54	87	39	14	3	0	146	2.0	1	75	55	0	971	11	2.4	+++	:	:	:	:	
821[1]	23	20	48	48	4	11	5	0	108	2.0	3	44	97	0	1157	24	1.8	:	:	:+	:	+	+
996[1]	62	19	43	47	19	26	13	0	310	6.0	32	48	77	0	876	19	2.8	+	:	:	:	:	
981	28	88	60	41	11	21	12	0	236	5.0	80	65	92	0	1150	28	8.9	:	+	:	:	:	
994	15	49	33	57	41	41	35	0	639	11.0	13	67	117	0	1617	28	6.3	++	:	:+	:+++	:++	++
1005[1]	31	27	51	33	24	2	0	0	77	2.0	11	50	83	0	1075	33	15.0	:	+	:	:	:	
1008	41	69	65	49	40	8	1	0	192	4.0	9	54	74	0	921	19	3.9	:	+	:	:	:	+
1013	46	27	40	63	40	26	12	0	345	5.0	11	54	102	14	1329	21	4.4	:	+	:	:	+	
1011	25	69	38	38	4	11	2	0	63	2.0	4	54	61	5	902	24	3.4	:	+	:	+ :	:	
1022	53	18	84	83	45	29	20	0	460	5.0	29	70	106	5	1397	17	20.0	:	+	:	:	+	

[1] Died within eight months of discharge.

TABLE 188.—THE TREATMENT OF THIRTY CASES OF DIABETES BETWEEN MARCH 19, 1916, AND JULY 19, 1916.

| Case No. | Age at onset, yrs. | Days in hospital | Weight in kilograms | | Average daily diet in hospital in grams | | | | | | | | | | | | Duration in years to Jan. 1, 1923, or to death. | Fasting. | Treatment began with exclusion of fat, preparatory treatment. | Acidosis. | | |
| | | | | | First week. | | | | | | Last week. | | | | | | | | | Present. | | Absent during hospital stay. |
			Entrance.	Exit.	Carbo-hydrate.	Protein.	Fat.	Alcohol.	Calories Total.	Per kilo.	Carbo-hydrate.	Protein.	Fat.	Alcohol.	Calories Total.	Per kilo.				Developed after entrance.	Decreased after entrance.	
9041	40	45	62	57	18	16	6	6	244	4.0	7	38	51	71	1137	20	16.0		+++	+		+++
1033	51	20	56	53	49	14	1	0	265	5.0	31	59	33	0	655	12	10.8					+
1024	69	41	55	55	28	12	0	10	235	4.0	18	57	57	12	1210	23	10.0		++			+
1028	29	24	59	55	6	18	4	9	198	3.0	38	63	42	8	886	16	2.3	++		+	+	
1029	33	17	53	51	0	9	2	1	127	2.0	21	59	74	0	809	16	4.6					
1030	64	23	75	71	21	30	12	0	312	4.0	73	69	129	0	1730	24	12.3					
1032	50	20	48	41	14	11	2	0	110	2.0	54	60	61	0	1012	22	17.0	++	+			+++++
327	40	16	78	75	18	20	9	0	228	29.0	59	78	84	0	1330	22	9.8					
1025¹	21	27	78	40	2	1	0	0	13	0.3	8	48	64	0	811	18	1.6				+	+++
1036	52	21	43	66	21	27	15	0	322	4.0	34	82	110	0	1451	20	6.0					
1038	37	22	74	74	19	17	6	0	191	2.0	73	51	75	0	1177	16	.2		+		:	
1041	59	20	78	52	20	23	7	0	234	5.0	32	61	87	8	1157	22	3.7					
1045	56	16	51	44	17	21	10	0	258	6.0	43	52	81	0	1165	27	2.4	++				
1046	41	22	45	42	14	8	2	0	105	2.0	51	67	76	0	1153	27	2.5		+			
1050	66	20	45	67	28	31	17	0	387	6.0	72	66	87	0	1120	28	10.0	++				
1052	57	25	68	72	53	49	34	0	716	10.0	55	64	121	0	1567	17	13.0	++				++++
1054	53	19	74	60	24	38	18	0	415	6.0	64	85	85	0	1343	22	7.1					
875	46	20	63	45	41	16	4	0	274	4.0	110	42	102	0	1531	34	4.0					
1066	38	20	46	32	21	11	0	0	129	3.0	29	56	76	0	1019	32	5.8	+++	++		:	
1058¹	39	20	32	33	26	101	2	0	166	3.0	28	51	69	0	937	18	1.1	+				
1055	41	20	59	57	32	12	0	0	173	5.0	30	42	66	0	879	13	21.0	+				
1063	71	25	73	67	59	123	2	0	300	2.0	31	78	119	0	1169	19	.2	+			+	
1061	47	19	63	61	26	9	0	0	142	5.0	51	74	118	0	1277	20	.2	+				+
1065	44	16	67	61	51	30	14	0	447	4.0	85	75	124	0	1753	18	3.4	+				
786	38	33	98	96	33	15	2	0	216	5.0	37	72	63	0	1004	22	2.1	+			:	++++
1079	54	17	49	56	19	17	10	0	230	4.0	71	48	73	0	1137	20	1.3					
942¹	30	48	59	56	28	7	0	0	140	4.0	8	41	54	0	677	18	0.8				+	+
1085¹	34	121	40	38	29	16	2	0	198	5.0	2	30	27	28	571	20	1.8	+	++		+	
1083	54	21	40	28	4	10	5	0	101	2.0	32	67	120	0	1476	27	1.8					++
1084	34	18	57	55	21	13	2	0	161	3.0	48	68	100	0	1377	23	3.0	++			:	

¹ Died within eight months of discharge.
² Untraced.

TABLE 189.—The Treatment of Thirty Cases of Diabetes between July 20, 1916, and February 2, 1917.

Case No.	Age at onset, yrs.	Days in hospital.	Weight in kilograms. Entrance.	Weight in kilograms. Exit.	First week. Carbo-hydrate.	First week. Protein.	First week. Fat.	First week. Alcohol.	First week. Calories. Total.	First week. Calories. Per kilo.	Last week. Carbo-hydrate.	Last week. Protein.	Last week. Fat.	Last week. Alcohol.	Last week. Calories. Total.	Last week. Calories. Per kilo.	Duration in years to Jan. 1, 1923, or to death.	Fasting.	Treatment begun with exclusion of fat, preparatory treatment.	Acidosis. Present. Developed after entrance.	Acidosis. Present. Decreased after entrance.	Acidosis. Absent during hospital stay.
1090	18	13	55	53	45	25	11	0	364	7.0	67	55	76	0	1169	22	4.8		+			+
1088	55	34	64	64	63	44	56	0	933	15.0	97	48	82	0	1276	20	6.7		+	+		+
1098	47	13	70	70	55	46	16	0	616	9.0	70	61	76	0	1182	17	14.0		+		+	++
479	35	29	54	52	38	8	0	0	185	3.0	9	79	112	0	1362	26	7.0		+			
1094	55	35	72	71	26	33	9	0	321	4.0	72	81	141	0	1891	27	7.9		+		++	+
1034	36	45	51	40	0	7	0	0	27	0.5	24	50	87	0	1078	27	7.0		:			
1101	51	41	53	54	25	18	3	0	203	4.0	14	66	125	0	1436	26	8.8		+		+++	
1099	51	15	60	60	23	30	11	0	313	5.0	40	71	109	0	1437	24	8.4	+	+		+	
1102	21	59	49	45	23	12	1	0	154	3.0	27	47	77	0	993	22	3.4		+			
1110	61	14	58	57	62	43	24	6	637	11.0	103	69	76	19	1368	24	9.0					
1114	27	34	49	50	1	7	6	0	78	2.0	2	68	79	0	1137	23	10.0		+		+	
1125	34	27	36	37	21	17	9	0	226	6.0	20	50	89	0	1087	29	2.9		:		+	+++++++++
1130	21	20	43	41	4	5	7	7	98	2.0	6	36	84	0	922	33	7.8					
815	59	16	55	57	15	32	68	0	799	15.0	38	59	159	0	1819	24	2.4	+	+		+	
1131	27	15	54	54	25	23	16	0	342	6.0	91	77	70	0	1303	32	4.7	+	+		+	
1134	24	35	67	64	25	16	16	0	344	5.0	167	92	115	9	2071	19	.1[1]	+	+		+	
1159	39	43	41	36	14	5	0	0	74	2.0	7	44	45	0	679	14	1.3	+	+			
1160	24	34	65	68	26	4	0	0	122	2.0	24	62	69	4	964	19	12.0	+	+			
1180	40	20	54	62	11	18	3	0	150	2.0	26	61	95	0	1199	23	19.3		+			
1157	59	20	82	57	32	34	25	0	535	10.0	32	64	102	0	1332	20	7.0		+			
1171	52	16	58	80	60	50	18	0	601	7.0	87	83	104	0	1619	18	6.2		+			
1164	42	26	34	54	26	35	24	6	470	8.0	38	38	75	0	985	28	15.0		+			
1195	39	34	44	35	20	8	0	13	113	8.0	31	45	76	0	982	25	3.6		+			
1196	49	69	68	44	0	27	29	9	463	11.0	4	65	77	0	1101	20	8.0		+			
1193	50	22	67	66	19	23	10	0	317	5.0	49	61	100	30	1338	25	.1[1]		+		+++	
1214	48	27	63	62	15	19	9	0	222	3.0	19	30	52	0	675	11	11.3		+	+		+
1217	55	13	39	62	49	31	26	0	553	9.0	44	53	75	0	1078	17	7.8		+		++	
1218	33	30	39	38	16	13	2	0	135	3.0	16	51	85	0	1030	27	2.7		+			+
1226	42	28	52	49	27	13	1	0	168	3.0	13	50	90	0	1103	23	1.5		+			
1228		27	56	52	49	55	75	2	1108	20.0	55	70	104	15	1544	30	6.5		+			

[1] Untraced.

TABLE 190.—THE TREATMENT WITH INSULIN OF THIRTY CASES BETWEEN FEBRUARY AND MAY, 1923.

Case No.	Age at onset, years.	Days in hospital.	Weight in kilograms.		Average daily diet in hospital in grams.												Duration in years to May, 1923.	Treatment begun with:	
			Entrance.	Exit.	First week.						Last week.							Test diets.	Insulin.
					Carbo-hydrate.	Protein.	Fat.	Total¹.	Per kilo.	Insulin, aver-age units, daily.	Carbo-hydrate.	Protein.	Fat.	Total.	Per kilo.	Insulin, aver-age units, daily.			
812	31	16	54.0	54.7	97	55	89	1409	26.0	5	107	62	119	1747	32.0	8	8.4	T.D. 2	2
1182	33	23	76.3	75.7	75	46	93	1321	15.5	9	111	74	123	1847	24.0	10	9.8	T.D. 2	2
1579	50	16	89.7	89.7	44	35	61	856	9.5	11	78	72	135	1815	20.5	6	3.8	S.T.D. 2¹	2
1609	11	15	37.8	38.6	49	32	52	789	21.0	11	48	49	113	1400	36.5	13	5.8	T.D. 2	3
1705	21	19	64.1	61.7	35	20	35	537	8.5	15	77	65	130	1740	28.0	15	3.5	T.D. 2	8
1887	15	26	24.6	26.7	50	32	58	853	34.0	14	51	43	114	1394	24.5	21	8.0	T.D. 2	10
1947	53	28	46.3	45.0	45	28	49	736	16.5	14	58	54	142	1730	38.5	17	3.3	T.D. 3	0
2266	58	19	35.0	36.0	44	32	68	915	11.5	8	48	47	103	1303	36.0	11	3.3	T.D. 3	0
2319	54	20	61.3	62.7	48	32	88	1207	20.0	7	50	57	139	1550	24.5	15	1.9	CaPF5	2
2420	51	16	38.3	40.1	50	56	79	1070	28.0	9	78	56	112	1544	39.0	13	8.8	Acidosis	30
2448	18	17	44.0	44.0	39	41	73	936	20.5	31	38	43	123	1433	29.0	28	2.1	T.D. 2	2
2476	32	36	56.1	57.9	40	39	76	1001	17.5	17	43	60	152	1782	30.5	14	1.5	T.D. 3	1
2588	33	14	33.1	30.6	44	35	71	972	30.0	9	56	46	105	1402	46.0	10	6.1	CaPF6	5
2793	65	14	67.6	70.6	69	48	96	1333	19.5	12	111	67	131	1894	29.0	9	2.0	Acidosis	0
2801	15	277	45.8	43.4	37	21	4	270	6.0	9	49	63	144	1744	40.0	35	0.8	CaPF7	3
2854	42	14	43.8	46.3	64	51	85	1215	27.0	9	88	64	115	1643	36.0	10	0.9	CaPF7	2
2955	64	29	45.6	47.8	72	51	101	1289	28.0	12	60	62	151	1847	45.0	14	3.3	Acidosis	3
3034	64	26	35.4	36.3	53	44	70	1099	30.5	10	66	54	102	1400	25.5	10	1.7	S.T.D. 1	3
3064	45	16	55.8	53.0	64	40	76	1053	19.0	13	48	50	110	1382	27.0	12	2.2	T.D. 1	3
3067	39	18	56.6	58.2	51	34	54	872	15.5	10	48	57	127	1558	45.0	12	1.7	S.T.D. 2	3
3068	10	18	24.5	25.4	56	31	50	781	31.0	9	65	45	80	1160	63.0	10	0.6	T.D. 1	3
3071	50	15	63.9	62.5	66	32	74	1010	63.0	6	68	81	130	1606	26.0	8	3.2	T.D. 2	3
3073	25	16	75.8	76.7	60	57	97	1368	17.5	11	72	64	142	2002	24.5	8	0.8	T.D. 2	5
3077	44	14	69.9	70.2	78	45	78	1098	15.5	5	100	71	131	1713	32.5	10	2.9	T.D. 2	2
3086	18	14	60.7	61.1	49	51	93	1266	21.0	9	87	48	108	1985	36.0	10	0.3	T.D. 3	5
3092	35	23	39.0	41.8	49	40	63	1033	26.0	13	68	49	131	1515	29.0	12	0.5	CaPF5	3
3096	61	26	55.1	56.3	39	38	79	911	16.0	0	89	65	130	1631	29.5	15	1.8	S.T.D. 3	3
3118	44	17	60.8	60.8	49	22	35	603	10.0	6	77	67	118	1675	27.5	15	0.2	T.D. 2	5
3121	26	16	55.3	54.0	39	22	39	593	11.0	9	89	67	108	1549	29.0	15	1.1		3
3124	38	23	60.2	59.2	27	23	41	563	16.0	13	60	63	134	1699	28.5		1.6		0

¹ S. T. D signifies Surgical Test Diets. These were similar to the Maintenance Diets which have now replaced them.

TABLE 191.—SUMMARY OF TABLES 190, 191, 192 AND 193 SHOWING THE TREATMENT OF FOUR GROUPS OF THIRTY CASES EACH OF DIABETES AT SUCCESSIVE PERIODS.

Group	Date	Age at onset, years	Average number of days in hospital	Weight in kilograms — Entrance	Exit	Gain or loss	First week Carbo-hydrate	First week Protein	First week Fat	First week Alcohol	First week Calories Total	First week Calories Per kilo	Last week Carbo-hydrate	Last week Protein	Last week Fat	Last week Alcohol	Last week Calories Total	Last week Calories Per kilo	Duration in years to Jan. 1, 1923, or to death	Treatment begun with: Fasting	Treatment begun with: Exclusion of fat. Preparatory treatment.	Acidosis Present — Developed after entrance	Acidosis Present — Decreased after entrance	Absent during hospital stay.
I.	April, 1915, to March, 1916	40	33	60	57	−3.07	19	17	11	2	243	4	26	54	76	1	992	18	8.6	12	18	7	15	8
II.	March, 1916, to July, 1916.	46	23	59	56	−2.87	25	24	6	1	234	4	43	60	82	4	1151	21	6.7	16	14	4	6	20
III.	July, 1916, to Feb., 1917	42	28	56	54	−1.60	27	24	16	1	356	6	43	60	90	3	1239	23	7.1	6	24	2	12	16

For Group IV the "Duration" column heading reads *Duration in years to May 1, 1923*, and the "Treatment begun with" columns become *Insulin, average units daily — First week / Last week*.

Group	Date	Age at onset, years	Average number of days in hospital	Weight — Entrance	Exit	Gain or loss	First week Carbo-hydrate	First week Protein	First week Fat	First week Alcohol	First week Calories Total	First week Calories Per kilo	Last week Carbo-hydrate	Last week Protein	Last week Fat	Last week Alcohol	Last week Calories Total	Last week Calories Per kilo	Duration in years to May 1, 1923	Insulin First week	Insulin Last week	Developed after entrance	Decreased after entrance	Absent
IV.	Feb., 1923, to May, 1923	37	19[1]	52.6	53.1	+0.50	53	38	67	..	965	21	71	58	123	..	1623	33.5	3.0	10	13			

[1] Not including No. 2801, who stayed in hospital two hundred and seventy-seven days.

The average duration of hospital stay of 100 cases treated without insulin, just prior to August 7, 1922, was 12 days and of 100 cases treated with insulin, prior to August 7, 1923, was 10 days.

2. **Body Protein.**—Desire to protect body protein by more protein attained some fulfilment, even in pre-insulin days. In the early group the protein per day per patient for the first week was but 17 grams, or less than 0.33 gram per kilogram body weight, during the last week it was 0.9 gram per kilogram body weight. In the two later series the figures change, and in the first week the protein almost reached 0.5 gram per kilogram body weight, and in the last week is fully 1 gram. The insulin cases in the fourth group received 1.1 grams protein per kilogram.

3. **Total Calories.**—The gain in calories given the patients in the last week of the third group was distinct. Writing in 1917, my comment was, "At the present time the patients certainly go home in better condition and with lower blood sugars than two years ago. Still the melancholy fact remains that the patients leave the hospital with 23 calories instead of a permanent, self-sustaining diet. A gain in 3 or 4 calories per kilo would mean everything to diabetic patients. The shortage in calories now is in great part due to the weekly 'fasting' day or 'half' day, and the 21 and 23 calories respectively per kilo which the last group of patients daily received on leaving the hospital were chiefly taken by them during six days." Who of us at that time dared to believe that insulin was so near? Looking at the insulin group the metamorphosis of diabetic treatment is apparent. The caloric intake of the diabetic has been raised 64 per cent over that in the first period, 1915, and 31 per cent over that of the third period ending in 1917.

E. FOLLOW-UP METHODS.

Almost any physician can get his diabetic patients sugar-free, but to keep these patients sugar-free and in good health is an art. A doctor's ambition should be not to see how large a number of diabetic patients he can have, but how many he can keep in good condition. The education of the patient is the basis for success along this line, and this must begin at the very start. Upon finding that the mortality among patients was largely due to ignorance the importance of this aspect of treatment became evident. Insulin makes education even more necessary.

Patients must be taught from the first that the preliminary treatment represents only a beginning of treatment; that treatment lasts for life; that whenever sugar or acidosis returns or unusual loss of weight occurs and they are unable to control these phenomena, they must report to a physician. The physician, too, must do everything in his power to keep in touch with his patients at regular intervals. Of course, this is quite difficult because he is laid open to the suspicion of seeking practice; but it is better to run the chance of a misunderstanding on this score in 1 case than to let 10 other cases perish. One of the chief advantages of modern treatment is that it is less costly than former methods, because when once trained, there is less necessity to consult the physician at frequent intervals.

Doctors who have patients temporarily under their care in hospitals owe it to their patients to keep the family physician in touch with the method of treatment employed. Formerly a copy of the chart at the end of the hospital stay was sent to the physician, but this is not sufficient. Weekly reports, made out by the patients themselves are preferable and should be sent home. It is just as essential, in fact even more so, to educate the doctor as the patient. If a physician sends a diabetic patient to a hospital for treatment, from the reports he receives he should gain enough help to enable him to treat other similar cases at home. A patient with exophthalmic goiter sent to the Mayo Clinic, prior to 1917, led to the receipt of *four* unsolicited reports upon her progress.

F. SPECIAL DIETETIC METHODS.

1. **High Carbohydrate Diet.**—The normal diet for an adult with moderate activity consists of about carbohydrate 5 grams, protein 1.25 grams, and fat 1 gram, or a total of 34 calories, per kilogram body weight. A common diet in diabetes would be carbohydrate 1 gram, protein 1 gram, and fat 2.5 grams, or 30 calories, per kilogram body weight. The Newburgh-Marsh diet on the contrary consists of carbohydrate 0.5 gram, protein 0.66 gram, and fat 3 grams per kilogram. Applied to the diet of a child the arrangement of the foods per kilogram body weight is somewhat different, but still the variations are striking. These various calculations are shown in Table 192. The diets for adults represent estimated and suggested diets by the author and the routine diet of Newburgh and Marsh from whose writings a diet for a child is taken. A diet is inserted for a child now treated by H. Gray and Holt's standard diet for children.

TABLE 192.—DIETS IN HEALTH AND DIABETES ARRANGED PER KILOGRAM BODY WEIGHT.

Condition.	Author.	Carbohydrate, gm.	Protein, gm.	Fat, gm.	Calories.
Adults.					
Health	E. P. J.	5.0	1.25	1.0	34
Diabetes	E. P. J.	1.0	1.00	2.5	31
Diabetes	N. and M.[1]	0.5	0.66	3.0	32
Children.					
Health	Holt	10.2	3.30	3.3	83
Diabetes	H. G.	7.8	2.90	3.3	73
Diabetes	Newburgh[2]	1.4	2.50	7.8	86

[1] Newburgh and Marsh: Loc. cit., p. 525. [2] Personal communication,

Oliver L. Sharp, M. D.

304-305 JEFFERSON BUILDING   GREENSBORO, N. C.

OFFICE PHONE 3766   RESIDENCE PHONE 4137

FOR... ADDRESS...

℞

Dear Dr Berry –
Appropos our conversation,
Please refer to page 462 + 514 –
which substantiate my argument
about the relative proportions
of Chlorophylls & Xanthins in
Chlorella butter — (?) _____

The radical modification of the diet which diabetes entails has always attracted my attention and in addition, during the last few years, the following considerations have been influential: (1) That in those countries where the diet consists largely of carbohydrate, the diabetes is mild; (2) that the diets of those diabetics who live longest, whether they show sugar or not, are those whose carbohydrate has never been long reduced to a very low quantity; (3) that as yet few cases have been published who have lived constantly, either in or outside of institutions, upon very low-carbohydrate and high-fat diets and attained an average duration of their diabetes equivalent to the six years recorded for my own 597 fatal cases since June, 1914. Of all my cases there is perhaps but 1, Case No. 632, aged thirty-three years, who has lived for the last six years on approximately carbohydrate 28 grams, protein 79 grams, fat 133 grams, alcohol 15 grams. Would he be better off today if the protein had been lower? (4) That, given a diabetic in the last stage of inanition, he may gain a considerable lease of life when carbohydrate and protein are given freely; but this, however, is soon shortened by coma if much fat is also added, (5) that if the liver can be made to harbor any carbohydrate it is a protective phenomenon (witness the giving of carbohydrate freely to children prior to tonsillectomies and the resulting avoidance of acidosis); (6) that upon analysis of cases of coma it will be found that usually preceding its onset carbohydrate has been lowered and the fat metabolized has been increased, whether from exogenous or endogenous sources; (7) that the work done by Benedict and the writer at the Nutrition Laboratory has shown that there is no diabetic so severe as to have completely lost the power of responding to carbohydrate by a failure to raise the respiratory quotient as a result of its administration; and (8) finally, that it is more rational to tend toward than to deviate from the standard diet of healthy people.

A high-carbohydrate diet preceding a test meal was found by Kageura[1] to lead to a lesser increase in the blood sugar than as if the preceding diet was composed exclusively of fat and protein. He also proved that this effect of the high-protein-fat diet was not due to acidosis.

My attention to a high-carbohydrate and low-fat diet has been drawn especially by a little boy, George B., Case No. 2007, an only child, who two years and six months after onset continues to keep sugar-free on a diet of carbohydrate 178 grams, protein 75 grams, and fat 44 grams. The diagnosis was made by Dr. John Lovett Morse in the course of a *routine* examination on December 1, 1920,

[1] Kageura: Jour. of Biochemistry, 1922, **1**, 333. Also ibid., 1923, **2**, 341.

at five and eight-tenths years of age, a few days after the beginning of symptoms, when the urine showed a specific gravity of 1.035. It was 1.028 on the following day. The percentage of sugar on December 3 was 4.4. Ten days after the onset of symptoms he excreted but 3 grams of sugar, although his diet consisted of the then Test Diet 2; carbohydrate 102 grams, protein 58 grams, fat none, calories 640, and he was sugar-free the next day on Test Diet 3; carbohydrate 64 grams, protein 33 grams, fat none. From that time on his carbohydrate has been gradually increased until he is now taking carbohydrate 178 grams. The protein has been raised from 33 grams to 75 grams—*i. e.*, 3.3 grams per kilogram body weight—but the fat has been constantly kept low, never having risen above 44 grams. This little boy, George B., has been sugar-free, except on a few occasions: November, 1921, when he had an infection with a temperature of 102° F. for three days, again in February, 1922, when he had a cold, and recently after the clinic at the New York Academy of Medicine. He has gained $5\frac{1}{4}$ pounds in two and a half years and 2 inches in height in a year and ten months. The diet has almost never been broken. The urine is examined five times daily. On June 7, 1922, two hours after a meal, the blood sugar was found to be 0.09 per cent, on September 20, two hours and a quarter after a meal, it was 0.14 per cent, on October 31, three hours and a half after a meal, 0.13 per cent, on December 4, four hours after lunch and one hour after orange 150 grams, 0.17 per cent, on January 20, 1923, four hours after lunch and one hour after orange 120 grams, 0.21 per cent, and on March 19, one and one-half hours after fruit, 0.15 per cent. Since writing this paragraph in July, 1923, the tolerance has dropped to about 120 grams. Perhaps insulin will prevent a further lowering.

The example of this case suggested similar treatment for other cases, but none of these other cases have done quite as well. Case No. 2140, aged twenty and eight-tenth years at onset, who originally showed 7 per cent sugar with acidosis and later acquired a tolerance for carbohydrate 186 grams, protein 89 grams, fat 75 grams, fell out of the race when he ate 9 doughnuts one night. Case No. 2052 thoughtlessly broke his diet by the addition of cream, and thus jeopardized his future. Case No. 2095 suffered from a tonsillitis. The diet of the little boy, George B., however, has been broken only on the rarest occasion, and not another one of my patients has had such close care. The future of this child, therefore, should disclose the merits of this form of treatment. It is, however, fully realized (1) that faithful supervision of a diabetic case, provided the diet is not distinctly bad—*i. e.*, excessive—is so great a factor in treatment that it largely overcomes many minor dietetic faults; (2) that this child's diabetes was discovered extraordinarily early, and (3) that this case too has an hereditary element in his grandparents. Whether the little boy, George B., Case No. 2007, is so very unusual, time will tell. (See p. 666.)

TABLE 193.—HIGH CARBOHYDRATE DIET.

Case No. 2052. Age at onset, November, 1920, seventeen years and six months.

| Date. | Fe₂Cl₆ | Sugar. | | Carb., gm. | Prot., gm. | Fat, gm. | Cal. | Insulin, units. | Weight, kg., net. |
		Urine, per cent.	Blood, per cent.						
1920.									
Dec. 7	..	..	0.23						
1921.									
Jan. 6	0	0	0.09						
24–25	0	0	0.10	67	54	35	799	...	53
31, Feb. 1	0	0	0.08	121	65	48	1176		
Feb. 12–13	0	0	0.09	200	71	62	1642	...	54
May	..	..		170	75	60	1520		
June	..	..	0.10						
Sept.	..	..	0.12	142+	57+	70+	1036+	...	57
Nov. 5– 6	0	0	0.09	138	69	71	1467	...	56
1922.									
April	..	..	0.12						
1923.									
April 20	++++	6.2	..	Effect of Christian Science					
20–21	++	4.0	..	121	26	25	813	0 1 2	52
21–22	+	4.0	0.18	101	35	43	931	3 4 5	
22–23	+	2.0	..	66	24	37	693	5 5 5	
23–24	..	Tr.	..	64	44	83	1179	5 5 5	
24–25	..	Tr.	..	74	52	88	1206	5 5 5	
25–26	..	0.1	..	84	61	94	1426	5 5 5	
26–27	..	0.3	..	98	65	106	1606	5 5 5	
27–28	..	Tr.	0.28	86	63	129	1657	5 7 5	
28–29	..	0	..	86	63	129	1657	7 7 5	
29, May 2	..	0	..	88	65	131	1781	7 7 5	
May 2– 3	..	0	..	98	66	132	1844	7 7 5	
3– 4	..	0	..	108	67	133	1897	7 7 5	
4– 5	..	0	..	135	80	135	2075	7 7 5	
5– 8	..	0	0.14	159	84	135	2187	7 7 5	
8– 9	..	0	..	159	84	135	2187	7 5 5	
9–10	..	Tr.	..	159	84	135	2187	7 4 5	
10–11	..	0	..	159	84	135	2187	7 4 7	
11–12	..	0	..	159	84	135	2187	7 2 7	
12–13	..	0	..	159	84	135	2187	7 0 7	
13–14	..	0	..	159	84	135	2187	7 0 7	
14–15	..	0	..	159	84	135	2187	8 0 5	
15–16	..	0	0.14	159	84	135	2187	10 0 5	53

Strangely enough by one of those coincidences so common in medicine, a case similar in many respects—Jack R., Case No.

2661, who has been under the care of another physician from the
beginning—I had the opportunity to observe for a few days soon
after George B. appeared. This little boy is also an only child,
his diabetes was also diagnosed promptly after onset of symptoms—
namely, in September, 1921—at the age of five and one-tenth
years. The first specimen of urine showed 8 per cent sugar in
October, 1921. On May 26, 1922, nine months after the onset
of his diabetes, his diet was carbohydrate 36 grams, protein 42
grams, fat 114 grams, making the calories 1338 or exactly identical
with those of George B. His fasting blood sugar was 0.09 per cent
on May 26, and on May 29, 0.07 per cent, and the blood fat was
0.71 per cent. His weight at onset was 17.1 kilograms and May
26, 1922 was 16.9 kilograms. The urine at that time contained
no sugar, but showed a positive test for acetone and for diacetic
acid. The average of the twenty-four-hourly analyses of ammonia
for five days was 0.53 gram and of nitrogen, 7.8 grams. Dr.
Alan Brown, of Toronto, reports that at present, May 17, 1923,
Jack R., is taking carbohydrate 70.6 grams, protein 70.07 grams,
fat 143.14 grams, calories 1850, with 17.5 units of insulin daily.
By July, he was able to reduce the dose. The blood sugar on May 1,
was 0.106 per cent. Since each child will be guarded by his parents
with equally scrupulous care, their careers will be watched with
aggressive vigilance.

It is only within this decade that diets have been accurately
controlled for months and years and the quantities of carbohydrate,
protein, and fat recorded, and only within the last eight years
that the total quantity of food has been at all closely limited. In
consequence it is only today that we are in a position to compare
the effects of various diets, only today that we can begin to discuss
how, for instance, it is best to distribute a given intake between
the three food-stuffs. In point are the two "only" children cases
described above. There are no two cases who are more likely to
afford crucial evidence regarding the optimal carbohydrate-fat
ratio, and as no data exist to prove which is the better of the diets
prescribed for these two boys, one is forced to prescribe empirically. Which child is on the better diet?

2. **Fasting Days.**—Only those who have cared for many patients
by the older methods can appreciate the advance which Allen
gave to diabetic therapy, with his introduction into general practice
of fasting and undernutrition. Many years ago Naunyn strongly
urged the use of starvation days in the treatment of diabetes.
He repeatedly called attention to the advantages derived therefrom, and said one should not fear temporary undernutrition if
thereby it was possible to remove the sugar from the urine. Over
and over again a day of starvation would render a patient sugar-

free when all else had failed. Such days were usually indicated in the treatment of the severest cases of diabetes, and in a case of moderate severity such a day would do what many days of low diet had failed to accomplish. Naunyn used these days not alone to render the urine free from sugar and to place the patient in a better condition to acquire tolerance for carbohydrates, but also to lower the acidosis in a striking manner. Von Noorden agreed with Naunyn that these days were never disadvantageous. He writes: "I make use of these, especially when there is high acetonuria. It is astonishing how strikingly the acetone falls on a hunger day. Its effect stretches out for a number of days later. In numerous severe cases a hunger day has been instituted every week with excellent results." A third reason existed which also accounted for the good effects of a starvation day, to wit: the patient's digestion was given a rest Naunyn, in an indirect way, protected the digestion of his patients by emphasizing the value of a low caloric intake. Hodgson, too, is precise upon this point. He says: "Again it should be stated that the quantity of all food, even if it is carbohydrate-free, must be greatly restricted. The number of calories that the body ordinarily requires is no safe criterion of the amount of food that should be given a diabetic. It is not the quantity of food that should be metabolized, but the amount that can be metabolized that should determine the quantity given to the patient. All in excess of what a patient can actually use burdens the already overtaxed excretory organs and retards improvement."

Hodgson should be given the credit of having published this article in 1911.[1] Guelpa[2] in 1910 reported his success in the treatment of diabetes by the employment of several days' fasting combined with purgation: "I do not pretend that this cure has been put as yet on a definite scientific basis. Much further and more generalized experience of it is required before we can arrive at clear conclusions as to the extent of its sphere of usefulness. From the observations I have already made, however, of the action of the cure, it is possible to draw certain inferences of capital importance.

"1. There is absolutely no danger and no serious inconvenience in abstaining entirely from food for three or four days, or even longer; the period of abstinence, also, may be repeated several times without risk or inconvenience, if each day a large dose of a purgative is given to insure intestinal disinfection.

"2. While there may be some slight discomforts during the period of abstinence, these never persist after food is resumed. On the

[1] Hodgson: Jour. Am. Med. Assn., 1911, **57**, 1187.
[2] Guelpa: British Med. Jour., 1910, **2**, 1050.

other hand, undoubted and durable benefits are always gained, in the shape of increased freedom of movement, greater clearness of ideas, amelioration of all congestive conditions, and a true feeling of general well-being. In a word, one is always better in all respects after the cure than before.

"3. The cure is a perfectly safe procedure if controlled by examinations of the blood and the urine. It insures the maximum of benefit being derived from any concomitant therapeutic measures."

Guelpa reports many cases of diabetes and the astonishingly good results which followed the method he employed. He deserves great credit for his originality and courage in applying this method as well as for his modesty, and his name should always receive a prominent place when fasting is mentioned.

The advantages of the fasting method at the outset of treatment are many: (1) It is a simple method and enables the practising physician to render all save exceptional cases of diabetes sugar-free and to keep them so. (2) The treatment is such that acidosis is almost invariably diminished rather than increased. (3) The method is suitable for a patient to learn, and he is thereby placed in a position to protect himself. (4) The expense of treatment to the patient is reduced because he can readily perform the urinary tests essential for treatment, and by keeping sugar-free, visits to a physician are rendered infrequent. (5) The responsibility of treatment rests upon the patient, and this makes the chances of his following directions far more probable. Others have employed fasting; Naunyn and Guelpa tried it extensively; Hodgson used a low diet with success, but Allen proved prolonged fasting efficacious. Before he treated any human patients by fasting, he demonstrated that his method was useful for animals. Allen's experience convinced him that the glycosuria of even the severest type of diabetes might be cleared up advantageously by one initial fast, though it might be necessary to prolong it exceptionally for eight or ten days. And he goes on to say: "Broadly speaking, freedom from glycosuria seems obtainable in all cases of uncomplicated human diabetes before there is danger of death from starvation. Even wasted and emaciated patients have borne fasting with apparent benefit, giving the impression that they have been suffering more from intoxication than from a lack of nutrition;" and in another place, "among the patients treated thus far during a variable number of months, in the hospital and at home, spontaneous downward progress has not yet been observed."

The method which I formerly found worked best when fasting seemed required was as follows:

Preparation for Fasting.—In severe, long-standing, complicated, obese and elderly cases, as well as in all cases with acidosis or in any case if desired, without otherwise changing habits of diet, omit fat, after two days omit protein, and then halve the carbohydrate daily until the patient is taking only 10 grams; then fast. In other cases begin fasting at once. It is not only more rational but it is easier to prevent acidosis than to treat it. This is the reason for the preparation for fasting. The majority of diabetic patients show little acidosis upon fasting if protected in this way because they gain carbohydrate tolerance in the process, or if acidosis has been present it will decrease. (Table 189, p. 510.) On the other hand, it is not always easy to predict[1] what will occur, and an acidosis which has not been present may appear or an existing acidosis may grow worse. Therefore it is safer to take pains to avoid the development of acidosis in those predisposed to it, for it is a sound rule of all treatment that patients coming to the physician in an endurable state must not be made worse or have their lives jeopardized by the therapeutic procedures adopted.

Individuals predisposed to acidosis are those in whom the disease is of long duration. Changes in the diet and regimen of such patients are always dangerous, and particularly so in the cases of extraordinary length. Treatment of such individuals should never be undertaken lightly nor without a full realization of the gravity involved. This has been illustrated by Cases 295, 304 and 310. These three were hereditary cases and this fact may have accounted for the long duration of their disease, which was nine, seven and nineteen years respectively. They finally came under my supervision in a much debilitated condition. Even at that time the danger of changing the diet was appreciated, and unusual care was taken to prevent a fatal issue. Ultimately the 3 cases died in coma, 1 upon a sea voyage, 1 after unusual exertion, and 1 for reasons unknown, in periods of two and a half years, two months, and five months respectively, after being seen. Consequently, when Case No. 887 came for treatment in 1915, with a duration of the disease of twenty-nine years, unusual apprehension was felt. For nine days the patient was not allowed to make the slightest possible change in the regimen for, although she was wretched, she was alive. She was then admitted to the hospital, but with much foreboding, although no alarm was felt by other physicians, experienced in diabetes, who saw her. Table 197, shows the progress of the patient.

Fasting for nine days except for 150 grams of 5 per cent vegetables on one day failed to rid the urine of sugar save upon the second day after admission; indeed upon the ninth day the quantity of dextrose in the urine was 17 grams. On the following day, August 8, 3

---

[1] Stillman: Am. Jour. Med. Sci., 1916, **151**, 505.

TABLE 194.—CASE No. 887. DIABETES OF LONG DURATION WITH DEATH IN COMA AFTER FASTING.

Date, 1915.	Volume, cc.	Diacetic acid.	NaCl, gms.	Nitrogen, gms.	NH₃, total gms.	D:N ratio.	Total gms.	Carbohydrate.	Protein.	Fat.	Alcohol.	Calories.	Carbohydrate balance, gms.	NaHCO₃, gms.	Naked weight, pounds.	Pulse.	Blood sugar, per cent.	Alveolar air, CO₂ mm Hg.
July 21		++		21.3			4% 72						−35	0				
26	3000	+++			3.7			37										
									Entrance to Hospital.									
30-31	1350	+++					24	0	0	0	20	140	0	0	132		0.23	32
31, Aug. 1	1250	+					0	0	0	0	16	112	−5	0	131			30
Aug. 1-2	1650	0					10	5	2	0	2	42	−13	0	131			28
2-3	1600	+++		6.5	2.4	1.85:1	13	0	0	0	0	0	−12	4	128			28
3-4	1500	++		8.6	2.8	2.79:1	12	0	0	0	25	175	−18	24	127		0.18	26
4-5	2400¹	+++		9.0	3.4	2.00:1	24	0	0	0	32	224	−11	24	128			28
5-6	3000	+++		11.2	3.7	0.98:1	18	0	0	0	32	224	−17	36	127		0.15	26
6-7	2800	+++		11.9	4.0	1.43:1	11	0	0	0	32	224	−17	36	127		0.19	29
7-8	2900	+++		11.2	3.8	1.52:1	17	0	0	0	8	56	−23	42	125			29
8-9	2950	+++		17.6	4.3	1.31:1	17	0	18	15	24	375	−14	30			0.28	28
9-10	3900	+++	4.3	6.5	1.7	2.15:1	23	0	26	18	12	350			122		0.21	29
10-11	1750	++++	2.8	11.0	2.7	3.73:1	14									84-144	0.43	14
11-12	2900	+++	4.6				41									136-172		
12							Death in Coma.											

¹ Notice increase in volume of urine presumably due to the washing-out of acid bodies coincident with the administration of sodium bicarbonate.

eggs were allowed; on August 9, 3 eggs, lean meat 30 grams; on August 10, 200 grams of orange, about 15 grams oatmeal and the whites of 3 eggs, but otherwise the patient took no food from her entrance to the hospital on July 30 to death on August 12 of coma.

March, 1917, comment on Case No. 887. This case constituted a distinct failure. The carbon dioxide tension of the alveolar air remained between 32 and 26 mm. mercury tension until the day of death when it fell to 14 mm. mercury pressure. The inferences which were drawn from the behavior of the alveolar air were misleading. No great change took place in the quantity of sugar excreted. The dextrose-nitrogen ratio at the beginning afforded an index of the severity of the disease, though this statement cannot be made without qualification, because the sugar was estimated by rotation instead of by reduction. Later it fell for two successive days as the quantity of ammonia rose, but this may have been related to the changing conditions brought about by the increasing doses of sodium bicarbonate. The D:N ratio was 3.73:1 the day before death. Two other features claim attention first, the change in weight of the patient from 132 pounds to 122 pounds in ten days, and the low excretion of salt. On the other hand, there was an increase in the output of nitrogen which rose steadily from 6.5 grams to 17.6 grams two days before death, indicating the drain upon body protein.

The patient was wretched, it is true, when she entered the hospital but she was not excessively weak. •With a gradual elimination of carbohydrate following the omission of protein and fat she might have shown a moderately large tolerance for carbohydrate. How could she have done otherwise if she had lived for twenty-nine years with the disease? With this modification of dietetic treatment and the omission of alkalis I should not anticipate a like catastrophe with a similar patient today.

The bowels must be thoroughly opened, but I do not believe in free catharsis. If the patient has not had a movement for several days, give an enema, followed by some simple cathartic or mild aperient, and another enema twelve or twenty-fours hours later, but do not purge the patient. Gain enough is obtained if a movement is produced once in twenty-four hours when it has only been taking place once in seventy-two. In other words, do not upset any patient who is in a tolerable state. Furthermore, allow the patient to move about his room or if having two-thirds of his maintenance diet and free from acidosis to go out-of-doors though prohibit a walk of more than a block, avoiding excess in any direction. Remember what happens to an old man who is suddenly confined to bed, and the discomfort which follows confinement after a fracture. Do not force a temperate man to drink against his will.

Fasting is never so rigorous as doctors or patients expect. Patients are more ready to undergo it than physicians to prescribe it. Quite as often it is as much a relief to the patient as it is discomfort. This is in part due to the gradual decrease in polydipsia and polyuria. Headache occurs less frequently than would be expected, and is usually dispelled by a cup of coffee. Nausea almost never occurs unless a patient is given alkali or alcohol. Children bear it more easily than adults. Case No. 899 with onset at eighty, shunned it rightly, but she became sugar-free, lived to eat pie without glycosuria and died of hemiplegia at eighty-three years. It is always desirable to avoid fasting in the old, and this can be accomplished usually by the help of preparatory treatment.

Fasting does not seem like fasting to the patients when they receive coffee, tea, cracked cocoa shells and broths, and are given an unlimited supply of water. Warm drinks are preferable. If the quantity of urine, as it often does, falls to less than normal, the patients are urged to drink water freely. Clear meat broths are a great satisfaction. An analysis of the 1220 cc of broths taken by Case No. 765, during three days showed the total amount of calories therein contained to be negligible. Contrary to my experience with digestive cases, broths do not stimulate the appetite in fasting diabetics; they relieve it. The advantage of broths is probably due in part to this, but to a considerable extent to the patient receiving salt by which he may maintain the equilibrium of body fluid.

It is surprising, though usually explainable, how variable is the period required to render the urine sugar-free. Frequently a urine which contains 7 per cent of sugar becomes free from sugar after fasting for four meals, and conversely, a urine with only 3 per cent of sugar may still retain traces after the patient has been deprived of food for three or four days. In general, cases seen soon after onset become sugar-free promptly, whereas the reverse is usually true for those of long duration. "In one case we may be dealing with fatigue; in the other exhaustion of an already weakened organ," according to Greeley.[1] However, Case No. 733, age at onset seventeen, was fasted twenty-six months later, when he showed 6.6 per cent of sugar and became sugar-free in two days. The explanation in this instance was apparently the fact that the case was remarkably mild, being of the obesity type; in fact, the patient's highest weight—196 pounds—was reached when he first came under observation, and during the preceding twenty-six months he had gained 26 pounds. Despite

---

[1] Greeley: Boston Med. and Surg. Jour., 1916, **175**, 753.

this improvement he died nine months later of coma. Children showing large amounts of sugar have also become sugar-free very promptly when the duration has been only a few weeks. Cases of long standing appear to become sugar-free more quickly with a gradually limited diet than with an immediate fast. This is probably due to the avoidance of acidosis.

Many clinicians of the old school advantageously fasted their diabetics one day a week and this has given the cue to intermittent fasting. Very few of my patients have been subjected to a fast of more than four days. No patient has undergone a fast exceeding nine days. Such a prolonged fast is unnecessary, and even if the fast is carried out, it is doubtful if the patient would always become sugar-free. Since the advent of insulin no patient has been fasted at all. Fasting, however, taught a great many useful lessons, because it untangled many complexities of diabetes.

The apparent reason for the persistence of sugar in Case No. 610, who fasted the nine days, was the presence of a vulvar abscess. This patient showed a carbohydrate tolerance of only 2 grams for the subsequent year, but upon readmission to the hospital in May, 1916, and the institution of routine treatment, she became sugar-free in one day and the tolerance rose to 55 grams carbohydrate and an equal quantity of protein, and the total calories rapidly increased to over 20 per kilogram body weight. The gain persisted until autumn, when it gradually decreased, but it returned temporarily with renewal of energetic treatment and the use of levulose.

Favorable results with fasting are recorded from Minkowski's Clinic by Gooke[1] and in France by Rathery,[2] who prefers to use Guelpa's purgation with the fasting.

3. **Treatment with Low-carbohydrate and Low-protein and High-fat Diets.**—(Newburgh and Marsh and Petrén.). "When a patient enters the clinic, he is placed on a diet containing from 900 to 1000 calories of which about 90 grams is fat, 10 grams is protein, and 14 grams is carbohydrate. After the patient has been sugar-free for one or two weeks, his diet is increased to about 1400 calories, of which 140 grams is fat, 28 grams is protein and from 15 to 20 grams is carbohydrate. In the case of small individuals this diet is sufficient for prolonged use, and some of them are discharged with instructions to continue it. For larger persons, after another period of trial, a second increase is made, reaching 1800 calories, containing 170 grams of fat, from 30 to 40 grams of protein, and from 25 to 30 grams carbohydrate. Further additions up to 2500 calories may be made to suit individual cases.[3]

---

[1] Gooke: Arch. f. Verdauungs-Krank., 1922, **78**, 853.
[2] Rathery: Bull. Acad. de Méd., 1921, **85**, 262.
[3] Newburgh and Marsh: Arch. Int. Med., 1920, **26**, 647; ibid., 1921, **27**, 699 (Blood Sugar); ibid., 1922, **29**, 97 (Urinary Nitrogen); ibid., 1923, **31**, 3 (Fat Lipemia); ibid., 1923, **31**, 455

"In order to prove that our procedure is an improvement over the usual method, we must show (1) that glycosuria is avoided in severe diabetes; (2) that this diet does not precipitate acidosis; (3) that nitrogen equilibrium is maintained; and (4) that the patients are able to lead at least a moderately active, comfortable life."

The courage of Newburgh and Marsh, and of Petrén in giving a diet of high fat, with low carbohydrate and protein should be recognized. They have demonstrated that diabetic patients protected by a diet of undernutrition even largely composed of fat will not develop coma. Even before ketogenic-antiketogenic ratios were promulgated they showed empirically the advantage of low protein in the prevention of acidosis. Their work has made me feel justified in allowing more fat to my patients. Their diabetic creed is sound. They believe the urine should be sugar-free, they endeavor to keep the blood sugar normal, and they do not give alkalis. In fact they record that no alkalis have been given to the diabetic patients under their care at the University Hospital in Ann Arbor since January, 1920, and that no deaths from coma have occurred. This is doubly gratifying first because it confirms our experiences without alkalis at the New England Deaconess Hospital and second because it is proof of the possibility of the avoidance of deaths from coma in hospitals. Petrén, of Lund, Sweden, likewise reports the same general results because he states that since he has followed his plan of treatment, which is similar to that of Newburgh and Marsh, no diabetic patient, who has been for fourteen days in his hospital, has developed coma. However he gives alkalis.

A decision regarding the usefulness of this diet is concerned as much with its safety as with the results achieved.

These results Newburgh and Marsh present in Table 195 and one wonders whether the advantages of their plan, as here shown, are quite as great as they would have us believe. The table shows that the percentage of deaths of patients who have been treated in Ann Arbor or in Boston is about the same. It requires a great deal of intelligence to live on a low-carbohydrate, low-protein, and high-fat diet. The dangers of breaking over such a diet by increasing fat are far greater than the dangers of breaking over a diet by increasing carbohydrate. The patient who breaks over only in carbohydrate pays an immediate penalty and is warned by increased urination; the patient who breaks over only in fat and protein is not warned and dies.

Undernutrition is the explanation of the success of the Newburgh-Marsh diet. A patient of 60 kilograms body weight, receiving their first diet of 900 calories, is on half rations. Only when one to two weeks of undernutrition with this diet has made the urine of the patient sugar-free, is he advanced to the next diet of 1400 calories, which is about sufficient for the requirements of basal metabolism. Thereafter those patients who can tolerate it are given an increased diet, ranging to 1800 calories or 30 calories per kilogram body weight or even more, but the carbohydrate is never raised over 40 grams.

TABLE 195.—NEWBURGH-MARSH DIETS.

Carbohydrate.	Protein.	Fat.	Calories.
14	10	90	900
15–20	28	140	1400
25–30	30–40	170	1800
			2500

The diabetic's complaint against the Newburgh-Marsh diet is based upon its inflexibility. "There has been no selection of cases—every patient entering the service has been placed on this regimen." In other words, the mild, the moderate, and the severe diabetic, the old and the young diabetic, the diabetic with and the diabetic without acidosis, all are subjected to the same treatment. It is true that this shows the safety with which undernutrition can be invoked, and temporarily undernutrition will not harm either the mild or the severe case. With this factor of the diet there can be no objection. The innocent diabetic can well register his complaint against being sentenced for life, and this might be for over twenty years, see p. 678, to a diet of 35 to 40 grams of carbohydrate. A life sentence takes away all hope, ignores the possibility of the patient's having a tolerance for a much higher quantity of carbohydrate as well as a restoration of tolerance for carbohydrate. This condemnation of the innocent with the severe diabetic is the reason why the writer is unalterably opposed to this one phase of the Ann Arbor regimen.[1]

In their original paper all patients entering the Ann Arbor clinic were placed on the same diet, but in a subsequent paper,[2] the writers modify their procedure "because of the small body mass of children, their total calories are reduced, but the portions of foodstuffs used are the same. After the adult patient is desugarized, his diet is increased by steps until he is receiving 0.67 gram protein and from 30 to 40 calories per kilogram body weight, or sometimes a little more than this. In children more protein and more calories per kilogram body weight are allowed. . . . In no cases in this series has the daily carbohydrate allowance been greater than 35 grams. After the patient has been found to tolerate a maintenance diet of this type during several days in the ward, he is discharged with instructions to adhere to it rigidly."

[1] From a personal letter received October 4, 1923, I understand that these authors do not adhere to this low carbohydrate value as tenaciously as their published papers imply.

[2] Newburgh and Marsh: Arch. Int. Med., 1923, **31**, 455; also idem, 1921, **27**, 699.

Adherence to the rigidity of the tenets of the above diet may not be quite as absolute as Newburgh and Marsh would imply. For example, in their original communication they give 5 examples of Diabetic Diet No. 1, which, according to their paper, should contain 10 grams of protein, but as a matter of fact none of the 5 diets published by these authors contains less than 18.22 grams protein, and 4 of their illustrative Diets No. 1 contain twice the quantity of protein which they recommend.

The abolishment of glycosuria was attained, according to Newburgh and Marsh, in all cases coming for treatment, save a few justifiable exceptions. Such a demonstration merits attention and shows how useful moderate undernutrition is when combined with the low carbohydrate and low protein.

The reduction of the percentage of sugar in the blood to nearly normal was also attained in the vast majority of cases. Exceptions to this rule are those diabetics complicated with nephritis and a minor group whose failure to respond to treatment may in part have been due to complications.

The fat in the blood decreased in 12 of the cases studied by Newburgh and Marsh during the period of observation while they were upon the diets of low carbohydrate, low protein, and high fat. The average fat in the blood at the time of the first observation was 2.1 per cent and at the last observation, 1.1 per cent, or about 25 per cent above Bloor's normal. The interval between observations averaged eighty-one days, being in one case three hundred and ninety-five days.

The ability of a diabetic patient to subsist upon a diet which does not exceed 35 grams of carbohydrate and 0.66 protein grams, per kilogram body weight, for a period of ten years, irrespective of the quantity of fat, has not been demonstrated. In my experience with considerable numbers of diabetics I have known of no patient who has lived upon as low a diet as 35 grams of carbohydrate for ten years, even though the protein has been considerably higher than $\frac{2}{3}$ of a gram per kilogram body weight. Case No. 632, has now had diabetes for eleven years and for six years his diet was carbohydrate 15 to 28 grams, protein 69 to 88 grams, fat 103 to 170 grams, and about 15 grams of alcohol.

The advantages of a low-protein diet in the treatment of diabetes have been shown to be most advantageous both in the Ann Arbor and Lund clinics. From both sources it has been demonstrated that diabetics can be in nitrogenous equilibrium when the protein falls to as low as 0.66 gram per kilogram body weight, provided certain other conditions are satisfied. These are the presence of sufficient total calories in the ingested food. Whereas carbohydrate is more efficient in sparing protein than is fat, it is possible to use fat in far higher quantities than was previously supposed to be possible. It has generally been believed that for fat to be effective in sparing protein the carbohydrate calories must not fall below 10 per cent of the total calories, but Newburgh and Marsh found only 3.8 per cent in the form of carbohydrate necessary. Their evidence is somewhat invalidated by the recent work of DuBois and Richardson who showed that it is not the quantity of carbohydrate, protein, and fat *given* the patient but that which is *burned*, as proven by calorimetric determinations, which is the deciding factor. Both Petrén and Newburgh and Marsh give extraordinarily low values for the urinary nitrogen excretion of their patients. These are sometimes hard to explain. Thus Newburgh and Marsh record that Case No. 4, weighing 92 pounds, ingested 4.49 grams nitrogen daily for five days. Of this but 1.21 grams were excreted in the urine and 1.15 grams excreted in the stools, there being a nitrogen retention of 2.13 grams. That an individual on 28.06 grams of protein should maintain a positive nitrogen balance for nearly one-half this amount daily appears inconceivable, as also the possibility of the excretion of nitrogen in the urine falling to approximately the same level as the excretion of nitrogen in the feces. There must be some unexplained factor which accounts for these low nitrogen values, because there are many such in the records of the clinics, both at Lund and Ann Arbor. There is no ground for doubting the analyses; those of Petrén are similar, but how they can occur shou'd be explained.

Petrén is fully as enthusiastic an advocate of an extremely low protein diet in diabetes. He combines this with a high caloric intake made up almost exclusively of fat. The carbohydrate in the diet however, is not as low as that prescribed by Newburgh and Marsh. In conjunction with his low-protein, high-fat diet, Petrén employs opium (!) and alkali (!) as a routine. Petrén is thoroughly convinced of the harmlessness of the abundant caloric intake in the form of fat. Although he does not completely deny the rôle of fat in the development of acidosis, he ascribes to it a very subordinate place and considers the protein as the chief ketogenic factor. Very likely his views would be changed had his book, which has recently appeared, been written after he had become conversant with the American contributions upon ketogenic-antiketogenic problems. Owing to the great kindness of Prof. Hilding Berglund of the Harvard Medical School, I am able to present comments upon Petrén's book[1] which otherwise would have been

---

[1] Petrén: Diabetes-Studier, Kopenhagen, Glydendalske, 1923. Various articles in medical journals by Petrén have appeared which are in French or German. Of these the following may be cited: Verhand. d. XXXIV Kong. d. Deut. Gesell. f. inn. Med., 1922. Acta Med. Scand., Suppl. **3**, 101, 112. Verd. v. Staff,-Krank,, 1923, **8**, 5.

34

impossible, because it is written in the Scandinavian language. Most of what follows is exactly transcribed from Prof. Berglund's notes, but as I have interspersed comments of my own, responsibility for the text must rest with me in case I have failed to interpret Petrén aright.

During his trials with a low-protein diet, Petrén reached the lowest figures so far obtained for urinary-nitrogen equilibrium per kilogram body weight, *i. e.*, for the quotient $\dfrac{\text{metabolized protein}}{\text{body weight}}$. In this quotient the protein is calculated in grams from the urinary nitrogen and the weight is expressed in kilograms. It will be remembered that 0.66 grams protein per kilogram body weight has been considered to be about the minimum protein required for nitrogenous equilibrium in the regular diet. In a patient with a body weight of 57 kilograms, Petrén obtained a quotient 0.14 gram for a twelve-day period, and the quotient 0.18 gram for a thirty-six-day period. The lowest quotient for a normal person in the earlier literature was Siven's 0.22 gram for a period of six days. Petrén's further results are shown in Table 196.

TABLE 196.—LOW PROTEIN METABOLISM IN DIABETES. (PETRÉN.)

Protein metabolized per kilogram body weight, grams.	Number of diabetic cases.
0.20	2
0.22–0.24	3
0.25–0.29	11
0.30–0.34	14
0.35–0.39	8
0.40–0.44	5

With the exception of the twelve-day period already mentioned all of the quotients shown in Table 196 were secured from periods varying in length from twenty to eighty days or even more.

In the experiments on normal subjects given in the literature in which an attempt has been made to obtain a low-protein metabolism, a diet high in calories and also rich in carbohydrates was administered to the subject and was considered essential. In most of Petrén's cases it is true a high caloric diet was given, but he found this unnecessary in all cases. Petrén's lowest quotients were obtained with a diet of less than 2000 calories and in 2 cases with about 1500 calories.

The most important difference, however, between Petrén's and earlier investigators' work is found in the carbohydrate intake. Of course there must exist, from a theoretical point of view, some carbohydrate minimum under which it is impossible to reach a nitrogen minimum. To calculate the level for such a minimum was formerly difficult. By Landergren, this was placed between 40 and 50 grams, but by Rubner 60 grams. Thanks to various Americans we know it can be less. In the majority of Petrén's cases with a low level of the protein metabolism the carbohydrate intake was higher than 50 grams. Table 197 however, shows a number of cases with an astonishingly low carbohydrate intake.

TABLE 197.

Quotient, metabolized protein, body weight.		Carbohydrate, intake, grams.
0.28 0.34 0.30	. . . .	15–20
0.25 0.28 0.26	. . . .	30–35

Elsewhere an explanation for results similar to those of Petrén with this surprisingly low carbohydrate intake has been given, based upon the work of Shaffer, DuBois, Richardson and McCann. From their researches it is evident that it is not the diet given, which must be used for a basis of conclusions, but the diet metabolized by the patients as proved by calorimetric studies. The work of the above authors was not available to Petrén when he formulated his theories. Undoubtedly he will study his patients anew with this aspect of the problem in mind and future results from his laboratory will be awaited with interest. Particularly would such studies appear indicated because of another finding which he records. In a certain number of instances upon fasting days, he discovered that the nitrogen output of the patient was lower than prior to the fasting. This occurred even in cases where the nitrogen elimination before the fast was already as low as 2 to 2.4 grams in the twenty-four hours. Prof. Berglund points out that this further decrease occurred when the diet immediately prior to the fasting was high in calories rather than at the lower level. This is in complete harmony with other observations of Petrén namely that when fat alone was given for a day, the nitrogen output decreased to the same extent or even with greater regularity than when the patient actually fasted.

From the simultaneous decrease of acidosis and nitrogen elimination, Petrén concludes that the protein is responsible for the acidosis. In every case of diabetes of any severity there exists according to Petrén's conception a certain "threshold for the nitrogen metabolism," above which acidosis occurs. A difference between the acidosis in normal and diabetic individuals exists and consists according to Petrén in a lack of sensitiveness to the level of the protein metabolism in the diabetic individual. Fat, according to Petrén, only increases the formation of acetone bodies when the fat intake approaches or surpasses 300 grams per day.

Commenting on Petrén's theories, Berglund writes that the considerable decrease in the specific dynamic action of the proteins, which the Petrén diet involves, favorably influences the carbohydrate tolerance to a larger extent than has been determined hitherto. And the considerable amount of carbohydrate which the Petrén diet contains, he considers to be the most important factor in the interpretation of the high-fat tolerance of his patients.

4. **The Oatmeal Treatment.**—The use of oatmeal as a special form of treatment in diabetes was introduced by von Noorden in 1903.[1] The sudden disappearance of sugar from the urine, despite the administration of so much carbohydrate, was at first looked upon with awe. Gradual'y with a better understanding of the storage of carbohydrate in the body, its utilization or non-utilization, as disclosed by the respiratory quotient, and recognition of the low protein content of the oatmeal "cure," the mystery began to disappear. The experimental problems associated with it are so many that it deserves extended discussion. Formerly I occasionally employed it in the treatment of very severe cases of diabetes, but the apparent lack of the utilization of oatmeal as disclosed by the respiratory quotient discouraged extensive use of the same. Notwithstanding this fact, and although I have not treated a case in this manner for several years, the oatmeal treatment has taught us much.

The "cure" was originally prescribed by von Noorden[2] as follows: "The oat cure, as now prescribed by me, consists in the daily administration of 200 to 250 grams of oatmeal, best given in the form of gruel every two hours, and 200 to 300 grams of butter, and often about 100 grams of vegetable proteid or a few eggs may be taken in addition. Otherwise, nothing else is allowed, except black coffee, or tea, lemon juice, good old wine, or a little brandy or whisky. Such a diet is often disliked by the patient, but I have always succeeded in getting over this difficulty. After three or four days upon it the purpose for which it was intended is often found to have been attained; in other cases the same program must be repeated two or three times. It is apparently advisable to precede the oat cure with a few days of restricted diet, or even one or two vegetables days, for when the cure immediately supervenes upon a mixed diet the desired effect follows rather late.

"At the commencement of the oat-cure treatment one notices, it is true, even in the most favorable cases, an increase of the

[1] Von Noorden: Berl. klin. Wchnschr., 1903, **40**, 817.
[2] Von Noorden: Diabetes Mellitus, E. B. Treat & Co., 1905, p. 190.

glycosuria; but after a few days the excretion of sugar diminishes and the acetonuria even more so. During the oat days the urine may often be quite free from sugar, and if it is not entirely free, one may be fairly certain that it will be so in the succeeding vegetable days. Table 198 gives the details of one such favorable case.

TABLE 198.—VON NOORDEN'S ILLUSTRATION OF THE "OAT CURE."

Diet.	Sugar, gms.	Acetone, gms.	Ferric chloride reaction.	Ammonia, gms.
1. Strict diet	50.4	2.1	++	3.2
2. Strict diet	48.3	2.4	++	3.8
3. Strict diet	58.9	3.1	++	4.3
4. Vegetable day	28.2	2.1	++	2.9
5. Vegetable day	20.3	2.1	++	2.8
6. Oatmeal day	38.3	1.9	++	2.4
7. Oatmeal day	40.3	1.3	+	1.6
8. Oatmeal day	30.0	0.9	+	1.5
9. Oatmeal day	20.1	0.6	+	1.1
10. Vegetable day	8.0	0.8	+	1.3
11. Vegetable day	2.3	1.2	+	1.8
12. Oatmeal day	18.3	0.5	−	0.9
13. Oatmeal day	5.6	0.1	−	0.9
14. Oatmeal day	0	0.05	−	1.0
15. Vegetable day	0	0.1	−	0.8
16. Vegetable day	0	0.1	−	0.8
17. Strict diet	0	0.15	−	0.7
18. Strict diet	0	0.18	−	1.0
19. Strict diet and 20 gms. bread	0	0.12	−	0.9
20. Strict diet and 20 gms. bread	0	0.13	−	0.8

"The estimations made before the oat cure was begun show plainly enough that it is a case of severe glycosuria combined with excessive acetonuria. With the most restricted diet it had not been possible to bring the sugar below 40 grams; even on vegetable days more than 20 grams were excreted. In the course of the oatmeal treatment the urine became free from sugar, and it remained so on the subsequent return to the restricted diet. It even appeared that small quantities of carbohydrate could be well tolerated, whereas for several months previously there had been no question of such a thing.[1]

"I believe that a glance at Table 198, which is only one out of a large number showing the same thing, will suffice to show that a result has accrued which formerly would have been deemed impossible to obtain. Unfortunately, however, there are only relatively few cases in which the result is quite so surprisingly beneficial; in many others it is incomplete, although still satisfactory; in others again no result at all is obtained. The following fact is noteworthy: Cases in which the results of the treatment were most

[1] From the data furnished in Table 198, this case would not appear severe today. This may be one reason why the improvement was so marked.

beneficial relate without exception to the very severe forms of glycosuria; many of them were in children or young people. On the other hand, the result was almost without exception a failure in cases of slight glycosuria, the exact opposite of what might a *priori* have been expected. The oat cure rendered me immense service in severe cases, and I may even say that I have often succeeded in fending off incipient coma by its use."

The positive proof of the value of an oatmeal day would be the demonstration that the carbohydrate in the oatmeal was oxidized in the body. As yet, such a proof has not been satisfactorily established. It does not suffice to show that the sugar represented by the oatmeal does not appear in the urine during the oatmeal period. One should demonstrate a rise of the respiratory quotient following the use of oatmeal. This would appear an easy problem. Thus my own respiratory quotient before breakfast on September 30, 1914, was 0.82, but forty-five minutes later, after I had eaten 60 grams carbohydrate in the form of oatmeal it rose to 0.9. With diabetic patients the results were irregular but the evidence on the whole suggested a slight utilization by rise in respiratory quotient though a marked increase in metabolism. (See p. 260.)

Allen and DuBois[1] in studies upon several severe diabetics find "no special influence of oatmeal in diabetes or special readiness of oxidation. . . . The respiratory exchange fails to account for all the carbohydrate that disappears. The behavior of the respiratory quotient showed no important difference on the first day and on the third day of the oatmeal treatment."

In the light of present knowledge the frequently striking successes of the oatmeal treatment in diabetes as practised during the last few years are seen to depend upon several factors of which the most important is the fasting or greatly restricted diet which preceded and followed the cure. A similar result could be obtained with any carbohydrate as Blum pointed out and as Klemperer's experiments with dextrose and Benedict's and my experiments with levulose show. During fasting the sugar level in the body is lowered and the body is therefore in a more favorable condition to store carbohydrate and possibly to utilize it than under ordinary circumstances. The fasting or semifasting which followed the oatmeal days may be of very great advantage. It is quite possible that carbohydrates stored for a long period in the body may ultimately be better oxidized than carbohydrates representing more nearly an overflow of the carbohydrate reservoir which escape quickly into the urine. With this in mind it is easy to understand why Blum found small quantities of oatmeal worked better than large amounts in

---

[1] Allen and DuBois: Arch. Int. Med., 1916, **17**, 1010.

severe diabetics. He also showed it was more successful in mild than in severe cases.

Von Noorden also made another observation which indicates that the oatmeal is simply stored. A patient showed no sugar during the two preliminary vegetable days and the three following oatmeal days, yet in the next three vegetable days 96, 106 and 32 grams of sugar were excreted respectively.

The quantity of protein upon the oatmeal days is extremely slight. Thus, whereas the carelessly treated patient in diabetes ordinarily consumes far more than 100 grams of protein, if he takes even the full quantity of oatmeal, namely, 250 grams, he will receive not over 40 grams. The low quantity of protein is undoubtedly an important factor in the success of the treatment. In his study of the oatmeal treatment, Falta observed that protein added to the oatmeal tended to the excretion of more sugar in the urine than could come theoretically from the added protein, and that meat was especially harmful as compared with vegetable protein. Indeed, some patients were more sensitive to protein than to carbohydrate. Bernstein and Falta[1] have shown that a carbohydrate-fat diet lowers the metabolism, and they explain this as a result of the attendant decreased protein metabolism. A lowering of the metabolism is therefore, according to them, to be expected in the oatmeal treatment, because of the small quantity of protein therein contained. This has been observed, but they point out that such a lowering is to be expected only when the carbohydrate is utilized and thereby body protein spared. This lowering of the metabolism in and of itself helps the diabetic.

A gain in weight is usually coincident with the employment of the oatmeal cure. This is not peculiar to oatmeal, and is said to occur as a result of any carbohydrate day. Attention has been called to this phenomenon of gain in weight on changing from a fat to a carbohydrate diet in normal individuals. (See p. 218.) Contrary to many observers, who have considered it a disadvantage that the patient develops edema, in most cases I think it is distinctly helpful. Patients with edema seldom, if ever, develop diabetic coma. Falta noted a remarkable retention of protein during the oatmeal cure. The significance of this has not been explained, but it is probably in some way connected with the retention of fluids by the body. A second explanation of the gain in weight may be the behavior of the kidneys, according to Barrenscheen. He injected human subjects intravenously with 20 cc of a 10 per cent solution of lactose, and upon each of the following two days he gave 250 grams oatmeal. On the third day he gave a mixed diet,

[1] Bernstein and Falta: Deutsch. Arch. f. klin. Med., 1916, **121**, 95.

together with a repetition of the injection. Upon the oatmeal days the excretion of the lactose was delayed from one to five hours, which Barrenscheen attributed to slight renal changes, not otherwise demonstrable, caused by the oatmeal. A third reason for the gain in weight may be the high caloric value of an oatmeal day. This is not generally appreciated. It is shown in Table 199.

TABLE 199.—NUTRITIVE VALUE OF AN OATMEAL DAY.

Substance.	Quantity.	Carbo-hydrate.	Protein.	Fat.	Alcohol.	Calories.
Oatmeal . . .	240	160	40	16	..	944
Butter	240	...	..	200	..	1800
Whisky . . .	60	...	..	...	30	210
Total	160	40	216	30	2954

A fourth cause of gain in weight upon an oatmeal day is the considerable quantity of salt taken by the patient. For example, in the preparation of 240 grams of oatmeal the usual quantity of salt added by the cook is 10 grams and the patient may take even more. If to the oatmeal an equal amount of butter is added, according to the original advice of von Noorden, the quantity of salt is increased by 6.3 grams, for butter contains on the average 2.51 per cent salt. It would therefore seem quite likely that the edema which is associated with the oatmeal treatment might in great part be explained by the unusual quantity of salt given upon that day, and it is conceivable that along with the salt a considerable quantity of the carbohydrate of the oatmeal might be retained as well. One should try a salt-free oatmeal day and study the result.

A striking characteristic of the oatmeal treatment is that carbohydrate is administered in only one form and it has been contended that this is one reason for its apparently better assimilation than the same amount of carbohydrate in several forms. This supposition may be true but there is little sound evidence behind it. Such a phenomenon might be explained by the simplicity and blandness of such a diet leading to very slight stimulation of the digestive glands in general, and the pancreas in particular. In fact Cohnheim and Klee have noted this peculiarity in oatmeal. This may explain why boiled oatmeal acts better than baked oatmeal. Allen has pointed out that if the external function of the pancreas is relieved of work the internal function may act more vigorously and the diabetic condition be correspondingly benefited. The explanation agrees with facts. Allen[1] cites the work of Cohnheim and Klee, who observed that the foods which caused the

---

[1] The literature on the oatmeal treatment is given by Allen: Glycosuria and Diabetes, 1913, 441.

greatest activity of the external pancreatic function are the ones which give rise to glycosuria, and the foods which stimulate the external pancreatic function least are the ones which have least tendency to glycosuria. These writers suggest that the internal function of the pancreas is strengthened by relieving the strain upon the external function. The duodenal tube should furnish information along these lines.

The acidosis frequently decreases or disappears following or during the oatmeal cure. If such a reduction was constant it could be used as an argument in favor of the utilization of oatmeal, but unfortunately it is not. With Case Nos. 591 and 707, the acidosis was so severe that the respiratory quotient reached our lowest recorded levels, 0.65 to 0.62. The tests for acidosis were far less accurate when the oatmeal cure was in vogue and consequently the data upon this point are not as complete as one would wish. Unfortunately, too, for settlement of this question the treatment was complicated by the use of fat in the form of butter which would act in a manner directly opposed to oatmeal.

The employment of oatmeal in the "oatmeal cure" has stimulated its use in smaller quantities, and it is undoubtedly one of the most valuable additions to the strict diet of diabetic patients. It can be given in many different forms, it serves well as a vehicle for butter and cream, and is useful as gruel in the treatment of indigestion or diarrhea. It subjects the patient to less temptation than bread though the carbohydrate value is similar. Oatmeal water gruel and orange juice are the foods best borne by the patient on the verge of coma.

In prescribing oatmeal the dry weight should be the measure employed. Different brands vary enormously in bulk and hence in content of carbohydrate when cooked, because of the water employed. How wide these variations are the following table illustrates:

TABLE 200.—WEIGHTS OF DIFFERENT VARIETIES OF OATMEAL UNCOOKED AND COOKED.

| Quantity, 1 gill. | UNCOOKED. | | | COOKED. | |
	Weight, grams.	Carbohydrate, content.	No. tablespoonfuls, heaping.	Weight, grams.	No. tablespoonfuls, heaping.
H-O oatmeal . .	32	19	4	353	3½
Quaker oats . .	37	22	5	325	4
Scotch oatmeal . .	81	49	5	851	10
American oatmeal .	84	50	3½	690	6½
Irish oatmeal . .	96	58	5	853	15

Other Carbohydrate Cures.—(*a*) **Wheat.**—Blum[1] believes wheat flour acts just as efficaciously as oatmeal in a carbohydrate cure,

[1] Blum: Semaine médicale, 1913, **33**, 313.

and Csonka[1] has observed no difference between the utilization of starch of wheat and the starch of oatmeal flour by completely phloridzinized dogs. Blum demonstrated that the effect of the oatmeal or wheat was most marked in the mild cases. He noted that patients having a positive carbohydrate balance of 70 to 80 grams could take 200 to 250 grams of oatmeal with a similar quantity of butter and occasionally three or four eggs or 50 to 75 grams of vegetable albumin, and after living upon the diet for the customary three days, and then having a vegetable day, the last trace of sugar would disappear. Should the diabetes be a little more severe he employed 125 to 150 grams of oatmeal, but the same amount of butter. In still severer forms of diabetes with acid intoxication only 100 grams of oatmeal were allowed for a day or two, then only 75 grams for a few days, and finally a vegetable day. In other words, he was fasting his patient to a moderate degree.

(b) **Potatoes.**—A potato diet was advocated years ago by Mossé,[2] and in fact was the first of the carbohydrate cures recommended in diabetes. From what is known now it is easy to understand why a potato diet frequently worked well. (1) The potato diet was an undernutrition diet because no emphasis was laid upon the simultaneous use of fat; (2) there is little protein in a potato; (3) potatoes are a bulky food, and so satisfy the patient's appetite. The claim that considerable quantities of alkali are thus introduced into the system does not rest upon a firm foundation. I have had little experience with potato, but in 2 cases (Nos. 765 and 806) in which it was employed, respiratory quotients gave no evidence that it was assimilated.

In small quantities potato, like oatmeal, is most valuable. It carries butter well, contains only about one-third the quantity of carbohydrate in bread, and is easily measured. A potato the size of an egg weighs about 60 grams, whether cooked or uncooked, and contains 12 grams carbohydrate. With a good many mild cases of diabetes it is advantageous to exclude bread entirely from the diet and to substitute potato, of which the quantity need be only slightly restricted. One hundred grams of carbohydrate in the form of 160 grams bread are quickly eaten, but it is not so easy to take the same 100 grams carbohydrate in 500 grams of potato.

Little potatoes, carefully cleaned, when baked are often eaten with the skins by patients with much relish, and with relief to their constipation as well.

(c) **Bananas.**—Bananas have been advocated by von Noorden as a substitute for oatmeal. Like potatoes they contain about 20 per cent carbohydrate. Most of the carbohydrate is in the form

---

[1] Csonka: Jour. Am. Med. Assn., 1916, **67**, 1114.
[2] Mossé: Rev. de méd., 1902, **22**, 107, 279, 371, 620. Cited by Naunyn.

of starch, but when the banana thoroughly softens and ripens this changes to sugar. Bananas are usually eaten in the starch stage. The average weight of 12 whole bananas was 141 grams, the range 119 to 167 grams. When peeled these same bananas weighed on the average 87 grams, the range 73 to 101 grams. The carbohydrate in 1 banana is about 20 grams and this partial standardization makes them superior to potatoes.

(*d*) **The Milk Cure.**—Milk was advocated as an exclusive diet for diabetic patients by Donkin[1] some years ago, and again attention has been again called to it by Williamson.[2] It has not come into favor. It was not intended by the original promoters of the milk cure that other foods should be simultaneously eaten, but, as so often happens, the original directions have been overlooked. More harmful than the indiscriminate use of milk is that of buttermilk. Buttermilk contains all the carbohydrate which is in ordinary milk, but the fat which contains so much nutriment for the diabetic has been removed.

Case No. 17, is the only one in my series who suggested an apparent tolerance for milk. Male, teacher, onset of diabetes at the age of fifty-five years; came under my observation in August, 1900, at the age of sixty years, having lost 27 pounds, 16 per cent from his highest weight. Upon a diet of 3000 cc milk, containing 150 grams carbohydrate, which he had employed with only trifling additions for a period of six weeks, the sugar in the urine was only 13 grams. During this period weight fell 1 kilo. I endeavored to make him sugar-free, and lowered the carbohydrates in the diet to 25 grams, but the sugar in the urine fell only to 9 grams. I well remember having greatly increased the protein and fat in the diet when the milk was omitted. Undoubtedly the secret of the favorable course of the patient upon the milk diet was the comparatively small number of calories which he obtained and, conversely, the harmful effect of the rigid protein-fat diet was due to the large number of calories it contained as well as to the acidosis which my records of twenty-three years ago show it brought on. How plain the explanation of this case is today, but for a long time it was a puzzle.

5. **Levulose, Its Clinical Use.**—(Marion L. Baker, Howard F. Root, Elliott P. Joslin.) Levulose behaves differently from the other sugars, both in normals and diabetics. Külz[3] and Minkowski[4] noted this peculiarity. Writers generally recognized an unusual utilization of levulose by diabetics, but, like von Noorden and

---

[1] Donkin: British Med. Jour., 1874, **1**, 838.
[2] Williamson: British Med. Jour., 1915, **1**, 456.
[3] Külz: Beit. zur. Path. und Ther. des Diab., 1874, 130.
[4] Minkowski: Ueber Diab. Mel., 1893, 80.

Naunyn, saw that this vanished when the levulose was given continuously. Folin and Berglund observed only a trifling increase in the blood sugar of normal individuals when levulose was administered. Offenbacher found that inulin raised the blood sugar in diabetes less than levulose or dextrose.[1] Students of respiratory metabolism, likewise, have perceived the peculiarities of levulose. In experiments at the Carnegie Laboratory, the unusual degree to which levulose raised the respiratory quotient in normals as compared with other sugars was demonstrated by Benedict and Carpenter,[2] and in our experiments this same power was proved to hold with diabetics. (See pages 297 and 299.)

More recently Desgrez[3] and his co-workers have reported favorable results when they prescribed levulose for patients in two eight-day periods each month combined with vitamin B and calcium phosphate. They believe that levulose wards off certain metabolic disturbances. Labbé[4] on the contrary doubts the advantage of levulose over other carbohydrates, and regards the absence of protein and fat as more effective in combatting diabetic acidosis than levulose or any carbohydrate. Linossier[5] recommends infusions sweetened with levulose during fasting. Davidoff[6] observed that his Russian patients took honey with improvement of glycosuria. An interesting point in this connection is that the amount of levulose in different kinds of honey varies according to the food of the bees.

From the observations at the Nutrition Laboratory, both with normals and with diabetics, the conclusion seemed justified that levulose instead of being burned wholly as carbohydrate was in many cases, particularly in the diabetic, to a greater or less extent first transformed into fat. Only in this way could a satisfactory explanation be offered for the high respiratory quotients sometimes obtained.

This last year an attempt has been made to utilize clinically levulose and inulin, its precursor with our patients at the New England Deaconess Hospital. Insulin, however, complicated a problem, already intricate, and impressions, therefore, rather than conclusions must be drawn from the work. The levulose used was especially prepared and purified by Mr. Bean in the laboratory of Prof. Otto Folin in order to prevent the diarrhea which had frequently occurred according to the testimony of past workers. The levulose was administered in several different ways. The

[1] Offenbacher and Eliassow: München. med. Wchnschr., 1922, **69**, 1508.
[2] Benedict and Carpenter: Carnegie Inst., Wash., Pub. No. 261, 1918.
[3] Desgrez et al: Bull. Acad. de Méd., Paris, 1922, **88**, 167 and 1923, **89**, 25.
[4] Labbé: Bull. Acad. de Méd., Paris, 1922, **88**, 189.
[5] Linossier: Paris Médicale, 1922, **12**, 265.
[6] Davidoff: Russki Vrach, 1915, **26**, 601.

first method consisted in giving 1.5 grams levulose per kilogram body weight in water by mouth to a patient in the postabsorptive state and then recording the changes in the metabolism which took place during the next six hours. Analyses of blood and urine were made during this period and in many instances during the twenty-four hours before and after the test. A second method adopted was to give to certain cases small amounts of levulose daily for periods of days or weeks. To one patient, and this represented a third method, a large quantity of levulose was given daily for three consecutive days.

Inulin was administered as artichokes to a group of patients, chiefly young children, over a still more extended period. The artichokes were supplied for this purpose through the courtesy of Honorable Joseph C. Sibley of Franklin, Pennsylvania. And from our lipemia retinalis Case No. 2842 we have received dahlia bulbs out of which Mr. Bean promises us inulin.

The Effect of the Administration of Levulose in a Single Large Dose.—Ten patients whose age varied from sixteen years to fifty years received a single large dose of levulose and the respiratory metabolism was at once determined. In some cases two or even three series of experiments were carried out with the same patient.

Case No. 866 acted as a control subject in a blank experiment which was designed to show whether the nervous strain of a six-hours' experiment would affect analyses. He was a phlegmatic diabetic in whom nervousness would be least expected, yet his blood sugar rose 0.02 per cent during the first hour of his metabolism test. His excretion of urinary nitrogen was also higher during the first hour of the experiment than during any other period of the six hours. The gradual fall in respiratory quotient and heat production which took place as the interval lengthened since his meal the preceding evening was accompanied by a fall in the percentage of blood sugar as the metabolism of protein and fat replaced that of carbohydrate.

Faithful adherence to diet for a prolonged period has distinguished Case No. 632 and thus has rendered him an ideal subject for tests with levulose. These were performed in 1916 and repeated in 1922. During these six years his weight declined from 11.5 per cent below standard in 1916 to 30 per cent below standard in 1922. Similarly his basal metabolism fell from 3 per cent below to 18 per cent below the Harris and Benedict standard. Likewise tolerance for both levulose and dextrose had decreased, yet his blood sugar was 0.14 per cent in 1922 as compared to 0.19 per cent in 1916.

The amounts of levulose given this patient per kilogram body weight were approximately the same in 1916 as in 1922. Consequently the metabolic responses made at the two different dates are comparable. In 1922, the respiratory quotient did not rise quite as high as in 1916 with levulose, but the heat production was greater both at the maximum and for the average. It is clear that in this subject the greater the loss of weight and the more severe the diabetes, the greater the heat production after levulose but the less the rise in respiratory quotient.

A summary of a series of observations of the metabolism after a single dose of levulose in 1 normal and 8 diabetics is given in Table 201. In this series as in the 51 experiments of the Carnegie Series earlier reported, p. 292, the respiratory quotients, both maxima and average, were highest in the normal, next highest in the mild, and least in the severe cases. On the other hand, the increase in heat production was greatest in the severe cases, less in the mild, and least in the normal control. In the Carnegie Series, see p. 292, there was an average increase in the metabolism of 17 per cent with a maximum increase of 32 per cent in contrast to an increase of 9 per cent for normals under similar conditions. This increase was chiefly in the first two hours. In the present series shown in Table 201 the increase in the metabolism of the normal subject at no time rose above 15 per cent, of the mild diabetics not over 12 per cent, but of 2 of the 9 diabetics reached 29 per cent and more.

Significant Features of Clinical Tests with Levulose.—1. The respiratory quotient returned to the basal level within two hours in only 3 cases, Cases Nos. 632, 2476 and 2801. With Case No. 2801 no rise occurred, and this patient died of coma August 18, 1923 while taking daily over 45 units of insulin. Case No. 2476 showed 7.04 per cent fat in the blood thirteen days before the levulose test, and Case No. 632 was a diabetic who had lived on a low-carbohydrate diet, 25 grams, for many years.

2. The respiratory quotient did not return to the basal level even at the end of six hours with Cases Nos. 2296, 2548 and the first experiment with Case No. 3001, all of whom were comparatively mild cases, but it did with the subjects Case Nos. 2448, 2729 and the second experiment with Case No. 3001. The first two of these patients, Case Nos. 2448, 2729, were at the time of the test moderately severe and Case No. 3001 was on the borderline between moderate and mild. Thus the severest cases showed the least rise for the shortest period. The remainder of the cases were not so easily classified, but it is significant that Case No. 3001 showed a greater and more prolonged rise in quotient in the second experiment when she had been receiving more carbohydrate.

3. The heat productions were at or below the basal level at the end of six hours in two instances, Case Nos. 3001 and 2801. The

Table. 201—The Effect of Levulose upon the Metabolism of 1 Normal Individual and 8 Diabetics.

Case No.	Severity[1]	Weight, per cent of standard.	H and B[2] ±, per cent.		Basal.	Time in half hours.											
						1	2	3	4	5	6	7	8	9	10	11	12
Normal	....	−10	−8	R.Q.	0.76	0.85	1.01	0.94		0.90				0.80			0.76
				Cals.	1246	1398	1361	1438		1361				1303			1233
				% Deviation		+12	+9	+15		+9				+5			−1
2548	Mi.	−22	+3	R.Q.	0.78	0.80	0.96		0.91		0.89			0.80			0.79
				Cals.	1259	1350	1408		1383		1344			1269			1306
				% Deviation		+7	+12		+10		+7			+1			+4
3001	Mi.	−21	−14	R.Q.	0.79	0.86	0.88		0.85		0.83				0.85		0.78
				Cals.	1076	1182	1116		1085		1069				1125		1058
				% Deviation		+10	+4		+1		−1				+5		−2
3001	....	−21	−14	R.Q.	0.80	0.90	0.95		0.89		0.93				0.86		0.84
				Cals.	1078	1164	1128		1115		1132				1115		1094
				% Deviation		+8	+5		+3		+5				+3		+2
2448	Mod.	−19	−15	R.Q.	0.78	0.82	0.85	0.87		0.84				0.87			0.89
				Cals.	1243	1279	1446	1430		1397				1356			1414
				% Deviation		+3	+16	+15		+12				+9			+14
2476	Mod.	−22	−18	R.Q.	0.74	0.84	0.85		0.67		0.72			0.73			0.73
				Cals.	1334	1628	1754		1732		1485			1292			1407
				% Deviation		+22	+32		+30		+11			−3			+5
2687	Mod.	−27	±0	R.Q.	0.83	0.94	0.90				0.88			0.82			0.83
				Cals.	1240	1450	1479				1404			1229			1293
				% Deviation		+17	+19				+13			−1			+4
2729	Mod.	−26	−36	R.Q.	0.77	0.98		0.90		0.80			0.82			0.78	
				Cals.	954	1083		1063		982			966			975	
				% Deviation		+13		+11		+3			+1			+2	
2296	Mod.	−21	−3	R.Q.	0.74	0.79	0.79		0.77		0.78				0.76		0.72
				Cals.	1293	1482	1535		1556		1505				1393		1345
				% Deviation		+15	+19		+20		+16				+8		+4
632	S.	−31	−18	R.Q.	0.76	0.78	0.79		0.73		0.71				0.76		
				Cals.	1115	1424	1444		1425		1242				1155		
				% Deviation		+27	+29		+28		+11				+4		
2801	S.	−25	+5	R.Q.	0.75	0.73	0.76	0.72			0.74			0.72			0.72
				Cals.	1338	1437	1442	1456			1362			1289			1250
				% Deviation		+7	+8	+9			+2			−4			−7

[1] Mi = Mild; Mod. = Moderate; S. = Severe.
[2] Per cent ± variation from Harris and Benedict standard.

greatest increases in heat production occurred with Case Nos. 632 and 2476, both severe. The persistence of high quotients and high metabolism is all the more significant when one takes into account that in the control experiment with Case No. 866 both quotient and metabolism had fallen definitely below the initial level at the end of six hours.

The above results confirm the impression that here we are dealing with a different type of metabolism than takes place with the mere oxidation of carbohydrate. This could be explained upon the theory that levulose was being transformed into and being burned as fat in certain of the cases, but that in the severest cases, such as Case No. 2801, even this transformation failed.

Levulose and Blood Sugar.—The influence of levulose upon the percentage of sugar in the blood in normal individuals, mild diabetics, and severe diabetics, both with and without insulin, is shown in Table 202. To each patient the quantity of levulose given was 1.5 grams per kilogram body weight.

TABLE 202.—THE EFFECT OF LEVULOSE ON BLOOD SUGAR WITH AND WITHOUT INSULIN.

	No. of cases.	Levulose, grams.	Blood sugar, fasting.	After levulose.					
				1 hour.	2 hours.	3 hours.	4 hours.	6 hours.	24 hours.
Normal . . .	1	85	0.08	0.11	0.10	....	0.08	0.10	
Mild diabetes .	1	77	0.10	0.16	....	....	....	0.08	0.10
Moderate and severe diabetes .	9	73	0.21	0.29	0.30	0.26	....	0.22	0.24[1]
Moderate and severe diabetes .	4	74 and 11 units insulin	0.21	0.24	0.21	....	0.17	0.13	0.19

The normal subject had a slight rise in blood sugar of 0.03 per cent one hour after the ingestion of 85 grams levulose. This may be compared with the rise of 0.02 per cent shown by the control Case No. 866, who received no levulose. The mild diabetics showed a higher rise, and the moderate and severe diabetics a much higher rise than the normal control and the hyperglycemia was more prolonged. It should be said that the twenty-four-hour value was obtained in the fasting state. When insulin was given at the same time as the levulose there was a much less rise of blood sugar at the end of one hour and a steady fall thereafter to the lowest point at the end of six hours. Three patients, 1 mild and 2 severe, received both levulose and dextrose. In each case dextrose raised the blood sugar to a higher point than did levulose.

[1] Average of only 4 analyses.

The urinary sugar excreted averaged 5.7 grams when three patients took 74 grams levulose in six hours, but when the same quantity of levulose was preceded in these patients by 10 units of insulin, the sugar excreted was 0.4 grams. With 3 cases after 71.6 grams levulose the sugar excreted in six hours amounted to 6.5 grams, but with the same patients after 69 grams dextrose to 21.3 grams.

Thus levulose produced less marked hyperglycemia and glycosuria than did dextrose. Insulin counteracted the hyperglycemia produced by levulose just as it does with dextrose.

Levulose and its Relation to Acidosis.—The criteria by which the effect of levulose upon acidosis was estimated in the different subjects were derived from analyses of the plasma CO_2—combining power and of the acetone in the blood and from the urinary ammonia as well as the NH_3 N : total N ratio. At the beginning of the experiments 4 of the patients showed acidosis and 5 did not. As a result of the administration of levulose there was a definite increase in acidosis as shown by a fall in the plasma combining power during the first and second hours after the levulose was taken, but a decrease in acidosis as shown by a fall in the NH_3 N:N ratio. Various interpretations may be placed upon these two opposing results. It is possible that the lowering of the plasma CO_2 was the result of a dilution of the blood rather than a true acidosis because in our experiments the levulose was given in a highly concentrated solution, the average dose of 75.1 grams being dissolved in 50 to 55 cc water. At any rate the CO_2 value returned to about its initial level at the end of the six hours, so if acidosis was increased during the first and second hours it had disappeared by the end of the period. Likewise an explanation may be offered for the fall in the NH_3 N : total N ratio in that this may have been caused by the increased excretion of nitrogen. At all events, the excretion of NH_3 nitrogen per hour remained essentially uniform.

The development of an acidosis after levulose could be explained if a formation of acid metabolites took place, or it would be reasonable to explain it on the ground that the levulose was transformed into fat via fatty acids. The withdrawal of insulin on the days of experiments seemed a factor, especially in the more severe cases. It must be remembered that the ingestion of 60 to 70 grams levulose makes available calories in excess of metabolic needs immediately. On *a priori* grounds one might expect in severe cases acidosis from such over-feeding. That some abnormality of fat metabolism occurred in 2 of these cases after the levulose seems clear, because the blood acetone increased. However, this increase was not consistent since in 4 of the cases showing acidosis at the beginning of the experiment there was a lowering of the blood acetone at its

35

conclusion. Two of these had lipemia. What relation this lipemia bears to the acetone, it is impossible to say. From this confusing picture at least this conclusion appears justifiable, namely, that it is preferable to give levulose in small rather than in large doses.

The patients without acidosis who received levulose with a single exception, did not develop acetonemia, although the plasma CO_2 during the first two hours fell as in the cases with acidosis. The one exception was Case No. 3001 who exhibited a marked acetonemia on the third day of her levulose experiments.

TABLE 203.—THE ADMINISTRATION OF 72.5 GRAMS LEVULOSE DAILY FOR THREE DAYS. CASE No. 3001. DIET, ANALYSES OF URINE AND BLOOD, AND THE METABOLISM.

Date.	Diet in grams.				Urine.		
	C.	P.	F.	Calories.	Sugar, gms.	N. gm.	Acetone.
Feb. 15	77	59	110	1532	1.8	8.8	0.58
Feb. 16	140	64	106	1768	43.4	11.1	
Feb. 17	77	59	106	1614	29.4	10.1	0.8

BLOOD.

ANALYSES OF ACETONE AND SUGAR.

Date.	Fasting.		1 hour.		2d hour.		6th hour.	
	Sugar, per cent.	Acetone mg., per 100 cc.	Sugar, per cent.	Acetone mg., per 100 cc.	Sugar, per cent.	Acetone mg., per 100 cc.	Sugar, per cent.	Acetone mg., per 100 cc.
Feb. 15 . . .	0.18	1.6	0.26	18.8	0.30	....	0.26	tr.
Feb. 17 . . .	0.36	tr.	0.38	2.5	0.37	12.2	0.31	26.7
Feb. 22 . . .	0.21	6.7	0.23	42.4	0.22	....	0.19	tr.

METABOLISM.

	Feb. 15.	Feb. 17.	Feb. 22.
Basal heat production, calories . .	1076	1078	1072
Basal respiratory quotient . . .	0.79	0.80	0.84
Levulose, grams	72.5	72.5	{ 72.5 and 10 units insulin
Average respiratory quotient . .	0.86	0.92	0.87
Maximum respiratory quotient . .	0.88	0.98	0.93
Average increment over basal heat production (six hours) . . .	2.6 per cent	4.2 per cent	3.8 per cent
Maximum increment over basal heat production	10 per cent	9 per cent	13 per cent

The experiments with Case No. 3001 are most interesting. For the preceding week she had been sugar-free on a diet consisting of carbohydrate 66 grams, protein 64 grams, and fat 105 grams with the aid of 12 units of insulin. On February 15 she received 72.5 grams levulose in the postabsorptive state, and observations were carried out during the next six hours. During the remainder of the day she received sufficient protein and fat to bring her diet for the day up to approximately her regular diet. On February 16 she received 72.5 grams levulose in addition to her regular diet. On February 17 she received again 72.5 grams levulose in the fasting state, and metabolism studies were carried out as on the first day. During these three days no insulin was given. From February 18 to February 22, insulin 12 units and her usual diet were resumed. On February 22 she received again 73.2 grams levulose and this time 10 units of insulin in the postabsorptive state. Table 203 gives the analytical results.

If we compare the results of the metabolism for the first day when she was given levulose with the results of the third day of levulose feeding, it is clear that the respiratory quotient was higher both at its maximum and throughout the entire six hours on the third day, February 17. The maximum increment of heat production was less, however, on this day, although the average increment was greater for the six hours. The blood sugar was at a high level during this second experiment and acetone increased in the blood. A rise in plasma lipoids occurred at the end of the sixth hour. (Table 204, p. 548.) The acetonemia, the prolonged increase in heat production, the prolonged high respiratory quotient and the rise in plasma lipoids are interesting subjects for speculation. The patient had received carbohydrate in excess of her tolerance. A plethora of carbohydrate molecules and presumably metabolites existed in the blood and tissues. Possibly a transformation into fat of a part of these substances was occurring. At the end of the sixth hour on February 17 the respiratory quotient was 0.83. If fat formation was taking place probably carbohydrate burning also was taking place, especially in view of the fact that the blood sugar had dropped from 0.37 per cent to 0.31 per cent. This persistence of a high respiratory quotient may as logically be regarded as due to forced burning of carbohydrate under the pressure of a high concentration of carbohydrate molecules in the blood, as to transformation into fat except for the acetonemia which certainly should not develop with so high a respiratory quotient and plentiful supply of carbohydrate. Fat formation and faulty oxidation seem strongly suggested.

Another bit of evidence in favor of fat formation from the levulose consists of the fact that on February 22 when the patient received 10 units of insulin the respiratory quotient was not so high nor the average heat production so great as on February 17. The sugar excretion in the urine was also less, so we can be certain that more sugar was actually utilized on February 22 under the influence of insulin than on February 17. The higher quotients on February 17 without insulin are difficult to explain except by fat formation from levulose.

The analyses of plasma lipoids under various experimental conditions are presented in Table 204, and for these we are indebted to Prof. W. R. Bloor.

TABLE 204.—PLASMA LIPOIDS AFTER INGESTION OF LEVULOSE WITH AND WITHOUT INSULIN. (BLOOR.)

	Levulose without insulin.				Levulose and 10 units insulin.		
Case Nos. . .	3001	3001	2296	2476	3194	2296	3001
Date, 1923 . .	Feb. 15	Feb. 17	Feb. 7	Apr. 4	Mar. 14	Feb. 13	Feb. 22
Levulose, grams	72.5	72.5	75.6	90.0	71.5	75.6	73.2
Fasting:							
Cholesterol	132	115	375	465	92	340	142
Fatty acids	292	282	825	830	325	900	325
Lecithin .	250	242	440	720	. . .	528	260
One Hour Later:							
Cholesterol	. . .	. . .	415	220	97	390	132
Fatty acids	. . .	. . .	750	850	400	750	325
Lecithin .	. . .	. . .	438	800	280	560	236
Two Hours Later:							
Cholesterol	132	115	367	450	125	500	102
Fatty acids	277	282	650	830	300	700	300
Lecithin .	224	236	472	400	300	484	260
Six Hours Later:							
Cholesterol	140	187	340	415	102	450	102
Fatty acids	600	370	625	1250	300	800	300
Lecithin .	260	300	390	720	360	484	256

Levulose and Blood Lipoids.—We have data on only 7 experiments, 3 of which are on one patient and 2 on another. Visible lipemia was present in Case Nos. 2296 and 2476, and in all cases an abnormally high lecithin: cholesterol ratio was present. The most interesting question with regard to these figures relates to the rise in fatty acids six hours after the taking of levulose, because the highest point in the curve of blood lipoids after eating fat also occurs at six hours. Only Case No. 2296 failed to show this rise. He was an unusual patient in that he had such an extraordinarily low blood sugar renal threshold that for some time he was suspected of being a renal glycosuric. Possibly he should not be included in this group. However, the results of the other 3 experiments raise for discussion the possibility as to whether the rise in lipoids, especially fatty acids, is due to withdrawal of stored fat or to the metabolism of fat formed from levulose.

In the 3 cases who had levulose and insulin a pronounced drop in the fatty acids in the plasma occurred during the first hour. A slight rise followed at the end of six hours without, however, reaching the initial level. Thus the reaction of the plasma lipoids was quite different when insulin was taken with the levulose. Possibly insulin induced oxidation of the levulose as carbohydrate and thus prevented its transformation into fat. Possibly insulin affects fat metabolism directly. What an entrancing field for further investigation!

The daily administration of levulose in small quantities for prolonged periods was studied in 4 patients. Five grams of levulose three times daily for one to eight weeks were added directly to the routine diet. In Case No. 632 insulin was begun at the same time and so the results are difficult to interpret. In Case No. 2729 the addition of 15 grams levulose seemed to activate the combustion of carbohydrate so that it was possible afterward to substitute other forms of carbohydrate. However, the patient's blood sugar rose during the period, and this was also true of Case No. 2448 and Case No. 2422. The levulose was well borne at first, but later hyperglycemia and glycosuria followed.

Inulin.—Inulin, the chief carbohydrate constituent of artichokes, gives levulose by hydrolysis. Apparently inulin is not hydrolyzed and absorbed under all conditions. Sandmeyer,[1] Dean,[2] Chittenden,[3] Goudberg,[4] and Okey[5] have studied this problem. We have not tested the absorption of inulin. Dumont[6] found artichokes useful, especially in treating a patient with carbuncle. He believes that the levulose formed from the inulin modifies the intestinal flora, and in some way improves the defensive forces of the body.

Twelve patients took an average of 92 grams Jerusalem artichokes in addition to their regular diets for periods ranging from one week to three months without increasing glycosuria already present or producing glycosuria in patients previously sugar-free. The average increase in carbohydrate was thus about 13 grams. The weights of these patients at the beginning of this experiment averaged 88 kilograms. The average weight at the end of the period was 91 kilograms. The average calories in their diets increased from 1395 before taking artichokes to 1477 calories at the end of the period, allowing 56 calories for the artichokes. The average dose of insulin before taking the artichokes was 17 units, and the average dose at the end of the period was also 17 units. One little boy had scarlet fever during this period and showed a trace of sugar in the urine only on seven occasions during his illness.

[1] Sandmeyer: Zeit. f. Biol., 1895, **31**, 32.
[2] Dean: Am. Chem. Jour., 1904, **32**, 69.
[3] Chittenden: Proc. Am. Phys. Soc., 1898, 17.
[4] Goudberg: Ztschr. exper. Path. v. Therap., 1913, **13**, 310.
[5] Okey: Jour. Biol. Chem., 1919, **39**, 149.
[6] Dumont: Bull. Acad. Méd., 1922, **87**, 721.

While we cannot state definitely that the artichokes were in any way responsible for these patients' improvement, this experience encourages us to recommend them to others for trial.

Summary.—Tentatively we are inclined to the opinion that levulose can be used with advantage in the diabetic diet in very small amounts daily for intermittent periods. In the presence of acidosis its favorable influence is best obtained by giving small amounts at frequent intervals. It will raise the respiratory quotient in a diabetic more than dextrose and the heat production as well. Levulose seems to cause a different type of metabolism from dextrose, and this may be due to the conversion of levulose in part into fat by the diabetic. Similarly inulin in the form of artichokes was taken by our patients with pleasure and benefit. The question of the usefulness of levulose and inulin is of such interest that we shall continue our studies at the New England Deaconess Hospital, and we hope that other investigators will also become attracted by this complicated problem.

6. **Rectal Injections of Sugar.**—The experiments of Arnheim in 1904 showed that glycosuria in diabetic patients was not increased after enemata of solutions of sugar. Simultaneously, acetonuria diminished, and this appeared to be good proof that the sugar was absorbed and oxidized. This favorable action was attributed to the slow absorption of the rectal injection. Since this time others have studied the problem, notably Bingel, Reach, Balint, Lüthje, Jahnson-Blohm and Petitti.[1]

The subject is, however, by no means settled. The whole matter should be re-investigated, for the conditions are now much more favorable for its solution. In the first place, it is questionable whether in former experiments one sufficiently considered the effect of fasting, and secondly, the possibility of carbohydrate storage following fasting. Finally, today the respiratory exchange is far more generally employed, and this is really the ultimate test. Experiments dealing with rectal alimentation of normal individuals will throw much new light upon the question, and these have been in progress for some time under the direction of Dr. Carpenter of the Nutrition Laboratory. According to his studies the absorption of the sugar is between 34 and 72 per cent. Nearly all of the respiration experiments showed a more or less positive rise in the respiratory quotient after the injection of the sugar solutions.

Lüthje[2] repeatedly witnessed the disappearance of acidosis during the treatment of patients with enemata of sugar. As evidence of the absorption of sugar, he observed an increase of the percentage of sugar in the blood, and controlled the observation by noting

[1] See Allen: Glycosuria and Diabetes, W. M. Leonard, Boston, 1913, p. 59.
[2] Lüthje: Therapie der Gegenwart, 1913, **54**, 193.

no such increase following the administration of salt solution. The slow absorption of the sugar did not account for its better utilization when given by the rectum, because when sugar was introduced into the body at the same rate by being slowly sipped, the difference in favor of rectal alimentation persisted. Lüthje found that with good technic patients may absorb 1 or 2 liters of solutions of sugar containing 5.4 per cent, and thus may get 50 to 100 grams a day. Ten patients were treated by him by this method.

Bergmark also showed that after enemata of dextrose there was an increase in the carbon dioxide production, and that the experimental acidosis diminished as well. Jahnson-Blohm found that with healthy subjects the instantaneous as well as the repeated doses by mouth gave inside of the first three and one-fourth hours a strong increase in the glycemia, which rapidly sank in several cases so far that hypoglycemia took place. Dextrose injected by rectum gave blood-sugar values which lay very near to those at the beginning, and inside the limits of error of the method. The experiments with the diabetic subjects showed a strong rise of the blood-sugar curve with ingestion of dextrose by mouth. As with the normal subjects, the rectal experiments gave no increase in the percentage of the blood sugar. An increase in the urinary sugar did not occur either with healthy or diabetic subjects after the rectal feeding. This work shows well the unsettled state in which the question now rests.

G. THE TREATMENT OF ACID INTOXICATION AND DIABETIC COMA.

Brilliant as are the therapeutic triumphs over acidosis and diabetic coma with insulin, these facts remain for the practitioner ever to consider—that acid intoxication is nearly always preventable and that actual coma almost invariably implies negligence or ignorance of the fundamental principles of diabetic treatment. How can this be otherwise in the light of the following reports? In the University Hospital, at Ann Arbor, according to Newburgh and Marsh,[1] 190 successive cases of diabetes were treated without a death from coma save 4 patients who entered with it, 1 who developed it during an infection and another while in extremis. Petrén[2] reports that no deaths from coma have occurred in his hospital with any of his cases after the patients have been in residence for two weeks. To the writer's service, at the New England Deaconess Hospital and Mrs. Leatherbee's, 555 cases of diabetes

---

[1] Newburgh and Marsh: Arch. Int. Med., 1923, **31**, 455.
[2] Petrén: Verh. d. 34 Kong. f. inn. Med., 1922, 363.

have been admitted between July 8, 1922, and September 8, 1923, and there have been but 2 deaths in coma. One occurred in a child, six hours after admission, who had omitted insulin for several days, and the other likewise in a child, and likewise six hours after admission. She had been kept at home and in coma, for one day while under the care of an irregular practitioner and then brought a long journey to the hospital. It is contrary to reason to conclude that mild and moderately severe diabetics alone are sent for treatment to Lund, Ann Arbor, and Boston. If it is unnecessary for coma to develop in a hospital, it is equally unnecessary for coma to develop in the home.

One must always be awake to the possibilities of the appearance of coma during fever and whenever radical changes in the diet are made, particularly in long standing cases of diabetes, in obese individuals, in elderly patients with vulnerable kidneys, in pregnancy, and in operative cases because of the attendant excitement, trauma and narcosis.

Diabetic coma develops when the quantity of carbohydrate burned is insufficient to offset the fat metabolized. The oxidation of carbohydrate and the lowering of the metabolism are both favored by undernutrition and this is promoted by a diet low in calories, low in protein, and rest in bed. Without the latter, undernutrition may fail of accomplishment, because the metabolism may be kept elevated by the consumption of body protein and fat. My test diets and the diets of Newburgh and Marsh are each undernutrition diets. Both ban overfeeding as well as extreme undernutrition. In mine the carbohydrate at first is comparatively high and the fat low, because I believe most diabetics are mild and I wish to furnish them carbohydrates for the increasing oxidation which I feel sure progressive undernutrition will allow to take place. When coma threatens, I prefer to give moderate quantities of carbohydrate—40 to 60 grams carbohydrate in the form of three or four oranges or 30 to 60 grams oatmeal, as water gruel—and trust to the body to furnish from its own stores the required quantities of protein and fat which one can be very sure nature will make minimal. Newburgh and Marsh give one-third as much carbohydrate with an equal quantity of protein, but considerable fat.

The symptoms of diabetic coma are notoriously vague and even to a doctor the diagnosis often proves elusive. The spectre of threatening diabetic coma should always haunt the physician, particularly when the patient is first seen. It is astonishing how insidiously coma steals over a patient, and I have given up expecting nurses, unless they have had great experience with diabetic patients, to recognize its approach. It is better to treat any symptom out of the ordinary as premonitory of coma and *for patients when they feel sick to begin coma precautions* than to run the risk of beginning treatment too late. Despite the only too large number of cases of diabetic coma which I have seen myself, more than once I have been chagrined at having failed to realize its onset. Any occurrence out of the ordinary should arouse suspicion, and one should instantly investigate any of the following symptoms: Anorexia, nausea, vomiting, restlessness, unusual fatigue, excitement, vertigo, tinnitus aurium, drowsiness, listlessness, discomfort, painful or deep breathing. In the presence of fever always be on the alert for coma. Indeed to-day throughout all clinics there is general agreement about the seriousness of infections in diabetes and particularly about their frequency prior to coma. Petrén gives several examples showing that even the slighest infections are able to produce enormous destruction of protein in severe diabetes, but in coma, uncomplicated by infection, Petrén does not believe the nitrogenous metabolism increased. In about 20 cases of coma Petrén found the blood sugar between 0.5 per cent and 1 per cent. In every case with a percentage below 0.45 per cent the high blood-sugar level was associated with a high protein metabolism. The case with a high percentage of blood sugar, due to excessive protein metabolism, is more resistant to dietetic management than the case with an equally high percentage of blood sugar due to carbohydrate alone.

The soft eyeball in diabetic coma is a sign of considerable value. It was originally described by Krause[1] and subsequently its importance emphasized by Riesman.[2] It is not due to blood-pressure changes, or is it agonal, for it is not present in persons dying from other causes. Krause observed it in 22 cases of coma. I have repeatedly observed it in coma and have noted its absence in coma of non-diabetic origin.

Rules for the prevention of coma consequently are taught to all of my patients to be followed whenever they feel indisposed from any cause whatsoever. These measures can do no harm under any conditions and by their adoption in the early stages of acidosis will avert it in all but the most desperate cases. The prompt use of simple means renders heroic measures unnecessary later.

[1] Krause: Verh. d. XXI Kong. f. inn. Med., 1904, p. 439.
[2] Riesman: Jour. Am. Med. Assn., 1916, **66**, 85.

PREVENTION OF COMA.

The rules which the patients at the New England Deaconess Hospital learn for the prevention and treatment of diabetic coma are as follows:

1. Go to bed whenever indisposed.
2. Secure some one to wait upon you.
3. Drink a glass of liquid each hour, such as coffee, tea, broths, diluted orange juice, water oatmeal gruel.
4. Move the bowels by enema and if liquids have not been retained by mouth follow the enema by an injection of 1 pint luke warm water containing a teaspoonful of salt.
5. For nourishment depend upon orange juice and water oatmeal gruel.
6. Send for the doctor, who if he finds the symptoms of diabetic coma are really present will give
7. Insulin,
8. Digitalis, caffein or other circulatory stimulants, and perhaps
9. Wash out the stomach or
10. Give salt solution under the skin.

With the above measures even without insulin and without as definite a dietary regimen and as early an administration of salt solution as would now be employed 15 patients with alveolar CO_2 18 mm. Hg. pressure or below have been saved from death in diabetic coma. In none of these cases were alkalis used. (See Table 14, p. 80.)

It is appropriate to discuss more in detail the rules above given.

1. *Rest in bed is essential.*—This reduces the metabolism which is always absolutely or relatively increased when acidosis is present. It is the overfed, not the underfed, diabetic who succumbs to coma, though today it is recognized that overfeeding may be endogenous quite as much as exogenous under certain conditions such as bodily exertion and fever. By preventing exercise the metabolism is reduced and less ketogenic molecules are set free. To minimize exercise, often involuntary due to restlessness, demands nursing, and from the start either the time of a nurse or someone in the home must be devoted entirely to the patient's needs. Rest in bed is also the standard treatment for fever and by its early employment many severe illnesses are aborted. Fever is so dangerous to a diabetic that it should be treated with energy from its very inception. It is the antecedent of coma in many a case.

2. *Nurse.*—An attendant is necessary to enable the patient to rest and thus get the benefit of a lowered metabolism. If coma threatens, the patient deserves the help of the entire household, because he is nearer to death's door than if he had typhoid fever.

There is much to be done for the patient and he should have careful attention. Warmth is essential because this is a struggle for existence at a time when the patient is receiving little or no food. Flannel bed clothes and heaters should be employed to prevent the body becoming chilled.

3. *Liquids.*—Desiccation of the tissues is an almost invariable accompaniment of the onset of coma.[1] No matter what else is done, the patient must receive sufficient liquids to counteract this and to enable him to void considerable quantities of urine. All of the famous cases of recovery from coma in the past have passed large quantities of urine, and though recovery takes place with the excretion of less urine today than formerly, partly because alkalis are not allowed and partly because of insulin, the necessity for a liberal supply of liquid remains. Foster has recently emphasized this point.

Salt solution should be given subcutaneously if the case is in the slightest degree urgent, because more can be accomplished for the case threatened with coma in the first hour of treatment than in the following twenty-three hours. With modern aseptic precautions no instance of abscess following a subcutaneous injection of salt solution in a diabetic in the hospital has come to my attention. But even before the apparatus is made ready to give salt solution in this manner, liquids should be introduced by mouth and by rectum. Liquids given a diabetic patient with threatened coma should be hot or at least not ice cold. The latter are agreeable but in the end lead to vomiting. The liquids may take the form most agreeable to the patient, tea, coffee, broths, orange juice, or water oatmeal gruel. A glassful of liquid an hour is about as much as any diabetic can take continuously, save perhaps for the first one or two hours. Rather than run the chance of vomiting with the subsequent impossibility of giving liquids further by mouth, I depend upon the coincident administration of salt solution by the rectum. Here again one should be content with moderate quantities rather than with a maximum amount. So often recovery of the patient has been shattered by his inability to take liquid that one cannot say too much in favor of the subcutaneous injection of salt solution in the premonitory stages of coma. In operations upon diabetics it is almost always the rule for the surgeons to give it to the patients before they leave the table and there should be always an endeavor to fill the patients with liquids before the operation.

4. *Constipation* should be relieved by enema. Cathartics work too slowly and though possibly more efficacious, on the other hand they eliminate the use of the rectum temporarily for the introduction of liquids into the body.

[1] See Ehrström: Cited in Jour. Am. Med. Assoc., 1922, **79**, 173.

5. *Food.*—The choice of nourishment to be given during coma admits of little discussion. Fat is unnecessary in this twenty-four-hour struggle between life and death. It is hard to conceive of any patient so reduced that he has not enough fat available to furnish body needs for twenty-four hours. Patients so emaciated that such a quantity of fat is unavailable may die from inanition, but if they die from coma, it is due to the ingestion of too much exogenous fat. Protein, similarly, in this twenty-four-hour period is not required. The metabolism is stimulated quite enough, and here again, if death is imminent from inanition, coma will not appear. It is because of too much exogenous or endogenous protein rather than too little protein that coma appears. The experience of all those believing in the high-fat, low-protein diet confirms this. Carbohydrate, therefore, is the only food whose administration must be considered. I confess that I was not, in pre-insulin days, in the habit of giving much carbohydrate to a diabetic at the beginning of coma. Already the blood sugar is elevated enough and it is not logical to increase the percentage of sugar in the blood just before threatened death when in all the years of life one has tried in every way possible to decrease the sugar in the blood. Furthermore, I believe it probable that an increase of the already high percentage of sugar in the blood in these patients may work deleteriously toward their recovery. Petrén has the same idea and there is a general undercurrent in the literature pointing in the same direction.

The administration of comparatively small quantities of carbohydrate, given in small doses, is allowable today because insulin will be given simultaneously to the patient and the carbohydrate furnishes material upon which the insulin may act. Yet the insulin should be utilized to burn up the surplus carbohydrate in the body first. Fear, usually a sign of ignorance, is the excuse for giving additional carbohydrate on the ground that there is not enough carbohydrate in the body, when burned, to offset the acidosis. In giving carbohydrates one may be helping a symptom, acidosis, but one is hurting the disease, diabetes, and thus breaking one of the fundamental rules of therapeutics. An improvement in the tolerance for carbohydrate is a cardinal principle in diabetes. It makes no difference how this is brought about, whether by fasting, low diet, the exclusion of fat, the decrease of protein, or the gradual elimination of carbohydrate. So soon as carbohydrates begin to be assimilated in increasing quantity, the opportunity for acidosis declines. All that has been said about the treatment of the disease as a whole applies here. The chance for improvement of many a diabetic patient in the past has been shattered by the physician forgetting that the best way to prevent or overcome acid poisoning is, first and foremost, the treatment of the diabetes itself, and only subsidiarily the acidosis. Some years ago Lüthje remarked, with much truth, that one need not worry about acidosis when sugar is absent from the urine, and this I impress upon my patients. Treat the diabetes and the acid poisoning will take care of itself.

The argument for the administration of large quantities of carbohydrate in former days had a distinct foundation, because it is almost never that a diabetic fails to oxidize some of the carbohydrate administered. The conception was held, and to some extent justifiably, that, if an enormous quantity of carbohydrate were given the diabetic, enough would be oxidized to overcome the imminent acidosis and the damage done by the carbohydrate could be corrected later. No excuse for that method of procedure holds today.

The best form of carbohydrate to give would appear to be that which contains levulose. No carbohydrate has been proved to be stored by a diabetic as readily as levulose. Consequently, my patients are given orange juice, because this is always available, it is refreshing and does not disturb the digestion. Oatmeal water gruel is also freely employed because it is so easily administered and is so well borne. The quantity of orange juice or of oatmeal gruel which a diabetic patient in beginning coma will take during the twenty-four hours is never very large and one need not worry about the total amount. One would certainly not want to give over 100 grams carbohydrate in the twenty-four hours, and 25 to 50 grams would be preferable. Diabetic patients, as DuBois and Richardson have shown, have more carbohydrate available for oxidation than has been supposed. If this is the case without the use of insulin, with insulin it holds all the more.

6. *The Circulation Must be Supported.*—Patients in diabetic coma have low blood-pressures.[1] The work involved in hyperpnea is considerable and the heart has difficulty in withstanding the demands made upon it. It must be protected in every possible way, and under no conditions be imperiled by the treatment adopted. The subcutaneous administration of salt solution helps and does not hinder the activity of the heart, but the intravenous administration of salt solution may kill the patient by producing cardiac dilatation. In somewhat less striking degree the heart is impaired by the giving of enormous quantities of liquids orally through the production of a dilatation of the stomach with its consequent reflex action upon the heart. This is the reason why lavage of the stomach is to be recommended in the early stages of diabetic coma. Frequently the coarse food of the diabetic diet, or the excess food which the patient has almost invariably taken preceding coma, may be retained and additional quantities of liquid will produce gastric

---

[1] This deserves more thorough investigation.

dilatation. A word of warning is here needed, however, because it has been called to my attention by a visitor at the hospital that he once saw a diabetic patient in the early stages of coma die suddenly during the rather strenuous manipulation involved in washing out the stomach. This only goes to show how cautiously, delicately, and tenderly one must treat the coma patient. The life of a diabetic in acidosis hangs by a thread.

Caffein and digitalis have been the cardiac stimulants employed.

7. *Insulin. The Use of Insulin in Diabetic Coma.*—Compared with all the useful measures hitherto described insulin stands preeminent in its efficacy in rescuing the diabetic patient from coma. Yet, paradoxical as it appears, the employment of insulin generally in the treatment of diabetes may easily increase the number of deaths from coma unless it is rightly controlled. Diabetic patients who receive insulin are the severest cases of diabetes. These patients when living upon a restricted diet are protected against coma, but with the help of insulin they receive diets which represent 30, 50 or even 100 per cent more food than they were able to metabolize without insulin. In consequence of this they are walking on insulin stilts and if the insulin is removed, death from coma can very shortly result. Insulin patients above all others must be taught to protect themselves from death by coma by instantly going to bed and curtailing the diet at least one-third if insulin is omitted. They must take no chances with the omission of insulin. They must protect themselves before the need becomes obvious and should not await the onset of symptoms. Little Thomas D., did not experience the full effects of the omission of insulin for over five days, and then, before he or his parents realized his critical condition, lapsed into coma.

The second danger from insulin in diabetic coma is its unnecessary employment. The measures hitherto recommended do no harm even if the coma is not due to acidosis. Not so with this powerful remedy—insulin. In one week 3 instances came to my attention of insulin being given to diabetic patients in coma when the coma was of other origin. In one of these cases the coma was caused by meningitis developing suddenly six weeks after a mastoid operation upon a diabetic, in a second instance the coma followed one hour after an operation for prostatectomy, not because of acid poisoning, though ether was the anesthetic used, but because of hemiplegia, and a third, because of uremia due to an unoperated prostatic obstruction. Later other cases have come to my attention in which the supposed coma was due to morphine and codeine.

All of us must realize that diabetic coma due to acidosis is decreasing in the community, but that with the increased duration of life of the diabetic patient of today coma in a diabetic, not due to acidosis, is on the increase. Make sure acidosis is the cause of the coma before giving insulin to a diabetic. Even the presence of sugar in the urine and a positive ferric chloride test for diacetic acid are not sufficient guarantees for its use. A differential diagnosis must be made. Perhaps the patient has had too much codeine or morphine.

The third danger in the employment of insulin in diabetes is the administration of too large a dose. There is no use in bringing a patient out of acidotic coma to plunge him into hypoglycemic coma. The quantity of insulin to be given a diabetic patient in diabetic coma has varied from a few units to about 300 units in twenty-four hours. As time goes on it is probable that smaller and smaller doses of insulin will be used. With smaller doses the danger of hypoglycemia will be avoided. There can be no advantage in giving a patient large quantities of carbohydrate requiring large quantities of insulin for oxidation so long as there is sufficient carbohydrate in the body the oxidation of which will offset the ketogenic properties of the fat and protein simultaneously metabolized. In the early days of insulin one was afraid to give the drug without protection against hypoglycemia, but with alert observation of the patient such dangers can be avoided. For the general practitioner, therefore, it is probably safer to run the risk of giving too little rather than too much insulin in his treatment of diabetic coma.

With some hesitancy I postulate advice about the treatment of diabetic coma with insulin because I have seen so very few cases. From an examination of the reports of others, kindly placed at my disposal, the safest plan would appear to be to give 10 to 20 units of insulin immediately upon diagnosis, and this is best given intravenously. The dose should be repeated at the end of one hour, and unless contraindicated by the rapid clinical improvement of the patient, or the decrease of evidence of acidosis as shown by analyses of blood, urine, and alveolar air, repeated in the third and fourth hour, but with each dose increasing scrutiny and study should be directed to the degree of acidosis still existent, because insulin is cumulative. The less the facilities for such study which the physician has at his disposal, the more cautious he should be. Methods safely adopted in the largest hospitals of the country under the supervision of diabetic specialists with a corps of assistants at hand are not necessarily advantageous in the home. Moreover in the home coma is almost invariably seen at an earlier stage than in the hospital and this constitutes an additional reason for cautious doses.

Promptness in action and early detection of the first symptoms of coma will lead to good results with comparatively small doses of insulin. No one will deny that 10 units given early will accomplish far more for the patient than 20 or 30 units after a delay of even two or three hours. We never shall succeed in the treatment of acidosis and coma unless we look upon these conditions as seriously as we regard the perforation of a duodenal ulcer.

After the fourth hourly dose, subsequent doses of 5 or 10 units each, depending upon the condition of the patient, should be given every two to four hours for the remainder of the twelve hours. There are very few cases in the literature with successful outcome from coma who required more than 80 units in twelve hours. The patients who received much above 80 units in twelve hours usually died.

Following insulin the blood sugar does not drop instantaneously and there may be a culmination of the effect of insulin in succeeding hours. This is the reason for the great caution advised in its use and for the caution to protect against hypoglycemia by the administration of half as many grams of carbohydrate as units of insulin, following the first 20 units, when laboratory facilities are not at hand.

If the blood-sugar estimations cannot be made, one can depend upon single urinary specimens, taken at frequent intervals. To be sure that the urine has been recently secreted it may be necessary to catheterize the patient at hourly intervals or even to insert a permanent catheter.

Insulin should be continued in liberal quantities for the days succeeding the recovery from coma. Most patients will require as many as 40 units daily. Failure to observe this precaution has frequently led to a relapse.

8. *Alkalis.*—Alkalis have been employed in the treatment of diabetic coma and of acidosis for a generation. I have given alkalis to about 1000 cases of diabetes and am fairly familiar with their effect. Since 1917, 2000 of my patients have been treated without alkalis and it can be said unhesitatingly that the condition of these patients, as proved by absence of acidosis, by infrequency of coma, and by duration of life, has been infinitely superior to that of the former group. (See Tables 14 and 29.) It is only fair to concede that the omission of alkalis is not wholly responsible for the more satisfactory condition of the latter group, because better dietetic methods, better hygiene, and better education of the patients are practised all the time, and in the second place, and quite as important a factor, in former days the quantity of alkali given was probably extreme and the damage done to the patient's stomach by oral administration of alkali or to the heart by its intravenous administration offset the good effect it might have produced. There are also other reasons. No diet is more predisposing to coma than a high-fat diet and yet no alkalis have been employed by Newburgh and Marsh. Bertnard Smith, of

Los Angeles, has had good results without alkalis since he gave them up in 1917.

A second reason against the administration of alkalis in diabetic coma is the demonstration that even when the alkalinity of the blood of a patient is brought back to normal, coma may persist. This applies not only to a patient but to the dog in diabetic coma. Allen in his Harvey Lecture said: "Aside from a possible, very brief rise in blood-pressure, sodium bicarbonate intravenously or otherwise brings no visible benefit to the dog dying of acidosis." However, too much weight should not be attached to the argument that the patient in diabetic coma whose blood alkalinity has been restored to normal has not recovered. It is quite possible that the reason for lack of recovery in these cases was due to the duration of the action of the oxybutyric acid upon the cells of the body. One can easily conceive that, whereas cells damaged for a short time with acid may recover, cells damaged for a long time cannot recover.

The third reason for not giving alkalis is the very simple one that alkalis are apt to upset the stomach. In this event medication and food must be given intravenously or subcutaneously. In a hospital where such methods are commonly in use the risk is not great, but in general practice the delays and dangers involved by such methods are considerable.

A fourth reason against the employment of alkalis is that they not infrequently do more harm than good in that they lead to convulsions as reported by Blum[1] years ago. So soon as we are given a standard mixture of alkalis which will make the use of sodium bicarbonate less dangerous, one can use these more freely. This raises the question of the part played by salts in the metabolism which has been so assiduously studied by Blum and others.

A fifth reason exists in that when alkalis are given to a patient with acidosis the quantity of β-oxybutyric acid and its derivatives removed through the kidneys is increased[2] and the volume of urine as well, because these acids are not excreted in concentrated form. With young individuals this is less important, but with adults it is serious because the acid is an irritant and their more vulnerable kidneys may be incapacitated thereby. Mrs. L., Case No. 2595 excreted 70 per cent of the phenolphthalein in a two-hour test and had a non-protein nitrogen value of 36 mg. per 100 cc in the blood three days before coma. During coma the non-protein nitrogen rose to 60 mg. and very little ammonia was excreted. Whether the anuria which formerly was seen so frequently in coma was due

[1] For Tetany after Soda. See also Harrop: Johns Hopkins Hosp. Bull., 1919, **30**, 63.

[2] Mosenthal, Killian and Myers: Jour. Am. Med. Assn., 1922, **78**, 1751.

36

to this cause, to an insufficient supply of liquids or to a failing heart is uncertain. The functional power of the kidneys during coma should be determined by the phenolsulphonphthalein and other tests. Added interest attaches to such an investigation because of the discovery of Benedict that ammonia is formed in the kidneys and not in the liver. Whether acids, latent and harmless in the body, are set free when alkalis are given and become dangerous is not proved.

The constant use of an alkali appears to promote the constant excretion of acid bodies. I have known a moderate acidosis of months' duration to vanish with the omission of soda. It is frequently to be observed that when an alkali is omitted in the convalescent stages of a diabetic cure that acidosis, as measured by the urine, entirely disappears, but will be brought back by resuming the alkali. A very small quantity of alkali may cause the appearance of a positive ferric chloride reaction in the urine. Patients have observed this after a Seidlitz powder, and one patient, Case No. 942, thought it followed the use of a brand of saccharin which was combined with sodium bicarbonate. In other words, the administration of an alkali may give a false idea as to the severity of the case if one is guided by the urine alone. This shows how necessary it is to study the blood. Van Slyke in the discussion of a paper by Fitz at the Association of American Physicians in May, 1917, pointed out that not only acids remaining in the body might do harm but also those excreted in the urine by removing bases. It is by no means, therefore, an unmixed blessing to favor the removal of acids from the body by the use of alkalis.

Woodyatt has called my attention to the necessity of clearing the mouth of alkali after it is given, and in this way preventing nausea. Frequently he says a diabetic's dry mouth is frosted by alkali and it is this that leads to the vomiting rather than the action of the alkali upon the stomach. A quart bottle of Célestins Vichy contains approximately 4 grams of sodium bicarbonate, and patients are often glad to take their alkali in this form. In some cases an additional 4 grams or more of the bicarbonate may be added to the chilled Vichy.

It is generally agreed that the sodium salts are preferable to the potassium salts if the doses given are to be large. Sodium bicarbonate was the alkali most commonly and advantageously used in my practice. Sodium citrate is of the same bulk as the bicarbonate, is said to be less irritating because carbon dioxide is not set free in the stomach, less apt to cause diarrhea and less disturbing to the appetite. The citrate is said to be oxidized in the body and in this oxidation to favor the combustion of acid products, but I question whether this property is of enough importance to outweigh the advantages of the use of sodium bicarbonate, which can be obtained so easily.

Sodium carbonate is too irritating, and, furthermore, on account of the water of crystallization, the actual amount of sodium which is contained in 100 grams of sodium carbonate is equivalent to only 58 grams of the bicarbonate. This is not generally recognized.

Magnesium citrate is an excellent preparation when constipation is associated with the acidosis, but naturally large amounts cannot be given in this form.

Chalk, calcium carbonate (creta preparata) is valuable because it will not only act as an alkali, but because it tends to render the sodium bicarbonate less irritating to the stomach and thus is less apt to cause nausea or diarrhea.

Alkali may be given by the rectum in the form of a 3 per cent solution of sodium bicarbonate in salt solution.

Sodium bicarbonate may be given intravenously. Unfortunately, at times following the intravenous administration of sodium bicarbonate, convulsions and collapse occur, so that one dislikes to resort to this method if others will suffice. The harmful effects attributed to the intravenous injection of alkalis may be connected in part with the late stage at which they are given. Sodium bicarbonate is the best form of alkali to give intravenously, and although 10 per cent solutions have been given, it is probably safer to use a 3 per cent solution. Young individuals present a much better prognosis than adults and much better than elderly individuals with damaged kidneys. Blum suggests that a second injection be avoided unless increased diuresis has shown that the body is capable of dealing with the first.

The sodium bicarbonate may be sterilized along with the salt solution. It is true that some of the carbon dioxide is liberated through sterilization, but this does no harm when injected intravenously. Under no conditions should soda solution be given subcutaneously. Magnus-Levy[1] pointed out that if a current of carbon dioxide should be passed through the solution of sodium bicarbonate after it has been sterilized and the sodium carbonate has been precipitated until the red tint with phenolphthalein disappears the sodium bicarbonate would be reformed. Sterilization, however, is probably not necessary. My former assistant, Dr. F. A. Stanwood, demonstrated by a series of experiments that if sodium bicarbonate was taken with a sterile spoon from a previously unopened Squibb's package, weighed in a sterile watch-glass, and then added to sterile salt solution, the resulting solution was sterile. He also found that if infected with staphylococci and typhoid bacilli the solution sterilized itself in three days.

[1] Magnus-Levy: Therap. Monatsschr., 1913, **27**, 838.

A sixth reason which can be raised against the routine employment of alkalis in diabetic coma is that no agreement exists among those who favor alkali therapy as to the quantity to be employed. Von Noorden and Woodyatt use comparatively large amounts. Allen uses but a few grams. Bock and Fitz recommend from 15 to 35 grams of sodium bicarbonate in twenty-four hours. They recommend the routine use of this quantity of alkali not because all patients require it, but because their studies in coma have demonstrated that a certain percentage of the cases of coma they have treated showed the disappearance of ketogenic acidosis but the existence of acidosis caused by an as yet unidentified organic acid. They therefore conclude it is safer to give alkalis to 9 patients needlessly than to with-hold it from 1 diabetic who might die without it.

I have great respect for the therapeutic results in coma which Bock, Fitz, Olmsted and Banting, Campbell and Fletcher of the Toronto School with all their several co-workers have attained. All of these clinicians use alkalis in amounts seldom in excess of 30 grams in twenty-four hours. It is hard for me to believe that two tablespoonfuls of sodium bicarbonate will save the life of a patient. However, there is much to learn about mineral metabolism in diabetes and the work of Blum and others who are engaged in this problem must be studied attentively. On the other hand, I have treated without alkalis 555 successive cases of diabetes at the New England Deaconess Hospital and Mrs. Leatherbee's with but 2 deaths from coma and for the present feel it my duty to continue this plan.

TREATMENT OF COMA, SEPTEMBER 15, 1923.

Case No. 3382 entered the New England Deaconess Hospital September 15, 1923, at noon, having had labored respiration for six days and complete coma for four hours. She had typical Kussmaul respiration, the pulse rate was 132, hands and feet cold and the rectal temperature was 95° C. The plasma CO_2 combining power was 10.9 volumes per cent. The blood sugar was 0.54 per cent and the non-protein nitrogen 65.5 mg. per 100 cc. The eyeballs were so soft that Dr. L. P. Tingley was unable to measure the tension with a tonometer. Eighteen hundred cc urine, obtained by catheter, contained 1.8 per cent sugar and gave a $+ + + +$ ferric chloride test.

The patient was immediately given 20 units of insulin by vein and 20 units subcutaneously, a subpectoral injection of 1200 cc saline, and an enema of 1 quart saline which she retained. A second dose of 20 units insulin subcutaneously was given one hour later and thereafter doses of 20 to 30 units were given at intervals of two to three hours until seven o'clock the next morning. Twenty grams of carbohydrate were given by mouth and 30 grams as rectal glucose during the first twenty-one hours. Fluids were given by mouth at the rate of 50 to 100 cc per hour. She vomited in the early evening and gastric lavage was performed at 11 P.M. Digitalis and caffeine were administered alternately every four hours for the first day and a half.

During the first eight hours of treatment four blood-sugar analyses varied from 0.50 to 0.59 per cent and the plasma CO_2 combining power rose to 29 volumes per cent.

At the end of twenty-one hours the patient had received 220 units of insulin, and (1) the urine was sugar- and acid-free; (2) the blood sugar was 0.17 per cent; (3) the plasma CO_2 combining power was 71 volumes per cent; (4) though very drowsy and weak, she was conscious and rational, and (5) the eyeballs were of nearly normal tension.

Four days later she was receiving 70 units of insulin, the urine was free from diacetic acid though containing 0.3 per cent sugar and the blood sugar was 0.25 per cent. The diet consisted of carbohydrate 84 grams, protein 51 grams, and fat 79 grams. Intraocular tension had returned to normal and recovery was assured.

Without insulin or alkalis, in 1921, Case No. 2366 with soft eyeballs, and plasma CO_2 combining power of 15 volumes per cent, recovered from partial coma. Therefore, at the New England Deaconess Hospital it has been demonstrated that both with and without insulin, recovery is possible without the use of alkalis or excessive carbohydrate by avoiding excess fluid by mouth through injections of saline solution subcutaneously, rectally or intravenously.[1]

H. TREATMENT OF COMPLICATIONS.

Intercurrent diseases, complications and sequelæ of diabetes are fully as important as the disease itself. In fact, they are responsible for as many of the deaths as those intimate complications of diabetes, coma and inanition, combined. The various maladies which may supervene or follow diabetes are dangerous, not so much because of their own severity, but because as in the case of infections, they make the diabetes more severe. To these changing conditions of the type of diabetes treatment must conform until recovery restores the diabetes to its former character. On every occasion treat the diabetes and then the patient will be kept in the best fighting trim, but do not think that the same type of diabetes is present in the same patient on successive days. It is the inadequately treated diabetic who develops many of the com-

---

[1] This case and another will be discussed and reported in greater detail by the Author, and by H. F. Root and G. H. Shedd in Med. Clin. No. Am., 1923, November.

plications and sequelæ of diabetes. Patients should remain free from complications because diabetics are, or should be, constantly under the doctor's eye and his prophylactic care.

The duration of life of diabetic patients in the past has been so short that the dangers which might result from peculiarities of treatment have been neglected, because in the space of five or six years these would not manifest themselves. Today with the duration of the disease so much prolonged, all these factors must be taken into account. It is a well-known fact that disease of the kidneys may occur in diabetics who have had diabetes for many years. Has this been brought about by the protein-fat diet? Those interested in the study of diseases of the kidney could ask no better experimental basis for the investigation of etiological dietetic problems than these patients. Here are experiments of a most accurate type going on before their very eyes, not for days or months, but for years.

1. **Infections.**—An infection makes a diabetic worse. If the infection is local, it should receive prompt surgical treatment; if it is general, the danger of acidosis must be realized, due largely to the fever with its resulting increase of metabolism. It is rarely possible to keep a patient sugar-free in the presence of an infection, whether local or general. This is where the family doctor has often scored on the supposedly wise consultant. The latter would order a fat-protein diet and death would result from coma. If the case is doing well, either leave it alone or make gradual changes and there will be more chances of having the individual for a patient during years to come than if brilliant dietetic orders are written. It is safer to undernourish than to fan the flame of metabbolism by overfeeding, and better to take an intermediate course and give not over 1 gram of protein per kilogram body weight. It is true that the patient may lose weight but so may a non-diabetic in fever, and it is wiser to trust to Nature to draw from the body the requisite stores of protein and fat than to insist on her taking in food that may be harmful. Empirically, in the past I followed this course in two quite different ways. The usual plan was to radically restrict the fat in the diet which lessened calories, though, at the time, it was done largely with the idea of diminishing acidosis. A second plan based upon the administrations of little protein accidentally adopted with an Italian who had typhoid fever at the Boston City Hospital in the sumer of 1908. He was given a diet composed exclusively of oatmeal and olive oil which he took with avidity until his recovery was complete.

Carbohydrate in the form of oatmeal gruel, orange juice and even as purée vegetables with protein as whites of eggs, oysters, fish and chicken, and fat in the form of cream will tide over many emergencies. In the hospital the nurse, in charge of the diabetic nursing, asks for the carbohydrate, protein and fat allowed and then arranges its administration according to the patients' whims. There is no reason for not giving what the full tolerance will allow.

When death results from an actual infectious disease, such as gangrene, pyelitis, pneumonia or appendicitis the blood-sugar percentage may be just as high as in coma. It seems strange to read that the highest blood-sugar percentage found by Petrén outside of coma, and not immediately followed by coma, was 0.42 per cent. These observations are distinctly at variance with our findings at the New England Deaconess Hospital. Thus Case No. 1887 with blood sugar of 0.5 per cent is alive six months after this determination. Case Nos. 2201, 2266, 2716, 2798 and 2870 showed blood-sugar percentages of 0.53, 0.54, 0.43, 0.45 and 0.64 and are alive from one to two and two-tenths years after these high determinations. I will acknowledge, however, that without cautious treatment such values are critical.

General Infections.—(*a*) *Pneumonia.*—Pneumonia has been by far the most important infection, if one can judge by its frequency in mortality tables. Fifty-two cases of diabetes out of a total of 887 have succumbed to it and as a cause of death it ranks with tuberculosis. Yet not all diabetic patients die who acquire pneumonia, as Table 205 shows. Doubtless others could be added to this list if the search were made.

The diagnosis of pneumonia must be often faulty in diabetes and the errors are probably both ways. An autopsy alone will satisfy the tenets of scientific accuracy. Coma may be blamed for a death which pneumonia has caused, Case No. 2446, and the reverse may be true, Case No. 3010. A pain in the chest at the beginning of coma by no means always signifies pneumonia. Among 33 deaths in hospitals since April 1, 1919, there were 3 deaths from pneumonia and the total number of cases of diabetes admitted to these hospitals on my service has been 1312.

TABLE 205.—RECOVERY FROM PNEUMONIA IN DIABETES.

Case. No.	Age at onset of diabetes, years.	Duration. Before pneumonia, years	After pneumonia, years.
8	60	12.5	1.1
19	47	0.6	9.0
36	42	7.0	3.3
46	62	20.0	0.3
131	37	12.5	4.0*
352	49	22.0	0.2
358	53	17.0	1.3*
435	33	23.0	6.0*
844	32	33.0	1.5
895	55	12.0	6.0*
911	57	7.0	2.3
1274	56	4.0	14.0*
1350	38	10.0	11.0

* Still living. Duration to July, 1923.

(*b*) *Other Infections.*—Influenza was credited with many deaths during the epidemic, but there have been none such recently. Tonsillitis, pertussis, dysentery and erysipelas are credited with a total of 3 deaths, and 1 patient in coma had diphtheria as proven by membrane and positive culture. Thus far, my cases who have had measles, mumps, scarlet fever, varicella, and whooping-cough have passed through these infections successfully, but it is customary to hear that the tolerance has been temporarily lowered and, one is happy to say, later regained. During an attack of herpes zoster the carbohydrate tolerance of Case No. 521 fell markedly. This is interesting because it suggests the infectious etiology of this disease.

Acute rheumatic fever seldom occurs in a diabetic despite his many infections. Case No. 694, a mild diabetic, had a slight attack in the Spring of 1917. Surely not more than 1 other such case has come to my attention in the 3300 diabetics under my care. Dr. Wilmot Marden of Lynn wrote me in January, 1921, that he had a woman of sixty-eight years whom he was treating who could be made sugar-free only with difficulty. She had a severe arthritis of the left knee and no local infection could be found in teeth, tonsils, ears, nose or elsewhere to account for it.

Local Infections.—These may be serious no matter whether they relate to an appendix, an abscess in the paranephritic region or to bad teeth with accompanying dangers of extraction. Under surgery, p. 611, these are more thoroughly discussed, and the desirability of surgical interference, as in non-diabetics, urged. Local infections are furthermost serious because they lead by no means rarely to a general septicemia. In fact septicemia is a far more common cause of death at the Deaconess Hospital than pneumonia. Hence prompt surgical intervention is demanded in every local infection in a diabetic.

2. **Tuberculosis.**—Tuberculosis formerly was responsible for about one-half of the deaths of diabetic patients, but today, in private practice, it seldom occurs. In Europe it is more frequent.[1] In Japan, according to a personal communication of Muryama and Yamaguchi, tuberculosis was diagnosed in 8.9 per cent of 633 cases and was the cause of death of 22 per cent of 49 fatal cases. Montgomery,[2] who has published an excellent critical summary of the literature upon diabetes mellitus and pulmonary tuberculosis, concludes that tuberculosis is not more frequent among diabetics than among the rest of the population of similar age. My statistics would support this view. At the moment I recall but 2 living cases of diabetes under my care with active tuberculosis. It is noteworthy that

---

[1] Labbé and Cumston: Diabetes Mellitus. Wm. Wood & Co., New York, 1922.
[2] Montgomery: Am. Jour. Med. Sci., 1912, **144**, 543.

in 1917, I knew of 6 living cases of tuberculosis in my group of diabetics in contrast to 2 such today. This is still more striking because the number of my diabetics is much larger and at present more of them proportionately go to the hospital, where constant supervision should make it easier to discover this complication. Undoubtedly this is due to the well-known decrease in the mortality from tuberculosis everywhere.

Von Noorden, writing later than did Naunyn, records a still lower percentage among his cases, though in Vienna von Noorden found it nearly twice as common among hospital diabetics as in Frankfort. This is a striking illustration and a warning against exposure of diabetic patients to tuberculosis. Case No. 838 died of tuberculosis in August, 1922, and his brother, Case No. 2314, who contracted diabetes in 1915 showed tubercle bacilli in the sputum in June, 1923.

Prophylaxis is important. Unfortunately a tuberculosis, latent for nearly a lifetime, may break out in the presence of diabetes, as it did in Case No. 629, at the age of sixty-nine years, and in Case No. 344, in whose family there had been much tuberculosis, though he himself had never shown recognizable signs of it. No matter how well the diabetic patient may appear, he remains a vulnerable individual.

The percentage of deaths due to tuberculosis to the total number (887) of diabetic deaths in my own series is 6 per cent. This percentage has been remarkably constant as the compilations have been made from year to year. They are shown in Table 31. The highest percentage has been 6 per cent, based upon 887 fatal cases of diabetes, and the lowest has not fallen under 4 per cent. Already the rarity of tuberculosis among the living cases has been commented upon. In this community, Massachusetts, the percentage of deaths due to tuberculosis to the total number of deaths was 6.9 in 1921 and the death-rate per 100,000, 84.2. It would, therefore, appear that tuberculosis was the same among my diabetics as among the population in general in this region.

A glance at Table 206 shows that the number of cases of tuberculosis was far more numerous among the early than among the late case numbers, another illustration of the disappearance of tuberculosis in the community and probably an illustration of the effects of treatment of diabetes, for I take it that in the last few years diabetic patients have not been so debilitated with the progress of the diabetes. On the other hand, an argument could be raised that recently diabetic patients have died prematurely of coma, whereas, according to the old regime, they would have lingered along and succumbed to some complication. This does not, however, appear likely, because the duration of life of my

TABLE 206.—TUBERCULOSIS AND DIABETES.

Case No.	Age at onset of diabetes, yrs.	Duration to death — Diabetes, yrs.	Duration to death — Pulmonary tuberculosis,[2] yrs.
10	39	12.0	1.0[3]
44	42	5.8	1.0[3]
56	44	7.7	2.3
68	42	0.3	. .
75[1]	35	6.0	12.0
106	31	9.0	. .
134	38	3.9	0.5
160	46	1.6	6.0
166[1]	52	4.0	4.0
200	61	5.2	1.0
205	51	5.0	1.0
206	41	7.1	6.0
209[1]	27	8.6	. .[3]
245	30	3.0	6.0
324	52	2.0	0.3
344[1]	40	8.4	. .[4]
353	53	2.5	. .[4]
403	55	6.1	1.0[4]
404	60	10.0	14.6[5]
443	55	13.5[5]	. .
453	49	4.9	. .
521	39	9.9	2.0
537	47	3.5	. .[3]
543	62	2.6	3.5[3]
559[1]	72	7.6	0.3
629	71	13.4	7.3
633	51	1.8	. .[3]
761	52	3.7	. .
810	27	2.9	0.1
861[1]	51	2.2	1.3
862	26	3.5	2.8
886	29	2.3	0.3
916	58	3.5	1.6
1002[1]	52	1.7	14.2
1023	44	3.2	0.1
1029	32	4.5	0.1
1060	27	18.4	2.0
1083	54	1.8	0.2
1101[1]	50	8.8	9.0
1221	50	8.0	7.8
1233	26	2.6	. .
1271	53	3.8	1.0
1319	27	2.2	0.3
1442	45	8.8	2.3
1512	39	20.0	0.2
1560	24	0.9	0.2
1569	28	3.8	0.8
1629[1]	32	2.4	0.3
1642[1]	54	7.4	1.2
1871	48	8.5	1.0
1890[1]	53	6.5	0.4
2158	32	1.6	0.2
2314[1]	37	8.3[5]	0.1[5]
2357	62	4.0	7.8
2541[1]	28	5.2	0.6
2670	25	5.0	0.3

[1] Tubercular heredity.

[2] The fixation of the onset of tuberculosis is, of course, to a considerable degree, uncertain. The statistics are so compiled that the onset is earlier rather than later than reported in this table. See footnote 5.

[3] Cause of death, coma.

[4] Cause of death, gangrene.

[5] Still living. Duration to July 1, 1923.

diabetics compares favorably with that of earlier writers and the percentage of deaths from coma has also decreased.

The duration of the diabetes of all my cases in whom tuberculosis has been demonstrated is shown in Table 206.

Six of the 54 fatal cases, or 11 per cent died in coma. This is far below the percentage of deaths from coma in the whole group of diabetics. It suggests that the diabetes decreased in severity, due to the emaciation and lack of food consumed. Forty-six patients apparently died in the ordinary manner of an uncomplicated tuberculous case. Among the 56 cases of tuberculosis, my records disclose that tuberculosis was present in only 13 instances in another member of the family.

Contrary to expectation, my records show that frequently tuberculosis occurred before the diabetes. Proof is not convincing, but my records indicate that this appeared to be true at the time I took the history of the individual. The explanation lies in the fact that the tuberculosis, though it existed for a longer period, was of a latent or mild type.

Tuberculosis comes on in diabetes even more insidiously than usual; more than once I have been surprised at discovering not only its presence, but the advance which it has made. Unless 3 cases had recently been detected suspicion would arise that other cases were being overlooked. Already 2 of these have died, 1 very suddenly despite insulin, and not caused by insulin, though several

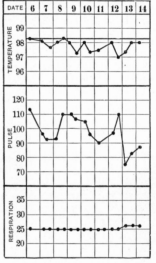

Fig. 29.—Insidiousness of tuberculosis in diabetes. The temperature, pulse and respiration chart of Case No. 916.

weeks earlier than the family were led to expect. One should always be on the watch for tuberculosis, taking for granted that it will not appear in an open manner, and therefore making complete physical examinations of all diabetic cases several times a year. Indeed, this is necessary for other reasons, for it is a very easy mistake for the physician to be so wrapped up in the treatment of the diabetes that he neglects the general condition of the patient. Loss of weight is attributed to the diabetes, and the characteristic absence of temperature throws the physician off his guard. Recollection of Fig. 29 has been of help in the diagnosis of many later cases. I can confirm older writers in the rarity of hemoptysis, though present in Case No. 861. A suggestive family history should always put one on guard. Perhaps soon in hospital routine all diabetics will have roentgen-ray examinations of the chest and teeth, and the elderly of the bloodvessels of their lower extremities.

It is frequently not easy to find the tubercle bacilli in the sputa of diabetic patients. Repeatedly a search has been necessary for several days in succession.

The presence of tuberculosis was first disclosed at autopsy in Case No. 633, in March, 1914. It was supposed by those of us in attendance that the patient's decline was wholly due to severe diabetes, ultimately culminating in pneumonia. The postmortem examination revealed extensive tuberculosis. Such a mistake is not extraordinary, for shortly after, bearing it in mind, a similar case in the wards of one of the best hospitals in the country was seen where this diagnosis had not been entertained. The diagnosis of tuberculosis was suspected, because the tolerance of the patient was gradually improving, but he was losing weight. On the other hand, an error was made in Case No. 1083 by neglect to observe the rise in temperature upon two days during his hospital stay. Since then temperature charts have been kept in plainer view.

The prognosis in diabetes complicated by tuberculosis is bad, but not immediately so. Yet tuberculosis, angina pectoris, disturbing arthritis, not rheumatic fever, which was relieved by the removal of bad teeth, old age, and diabetes are compatible with a useful life and a fair degree of health. In Case No. 629 diabetes developed at the age of seventy-one in 1909, tuberculosis became active at seventy-five, and angina pectoris at seventy-seven. The patient was first seen in July, 1913. Six months later tubercle bacilli were found, though previous physical examinations had disclosed no lesions. Undoubtedly tuberculosis had existed in latent form since youth. Under the close supervision of a devoted nurse, thoroughly trained in diabetes, the patient attended to active duties, and was living in comfort at the age of seventy-nine, not yielding to death by tuberculosis until March, 1922. In his last years he remained sugar-free on carbohydrate 69 grams, protein 42 grams, fat 94 grams. He was an illustration of the hopefulness which one is justified in assuming even in the presence of diabetes, tuberculosis, and angina pectoris. My friend did not enjoy fasting; his nurse and he taught me it was unnecessary and consequently inadvisable in the elderly.

Case No. 861, male, aged fifty-two years, developed diabetes while traveling in Europe in 1914. Tuberculosis superimposed itself upon the diabetes, but apparently neither was discovered until considerable progress had been made in both. The patient was seen by Dr. Lawrason Brown, and it is gratifying to record that after less than a day of fasting he became sugar-free, and gradually acquired a tolerance for 67 grams carbohydrate, and hemorrhages ceased. He subsequently succumbed to tubercular meningitis. In the intervening eight months the weight increased 20 pounds. How extensive an improvement can take place in pulmonary tuberculosis complicated by diabetes is shown by Dr. Brown's letter: "The patient presented dulness with broncho-vesicular breathing and increased vocal resonance below the fifth vertebral spine on the left side. There were also numerous moderately coarse rales. Over the right side there were moderately coarse and fine rales. Five months later the lesion at the left base cleared up almost completely. There were a few fine rales to the third vertebral spine, when he left, on the left side and possibly below the fifth rib. The right side still showed signs over most of the side."

The improvement in the last 2 cases is not exceptional. Naunyn records a case of a physician, aged fifty-three years, with diffuse pulmonary tuberculosis, and also a small ulcer on the left vocal cord, in whose urine was found 4 per cent of sugar. Careful treatment of the diabetes and the tuberculosis gradually brought about a gain, although some months after the beginning of the treatment there was slight hemoptysis, with tubercle bacilli present. The condition, however, kept improving, and sixteen years later both diseases were apparently arrested.

Case No. 443, a woman, aged fifty-five years, first seen on September 20, 1911, gave a history of congestion of the lungs at the age of twelve, hemoptysis at sixteen, and again to a marked degree at the age of twenty-four. Tuberculosis was confirmed by Drs. Flint and Loomis, of New York. Tubercle bacilli were never found, but the evidence of tuberculosis was undoubted. A roentgen-ray examination on September 21, 1911, showed general peribronchitis with numerous broken-down glands with healed borders, increased density and mottling with an appearance of healing at the right apex, small area of calcification, slight emphysema. The patient was sugar-free in September, 1911, and is still living and well, July, 1923. Case No. 1861, a mild diabetic, showed tubercle bacilli in the sputum in 1910 and again in 1920, yet now is in good health and actively engaged in business.

The explanation for the rarity of diabetes in sanatoria for tuberculosis is shown by the course of the case described in the following paragraphs. (Case No. 344, p. 577.)

TABLE 207.—CASE 344. ILLUSTRATION OF THE OLD-FASHIONED TYPE OF TREATMENT OF DIABETES. SEVERE ACIDOSIS, DECLINE IN CARBOHYDRATE TOLERANCE, DEVELOPMENT OF PULMONARY TUBERCULOSIS WITH IMPROVEMENT IN TOLERANCE COINCIDENT WITH EMACIATION. DISAPPEARANCE OF ACIDOSIS. (See page 577.)

Date	Volume of urine, c.c.	Specific gravity	Diacetic acid	β-oxybutyric acid, gms.	Nitrogen, gms.	Ammonia		Sugar		Diet		Carbohydrate balance, gms.	$NaHCO_3$ gms.	Body weight without clothing, kilos.	Remarks
						Total gms.	NH3-N/Total N per cent.	By copper reduction, gms.	By rotation, gms.	Carbohydrate, gms.	Alcohol, gms.				
1908.															
April 13-14	2000	1033	Trace		23.6	1.1	3.8		38	15±		− 25			Strict diet.[9]
17-18	1600	1026	Trace						5	10		+ 5		63.9	Vegetable day.
18-19	1700	1025	Trace		6.6	0.6	3.9		5	10		+ 10			Vegetable day.
19-20	1650	1022	Trace		6.4	0.3	3.6		5	180±		+ 175		64.8	Oatmeal day.
20-21	1900	1018	0		5.9	0.4	5.0		8	180±		+ 170			Oatmeal day.
21-22	2000	1016	0		9.9	0.6	4.7		7	180±		+ 175		65.3	Oatmeal day.
22-23	2900	1019	0		12.3	0.7			0			− 5			Vegetable day.
23-24	1840	1025	++		14.1				15	10		+ 10		64.8	Vegetable day.
24-25	1900	1024	Trace		10.6	0.3	2.3		2	10		+ 5		65.2	Strict diet; meat once.
29-30	1880	1024							3	10±		+ 10			Vegetable day.
April 30) / May 1)	2000	1024	+		12.8	0.5	2.6		2	10±		0		65.4	Strict diet; meat once.
6- 7	1600	1036	++			0.4			46						Vegetable day.
7- 8	1600	1027	++						9						Vegetable day.
1909.															
Jan. 2- 3		1024						0.5^2							Rarely a hyaline cast.
Dec. 27-28		1026						0.9^1		50					Vegetables and eggs.
1910.															
June 19-20	2100	1029	+++	8.7	22.5	2.6	9.5	91	38	10±	0	− 40	14	60.5	Strict diet; vegetables in 5-6-10 per cent. groups, cream 250 c.c., half grapefruit.
28-29	1720	1034	+++	30.1	19.6	4.6	19.3	48	37	10	0	− 40	14	58.5	Strict diet; vegetables 5-6-10 per cent., cream 250 c.c., half grapefruit, oatmeal 36 gms., peas 1 tablespoonful.
July 4- 5	2240	1027	+++	28.9	22.5	5.7	20.8	52^3	73	20	0	− 85	24	58.2	
6- 7	3340	1028	+++					107							
10-11	2975	1028	++++	21.7	19.3	4.8	20.5	107	83	50	0	− 55	24	58.9	Strict diet; vegetables 5-6-10 per cent., cream 375 c.c., half grapefruit, oatmeal 36 gms., peas 1 tablespoonful.
17-18	2960				18.8			88							
24-25	2780				16.5			81							
31)	2680				22.0			116							
Aug. 7- 8	2630	1028	++	28.4	15.0	2.2	12.1	90	68	55	15	− 35	24	59.0	Strict diet; vegetables 5-6-10 per cent., cream 375 c.c., half grapefruit, oatmeal 36 gms., peas 1 tablespoonful.
14-16	2800	1029	+++	31.9	18.3	4.5	20.0	105	67	55	15	− 10		57.6	Diet for Aug. 22-23 same as for Aug. 7-8.
22-23	2800		+++		18.5			88							
23-24	2320	1027	++++	26.1	16.7	3.8	18.7	64	46	20	15	− 45	24	58.2	Vegetables 450 ± gms., cream 250 c.c., 14 eggs, bacon 215 gms.
24-25	3020	1024	++++	21.6	15.9	3.0	15.5	36	12	15	10	− 20	24	58.1	Vegetables, broths.
25-26	3030	1027	++++	33.6	15.1	3.3	15.1	79	73	55	15	− 25	24	57.4	As August 8.
28-29	2840	1032	++++	31.6	17.3	2.3	10.9	108	85	70	15	− 55	24	57.9	As August 8.
Sept. 7- 8	3760	1030	++++	32.9	20.6	4.5	18.0	122	98		15	− 50	24	56.7	Strict diet; cream 250-375 c.c., half grapefruit, vegetables 5-6-10 per cent. peas...

Date															Diet
1910.															
Sept. 14–15	2560	1029	++++	32.8	16.8	4.1	20.1	63	41	20	8	−45	20	57.2	250 c.c. cream, 6 eggs, vegetables 450 gms., bacon 150 gms., claret 75 gms.
15–16	3250	..	++++	27.6	12.9	.	.	119	.	125[4]	40	+6	20	56.8	Oatmeal 180 gms., cream 300 gms., eggs 3, brandy 60 gms., claret 90 gms., butter 262 gms.
16–17	2900	1027	+++	38.5	11.7	4.4	30.9	69	46	20	30	−50	20	57.1	Cream 125 c.c., vegetables 500 gms., eggs 6, bacon, bouillon, much butter.
17–18	3200	1028	++++	19.6	13.6	5.0	30.2	92	64	45	23	−45	14	56.1	Strict diet; oatmeal 36 gms., cream 375 c.c., half grapefruit, vegetables 200 gms.
21–22	3340	1020	++++	40.7	18.4	4.2	18.8	113	80	55	23	−60	20	55.8	As August 8.
Oct. 5–6	3370	1029	+++	37.0	17.2	3.9	18.6	128	96	70	30	−60	20	55.8	Strict diet; vegetables 5-6-10 p.cent.groups,1 tablespoonful 15 per cent., oatmeal 36 gms., cream 250 c.c., half grapefruit, potato 90 gms.
Nov. 30–31	3230	1029	.	.	19.2	.	19.9	111	70	20	30	−60	20	57.2	Vegetables, eggs 7½, bacon, cream, 300 c.c.
6–7	3175	1028	+++	29.3	17.4	4.2		82							
16–17	3625	1031	.++	42.3	22.4	6.2	27.6	143	110	70	30	−60	20	54.8	Butter, 7 eggs, vegetables, bacon, cream, alcohol.
Dec. 27–28	3380	1030	++	42.6	18.5	5.1	26.5	132	56	20	30	−55	20	56.1	Butter, 7 eggs, vegetables, bacon, cream, alcohol.
7–8	3500	1025	++++		15.8			77							
26–27	2800	1027	++++	26.8	14.7	2.8	15.7	64	50	20	30	−45	20	58.0	Butter, 7 eggs, vegetables, bacon, cream, alcohol.
1911.															
Jan. 11–12	4130	1024	+++	39.6	17.0	4.2	20.3	74	58	20	30	−55	20	57.6	Butter, 7 eggs, vegetables, bacon, cream, alcohol.
25–26	4130	1029	++++	48.4	19.3	7.4	31.5	145	124	90	30	−55	20	.	Strict diet; vegetables 5-6-10 per cent., groups, 1 tablespoonful 15 per cent., oatmeal 36 gms., cream 300 c.c., half grapefruit, potato 90 gms., bread 30 gms.
Feb. 19–20	4500	.	++	.	19.2	8.0	34.3	.	153	125	30	−30	20	.	Strict diet; vegetables 5-6-10 per cent., oatmeal 18 gms., potato 90 gms., bread 60 gms., cream 500 gms., grapefruit, half orange, bananas 45 gms., macaroni 60 gms.
Mar. 5–6	5120	1029	+++	52.7	18.3	6.1	27.4	200	174	125	30	−75	20	56.3	Essentially the same.
16–17	4380	1027	+++	26.3	19.5	7.1	29.9	180	158	125	30	−55	20	.	"
April 2–3	4475	1030	+++	51.0	14.8	4.4	24.5	139	111	125	30	−15	20	55.9	"
26–27	4500	1028	+++	42.4	16.3	6.3	31.8	185	162	130	30	−55	20	55.7	"
May 10–11	5448	1028	+++		13.2	5.3	33.0	158	133	125	30	−35	20	.	"
12–13	4220	1026	.++	49.8	2.6	.	.	.	152	125	30	.	20	55.3	"
28–29	3150	1027	+++	18.9	11.4	6.0	.	186	126	125	30	−60	20	54.5	"
July 5–6	3900	1026	+++	36.2	14.1	5.1	29.8	117	125	30	.	+10	20	56.5	"
30–31	.	1023		.	.	.	.	2.5[2]	1.6[2]	20	30	.	23	55.7	4 eggs, cream 375 c.c., bacon, vegetables 5-6-10 per cent.
Aug. 9–10															

TABLE 207.—CASE 344. ILLUSTRATION OF THE OLD-FASHIONED TYPE OF TREATMENT OF DIABETES, SEVERE ACIDOSIS, DECLINE IN CARBOHYDRATE TOLERANCE, DEVELOPMENT OF PULMONARY TUBERCULOSIS WITH IMPROVEMENT IN TOLERANCE COINCIDENT WITH EMACIATION. DISAPPEARANCE OF ACIDOSIS.—(Continued.)

Date.	Volume of urine, c.c.	Specific gravity.	Diacetic acid.	β-oxybutyric acid, gms.	Nitrogen, gms.	Ammonia, Total gms.	Ammonia, NH₃-N/total N per cent.	Sugar, By copper reduction, gms.	Sugar, By rotation, gms.	Diet, Carbohydrate,[1] gms.	Diet, Alcohol, gms.	Carbohydrate balance, gms.	NaHCO₃, gms.	Body-weight without clothing, kilos.	Remarks.
1911. Aug. 10-11	3140	1027	++	36.3	9.8	4.8	40.3	122	94	95	30	− 25	23	55.8	Oatmeal 120 gms., cream 250 c.c., vegetables 5-6-10 per cent.
11-12	3600	1024	++	46.7	8.7	4.7	44.4	97	86	95	30	0	13	56.3	Oatmeal 120 gms., cream 250 c.c., vegetables 5-6-10 per cent.
12-13	3310	1020	∶∶∶	51.5	8.6	4.6	44.0	46	26	20	30	− 25	27	56.2	As on August 9-10.
16-17	3500	1029	+++	39.9	11.3	4.6	33.5	126	119	125	30	0	23	55.6	As on February 19-20.
Sept. 6-7	3420	1029	+++	38.3	13.2	4.1	25.5	150	137	125	30	− 25	23	55.4	As on February 19-20.
17-18	3800	1029	+	52.0	12.6	4.5	29.4	141	106	130[6]	30	− 10	23	55.0	Vegetable protein only, except protein in 3 eggs and 300 c.c. cream with usual carbohydrate.
27-28	3030	1032	+++			4.6	…	158	127	177[6]	30	+ 50	23	55.7	As on February 19-20.
28-29	2980	1031	+++++			4.4	…	143	113	130[6]	30	− 15	23	55.6	As on September 17-18.
29-30	3870	1028	+++++			5.2	…	155	116	130[6]	30	− 25	23	55.2	As on September 17-18.
Oct. 30 }	3800	1031	+			5.5	…	182	152	126	30	− 55	23	54.7	As on February 19-20.
8-9	3800	1030	+++	34.9	14.2	5.5	41.1	190	152	135	30	− 55	23	54.6	Same,+10gms.carbohydrate.
22-23	4000	1027	+++	52.0	13.0	7.1	34.8	180	144	135	30	− 45	23	53.8	Same,+10gms.carbohydrate.
Nov. 12-13	4400	1027	+	34.6	17.0	5.0	26.1	198	158	135	30	− 65	23	54.3	Same,+10gms.carbohydrate.
14-15	3800	1028				5.4		141	122	115	60	− 25	23	54.1	Butter 60 gms., oatmeal 150 gms., 2 cups broth, 600 c.c. cream = 180 gms. fat.
15-16	3800	1028	+++		11.4	5.4	39.0	144	114	130	45	− 15	23	54.2	As on September 17-18.
Dec. 30 }	4200	1028	++	46.2	13.4	5.2	31.9	168	151	135	45	− 35	23	53.7	As on October 8-9.
25-26	4700	1027	+++	54.8	14.5	6.3	35.7	188	160	135	45	− 55	23	50.4	As on October 8-9.
1912. Jan. 9-10	4840	1028	++		13.8	6.5	30.4	198	194	150	45	− 50	23	53.2	Same,+15gms.carbohydrate.
14-15	4000	1029	++		9.9	5.1	39.9	132	120	100	45	− 30	30		
15-16	3860	1029	+++		10.8	4.8	34.3	154	154	170	60	+ 15	30		
17-18	4945	1024				4.5		124	109	105	60	− 20	30		
Feb. 4-5	5270		Slight		17.3	5.2	24.7	198	183	150	45	− 50	30	53.1	
6-7	4820	1029	Slight		16.0	6.2	31.9	184	146	150	45	− 85	25	49.9	
12-13	4864	1027	++		14.3	6.2	35.7	191	176	100	85	− 40	25		
25-26	5175	1027	+++		9.6			126	134	150	4.57	− 25	25		
Mar. 14-15	4200[8]	1020	0		9.1	0.9	8.1	82	82	150	4.57	+ 70	25		
17-18	2940	1026	0	6.1	12.1	1.3	10.8	135	118	150	4.57	+ 15	15		
22-23	2700	1020	0	6.3	9.9			134	115	150	4.57	+ 15	15		
26-27	2400	1032	0	2.6				105	105	150	4.57	+ 45	10		
April 2-3	2100	1030	0		11.6			134	105	150	4.57	+ 45	5		
7-8	1680	1033	0					99	87	160	4.57	+ 60	5	34.5	

¹ Carbohydrates in diet up to June 29, 1910, are only approximately correct,   ⁵ Not twenty-four-hour urine,

The advent of diabetes upon tuberculosis is seldom observed, from reports of cases of tuberculosis treated in sanatoria. Montgomery[1] found that of 31,834 cases of tuberculosis treated in sanatoria there were 101 cases, 0.3 per cent, of glycosuria and 51 cases, 0.16 per cent, of diabetes, and he states that practically not a case of diabetes following tuberculosis has occurred at the Phipps Institute, in sanatoria or under the care of physicians with whom he is acquainted. Combining the data for glycosuria and diabetes we have 0.5 per cent incidence among 31,834 individuals. If this percentage among the tuberculous was applied to the population of the entire United States it would indicate half a million glycosurics and diabetics, a figure which is more consistent with my surmise than some other data suggest.

Diabetes, even of the severest grade, may practically disappear when tuberculosis intervenes and reaches an advanced stage. Many writers have observed such instances and it has repeatedly come to my attention. Unexplained improvement in the tolerance of a diabetic for carbohydrates always awakens suspicion. The patient whose course is here and elsewhere described, see pp. 574–7 and 453, is fundamental in this regard.

Case No. 344, cited hitherto as having an extremely severe type of diabetes, developed tuberculosis after eight years. Eventually the acidosis, which had amounted to the most extreme grade which I have met outside of coma, completely disappeared, and a minus carbohydrate balance of 40 grams, which had existed for months, changed to a positive carbohydrate balance of 60 grams. The complete record of the case is given in Table 207.

The disappearance of the acidosis is explained by the development of a positive carbohydrate balance. The explanation of the body's regaining power to utilize carbohydrates was difficult until I showed the records of the case to Dr. F. M. Allen and told him that if he could explain the improvement of the diabetes, which was coincident with the development of tuberculosis, a key to a valuable method of treatment of diabetes would be found. A few days later he said to me that he believed he could duplicate the case with his depancreatized dogs. At the time he gave no inkling of his plan, but how well he succeeded is known everywhere today by his experimental work upon animals, which showed that fasting and loss of weight will improve the tolerance of even the severest diabetic patients. Even if one does not make a discovery, it is a satisfaction to record the facts which may help another to do so.

Older writers laid emphasis upon the rapid extension of the tuberculosis in diabetes after it first appeared, and for this reason gave

---

[1] Montgomery: Am. Jour. Med. Sci., 1912, **144**, 643.

an especially unfavorable prognosis. Examples of this character are only too many, but while they are not encouraging from the therapeutic point of view, they should not be considered too discouraging. It is possible, indeed probable, that many of these cases had poor treatment not only for the diabetes but for the tuberculosis as well. The duration of the tuberculosis as well as of the diabetes in my cases absolutely controverts this former pessimistic view. Of the 46 cases in which the duration of the tuberculosis is recorded, in only 18 instances has the patient died during the first year of the tuberculosis. In one instance only did the diabetes last for less than one year.

The treatment of diabetes complicated by tuberculosis is the same as for diabetes alone. Adherence to the principle of treating the diabetes first and the tuberculosis second was put to a severe test when undernutrition was first employed. That Janney and Newell from a diabetic standpoint and Landis and Funk[1] and Montgomery from the standpoint of tuberculosis found their best results were achieved when undernutrition was employed is good proof that one should treat the diabetes as the primary disease.

Even though one hesitated to employ undernutrition in a wasting disease like tuberculosis the diabetes responded so favorably to it that soon undernutrition could be discarded and the patient fed a liberal amount of food. Insulin will aid in the maintenance of a generous diet, but advanced cases of tuberculosis will proceed to a fatal termination in quite the same manner as without it. There is this comfort in treating tuberculosis in a diabetic, namely, that with the progress of the tuberculosis the patient can eat more and more freely without glycosuria and yet keep himself free from diabetic symptoms.

3. **Arteriosclerosis.**—**Diseases of the Heart.**—**Bright's Disease.**— Arteriosclerosis is of common occurrence in protracted cases of diabetes. It is of the senile type. It seldom occurs even in the severest cases of diabetes in youth and not frequently before the age of fifty years—a strong argument against diabetes being a direct causative factor of arteriosclerosis. The comparative rarity of diabetic gangrene under the age of sixty years is also evidence in the same direction.

A study of the blood-pressure of a series of my diabetic cases favors the view that the presence of sugar and acid in the urine does not injure the arteries or kidneys. Thus, only 18.5 per cent of the cases occurring between the ages of twenty-one and fifty exhibited a blood-pressure over 150 mm. Hg. and but 32 per cent of the patients over the age of fifty years. When a later series was compiled for the years since April, 1919, it became evident

---

[1] Landis and Funk; Jour. Am. Med. Assoc., 1922, **79**, 1073,

that the figures were not greatly altered. Thus, of the cases under fifty years of age 14 per cent had a blood-pressure above 150 mm. Hg. and of the cases above fifty years of age, 40 per cent. When one considers the varying conditions under which blood-pressure readings are made in relation to meals, time of day, and calories in the diet for the preceding days, one must be cautious in arriving at conclusions. I am led all the more to this belief because the limitation of the diet of 11 healthy young men[1] to 1400 calories for one week lowered the systolic pressure from 120 to 102 mm. Hg. and the diastolic, from 83 to 69 mm. Hg.

The blood-pressure in diabetes is slightly below normal until the age of thirty-five years is reached; it then changes to slightly above normal and the interval between diabetic and normal widens as age advances. The above statements are based upon data secured from diabetics since April 1, 1919. Previously, the blood-pressure of diabetics was a trifle higher. Whereas the average normal blood-pressure based upon 19,339 normals between the ages of fifteen and fifty years according to Fisher[2] average 127, that of diabetics prior to April, 1919 was 139 and since that date, 129. (Tables 208, 209.)

Janeway's conclusions[3] coincide with my data. He wrote: ". . . .it is clear from my own observations and those of Elliott[4] that diabetes itself is without influence on the arterial pressure. Hypertension is therefore presumably an expression of the well-known tendency of diabetics of suitable age to develop arterial disease; or possibly in some cases arterial disease is the cause of the lesions responsible for the diabetes."

Rosenbloom's[5] experience is also similar because in every case in which the blood-pressure was found high in his diabetic patients there was a complicating nephritis, arteriosclerosis, or aortitis. In the uncomplicated cases of diabetes the blood-pressure was normal or subnormal.

A distinction in the .increase in blood-pressure in diabetes has been observed by Kylin.[6] In the 97 cases of diabetes studied by him since 1919, a high blood-pressure of a purely arterial type was found. In this type the blood-pressure drops toward normal during sleep and there is no high capillary blood-pressure. He considers that this special type of blood-pressure and the diabetes are the resultant of some common cause. Among my patients, at the New England Deaconess Hospital with diabetes and hyperten-

[1] Benedict, Miles, Roth and Smith: Carnegie Institute, Washington, 1919, Pub. No. 280, p. 373.
[2] Fisher: Jour. Am. Med. Assn., 1914, **43**, 1752.
[3] Janeway: Johns Hopkins Hosp. Bull., 1915, **26**, 341.
[4] Elliott: Jour. Am. Med. Assn., 1907, **49**, 27.
[5] Rosenbloom: Jour. Lab. and Clin. Med., 1922, **7**, 392.
[6] Kylin: Zentralblatt f. inn. Med., 1921, **42**, 873.

TABLE 208.—THE BLOOD-PRESSURE IN DIABETES.

Period.	Age, group, years.	Total cases.	Blood-pressure.									
			100–125		126–150		151–175		176–200		Above 200	
			No. of cases.	Per cent.	No. of cases.	Per cent.	No. of cases.	Per cent.	No. of cases.	Per cent.	No. of cases.	Per cent.
Before April, 1919	21–50	448	174	39	191	43	56	12	19	4	8	2
After April, 1919	21–50	356	161	45	147	41	35	10	10	3	3	1
Before April, 1919	Over 50	675	172	26	283	42	129	19	62	9	29	4
After April, 1919	Over 50	522	119	23	196	37	124	24	53	10	30	6

sion Root, Thompson and White[1] found an average fall in systolic blood-pressure between 5 P.M. and 8 A.M. of 41.4 mm. Hg. The corresponding drop in diastolic pressure was 17.4 mm. Hg. Patients with diabetes and no hypertension showed a slight rise in both systolic and diastolic pressures during this same period. Counts of the red corpuscles in capillary and venous blood showed in the patients with hypertension evidence of capillary stasis in the afternoon and a fall in the capillary count during the night. This finding may be related to the occurrence of gangrene in that it shows stasis in the terminal blood supply when the patient is active.

TABLE 209.—THE AVERAGE BLOOD-PRESSURE OF NORMAL AND DIABETIC INDIVIDUALS.

Ages.	Number of individuals.			Average blood-pressure, mm. Hg.		
	Normals, Fisher.	Diabetics, Joslin.		Normals, Fisher.	Diabetics, Joslin.	
		Before April 1, 1919.	After April 1, 1919.		Before April 1, 1919.	After April 1, 1919.
15–20	281	38	50	120	124	117
21–25	785	33	50	123	122	117
26–30	791	56	50	124	121	121
31–35	689	39	50	124	120	119
36–40	2111	64	50	127	125	126
41–45	6740	75	50	129	139	131
46–50	4471	116	50	131	143	135
51–55	2371	127	50	132	154	146
56–60	1100	103	50	135	154	153
Over 60	. . . .	163	50	. . .	156[2]	155[2]
	19,339	814	500	127	139	129

Low blood-pressures are frequently encountered with diabetic patients. It would appear as if the number of such cases had become greater in the period since undernutrition was introduced and prior to treatment with insulin. Thus, 35 cases were found among 500 cases.

TABLE 210.—CASES OF DIABETES WITH BLOOD-PRESSURE OF 100 MM. HG. OR BELOW.

Age.	15–20.	21–25.	26–30.	31–35.	36–40.	51–55.
	1130	1143	1005	1085	1066	1101
Case	1227	1102	1018	1215	1073	
	. . . .	. . . .	1159	. . . .	1155	2835[3]
	2037[3]	2042[3]	1196	2200[3]		
	2052	2391	1232	2259	2496[3]	
Nos.	2220	2406	1259	2360	2513	
	2432	2416	. . . .	2476	2852	
	2684	2516	2079[3]	2582	2868	
	2801	2687	2156	2611	2909	
	. . . .	2696	2206	2656		
	. . . .	. . . .	2340	2669		
	. . . .	. . . .	2808	2702		
	. . . .	. . . .	2948	2943		
No. of cases	8	9	12	12	8	2

[1] Root, Thompson and White: To be published.
[2] Not included in average.
[3] This and subsequent cases taken from a group of 500 since April 1, 1919.

Case No.	Age at onset, years	Under 1	||| Duration since onset in years																									Greatest rise	Greatest fall	Greatest variation from first to last
			1	2	3	4	5	6	7	8	9	10	11	12	13	14	15	16	17	18	19	20	21	22	23	24	25	30			
8[1]	60										150			210	220														70		70
29	29																				130				120			125			10	5
70	42			135		135			150			160	165	170	155									150						35		20
155	38	135	145						170		160	155	135		155															10	15	0
163	45	135						185		210	200											135								35	35	0
173[1]	65						120							160			160	155	140										75		65
176[1]	48									120	115	120	125	115	118	140		140	140						138			40		40
177	44					135	135		130	150	115	115	110				135												20	5	18
179[1]	54					105	135		110	100	115																		20	5	15
181[1]	43																												10	0	5
182	46			150												120	150											140		0	0
184	44			150					120	180				180	110										150					10	10
190[2]	55	178	150			130	170	163	170				150		140														10	10	0
198	48		170			130					130	160																	2	40	30
215	45															174													0		2
239	43				115									182	160	205													35	0	0
240	44	130				115	140	140								110													10	0	0
263	34	125	125										130	122	122														15	31	4
265	37	120											140	120	120														0	30	20
268	35	180	200											120	120		180	180													15
293[1]	69			178			180								115					140	160								20	0	0
309	35						160				118			115	115		160		140	190	160								45	22	45
321	51													170	150	160	160	180											30		30
329[1]	58										118			110															30		10
331	34	100		100			110	115		175				145	140		145												18	20	10
348	42			140			160	160	150	160				145	140		145												35	35	5

Table of cases — blood-pressure readings and amount of sugar.

No.	Age	Blood-pressure readings (earliest → latest)	Sugar (successive observations)
352	37	100, 110, 100, 110	10, 10, 10
359	33	105, 100, 160, 155	5, 15, 10
392	47	105, 130, 130, 150, 160	10, 10, 10
399	46	120, 130, 130, 140, 120, 110, 115	10, 10, 20
406	41	120, 180, 140, 130, 230, 180, 260, 225, 120, 125, 115, 110	10, 30, 80
416[1][2]	54	230, 180, 225, 120, 115, 110, 150	45, 35, 5
428	28		5, 15, 30
435	32	120, 120, 122, 105, 110	30, 0, 20
436	20	95, 120, 110, 110, 110	10, 30, 20
444	42	95, 120, 110, 105, 110	20, 5, 15
445	38	150, 150, 190, 180, 170, 180, 115, 115	15, 15, 0
450	43	150, 140, 190, 180, 190, 160, 130	0, 10, 10
455[1]	64	135, 165, 170, 165, 180, 160, 130	15, 20, 5
457	50	190, 110, 110, 120, 115	5, 5, 20
459	51	170, 170, 180, 180, 130	20, 10, 20
462	38	110, 120, 110, 100, 115, 130	15, 20, 30
468[1]	38	140, 145, 140, 160, 160, 115, 110, 115, 150	10, 20, 20
481	49	125, 145, 155, 140, 155, 120	20, 10, 15
488	60	140, 145, 160, 95, 145	5, 20, 20
503	30	125, 100, 200	30, 5, 5
507	46	130, 130, 140, 160, 160, 180	20, 30, 0
632	30	220, 160, 150, 130, 140	10, 60, 30
727	51	125, 130, 140, 130, 120, 120	5, 40, 10
748[1]	61	140, 130, 160, 135, 240, 220, 240, 225, 180	10, 5, 10
778	58	140, 178, 180, 100, 240	60, 22, 0
780[1]	64	200, 190	0, 60, 40
805[1]	49	190, 130, 140, 105, 105, 130, 120, 180	10, 40, 0
866[1]	31	100, 130, 140, 100	15, 10, 40
882[1]	59	130, 130, 150, 150, 120, 130	9, 15, —
907	52	165, 160, 155, 120, 120	0, 15, 24
941	47	165, 140, 132, 136, 120, 164	10, 0, 0
972[1]	55	130, 130, 130, 120	15, 15, 8
1182	36	140	10, 0, 10

[1] Fatal.
[2] Cases in which blood-pressure fell with disappearance of sugar.

Another source of information upon the influence of diabetes on blood-pressure can be found by comparing the blood-pressure of a series of diabetics during subsequent stages of the disease. In Table 211, the changes in the blood-pressure are recorded for 59 cases during intervals of five to fifteen years. For the majority (34) of the cases the blood-pressure remained within 10 mm. below or above the original observation; in 16 cases it rose over 11 mm., and in 9 cases it fell more than 11 mm. The greatest rise in blood-pressure was in Case No. 8, (70), and the greatest fall in Cases Nos. 727 and 805, (60). The greatest variation between the first and last observation was 70 mm., Case No. 8. This patient lived fourteen years after the onset of diabetes.

TABLE 212.—CHANGES IN BLOOD-PRESSURE DURING NINE YEARS OF TREATMENT FOR DIABETES. BENEFIT FROM INSULIN. CASE NO. 727.

	Sugar, per cent.	Diet in grams.				Insulin, units.	Weight, lbs.	Blood-pressure, mm. Hg.
		C.	P.	F.	Cals.			
1914.								
May 14 . .	7.6	...	..	...	....	...	...	220
17 . .	6.2	188	..	...	....	...	114	
25 . .	2.2	103	..	...	....	...	113	
June 4 . .	0	10	..	...	....	...	111	
Aug. 13 . .	0	45	..	...	....	...	122	180
Nov. 17 . .	0	0	..	...	....	...	127	170
Dec. 31 . .	0	70	..	...	....	...	128	160
1915.								
Mar. 29 . .	0	70	..	...	....	...	128	160
July 22 . .	0	70	..	...	....	...	125	150
Nov. 2 . .	0	...	..	...	....	Attack	of gall	stones
1916.								
Feb. 23 . .	0	70	..	...	....	...	123	180
1917.								
Mar. 1 . .	1.0	...	..	...	....	...	123	160
1922.								
June . .	Broke	knee.	Bone s	utered.				
1923.								
May 16 . .	2.4	...	..	...	....	...	116	200
June 7 . .	1.0	63	46	43	823[1]	...		
7– 8 .	0.2	104	53	55	1123	0–1–2	...	180
8– 9 .	0.2	84	61	94	1426	3–4–3		
9–10 .	0.1	84	61	94	1426	3–3–2		
10–11 .	0	84	61	94	1426	3–0–3		
11–12 .	0.1	84	53	89	1349	3–0–3		
12–13 .	0.1	84	53	89	1349	3–0–3		
13–14 .	0.3	86	63	106	1550	3–0–3		
14–15 .	0.2	86	63	106	1550	3–0–3		
15–16 .	...	86	63	106	1550	3–0–3		
21–22 .	...	86	63	106	1550	3–0–3	114	

Case No. 727, with onset of diabetes at the age of fifty-one years, showed 7.6 per cent of sugar when she was first seen at the age of

[1] Approximate.

fifty-five, May 14, 1914. The systolic blood-pressure was 220 mm. (Riva Rocci). The changes in the urine and in the blood-pressure during the course of treatment are given in Table 216. She did remarkably well and like so many of such cases evidence of disease of the gall-bladder was demonstrated. Later a suture of the bones of the knee resulted successfully, and happily this summer she has been rewarded for her faithfulness in the past by the use of insulin. Her diet satisfies her and she is better than for years. The extraction of sixteen teeth under local anesthesia at two sittings was undergone without event. This patient shows both a rise and a fall in the blood-pressure during the course of treatment.

Maranon[1] has noted such a fall of blood-pressure quite commonly as the duration of the diabetes progressed. Conversely, he has observed that a high blood-pressure may precede the onset of diabetes, as it did with Case No. 872.

It is possible that in the past the excessive feeding of diabetic patients and particularly the excessive quantity of protein may have predisposed the diabetic patient of advancing years to an earlier appearance of vascular changes. With the advent of under-nutrition in 1914, it was thought that light would be shed upon this feature, but such is not the case. From Table 62 it is clear that there has been a general advance in the duration of life for all decades since 1914, and that this increase of nearly one and a half years has been among the younger as well as the older diabetics who would be more prone to show arterial changes.

Arteriosclerosis, on the other hand, may play an important rôle in the production of diabetes. Many pathologists have pointed out the presence of arteriosclerotic changes in the vessels of the pancreas, liver and brain, and have called attention to the resulting degeneration of these organs which might lead to diabetes. This view appears most reasonable. According to Naunyn's conception of diabetes, those individuals with an inherent though mild tendency to diabetes would be prone to develop the disease when degenerative bodily changes begin to appear.

An illustrative case is No. 629, who, after several years of circulatory symptoms with annoying angina pectoris, developed diabetes at the age of seventy-one, and also Case No. 872 who had a blood-pressure of 250 at the age of sixty-five without quantitatable sugar in the urine, but in whose urine three years later 5.2 per cent of sugar was found. After treatment of the diabetes sugar disappeared, and the blood-pressure fell in succeeding years to 230, 220 and 210. Coincidently there has been marked amelioration

---

[1] Maranon: Zentralblatt f. inn. Med., 1922, **43**, 169.

of the anginal pains, and the patient says he feels better than for years. The improvement may be due to the gradual loss of weight which occurred following the onset of the diabetes.

A considerable number of my cases have suggested the development of diabetes as a result of arteriosclerosis, because the diabetes has appeared insusceptible to improvement. It is hard to understand however, why it should come on so suddenly with so slow a process as arteriosclerosis as a cause, but its onset in some of these cases is certainly analogous to the onset of diabetes in youth. However, a change in less than 1 gram of islands would amply suffice. On the other hand, if arteriosclerosis is a cause of diabetes why do not many more arteriosclerotics have it?

No reciprocal relation between the level of sugar in the blood and the height of blood-pressure was found by Härle.[1]

Syphilis.—Few cases of arteriosclerosis in diabetic patients appear to result from syphilis. There were 55 cases with a history of syphilis among a total of 3200 patients. Wassermann tests are performed upon my patients as a routine, but special pains are taken to have the test made and repeated in suspicious cases. Yet of 1000 patients whose blood was tested, only 16 gave a positive result. This is confirmatory of clinical and pathological observation that the type of arteriosclerosis which one sees in diabetes is not that which is usually attributed to syphilis.

The symptoms of which diabetic patients suffering from arteriosclerosis complain are chiefly related to the lower extremities and the heart but less commonly to the brain—characteristic symptoms of senile rather than syphilitic arteriosclerosis. Pains and numbness of the legs and cold feet are very common. Intermittent claudication occurred in Case No. 8 one year before a cerebral hemorrhage. The whole train of symptoms leading up to gangrene often extends through a period of months, and these patients suffer more than those with actual gangrene.

Diseases of the Heart.—The cardiac symptoms from which diabetic patients suffer are more of the order of angina pectoris than of cardiac incompetency. Indeed, angina pectoris is fairly common, though my records show only 19 cases in which there was sudden death from this cause, Cases Nos. 11, 66, 100, 285, 355, 415, 449, 475, 705, 759, 782, 1027, 1128, 1196, 1203, 1252, 1784, 1941 and 2374. Case No. 11, whose brother died of diabetes at fifty-two years, developed diabetes at fifty-eight and came under my observation six years later when I was called to see her during a midnight attack of angina pectoris. Some weeks later she went through a course of restricted diet, became temporarily sugar-free, but

[1] Härle: Ztschr. f. klin. Med., 1921, **92**, 124.

ultimately sugar returned. After three months death occurred in a second attack. At the time I was self-condemnatory and inclined to attribute the final attack of angina pectoris to the change in diet, but in the subsequent twenty years this experience has not been duplicated, until the death of Case No. 705 presumably due to this cause. Case No. 127, elsewhere cited, see p. 629, developed symptoms of angina abruptly with a coronary thrombosis and attacks have been frequent during the last two years. With Case No. 2056, the pain was so severe that it was necessary to keep him in bed for several weeks and this treatment resulted in relief. One of my doctors, who had gout, had angina pectoris, too. He was fat!

Sudden cardiac failure in diabetes has been frequent in Williamson's[1] experience and in fact such deaths stand third in frequency in his causes of death. Thus, there were 59 cases of coma, 17 of tuberculosis, and 7 of sudden cardiac failure. In these patients there were no previous signs of valvular disease.

Cardiac incompetency is rare. Case No. 354, with onset of diabetes at fifty, died with such symptoms at the age of seventy, but for the preceding one or two years the sugar in the urine had been replaced by albumin. Case No. 234, who developed mild diabetes in addition to his obesity at the age of seventy-seven, died with symptoms of heart failure. But two cases of decompensation due to myocardial disease have occurred in approximately the last 1000 cases of the series treated at the New England Deaconess Hospital. Relief of decompensation by digitalis in one case, Case No. 1922, seemed to improve the glycosuria remarkably. This suggests a relation to the disturbance in glycogenesis which is said to occur in cardiac decompensation. Cardiac weakness due to coronary disease or arteriosclerosis was fairly common among the elderly diabetics. The cardiac asthma often referred to in the older diabetic literature has not been recognized by me.

Rheumatic heart disease is of extraordinary rarity. In 1917, I could recall no case of diabetes under fifty years of age in which the patient complained of shortness of breath or presented the signs of an incompetent heart due to valvular disease of definite and unquestionable rheumatic origin. This circumstance, Root points out, suggests the infrequency of local infections of tonsils and teeth or other infections as an etiological factor in diabetes. Recently, the exceptional case appeared in Mr. P., Case No. 2989, who entered the hospital with 5.3 per cent sugar and diabetes of two months' duration. His heart showed double mitral and aortic murmurs. He was placed upon the routine of Test and Mainte-

[1] Williamson: Practitioner, 1922, **109**, 279.

nance Diets when it was discovered from the discomfort thereby caused that he had a duodenal ulcer with pyloric obstruction. Under local anesthesia a gastro-enterostomy was performed by D. F. Jones with complete recovery, though the patient's heart fibrillated for some days following it. He returned to work in five weeks. This is 1 of the only 2 cases which F. G. Brigham, H. Gray, A. A. Hornor, H. F. Root, or I remember among all my cases.

Myocardial disease in contradistinction to valvular disease is not infrequent among the diabetics. The diabetics in fact present a favorable field for the study of such lesions. Three autopsies within two years have revealed extensive myocardial disease probably secondary to coronary sclerosis. Two of these patients, Cases Nos. 870 and 2479, died within a few weeks of operation, thus emphasizing anew the importance of searching for evidences of myocardial weakness in elderly diabetic patients. The lack of symptoms resulting from the comparative inactivity of the patients sometimes is deceptive, and occasionally the electro-cardiograph and roentgen-ray give important aid to the clinical findings.

Severe diabetes in two elderly patients with marked arteriosclerosis deserves citation.

Mrs. L., Case No. 2716, with onset of diabetes at the age of sixty years in 1920, lost 96 pounds, chiefly during the year preceding July 12, 1922, when she first came under observation. The sugar in the urine was 8 per cent, in the blood 0.43 per cent, and the plasma was creamy, containing 3.9 per cent fat, Bloor. There was marked arteriosclerosis, the blood-pressure, 145–90. Five days later following sharp restriction of diet the blood sugar fell to 0.03 per cent, analysis checked by three observers using two standards, and the blood fat was 1.94 per cent. The patient was rescued from a death in hypoglycemia by the alertness of H. F. Root, who supplied her liberally with carbohydrate. Later even when the patient's diet contained carbohydrate 36 grams, protein 34 grams, and fat 77 grams, calories 964 or 28 calories per kilogram body weight, the sugar in the urine amounted to 11 grams and the blood sugar, fasting, varied between 0.2 and 0.27 per cent. This elderly diabetic therefore was distinguished by (1) marked loss of weight, 53 per cent; (2) high glycosuria, 8 per cent; (3) high blood sugar, 0.43 per cent; (4) high blood fat, 3.9 per cent; (5) marked hypoglycemia, 0.03 per cent, coming on acutely but with recovery and (6) intractability to dietetic control. With insulin and orthopedic treatment for the contractures which had developed during months of invalidism the patient is able to be up and about September, 1923.

A man, Case No. 2241, with onset of diabetes in January, 1921 at the age of sixty-nine years, came under observation five months later having lost approximately one-third of his weight and then weighing 43 kilograms. With carbohydrate 33 grams, protein 54 grams, and fat 91 grams, or 27 calories per kilogram body weight his fasting blood sugar was 0.21 per cent and rose to 0.31 per cent with carbohydrate 32 grams, protein 46 grams, and fat 86 grams. He developed edema and died December, 1921, of asthenia. Here again there was slight response to treatment in a diabetic of advanced age.

Bright's Disease.—Albuminuria is frequently observed in the urine of diabetic patients, but actual Bright's disease, like arteriosclerosis, is practically unknown except in cases past fifty years of age. It appears safe to conclude that diabetes does not lead to the type of nephritis we include under the name Bright's disease. The association of the two diseases in the latter part of life is not uncommon, but the underlying cause of both appears to be the arteriosclerosis of advancing years. It is seldom that one sees death from uremia in diabetes. Confusion rarely exists between uremic and diabetic coma except in cases of pregnancy. In other words, the renal complications of diabetes have been unimportant in the past. With the prolongation of life which modern treatment is bringing about they may deserve more attention.

Cerebral Arteriosclerosis (including under this term such diagnoses as cerebral hemorrhage, apoplexy, hemiplegia, or paralysis) was responsible for the death of 33 cases.

Treatment.—The treatment of diabetes in the presence of arteriosclerosis, whether general or primarily localized in the kidney, must not be undertaken lightly. Years ago this was impressed upon me by Case No. 347, who became sugar-free under the old regimen of restricted carbohydrate and increased fat-protein diet. Soon after discharge from the hospital, however, acidosis increased, and coincidently with this a latent nephritis broke out, and death in coma followed. The greater sensitiveness of patients with diseased kidneys to acidosis was pointed out by Goodall and Joslin.[1]

It should also be remembered that an acidosis develops in the course of Bright's disease quite independently of the acidosis which occurs in diabetes. This was noted by Frothingham.[2]

That marked changes in the diet seriously affect the circulation I am also led to believe by Case No. 859, who, in the course of fasting treatment, developed symptoms in which was indicated marked disturbance of the cerebral circulation, though no actual paralysis developed. These examples show how careful one should be in attempting to better the condition of arteriosclerotic patients who

[1] Goodall and Joslin: Boston Med. and Surg. Jour., 1908, **158**, 799.
[2] Frothingham: Arch. Int. Med., 1916, **18**, 717.

have diabetes. They furthermore show why the older generation of doctors hesitated, and at that period with good reason, to alter the diet of such of their elderly patients who were leading tolerably comfortable lives. Today the dangers attending the beginning of treatment of such individuals are less, because acid poisoning is so readily avoided at the beginning of treatment. Indeed, the rational treatment of diabetes differs little from the rational treatment of hypertension and nephritis save that fat is used more freely than carbohydrate. In all the protein is kept as low, if not lower, than 1 gram per kilogram body weight and in all salt is restricted to a greater or less degree.

It should be remembered that there is no need for hurry in the treatment of diabetes in the presence of arteriosclerosis, because the diabetes has probably existed for a long time, and under treatment it is hoped that the patient will continue to live for many years to come.

The improvement in the condition of patients showing Bright's disease and diabetes combined is often striking. So frequently is this circumstance noted that it cannot be lightly passed over. Presumably the restricted diet and the low protein in the modern diabetic treatment conduce to this result, quite apart from the fact that the Bright's disease has previously been made worse by the diabetes. Repeatedly patients with Bright's disease acquire an increased tolerance for carbohydrate as the Bright's disease increases in intensity. This often is quite a comfort to the patient, and the physician should be always on the watch for it, so as to give these individuals the benefit of the freedom of diet of which they have so long been deprived. The possibility of renal "block" should be borne in mind.

The surprising improvements which occur in the circulatory symptoms of these patients quite likely may be due to the decrease in weight which ensues upon the restricted diet. Thus along with the treatment of diabetes very desirable treatment of the arteriosclerosis is accomplished.

4. **Care of the Skin.** — **Pruritus.** — **Furunculosis.** — **Carbuncles.** — Cutaneous eruptions due to the presence of hyperglycemia may be divided into two main categories: (1) The toxidermata, conditions due solely to the presence of a chemical irritant in the skin, and (2) conditions due to the action of various bacteria or higher vegetable species finding a favorable medium for growth in this sugared soil.

In the first group we include anidrosis or asteatosis, a dried-up condition; pruritus, a generalized or localized itching; chronic urticaria, an intractable and usually papular form of hives; eczema, sometimes generalized but generally confined to the vulva and the mons Veneris in women and to the glans penis and prepuce in men; purpura, a rare type; a somewhat universal deep pigmentation, the *diabète bronzé* of the French; perforating ulcer; lastly, the diabetic xanthomata, the often brilliant yellow tumors associated with a red periphery which differentiate them from all other types of xanthomata.

In the second group we find impetigo, a superficial and streptococcic infection; ecthyma, a somewhat deeper and larger and more obstinate staphylococcic type; folliculitis, furunculosis and carbunculosis, the deepest variety of staphylococci, differing only in size and multiplicity of foci; paronchyia, the so-called "run-around" and gangrene.

In this group we place the examples of epidermophytosis and tricophytosis, especially of the genital regions, and the yeast eruptions found in the webs of fingers. This latter type seems to be practically limited to women of the Russian-Jewish race.

In enumerating this second group of diabetic dermatoses we wish to make ourselves clearly understood. Each disease has its own bacterial or hyphomycetal cause and exists very largely independently of diabetes mellitus; but when excessive sugar is present in the cutaneous tissues these same organisms find a more favorable soil for growth and objectively flourish accordingly.[1]

Pruritus pudendi frequently occurs in diabetes and will usually vanish within a few days, but occasionally not until two weeks after the disappearance of sugar from the urine. General pruritus, on the other hand, is exceptional, may be annoying and persist for weeks. It does not occur in young diabetics. If pruritus pudendi does not clear up promptly, as the urine becomes sugar-free, an examination will probably disclose a prolapse, leucorrhea or urinary incontinence. Rest in bed, absolute cleanliness, simple douches and the simplest of ointments are indicated. The free use of oil to prevent irritation during micturition is helpful. Patients with chronic nephritis are often relieved of pruritus when the protein and salt in the diet are reduced. There may be cases where $\frac{1}{4}$-skin unit doses of roentgen-ray becomes necessary to allay the itching.

Infections of the skin are less common now than formerly and this may be attributed to the improved hygiene. Such infections are and should be rare in diabetic patients under treatment. They demand immediate, thorough, yet gentle, treatment. One of the first duties of the physician is to tell diabetic patients to keep the skin exquisitely clean and to report the beginning of an infection at once. Patients should be warned of the danger from

---

[1] I wish to acknowledge help received from Professor C. J. White who with Dr. Greenwood has undertaken an investigation of the diseases of the skin of diabetics at the New England Deaconess Hospital.

slight wounds, should specifically be advised not to allow manicurists or chiropodists to draw a drop of blood and cautioned to
report promptly any injury to the skin. Finger and toe nails
should be cleaned with a blunt—not sharp—tipped file or, better,
an orange stick. Absolute cleanliness of the body is essential.
Formerly the increased percentage of sugar in the tissues was held
responsible for the presence of infections, but recent work has
tended to disprove this theory. Von Noorden has observed such
infections to be more common soon after the development of
diabetes than when the cases were well established. One would
expect the reverse if either the sugar or acid in the tissues predisposed to infection, because these tend to increase as the diabetes
progresses. Subcutaneous injections can be given as in any normal individual, but scrupulous asepsis should be practised.

If there is the slightest tendency to furunculosis at once adopt
simple measures analogous to those described by Bowen.[1] The
patient is advised to wash the whole body twice a day with soap
and water, using a fresh piece of sterilized gauze and powdered or
liquefied soap and to dry the skin with a freshly boiled towel without rubbing, so as to avoid breaking open any pustule; the whole
body is then bathed with a saturated solution of boracic acid in
water, with the addition of a small proportion of camphor water
and glycerin. I have often advised a solution of 2 parts medicated alcohol No. 1 and 1 part water to advantage, but I notice
that Bowen, in his second paper, still prefers the boracic acid.
Individual furuncles may be treated with the following ointment
according to Bowen:

Boracic acid	4
Precipitated sulphur	4
Carbolated petrolatum	30

One should be careful, however, not to overtreat the skin. Harm
may result from frequent dressings. The simplest lotions should
always be employed. In severe cases the patient should be put to
bed, all linen changed twice daily and the patient treated in as
aseptic a way as possible. In a few cases vaccines have appeared
to be of a marked benefit. "This procedure—thorough bathing
and soaping, the application of the borated solution and the dressing
of the individual furuncles—is repeated, as has been said, morning
and night. A further point of vital importance relates to the
clothing that is worn next to the skin. Every stitch of linen worn
next to the skin should be changed daily, and in the case of extensive furunculosis all the bedclothing that touches the individual,

[1] Bowen: Jour. Am. Med. Assn., 1910, **55**, 209; Boston Med. and Surg. Jour.,
1917, **176**, 96.

as well as the night-clothing, should be subjected to a daily change. Naturally, this treatment must be continued for several weeks after the last evidence of pyogenic infection has appeared, and this fact must be emphasized to the patient at the outset" (Bowen). Stannoxyl, 1 pill with water after each meal, is well worth a trial.

For the management of infections and carbuncles in diabetes, see pages 566 and 631.

Impetigo Contagiosa.—Impetigo contagiosa occurred in a young woman with severe diabetes (Case 2218, elsewhere described). Dr. C. J. White wrote me as follows: "She has a remarkable impetigo contagiosa circinata—remarkable in the extraordinary number of synchronous foci of infection. It would be possible to produce such a condition, I would suppose, by the forceful use of an infected towel in a susceptible individual—in this case a diabetic." Under his care recovery was prompt.

Xanthoma Diabeticorum.—Xanthoma diabeticorum is a disease of considerable frequency in a diabetic clinic, but apparently not very common in dermatological clinics. Thus, C. J. White, in 1920, wrote me he had encountered but 3 or 4 cases.

The presence of xanthoma is recorded in 6 of my patients, but I suspect there have been at least five times as many instances of it. Three of these cases, Cases 1705, 2245 and 3017, were males, and 3 Cases 1753, 1936 and 2980, females. The age of the youngest patient was twelve years. The duration of the diabetes when the patient was first seen varied between three and eight years. Of these cases, 1 died of coma six months after the first visit, making the total duration of the disease in his instance five and a half years; the other 5 cases are probably alive in 1923. The blood fat was 1.1 per cent and 1.4 per cent in 2 cases, and the blood sugar in 5 cases ranged from 0.22 to 0.35 per cent. All of the cases belonged to the moderately severe type of diabetics.

The blood fat in xanthoma diabeticorum is usually reported to be increased. In the 2 cases observed by Nicholson,[1] among his 600 diabetics, the cholesterol was 1.26 per cent with 1 and the creamy blood of the other showed 4.4 per cent (Bloor) blood fat. The latter case confirms C. J. White's favorable prognosis of the condition in that, with the improvement of the diabetes, there was a disappearance of the xanthoma. Later on this returned when the diet was relaxed and subsequently the blood fat rose to 7 per cent and the patient died in coma.

Epidermophytosis.—Epidermophytosis occurs in those diabetic patients who are distressingly neglected, in the form of an angry eruption. This is most frequently seen in women about the geni-

[1] Nicholson: Clifton Med. Bull., 1923, **9**, 12. Lyon: Edinburgh Med. Jour., 1922, **28**, 168. Griffith: Jour. Am. Med. Assn., 1922, **78**, 1836.

38

tals. Case 1217 was the first patient of this type whom I sent to C. J. White, who taught me the correct name of the disease and cured the case. He describes the condition, and from his article[1] I abstract a few sentences:

"*Anus and Intergluteal Fold.*—The clinical appearances are almost identical in these neighboring tissues and consist of redness, moisture and at times a decided maceration which results in a lusterless, dirty-white center and a narrow, angry, red, moist periphery.

"*Labia.*—The results of epidermophyton infection here are unusual. The most marked feature is the intense itching which is really cruel. The skin remains dry, dull red, perceptibly thickened and possibly furfuraceously scaling, but nothing more. One cannot appreciate any such appearances as usually exist on the contiguous thighs. The plant probably runs over onto the mucous surfaces. . . . The infectious agent in the disease under discussion is at times the epidermophyton inguinale, first definitely proved and established by Sabouraud, in 1910, but more often the trichophyton. . . . The disease on the thighs, on the pubes and in the axillæ will rapidly disappear after the application of an ointment containing precipitated sulphur, 2; salicylic acid, 2; and benzoated lard, 30; plus rigid but gentle antisepsis; but care must be taken that the skin of the penis and the scrotum is not overstimulated, and that the treatment must continue long enough to kill the plant in the horny layer as well as on it. The disease elsewhere, so far as I know, will not yield to this ointment or easily to any other combination of the ordinary drugs. Whitfield's modified ointment (*i. e.*, salicylic acid, 1; benzoic acid, 1.65; soft paraffin, 10; cocoanut oil, 22) is probably the most successful ointment for the dry types of the disease, and a 1 per cent aqueous solution of permanganate of potash is perhaps the best means of conquering the vericular and moist phases of the process."

5. **Care of the Teeth.**—Approximately 41 per cent of 300 diabetics had either poor or false teeth. Poor teeth are by no means necessary, even in diabetes of long duration. Cases which are carefully treated from the outset and are cautioned about care of the teeth have little more trouble than healthy individuals. Then, too, patients with diabetes of long duration are occasionally seen with perfect teeth. This may happen even though they have not dieted strictly.

Bad teeth should be removed and all pockets of pus drained, but the dentist should not be too radical because over and over

---

[1] White: Jour. Cutan. Dis., 1919, **37**, 501.

again, as a result of constitutional treatment, the condition of the mouth improves and loosened teeth become firm. The time spent by the patient in the hospital should be utilized to have the mouth put in perfect condition.

The extraction of teeth has probably often resulted in the death of the patient, due presumably to the anesthetic. In illustration of this point, and as an example *par excellence* of a needless diabetic death, I would cite Case No. 729.

Death Subsequent to Extraction of Teeth (Ether Anesthesia.)— Case No. 729, female, married, teacher; first seen, May 16, 1914; no diabetic heredity. Greatest weight, 163 pounds; but 124 at the first visit. One child born in 1905 and well. In September, 1907, sugar first found, while five months' pregnant. Confinement was normal, and the child is living and well. The patient became sugar-free and remained so until January, 1911, when she was again pregnant, but miscarried in the following March. In July, 1911, she became pregnant and the child was born at term and is also well. Sugar was absent at this time, but it soon came back and persisted. A miscarriage occurred in February, 1914, and there was a history of two other miscarriages. Under dietetic treatment at the New England Deaconess Hospital in June, 1914, the sugar decreased from 6.2 per cent to zero, and the patient acquired a tolerance varying between 15 and 45 grams. On April 26, 1915, three months after her last visit to me and without my knowledge, all her teeth were taken out with ether as an anesthetic. The extraction took place at the dentist's office. "She was very sick after getting home, and all that night and the next day complained of the awful weakness and pressure, so that it was hard for her to breathe. April 28 her mind was wandering, and it was difficult to bring her back to consciousness." She died in coma, April 30, 1915.

In contrast to the above, see Case 727, page 585, who had sixteen teeth removed under local anesthesia.

The same rules which govern the use of anesthetics in surgery apply in dentistry. Gas or gas and oxygen are undoubtedly the best anesthetics. Novocaine may be advantageously employed and obviates in these days the dangers of general anesthesia, but it should be used with caution because the infiltration of the tissues may be distinctly harmful. Ether might be employed if the occasion demanded, because the patient could be protected from hyperglycemia and acidosis by means of insulin.

The teeth and tonsils of all diabetics coming under observation are as sedulously cared for as with non-diabetics. One would like to conclude that subsequent gains in tolerance for carbohydrate in these patients are directly due to removal of these infecting agents, but proof is often lacking because the dietetic treatment of the disease begins coincidently with local treatment. Higgins,[1] however, reports an excellently studied case with a rise in tolerance from 60 grams of carbohydrate before operation to 100 grams after operation.

6. **Constipation.**—Constipation is the rule in diabetic patients. It is helped by restricting their diet more often than by the traditional forcing of vegetables. The latter method might secure better results were more care taken to choose those vegetables which lead to the formation of gas, because this prevents hard fecal masses. Thus one of my patients who has a diabetic garden regulates his bowels by beginning his breakfast with a slice of raw cabbage. More efficient than coarse vegetables are bran muffins, and better still are agar-agar jellies (see page 734).

Physical exercise is the best of all treatment for constipation. Since patients have been encouraged to walk outdoors several times a day and to take up other forms of exercise, there has been less need of drugs. The constipation of Case 348, whose prostate was successfully removed by Chute, in July, 1915, vanished when he began to saw wood, and he keeps it up.

Massage.—Mr. Gustaf Sundelius, who has been of so much help in giving massage and exercises to my patients with inanition and gangrene, and in training them to massage and exercise themselves, has furnished me the following sets of exercise for the relief of constipation. These are easy to execute and suitable for weak and elderly people:

1. *Abdominal Kneading and Stroking.*—*Kneading.*—Lying down, with knees slightly drawn up. Place hands one on top of the other on the abdomen at the right groin; with small circular movements and deep pressure work upward until the ribs are met, then across toward left, following the boundary line of the chest, then downward to the left groin. Repeat twenty to fifty times. *Stroking.*—With hands similarly placed, make long, steady and deep strokes following the same route. Repeat twenty-five to one hundred times.

2. *Leg Rolling.*—Lying down, take hold of both legs just below the knees, press the knees up close to the abdomen, then carry them apart, then down and inward until they meet again, thus letting the knees describe two circles. Repeat ten to twenty times.

3. *Abdominal Compression.*—Standing against the wall with hands clasped behind neck, draw the abdomen forcibly in, using the abdominal muscles, hold a second, then let go. Repeat ten to forty times.

[1] Higgins: Cincinnati Jour. Med., September, 1922.

4. *Trunk Rolling.*—Standing with hands on hips, feet apart and legs well stretched, roll the upper body in a circle on the hips by bending forward, to the left, backward and to the right. Then reverse, and repeat six to twelve times each way.

Mineral oil, salts and enemata can be used when active treatment is necessary, but when daily measures are required one should attempt to depend upon the diet. If the patient's tolerance allows the use of an orange in addition to 5 per cent vegetables, frequently nothing more is necessary. Great pains, however, should be taken to impress upon the patients the necessity of preparing coarse vegetables in a simple manner. It is perfectly possible to cook cabbage, cauliflower, turnips, parsnips, radishes, cucumbers and onions so as to be unirritating to the digestive tract and yet preserve their laxative qualities. Patients whose tolerance allows potatoes are encouraged to eat them with the skins on. Diarrhea should be carefully avoided.

Drugs which I have found most satisfactory have been cascara sagrada, compound rhubarb pills, aloin, strychnin and belladonna tablets or aloin alone. If compound rhubarb pills are employed, one must be on the watch for a false diacetic acid reaction with ferric chloride, due to the oil of peppermint which they contain.

Mineral oil may be advantageously employed and most pleasantly as a salad dressing (see page 747). The various aperient waters may be given, but loose movements should be avoided. Sodium or magnesium citrate in doses of one or two teaspoonfuls helps to relieve the constipation, but the alkali which it furnishes may prolong the presence of a diacetic acid reaction. Bran bread and agar-agar jellies are helpful (see page 729).

7. **Diarrhea.**—Diarrhea is a most serious complication. Rest in bed, fasting and preservation of body warmth should be carried out from beginning to end of the attack. Hot water, solutions of hot, weak tea or cracked cocoa may be given. If the water content of the body is threatened give salt solution subcutaneously. When the indication is plain the bowels should be cleared out with castor oil or, even better, a Seidlitz powder. Avoid strong cathartics because diabetic patients with diarrhea are usually too feeble to withstand their action. Should the cause of the diarrhea be low down in the intestinal tract give enemata. If any drug is employed it should be opium. The return to the diabetic diet is rendered easy by the use of lean meats, oatmeal gruel, milk, cream, biscuits, eggs, purée vegetables. The carefully prepared, tender vegetables are frequently better borne than a diet containing considerable quantities of albuminous and fatty food.

Insulin may be dangerous in diarrhea, possibly because of the small quantity of carbohydrate which the patient is taking. An instance in point is Case 2909 (page 72).

The tolerance of a diabetic may increase during an attack of diarrhea. This has been marked on several occasions and it has also been noted that when the diarrhea has ceased the tolerance has again fallen. Guelpa gave diarrhea along with fasting when he prescribed salts. Hirschfeld[1] mentions the favorable effect of diarrhea and he cites Külz as having observed this. Sugar was not found in the feces.

Case No. 2909, just mentioned, experienced a rise in tolerance from 63 grams carbohydrate on October 22, 1922, to 113 grams carbohydrate on November 8, 1922. Another patient, Case No. 2099, whose tolerance had been as low as 6 grams carbohydrate in February, 1921, during an attack of diarrhea in August, 1921, was able to take 45 grams carbohydrate without glycosuria. This is the patient who before coming for treatment took a gallon of olive oil in the course of some weeks instead of taking mineral oil and developed acidosis. In June, 1923, I learn that with 36 units insulin she is sugar-free on a diet of carbohydrate, 50 grams, protein, 50 grams, and fat, 100 grams, and that her weight has risen from 57 pounds in 1921 to 86 pounds.

The circulation of a diabetic is woefully weak when he is attacked with diarrhea. Death from inanition and asthenia might easily ensue.

8. **Neuritis.**—Neuritis is most uncommon among my patients. The explanation is simple, because three of the common causes of neuritis have been infrequent. In twenty-five years, I have attended but 2 of my diabetic patients for acute alcoholism and have seldom prescribed alcohol. Syphilis has been diagnosed in only 55 of 3200 cases and of the last 1000 Wassermann reactions, there have been but 1.6 per cent positive. Tuberculosis has caused but 6 per cent of 887 deaths. Neuritis yields as obstinately to treatment in diabetes as when it occurs in association with other diseases. Fortunately it is rare, but unfortunately it does not always disappear with the removal of the glycosuria. This cannot be due to the increased quantity of sugar persisting in the blood long after it has disappeared from the urine, because hyperglycemia of many years' duration is so seldom accompanied by neuritis. Indeed, primary "neuritis" in diabetes is rare, usually a misnomer, or is secondary to some form of circulatory obstruction or some form of arthritis. Sciatica is the most frequent type of neuritis which occurs in diabetes. From the help which modern orthopedic treatment has afforded my patients, it appears probable that the

[1] Hirschfeld: Ztschr. f. klin. Med., 1896, **31**, 219.

sciatica is not at all the result of the diabetes, save in so far as such a complication may appear in any individual who has lost weight and whose muscles afford only lax support to the large joints. Just as loss of weight may be harmful and cause sciatica in that it promotes sacro-iliac disease, the loss of weight may be beneficial and cure sciatica by relieving the strain on the back of a pendulous abdomen or relieve flat feet. A fibroid tumor was the cause of the sciatica in one diabetic woman. To treat the modern diabetic successfully the knowledge of an all round general practitioner is essential.

Hydrotherapeutic measures avail much in neuritis, but when this is an indirect result of an arthritis, fixation of the part, and in sciatica fixation of the sacro-iliac joints, brings most relief, as my orthopedic friends have been able to demonstrate upon intractable cases. In some cases of this type symptoms persist despite such treatment, but sometimes these can be explained as habit pains. Moist flannel applications changed every one or two minutes almost invariably give comfort. These are applied by placing a dry flannel upon the skin, for the sake of protection, with the moist, hot, freshly wrung-out flannel laid over it and the protruding ends of the dry flannel covered over the moist to retain the heat, while a third flannel is kept in hot water for future use. Dry heat is less efficacious.

Mental diversion, brought about by change in surroundings, often produces good results. Similarly, the improvement in the general condition which follows rigorous dietetic and physical treatment is of great advantage. Such cases are particularly helped by a brief stay in a hospital, or by having a well-trained diabetic nurse in the home.

The type of neuritis most commonly encountered has occurred in the lower extremities. When diminished sensation, pain and tenderness exist there is always doubt whether the condition is a true neuritis or simply the result of poor circulation. It is certainly true that a pure type of neuritis in other parts of the body in diabetes is seldom seen. For this reason I am inclined to believe that the poor bloodvessels of the lower extremities are the chief offenders. On account of this fact it is well to instruct all diabetics after the age of sixty to exercise the bloodvessels of their legs. They should not remain long in one position, should walk frequently, get in the habit of flexing and extending the feet on the legs, easily accomplished by rising on tip toes and standing on heels, when the clock strikes. It is remarkable what persistent effort will accomplish, combined with the stimulus wrought by improvement in the state of the diabetes. One must never despair of these cases.

Multiple neuritis occurred in a single patient, Case No. 2182, and alcohol was ruled out as a factor with reasonable certainty. The case has been described in detail by H. F. Root,[1] The neuritis developed seven weeks after the supposed onset of the diabetes. There was eventual improvement.

Alcohol was formerly an important etiological factor in neuritis, but today cases of alcoholic neuritis are rare.

The changes occurring in the posterior roots of spinal nerves have been described by Krause.[2] He considers them not uncommon.

Epilepsy has not been encountered in my group of diabetics.

Hay fever, typical in character and of the rag-weed type, ceased when the diabetes in Case No. 2383 began.

Asthma has been very rarely observed. I remember but 2 cases. W. R. Ohler in a personal communication states that 14 asthmatics had sugar tolerance tests which were found to be abnormally low. A. A. Hornor tells me that he has seen 2 diabetic asthmatics. The asthma improved not with the development of the diabetes, but rather with the institution of dietetic treatment. One of the patients had taken adrenalin chloride subcutaneously for sixteen years, at no time less frequently than every forty-eight hours, but since becoming sugar-free in July 15, 1923, has required it but twice and then when unloading a car load of horses.

Dr. F. M. Rackemann who treats many cases of asthma, has met with no instance of its association with diabetes, and Dr. I. C. Walker, in a personal communication, reports that he has seen but 2 cases of diabetes among 2500 to 3000 asthmatics.

9. **Eyes.**—Ocular complications in diabetes are frequent. Von Noorden reports that of 279 patients, 58.3 per cent had trouble with the eyes attributable to the diabetes, and of those patients over fifty years of age, 80 per cent. He summarizes the results of the examination of the eyes of 477 diabetics, taken in succession. Defects were found in 279 instances; in 259 of these cases there was no etiological cause other than the diabetes. A summary of the data is given in the following table:

TABLE 213.—OCULAR COMPLICATIONS IN DIABETES (VON NOORDEN[3]).

	No. of cases.
Retinitis	81
Retrobulbar neuritis	23
Atrophy of the optic nerve	18
Cataract	62
Iritis	2
Amblyopia without organic change	33
Diabetic myopia	21
Other conditions	39

[1] Root: Med. Clin. North America, 1922, **5**, 1433.
[2] Krause: Med. Clin. North America, 1920, **4**, 225.
[3] Von Noorden: Loc. cit., p. 217.

Fortunately complications often vanish after the patient has been free from sugar and acidosis for a few weeks. If treatment will accomplish so much when complications have appeared, how much it must accomplish in prevention of complications. One cannot too frequently impress upon the patient that treatment is instituted not simply to keep sugar out of the urine, but to save him from a great variety of serious incidental diseases. I have been told by an oculist friend that ocular complications in diabetes are less frequent than formerly. The subject deserves attention, and I shall endeavor to have my series of cases studied from this point of view as also the complications of the circulation and skin. Diabetic patients live so much longer today that there is more time and more cause for complications.

Conversely, with the institution of progressive treatment the eyesight often temporarily fails, and more than once patients in the course of a few days have become unable to read, and once even to recognize individuals. The explanation of this condition is undoubtedly due to changes in the water balance of the body and the disappearance of sugar. These incidentally involve the lens, causing refractive changes. Elschnig[1] describes such a case in which one lens had been removed for cataract. The diabetic hypermetropia occurred only in the other eye. One can always reassure such patients with the statement that the return of their former eyesight and even an improvement in the same will eventually take place. It is remarkable to how great an extent the eyesight may return in a long-standing, but neglected case of diabetes. Case No. 181 was unable to read his name when he entered the hospital, but after three weeks' stay he was able to do so. Case No. 924 showed marked failure of eyesight on October 28, 1915. Her eyes were examined at this time by Dr. F. M. Spalding, who reported a shrinking and flattening of the lenses. With a convex lens ($+2$) in front of each eye the vision later came up to normal.

Cataracts have not been frequent in my series, though, unlike many of the ocular complications, more are seen today. This is as one would expect because of the greater duration of the disease, but more especially because of increasing attention given to the eyes in this clinic by H. F. Root. One can easily understand that the ophthalmologist, Graefe, found cataracts in one-fourth of all his diabetics, whereas Frerichs, in 400 patients, discovered only 19 cataracts, and Seegen in only 4 per cent of his series. It is interesting that the haziness of the lenses in beginning cataract may diminish with constitutional treatment and improvement of the diabetes.

---

[1] Elschnig: Med. Klinik., Berlin, 1923, **80**, 968.

Cataracts must have a definite relation to the hyperglycemia, because they occur in young diabetics who have had the disease many years. At Dr. Allen's Clinic a boy lived for several years with double cataracts, who had been operated upon, was happy and had secured partial restoration of vision. In one of my cases there were double cataracts which developed in a child. This little girl, Case No. 1898, was the daughter of an ophthalmologist and became diabetic at the age of eleven years and eleven months, showing at one time 10 per cent of sugar and a blood sugar of 0.9 per cent. This value for the blood sugar was checked in two laboratories. She died in coma three years and four months after the onset of diabetes, but the cataracts were discovered at the detection of the disease which was five months after the onset. Her father wrote: "She had cataracts, which at that time were mostly in the posterior poles of the lenses, although there were scattered opacities throughout the lenses. The vision at that time came up with a weak cylinder to 20/20, but since then they had steadily increased until the vision dropped to 15/200, but as the opacities were to a great extent central and to a limited extent peripheral, she managed to get along fairly well by looking over them. In the twenty-five years that I have been engaged in the line of ophthalmology, that is the first time I have seen diabetic cataracts in the case of a child. . . . Four days before she died she was as well as she had been for a long time; she had suffered very little from fatigue, and at no time was she depressed; in fact she was always singing and laughing, quite in contrary to the majority of diabetics." Nicholson[1] describes a seventeen-year old boy in whom opacities over both lenses showed marked improvement one month after insulin was begun only to reform later.

One instance of paralysis of the abducens muscle I distinctly recall, though I cannot identify the record.

Case No. 806, cited on page 538, showed a retrobulbar neuritis, but it was probably due to syphilis and not to diabetes.

Operations for cataract have been successful as well as uneventful. Insulin has helped with a recent case, Case No. 3192, under the care of F. M. Spalding, but the others did well without it and have been operated upon during the course of years by G. S. Derby, F. E. Jack, L. P. Tingley and E. R. Williams. It is usually easy to arrange to have the patients in excellent condition from the diabetic standpoint prior to operation.

Lipemia retinalis occurs not infrequently, though is generally unobserved. Gray and Root,[2] in my clinic, have discovered and reported cases (Case Nos. 2216 and 2842). They found less than 30 cases recorded in the literature which they give *in extenso*.

[1] Nicholson: Clifton Med. Bull., 1923, **9**, 54.
[2] Gray and Root: Jour. Am. Med. Assn., 1923, **80**, 995.

The condition disappears with modern dietetic treatment and insulin in *hours* instead of in many days, weeks or months, as shown in Table 214.

TABLE 214.—DIMINUTION OF BLOOD FAT IN LIPEMIA RETINALIS.[1]

	Blood fat, per cent.	Interval.
White	...	2 months
Köllner	26.25–13.50	Not stated
Hardy	9.50– 2.90	2 weeks
Benedict	8.50– 3.50	Not stated
Wagener	8.20– 1.90	24 days
Gray and Root	6.30– 2.95	96 hours

I. ULCER—GASTRIC OR DUODENAL.

Hunger is a characteristic symptom in diabetes, but not until this year did the many sources of diabetic hunger come to my attention. (1) There is the hunger of the untreated diabetic, due to the excretion of enormous quantities of sugar in the urine with attending polyphagia. (2) There is the hunger of under-nutrition, which came to the fore when this type of treatment was introduced in 1914. (3) There is the hunger accompanying the hypoglycemia caused by an overdose of insulin. And finally (4), there is the hunger which is often a symptom of gastric or duodenal ulcer, and with this we are now concerned.

Of the first 2700 cases coming for treatment no instance of ulcer of the stomach or duodenum, developing after the onset of diabetes, was recognized, until in the last year striking examples have appeared. Of these Case No. 564 was the most pathetic. With severe acidosis and 3.4 per cent of sugar he entered the hospital in December, 1912, and only became sugar-free three months later through the help of a diabetic nurse at home. Courageously he went through boarding school and entered college, invariably keeping sugar-free, demonstrating that if adherence to a weighed diet is absolute, daily examinations of the urine can be omitted and reliance placed upon monthly blood-sugar tests. On November 15, 1922, he suddenly developed pain, succumbed in three days, and an ulcer of the stomach was found to have perforated.

The second instance was almost as tragic. Case No. 2559 developed diabetes at the age of fifty-four years, came under treatment in March, 1922, became sugar-free, acquired a tolerance of carbohydrate 96 grams, protein 71 grams, and fat 99 grams, and returned to business. Without ever having had a symptom of indigestion, so far as his family recall, in July, 1922, he suddenly had a violent hemorrhage, and despite transfusion, died within two days. At autopsy there was a double ulcer of the duodenum.

---

[1] Gray and Root: Loc. cit.

The third case was a delight. Case No. 2989, a working man of forty-seven years, with eight children, entered the hospital on February 24, 1923, with 5.3 per cent of sugar. Distress in the stomach led to examination, which disclosed retention of food, the presence of blood, and, by roentgen-ray, pyloric obstruction. The Wassermann reaction was negative. Double aortic and mitral murmurs were to be heard in the heart. Auricular fibrillation was present at times. Notwithstanding all, the patient became sugar-free with the help of insulin, acquired a tolerance for carbohydrate 75 grams, protein 48 grams, and fat 85 grams, and with novocaine anesthesia underwent at the hands of D. F. Jones a successful gastro-enterostomy. For nearly a week after the operation the heart fibrillated with a pulse-rate of 180, but five weeks later the man was back at light office work and sugar-free with the aid of a few units of insulin.

A fourth case of duodenal ulcer, Case No. 2350, occurred before the patient developed diabetes, and indeed the diabetes is of slight degree as it is with a fifth patient, Case No. 2890, who had had indigestion all his life. The sixth patient, Case No. 1122, also gave a history of a duodenal ulcer, the first symptoms of which began in 1910, at the age of twenty-eight years. From then on he was troubled more or less constantly, experiencing three distinct attacks, during the last of which, in 1913, he had rigorous treatment. Diabetes began three years later, in 1916, and he showed 8.4 per cent of sugar when he first came under my observation. With a carefully planned diet, faithfully carried out under the supervision of B. H. Ragle, his existence has been prolonged, and he is trying to come back to life with insulin. The sixth patient, Case No. 2600, is the only female in the group. Her diabetes began in December, 1920 and symptoms of ulcer in the same year. The roentgen-ray shows this to be located in the duodenum. With suitably adjusted diet and insulin, she has made marked improvement, gaining eight pounds.

When searching a series of 300 non-diabetic records for the presence of transient glycosuria, it was found that this was present in 50 (16 per cent) and the sugar could be quantitated in 25 of this number. Of these latter there were 6 instances in which the glycosuria was associated with disease of the stomach, duodenum, pancreas, or gall-bladder. Possibility of a more frequent association of sugar in the urine with lesions in the region of the duodenum should lead to the re-investigation of such patients for diabetes.

The diet of the diabetic furnishes ample reason for the development of an ulcer of the stomach or duodenum. It is a coarse diet. It is often associated with the use of highly seasoned food, with hot food, and oft-times is distinguished by an abundance of meat. That in the past ulcers of the stomach and duodenum have not been noted frequently with diabetics is not strange because in the past diabetics lived too short a period to develop and die of such conditions.   In his tabulation of the causes of death of 292 diabetic patients von Noorden[1] records 1 death from ulcer of the stomach with hemorrhage.   Although it must be acknowledge that with the cases above cited the duration of the diabetes was not long, yet in the care of diabetic patients in the future one will do well to remember that the causes for hunger are four.

J.   SYPHILIS.

The Wassermann test has been positive in 1.6 per cent of 1000 diabetic patients and negative in 98.4 per cent.   Among the number counted as negative there were 10 cases in which the first report was positive, but negative shortly afterward without any special treatment for lues.   In my total of 3200 cases of diabetes there was a history of syphilis or signs of syphilis in 55 or 1.7 per cent.   At the Bacteriological Laboratory of the Boston Board of Health, where I have been fortunate enough to have my Wassermann tests performed, the percentage of positive Wassermann tests for 1923 up to September, is 15.5 per cent.   Walker and Haller[2] at the Peter Bent Brigham Hospital report that 8 per cent of 89 diabetics gave a positive Wassermann reaction and that this was about one-half the incidence for the general hospital population.   Williams[3] found the Wassermann test in 144 diabetics to be positive in 4, absent in 126, doubtful in 1, and 13 cases anti-complementary.   Mason[4] among 168 diabetics discovered 2 strongly positive Wassermann reactions but without the history, symptoms, or signs of syphilis. These patients when treated for a short time for their supposed syphilitic infection showed marked and rapid *decline* of carbohydrate tolerance.

Table 215 shows the incidence of syphilis based on history and physical signs.

TABLE 215.—FREQUENCY OF SYPHILIS ACCORDING TO CASE HISTORIES AND PHYSICAL SIGNS OBSERVED.

Case Nos.	Total cases of syphilis
1– 400	7
401– 800	8
801–1200	6
1201–1600	6
1601–2000	5
2001–2400	10
2401–2800	6
2801–3200	7

[1] Von Noorden: Loc. cit., p. 342.
[2] Walker and Haller: Jour. Am. Med. Assn., 1916, **91**, 488.
[3] Williams: Jour. Am. Med. Assn., 1918, **70**, 365.
[4] Mason: Am. Jour. Med. Sci., 1921, **162**, 828.

The presence of diabetes does not interfere with the Wassermann reaction. Van Saun[1] reports that of 10,000 Wassermann tests the specimens in 73 instances were obtained from patients who were known to have diabetes. "Only 1 serum gave a positive reaction, 51 were negative, 2 doubtful, and in 19 the serum controls failed to hemolyze so that no readings could be made. All the sera giving the so-called anti-complementary results were chylous.

"The 1 serum which gave a positive result had been obtained from a patient who had also a history of syphilis.

"The sera with which doubtful reactions were obtained gave only weak fixation. One of these sera was obtained from a patient who gave a history of a chancre twenty-six years previously. The other patient gave no history of syphilis.

"These results with sera from cases of undoubted diabetes would seem to dispose of the contention that diabetic sera give readable positive reactions with Wassermann antigens when there is no clinical evidence of syphilis. It would seem that with carefully controlled tests non-specific fixations can always be checked. The 19 sera giving non-specific reactions in this series of tests might easily have been supposed to be positive had not their anti-complementary qualities been fully demonstrated by the double, as well as the single serum controls."

Labbé and Tauflet[2] give an exhaustive review of the literature and conclude that syphilis is rare in diabetes.

Warthin and Wilson[3] have strikingly different views from the above regarding the frequency of association of diabetes and syphilis. They find disease of the pancreas almost universal in cases of latent syphilis and also syphilitic lesions in 6 patients with diabetes at autopsy. As yet other investigators have not substantiated the work of these authors.

Lemann[4] has sought to throw light upon the question of the dependence of diabetes upon syphilis by comparing the frequency of diabetes in the white and negro patients of the Charity Hospital in New Orleans along with the frequency of syphilis. Despite the greater frequency of syphilis in the negro he demonstrated that diabetes is not as frequent in that race as in the white. Thus, between the years 1898 and 1909 the negroes furnished 40 per cent of the admissions, but only 30 per cent of the diabetics. The total incidence of diabetes was 0.63 per 1000, among the whites 0.72 and among the negroes 0.47 per 1000. Between 1910 and 1919, 160,044 patients were admitted to the hospital and of this number

[1] Van Saun: Jour. Med. Research, 1917, **37**, 205 (new series, **32**).
[2] Labbé and Tauflet: Annal. de Méd., 1923, **13**, 367.
[3] Warthin and Wilson: Am. Jour. Med. Sci., 1916, **152**, 157.
[4] Lemann: Am. Jour. Med. Sci., 1921, **162**, 226.

the negroes constituted 43 per cent, but only 30 per cent of the diabetics in the hospital. An increase in the incidence of diabetes took place in both races alike. Thus, the incidence for diabetes rose among the whites to 1.4 per 1000, and among the negroes, to 0.86 per 1000, whereas the negroes furnished more than 50 per cent of all the syphilitic diseases. The discrepancy between the incidence of diabetes in the two races might be explained by differences in the average ages of the whites and negroes. Perhaps the average age of the negroes in these series is less than that of the whites.

The rarity of syphilis among diabetics is also commented upon by Labbé.[1] He also records that in 7 diabetic patients with a history of inherited or acquired syphilis the treatment of the disease was without favorable results upon the diabetes and elsewhere he says that he knows of no case in the literature in which treatment of the syphilis improved the diabetes. This view was expressed in the discussion of a report of a patient treated by Pinard and Mendelsohn[2] whose diabetes had been greatly helped by the accompanying treatment of syphilis.

The absence among diabetics of the common sequelæ of syphilis —tabes dorsalis, paresis, aortic insufficiency and aneurysm—is confirmatory evidence of the infrequency of syphilis as an etiological factor in diabetes. Absolute data I cannot give, but since April 1, 1919, my former and present associates, Brigham, Hornor, Gray, Root and I can remember but 2 cases of tabes in my entire series of diabetics, 1 case of paresis, 1 case of aortic insufficiency and 1 case of aneurysm. Indeed I recall but 6 patients among the 3300 diabetics who have ever been sent to an insane asylum or required treatment for insanity.

Many of my diabetic cases with a syphilitic history have been of long duration. This type of the disease has occurred so frequently in connection with known syphilis that one must suspect the presence of syphilis in mild diabetes. (See Table 216.) In illustration of the above I would cite the following instance: Case No. 503 acquired syphilis at the age of sixteen years, and was energetically treated by the older methods. Fourteen years later, in May, 1912, when about to undergo an operation for appendicitis, sugar was found at a routine examination, and the Wassermann reaction, which had not previously been tried, was demonstrated to be positive. He was given a thorough course of treatment with salvarsan, and the Wassermann reaction has remained negative. Under dietetic treatment sugar decreased and gradually a marked carbohydrate tolerance was acquired. No further antisyphilitic

---

[1] Labbé: Bull de l'Acad. de méd., Paris, 1923, **89**, 53; Bull. et mém. Soc. méd. d. hôp., 1922, **46**, 400.

[2] Pinard and Mendelsohn: Bull. et mém. Soc. méd. d. hôp., 1922, **46**, 400.

treatment has been given. On August 19, 1915, the urine contained 0.5 per cent of sugar and the carbohydrates in the diet amounted to 140 grams. The blood sugar amounted to 0.16 per cent fasting. On August 7, 1922, the urine contained 0.5 per cent sugar, the blood sugar was 0.13 per cent, five hours after a meal and the Wassermann reaction was negative. The father, Case No. 711, of the patient developed mild diabetes, but his Wassermann reaction was negative.

A positive reaction has been found on 11 different occasions during three and nine-tenth years with Case No. 630. Acquirement of syphilis is denied by the patient and he presents no stigmata of it. The disease is mild, amenable to diet, although the urine has contained 5 per cent sugar. The diabetes has lasted fourteen years and at its onset the patient's expectation of life was but nineteen years. The individual is in full vigor.

The duration of syphilis and of the diabetes is shown in Table 216.

It would seem as if syphilitic diabetes was an ideal object for etiological treatment, but all writers agree that this is not usually the case. It is true that occasionally a case has been strikingly helped. For instance, Umber[1] recorded a case of diabetes, male, aged forty-eight years, with syphilitic infection in 1898. During 1909 indigestion, pain in epigastrium, thirst, transitory jaundice, loss of 18 pounds, and gastric tumor occurred. Upon a diet of 147 grams of carbohydrate, 113.4 grams of sugar were eliminated. Fatty stools, blood sugar 0.43 per cent, Wassermann reaction positive. Following the use of 0.4 gram of salvarsan the tumor decreased in size and the stools became less fatty. There was a continuous gain in weight for one year, and at the time of recording the case the patient lived without restriction of carbohydrate and no tumor was to be felt. Revillet[2] reports a cure with mercury.

Walker and Haller report that energetic treatment of 1 case of diabetes developing six months after the initial lesions was without any influence on the diabetes. The blood Wassermann became much weaker, but never negative and the patient finally died in coma.

Remarkable improvement in the diabetes of a young woman with syphilis, considered to be of congenital origin, though the Wassermann of the mother was negative, was noted by Dr. J. E. Paullin and Dr. H. M. Bowcock who have placed the following notes at my disposal. The patient, aged twenty-one years, was first seen in March, 1921. Her father died of apoplexy at sixty-three years. She had always been delicate; catamenia began at fourteen, but ceased seventeen months before the first visit. The greatest weight was 115 pounds at fifteen years of age but decreased to

[1] Umber: München. med. Wchnschr., 1911, **58**, 2499.
[2] Revillet: Lyon méd., 1916, **125**, 374.

85 pounds. Cramping pains in the epigastrium after meals were the chief complaint in 1921, from which she obtained relief by vomiting. Upon physical examination there was thoracic scoliosis, enlarged cervical glands, rales at the apices, pupillary and patellar reflexes normal, tenderness in the hypochondrium. The red blood

TABLE 216.—DURATION OF DIABETES IN PATIENTS SHOWING A POSITIVE WASSERMANN REACTION OR PRESENTING A POSITIVE HISTORY OF SYPHILIS.

LIVING CASES.

Case No.	Age at onset. Syph-ilis.	Dia-betes.	Duration of diabetes to July 1, 1923. Years.	Case No.	Age at onset. Syph-ilis.	Dia-betes.	Duration of diabetes to July 1, 1923. Years.
IV	26	46	13.5	XXXII	19	38	1.1
VI	16	30	6.7	XXXIV	49	44	5.3
IX	28	44	10.9	XXXV	32	51	1.4
XII	..	46	8.4	XXXVI	29	20	9.5
XIV	Under 42	42	19.7	XXXVII	36	51	10.2
XVI	31	32	28.6	XXXVIII	42	42	3.1
XVII	31	44	8.2	XXXIX	40	61	2.9
XVIII	35	54	7.6	XL	..	65	7.0
XIX	27	58	12.6	XLI	20	54	6.3
XX	54	47	17.6	XLII	38	49	0.3
XXI	32	34	34.6	XLIII	34	46	0.2
XXII	43	31	15.0	XLIV	25	51	1.3
XXIII	22	49	3.6	XLV	30	39	11.0
XXIV	51	54	3.8	XLVI	..	43	5.8
XXV	..	8	3.8	XLVII	47	75	4.4
XXVI	17	8	1.8	XLIX	..	36	13.8
XXVII	22	21	2.2	LI	46	41	7.0
XXVIII	49	46	3.9	LII	50	40	7.0
XXIX	24	23	2.2	LIII	23	29	5.2
XXX	57	49	9.0	LIV	49	57	4.2
XXXI	12	53	9.2				

Total average age and duration Av. 34 Av. 43 Av. 7.9

FATAL CASES.

Case No.	Age at onset. Syphilis.	Diabetes.	Duration of diabetes, years.	Cause of death.
I	..	42	10.6	Pneumonia
II	25	54	19.0	Coma
III	39	54	14.0	Cardiac
V	36	42	....	Cannot trace
VII	38	41	1.6	Coma
VIII	38	47	6.8	
X	..	51	7.5	Coma
XI	..	38	1.1	Coma
XIII	..	39	1.0	Coma
XV	..	54	7.8	Coma
XXXIII	57	55	7.7	Coma
XLVIII	26	28	6.7	Tuberculosis
L	54	53	1.8	
LV	59	48	11.8	

Average 41 Average 46 Average 7.4

39

corpuscles numbered 2,210,000, hemoglobin 50 per cent, Wassermann was four plus in two laboratories. The roentgen-ray showed a typical syphilitic stomach. The patient was treated with neo-arsphenamine 5.85 grams in 10 doses, later 6.3 grams in 7 doses and in addition iodide of mercury. The Wassermann being positive in

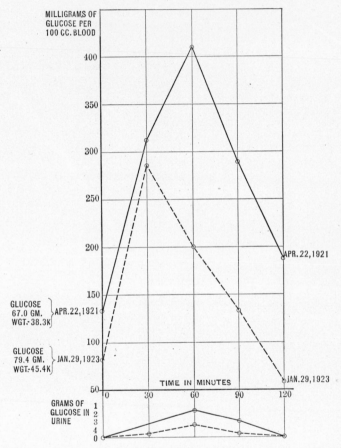

Fig. 30.—Glucose tolerance tests in a diabetic, before and after anti-luetic treatment. (Paullin and Bowcock.)

1923, she is again having arsphenamine. The roentgen-ray shows improvement of the stomach and menstrual periods have returned. The sugar in the urine amounted to 1.1 per cent March, 1921, and in March, 1923, she became sugar-free with unrestricted diet. The two blood-sugar curves in April, 1921, and January, 1923, after glucose tolerance tests are to be seen in Fig. 30 and indicate the improvement.   Dr. Bowcock adds, "We do not feel that this is an absolutely typical case of diabetes, or a typical case of pancreatic insufficiency." I expect that a more complete report of this remarkable case will appear elsewhere in the literature later.

Rosenbloom[1] has reviewed the literature upon the relation between syphilis and diabetes.   The possibilities of syphilis as an etiological factor are numerous.   The process might produce actual leutic lesions in the brain or spinal cord, and particularly of the medulla or secondarily through arterial disease.   Similarly the pancreas might be affected directly or through disease of the bloodvessels. In 139 of his own cases of diabetes he found 16 with a positive Wassermann but only 8 of these showed signs of arteriosclerosis. These 8 cases were intensively treated without increase in their tolerance for carbohydrate.

The occurrence of glycosuria in the course of tabes or general paralysis does not necessarily signify diabetes.   Urechia and Joseph[2] record that Siegmond found glycosuria in 27 cases out of 100 of general paralysis and Bond in 3 out of 62 such cases.   They also quote Nonne as reporting a case of cerebral syphilis in which the glycosuria disappeared with antisyphilitic medication, but without any antidiabetic regime.   In their own series glycosuria appeared in a proportion of 5 to 7 per 100 with disease of the brain and spinal cord.

K. SURGERY AND DIABETES.

Diabetic patients stand in need of the surgeon far more than the same number of non-diabetics or those suffering from most other chronic diseases.   As there are a million diabetics more or less in the country, the surgery of the diabetic becomes an everyday problem.   The frequent occurrence of gangrene and carbuncles is the chief reason for diabetic surgery.   The hospital diabetic is apt to be a surgical diabetic.   Fourteen per cent of 386 diabetics consecutively treated at the Massachusetts General Hospital required surgical intervention, according to Fitz,[3] and of the writer's 903 cases treated in hospitals between April 1, 1919, and December 31, 1922, at least 11 per cent required surgical aid.   In the past the mortality following surgical interference, whether for the relief of diabetic complications already alluded to or for surgery in general, was relatively high, so that the rule has been universal to avoid surgery whenever possible in the presence of diabetes.   But even without insulin the mortality following surgical

[1] Rosenbloom: Am. Jour. Syphilis., 1921, **5**, 634.
[2] Urechia and Joseph: Ann. de méd., 1921, **9**, 94.
[3] Fitz: Am. Jour. Surg., 1922, **36**, 46.

operations upon diabetics has decreased in the last few years, and now with insulin any condition in a diabetic which is remediable by surgery and at the same time lowers a diabetic's tolerance for carbohydrate should receive the benefit of prompt surgical intervention. In pre-insulin days I had almost reached this same conclusion, because so many diverse operations upon my patients had resulted favorably. The abdomen had been safely explored and gall stones or an appendix removed, resection of a portion of the stomach, intestine, or bladder, hysterectomies for cancer or fibroids carried out, and hernias of all varieties closed. Operations had also been successfully accomplished upon cancers of the breast and a tumor of the lip, upon the mastoid, tonsils, and teeth, and the lung had been incised and drained for an abscess. The operations for gangrene of the feet exceeded all others and those upon carbuncle were frequent. My optimism regarding diabetic surgery perhaps grew so steadily from the fact that my private patients were on the whole better risks than those diabetic patients entering large general hospitals, second because a few surgeons rather than a multitude of surgeons operated upon them, and third because the cases were all grouped together under the care of most highly trained diabetic nurses.

Before undertaking an operation upon a diabetic patient, the surgeon should thoroughly appreciate the dangers with which the patient has to contend and the elements which favor surgical success. The diabetic in the past has been a poor surgical risk, (1) because he was usually old and old tissues heal slowly, (2) because of the disease, which possibly made him liable to infections, or at least was made worse by infections, and (3) because of the frequent development of coma after the operation.

Age and slow healing often unite in prolonging convalescence, and unless one is ever alert the frail old man slips away from exhaustion. For such a result the physician more frequently than the surgeon is responsible. The age of the diabetic is largely accountable for the poor reputation he has acquired at the surgeon's hands. (See Table 217.) Gangrene, carbuncles, and gall stones—the common diabetic surgical ailments—are conditions which attack the elderly. Sixty-three per cent of the surgical cases in my series were above the age of fifty at the time of operation, and the average age of the gangrene cases was sixty-one years. Operate upon a series of non-diabetics of similar age and for similar conditions and the mortality likewise would be high. With the greater freedom exercised in advising operations upon diabetics today this handicap of age will decrease. It will be particularly reduced by the frequency with which tonsillectomies upon young children will be performed. The prevalence of damaged hearts, arteries, and kidneys among the patients is to be blamed for the serious prognosis equally with the diabetes. Recognition of these handicaps of age should lead to their appropriate preoperative and postoperative treatment and contribute to a better prognosis. Everyone knows the risk run by the old man with a broken hip who is forced into bed. The diabetic with a gangrenous toe runs still more risk, because in addition he needs exercise to help burn up his sugar. Deprive him of it and his disease gets worse. Therefore, teach him a set of movements to perform whenever the clock strikes the hour. Show him how to protect his lungs by long breaths and turning over in bed. In short, keep him busy getting well. A masseur may be of great help to an elderly diabetic, especially if he combines massage with resistant motions, but self massage is cheaper. Too often the pathetically low level to which these poor old men and women have been reduced is quite forgotten, simply because the laboratory reports a positive diacetic acid reaction or a trace of sugar in the urine. Be careful! Don't treat the laboratory test instead of the patient!

TABLE 217.—AGE AT TIME OF OPERATION OF 95 SURGICAL DIABETICS.[1]
APRIL 1, 1919 TO DECEMBER 31, 1922.

Age by decades.	No. of cases.	Per cent of whole.	Age by decades	No. of cases.	Per cent of whole.
0–10	1	1.1	41–50	20	21.0
11–20	0	..	51–60	29	30.5
21–30	6	6.3	61–70	27	28.4
31–40	9	9.5	71–80	3	3.2

The danger of a clean wound in a diabetic becoming infected is slight. Think of the thousands of intravenous punctures practised by medical men upon diabetics without the sign of an infection, the thousands of injections of insulin by unskilled patients, the 13 subcutaneous injections of salt solution given to Case No. 1650, by a nurse at the Corey Hill Hospital in the space of three weeks. Today one does not see and does not expect in a diabetic that susceptibility to infection which the older literature taught us to dread. Just as formerly tuberculosis claimed many diabetics but, with the lessening opportunity to contract it, has become infrequent; for much the same reason sepsis subsequent to an operation upon a diabetic is rare. Given an infection, it is freely granted that the disease becomes worse; prevent the infection and healing is prompt. In so close a relation do both stand to each other that a loss of tolerance for carbohydrate may be recorded on the diabetic chart before the wound discloses a retrograde course. Allen did

---

[1] Tonsillectomies are not included. Of these there have been about 20 and all without event.

not find sepsis a frequent condition in his operations upon animals, and through experimental work he showed that the presence of an excess of sugar in the blood was not deleterious. No work that I recall, however, has been done upon the possibly harmful effect of an excess of β-oxybutyric acid and the other acid bodies in the blood. Such studies are needed. The more one sees of diabetic surgery the less difference is observed between it and the surgery of the non-diabetic.

Coma is the third menace involved in an operation upon a diabetic. Old time surgery courted it (1) by the use of chloroform and ether; (2) by their administration, only too frequently, by untrained hands; (3) by the sudden restriction of carbohydrate prior to the operation with the desire to lower the glycosuria; (4) by the attempt to relieve the patient's hunger thus caused with an excess of protein and fat, wholly unmindful that in so doing acidosis was favored; (5) by large doses of sodium bicarbonate which upset the digestion, making it still more difficult for the postoperative patient to take liquids or food freely, besides possibly releasing latent acid bodies whose excretion would irritate the kidneys. Today, one guards against acidosis long before the operation, removes it if the condition is aseptic, but if the case is infected, operates at once knowing that the elimination of the infection is a far better cure for acidosis and glycosuria than many days of medical treatment.

The factors which favor surgical success in diabetes are first of all an early diagnosis and an early decision to operate. If surgical delays are dangerous under ordinary circumstances, in diabetes they are disastrous. The physician who presents the facts to his patient so clearly that he will recognize the necessity of being operated upon at once is lowering surgical mortality just as much as the surgeon who operates gently, rapidly and deftly. When consulted about the admission to my service of a diabetic whom I suspect requires immediate surgical intervention, I do not hesitate to set a time limit before which he must arrive. I consider this only a fair return to my surgical colleagues who are so prompt in asking me to see their surgical cases and in responding to my requests for advice or operation. The principle must be recognized that the surgical necessity determines the day (or night) and hour of operation. Too often valuable time has been lost by the surgeon waiting for the doctor. To the surgical condition the medical treatment must conform. Hitherto this has not been possible, because the physician did not know how to adjust the medical treatment to fit the surgical emergency. Today medical treatment is far more labile and can be adapted to the condition in hand, and the convalescence from the surgical complication utilized to free the patient from sugar and acidosis. The realization of this changed attitude toward the surgical diabetic leads to an appreciation of the advance which has taken place in the medical treatment of diabetes. The patient should be treated for the operation rather than for the diabetes. Get him successfully through the operation first, and then if you like, treat him for the diabetes the rest of his life. If you treat him first for the diabetes and second for the operation, the duration of that case of diabetes is apt to be brief.

The seriousness of operating under unfavorable diabetic conditions must not be overlooked, but they need not defer operation. I am aware that Foster[1] takes a somewhat different view. He writes that "Patients with hyperglycemia of more than 0.35 per cent, or a carbon dioxide combining power of the blood plasma of less than 40 volumes per cent cannot be expected to survive any operative procedure. Patients with hyperglycemia above this amount and without acidosis often die of postoperative infection. Patients without hyperglycemia but with more than this amount of acidosis are inclined to pass into coma." In order to confirm or disprove these categorical statements my records have been searched. Instead of finding a good many cases with a blood-sugar percentage of 0.35 per cent or over and severe acidosis as I anticipated, the search revealed only 5 patients who were operated upon whose blood sugar was as high; of these 4 survived. The postoperative blood sugar was above 0.35 per cent in 9 cases, and in this group there were 3 deaths. There were 77 cases in my series whose acidosis was recorded and of these it was absent in 64. Foster's statement need not necessarily postpone an operation, but it is a challenge which demands our best efforts.

The *second factor* which favors success in diabetic surgery is the *adjustment of the diet to the surgical requirements*. If there is no need for haste, any of the well-recognized systems recommended to get the patient free from sugar and acidosis will suffice. One physician may adopt Allen's method, another that of Newburgh and Marsh, another that of Woodyatt, and others my Test and Maintenance Diets. The point is to adopt a plan and then cling to it. All of these diets agree in slightly under- rather than in slightly overnourishing the patient. Such methods conduce to the patient being brought to the operating table with his highest tolerance for carbohydrate, and this means his greatest safeguard against acidosis. It is a great advantage to store carbohydrate in the body and particularly to fill the liver with glycogen before an operation. Throat specialists have known this empirically for

[1] Foster: Annals of Surg., 1920, **71**, 382.

a long time.   They avoid acidosis in the treatment of children by prescribing liberal quantities of carbohydrate the evening before they operate.   If the liver is stored with glycogen, or even partially stored, less harm results from the anesthetic and the almost inevitable postoperative curtailment of nourishment.   Not only is the liver protected thereby, but carbohydrate is available to aid in the combustion of fat after the operation which is just the time when the patient needs it most.   Therefore, feed the patient up to the last hour possible before the operation begins, and never fast a patient before a surgical operation.   He will most likely fast altogether too much afterward.   As a corollary to the above advice begin the administration of food as soon as possible after operating.   Our observations upon basal metabolism tell us the effect of a liberal meal is gone in fourteen hours.   Therefore, especially with diabetics whose carbohydrate stores are invariably low, one should begin the introduction of more carbohydrate before these fourteen hours have elapsed.

The forcible introduction of *liquids* into the patient after a surgical operation is a familiar sight in any hospital; it is wiser to anticipate the patient's need by liberally supplying him with liquids beforehand.   The genito-urinary surgeons do this as a routine, but it is not so common to see this practice followed before other operations.   For the diabetic, during the day prior to the operation, the freest possible administration of liquids should be favored. These should include broths on account of the salts therein contained, coffee, tea, water, and if necessary, salt solution or tap water by rectum.   If there is doubt about administering liquids and food soon after an operation, it is a safe, routine procedure to inject salt solution subcutaneously before the patient leaves the operating table and recovers from the anesthetic.   Especially is this desirable if ether is used, because ether diminishes the excretion of urine, nitrogen, and glucose, and what is still more important diminishes the excretion of acetone bodies.   There are few diabetics who do not need an intravenous or subcutaneous injection of salt solution at the time of an operation, and seldom one who is safe without salt solution by rectum.   If you want water to remain in the body, give isotonic solution, such as Ringer's solution or salt solution: if you want it for excretion, give as tap water.[1]

Of what shall the *diet for surgical diabetic patients before and after operation* consist?   If the case is one which is to be prepared leisurely for operation, no special change need be made in the regular program to free the urine from sugar and acid, save that the food should be prepared in simpler form.   The skill of those in the diet

---

[1] Starkenstein: Arch. f. Exp. Path. u. Pharm., 1922, **92**, 339.

kitchen should be utilized to serve the coarser vegetables as purées. Coarse diabetic substitute foods such as bran biscuits and agar-agar jellies should be omitted. If the situation is acute, and but a day or a few hours are available, sudden restriction of carbo-hydrate, particularly when dealing with severe diabetes or elderly patients, must be avoided, and great care taken not to upset the stomach. The simplest foods are, therefore, the best. Oatmeal gruel made with water is excellent, or, if this is not desired, orange juice with whites of eggs is a good alternative, and it will be difficult for the patient to take too much of either. These are first-rate preparations to employ as a routine in the few hours preceding and following any operation, just as they are in the treatment of coma. When more food can be borne, in substitution for the routine diabetic diet of 5 per cent vegetables, one can introduce gradually in sequence a few ounces of milk, an occasional Uneeda biscuit (5 grams carbohydrate) eggs, chicken, soft sieved vegetables, grapefruit. Eventually the patient returns to his former diet or very likely to a more liberal diet utilizing the Maintenance Diets for this purpose. (See Table 493.) If the food is not forced during convalescence, and indeed it is one of the advantages of convalescence that it cannot be forced, and if calories are kept at 15 to 20 per kilogram body weight, most any middle-aged adult diabetic will become sugar-free before he recovers from his surgical lesion. In fact, I look upon the surgeon as one of the greatest helps in medical treatment, and a surgical operation is ofttimes a blessing rather than a curse. Case No. 177 never once became sugar-free in the fourteen years I treated him until R. C. Cochrane kept him out of mischief by cutting off his leg. (Table 218.) The course of this patient was like that of many others in that the sugar in the urine became steadily less. There was, however, a temporary increase of glycosuria, though without acidosis, after the operation, but this fleeting increase was expected and likewise disregarded. A transient increase of sugar in the urine after an operation is a regular occurrence. It is important to remember this or the patient will be restricted in his diet needlessly. Within a few days the sugar usually disappears of itself. Aside from his gangrene, this patient had gall stones, angina pectoris, retinal hemorrhages, and had used morphine for years. The removal of a gangrenous leg is a boon to the patient apart from its effect upon the diabetes. The renal function test of Case No. 2173 rose from 12 per cent to 60 per cent during the seven months after the operation.

The *diet after operation* should certainly contain the minimum of $\frac{2}{3}$ of a gram of protein per kilogram body weight and more often a full gram of protein per kilogram body weight. Were it not for the possibility of glycosuria appearing with more protein, it might be advantageous to increase the amount, because of Clark's[1] experiments upon wound healing in dogs. He showed that with protein-fed dogs the length of the quiescent period was zero, but might reach six days in the fat-fed animals. Consequently, protein feeding shortened the date of final healing by five days.

TABLE 218.—UTILIZATION OF PERIOD OF CONVALESCENCE TO TREAT THE DIABETES.

(Case No. 177. Onset of diabetes at forty-four years. Operation for gangrene at sixty-six years, by R. C. Cochrane.)

Date.	Vol. cc.	Di-acetic acid.	Sugar in urine			Diet in grams			Blood sugar, per cent.
			Reduction, per cent.	Total grams.	Carbohydrate.	Protein.	Fat.	Calories.	
June, 1922									
4	Ssp.	sl. +	1.9						
4– 5	500	0	3.8	19	63	25	0	352	
5– 6	1200	0	1.6	19	102	58	0	640	0.23
6– 7	..	0	2.2	..	51	30	14	450	
	Am	putation.		Spinal	anesthesia.				
7– 8	1800+	0	4.0	72	57	38	30	650	
8– 9	2125+	0	1.8	38	42	36	29	573	
9–10	2800+	0	0.3	8	42	36	19	483	
10–11	2800	0	0.1	3	42	36	29	573	
11–12	3250	0	0	0	42	42	35	651	
12–13	2500	0	0.1	3	53	45	42	770	
13–14	2050	0	0.2	4	44	44	47	775	
14–15	1900	0	tr.	..	44	46	52	828	
15–16	2600	0	tr.	..	44	46	60	900	0.20
16–17	1800	0	0	0	44	46	69	981	
17–18	1260	0	tr.	0	44	46	78	1062	
18–19	1200	0	0.1	1	44	48	82	1106	
19–20	1750	0	0	0	44	52	92	1208	
23–24	2150	0	0	..		52	53	90	1230	0.16
July									
30– 1	1425	0	0	0	65	56	97	1357	0.17
3– 4	2200	0	0	0	65	56	97	1357	
4– 5	1200	..	..	..	65	56	97	1357	0.15
Sept., 1923									
6			Living	happily.					

When dealing with infections, a rigorous attempt should not be made to get the patient sugar-free either before or after operation. That is seldom possible and, even if attained, is secured at too great a loss of body tissue. Spencer[2] as long ago as 1892, urged that it was useless to attempt the reduction of the sugar by drugs

[1] Clark: Johns Hopkins Hosp. Bull., 1919, **30**, 117.
[2] Spencer: British Med. Jour., 1892, p. 1305.

and diet when a severe inflammatory lesion was present. It is better treatment to remove or give vent to the infection and then the tolerance for carbohydrate will improve. It is painful to look over the protocols of cases suffering from infections, in years gone by, who were terribly undernourished with the purpose to make them sugar-free. (See Case No. 513, p. 632.)

No method of treatment save with insulin could be expected to yield satisfactory results under such conditions. Even 80 units of insulin failed to free the urine of sugar in a diabetic suffering with a carbuncle in September, 1923.

If *acidosis* exists either *before or after operation* a vigorous attack upon it already has been made by the inauguration of a restricted diet containing a small amount of carbohydrate. If the acidosis is extreme, it is well to employ certain standard measures which apply to all diabetics in any danger whatsoever of coma. They have been summarized upon p. 553.

Insulin, a third factor promoting success, has been little mentioned thus far in the treatment of surgical diabetes because all the measures hitherto advocated should be adopted irrespective of the use of insulin. Insulin is an added safeguard, an insurance for the diabetic, which allows operations to be performed with less hazard to the patient and with far less trepidation for the surgical and medical attendants, but it does not displace any part of the treatment advised. Experience with insulin will allow it to be used most advantageously, but if one is not versed in the care of diabetic cases or of insulin, it must be employed with caution. It is seldom that a novice should give as much as 5 units every four hours or even 10 units before each of the three meals, and this should be done only when the urine collected before each dose contains sugar. Even under these circumstances it would be desirable to be assured that the patient was taking 1 gram of carbohydrate for each unit of insulin injected. Those acquainted with insulin can employ it with more freedom both to clear up an existing glycosuria and acidosis, and to counteract the hyperglycemia of ether. For the latter purpose I have utilized insulin successfully when the tonsils were removed from 2 children by D. Crosby Greene. The operations lasted, it is true, but a few minutes, and therefore, are hardly a test of insulin, but I should have dreaded ether without it. Both patients received slightly more than their regular quantity of carbohydrate on the day before the operation, received insulin and were fed within three hours of anesthetization. Despite these precautions 1 of these cases, Alice S., Case No. 2802, described on p. 56, showed increased glycosuria and acidosis the afternoon of the operation, but her subsequent convalescence was uneventful. In the earlier pages of this book the use of insulin is described at length.

The *anesthetic* including its method of application is the fourth agent which contributes to the fortunate outcome of a surgical operation upon a diabetic. Every effort should be made to shorten the period of anesthesia, irrespective of the type of anesthetic. If a preliminary injection of morphine is given, this should be small or else the respiration may be depressed too much. Avoid apprehension and excitement on the part of the patient. It is just as valuable to have an anesthetist, accustomed to diabetics, as it is in thyroid operations to have one accustomed to their peculiarities. Details count and in diabetic surgery there is need to be meticulous.

1. **Anesthesia.**—(*a*) **Chloroform.**—All agree that chloroform is harmful to the patient in diabetic surgery. Its use is accompanied by hyperglycemia. (Blum.) Either directly or indirectly through its interference with the metabolism of carbohydrate it must alter the fat metabolism, because after chloroform, acidosis resulting in coma is said to be common. Blum[1] points out that β-oxybutyric acid injected under the skin of a dog is burned without the formation of diacetic acid and acetone, but if the same experiment is repeated upon the same animal under chloroform narcosis, one will find a very definite acetonuria. This does not take place with ether narcosis. Chloroform is employed so rarely in this locality that I have had almost no experience with it. With little Buddy H., Case No. 2084, four years of age, 37 drops worked admirably when several abscesses were incised and for such short operative procedures I am surprised it is not employed more. The effect of anesthetics in the presence of diabetes deserves continued investigation. Unsatisfactory dietetic preparation of the patient in the past may have been as harmful as the anesthetic.

(*b*) **Ether.**—Ether administered to phloridzinized dogs leads immediately to hyperglycemia, according to Sansum and Woodyatt, and they explain this as due to the transformation of liver glycogen to sugar under the stimulus of asphyxia. During etherization the formation of glycogen is said to cease. Bloor has shown that ether given to normal dogs results in a marked rise in the concentration of the blood-fat, and this has been explained on the basis of an increased solubility in the blood-ether mixture of fatty substances in the tissues. Perhaps interference with the carbohydrate metabolism might be as important a factor. As with dogs, ether given to normal individuals gives rise to hyperglycemia and acidosis and, what is most serious to the diabetic, temporarily diminishes the excretion of urine, nitrogen, glucose, and acetone bodies. Katsch and von Friedrich[2] found that ether was a stimulus to the external

[1] Blum: Paris Méd., 1919, **9**, 341.
[2] Katsch and von Friedrich: Klin. Wchnschr., 1922, **1**, 112.

secretion of the pancreas. Might not the internal secretion be lowered in consequence?

The harmful effects of ether upon the metabolism of the diabetic are by no means confined to the observations reported above. The nausea which so frequently ensues after the administration of ether is of even greater importance, because it interferes for many hours with the intake of food and even of liquids. Furthermore, preceding ether the patient goes longer without food than preceding gas-oxygen, spinal anesthesia or novocaine, and when this period of fasting is combined with the longer fasting interval after the anesthetic, the period without food becomes considerable. It is quite probable that this period of fasting is more detrimental to the diabetic than the drug itself. Particularly in the presence of acidosis is a period of abstinence from carbohydrate and liquid to be deplored and when ether is employed, this period is greatest.

The explanation why the Mayo Brothers have been so fortunate in the use of ether with their diabetic patients is readily seen when one compares the quantity of ether given at Rochester and the duration of the anesthesia per patient. This has been tabulated by Fitz in a recent article for two series, each of 100 abdominal operations, the first in the Mayo Clinic and the second in a control group. The data are shown in Table 219. Not only was 36 per cent less ether given at the Mayo Clinic, but the period of anesthesia was 53 per cent shorter.

TABLE 219.—ETHER IN 100 ABDOMINAL OPERATIONS.[1]

Averages per patient.	Mayo Clinic.	Control group.
Body weight	64.5 kg.	61.3 kg.
Ether, quantity	170 cc	267 cc
Duration of anesthesia	48 minutes	102 minutes

Yet a case illy adapted for ether may do well. Case No. 2311, a man, aged fifty-eight years, had marked osteoarthritis and an attempt at spinal anesthesia failed; subsequently gas-oxygen proved to be inefficient. Ether was at length employed and, despite poor kidneys, a phenolsulphonephthalein excretion 19 per cent, with renal fixation between 1006 and 1010, and marked diabetes, a successful result was obtained. Ether has many times been used with success, but it is often dangerous. The statement will bear repetition that ether anesthesia is a burden which a light case of diabetes may easily bear, which may change a moderate to a severe case, and to a severe case prove fatal.

(c) **Gas-oxygen.—Nitrous Oxide.**—Both of these methods of anesthesia have worked excellently with various patients. Gas-oxygen anesthesia has repeatedly been employed in long operations.

---

[1] Fitz, R.: Am. Jour. Surg., 1922, **36**, 46.

Occasionally the gas-oxygen has been supplemented by a few cubic centimeters of ether, but there has been an effort in the last six years not to use ether at all. On two occasions gas-oxygen was ineffective. In the first instance this was probably due to the previous administration of morphine to an old man, Case No. 855, which markedly depressed the respiration, so that it was so superficial he was etherized with difficulty. Recourse was then taken to ether, but he survived only a few days after the operation for purulent appendicitis. In the other instance it was resorted to when spinal anesthesia was impossible on account of marked hypertrophic osteoarthritis. The outcome with this patient, Case No. 2311, was more favorable and has been related in the preceding paragraph.

With a diabetic operated upon for empyema and studied by Fitz gas-oxygen anesthesia was apparently accompanied by hyperglycemia and increased excretion of acetone bodies, but without signs of acidosis in the blood. Fitz suggests that it is possible that the carbohydrate diet on the day of operation was a factor in the case and that the administration of oxygen made it easier for the body to burn acetone bodies and that thus acidosis was actually prevented.

Illustrations of the harmful effects of ether and the comparatively harmless effect of gas-oxygen in a second operation on the same patient can be seen in Table 221, p. 623.

Case No. 348, male; age at onset of diabetes forty-two years; operation for removal of the prostate at forty-nine years of age, seven years later, in 1915, when light etherization was employed. A positive carbohydrate balance of 20 grams before the operation changed to a negative carbohydrate balance of 33 grams after the operation, and the acidosis became extreme. The patient fortunately made an uninterrupted recovery and continues well and active in 1923. (See Table 220.)

TABLE 220.—CASE NO. 348. MODERATELY SEVERE DIABETES. REMOVAL OF PROSTATE IN 1915. ETHER WITH SUBSEQUENT ACIDOSIS.

	Urine.				Diet.			
Date.	Diacetic acid.	NH₃, gms.	Total sugar, gms.	Carbo-hydrate, gms.	Pro-tein, gms.	Fat, gms.	Carbo-hydrate balance, gms.	Sodium bicar-bonate, gms.
1910								
July 21	0	..	160					
1915								
July 9	0	..	0	45	..	..	+45	
11–12	0	..	0	20	30	50	+20	0
July 11, operation—removal of prostate; Dr. A. L. Chute; anesthetic, ether.								
July 12–13	+ +	..	37	0	0	0	−37	0
13–14	+ +	..	33	0	0	0	−33	0
14–15	+ + +	3.3	41	0	0	0	−41	0
15–16	+ + +	3.2	36	5	0	0	−31	8
Aug. 1– 2	0	..	0					
1923								
Jan. 27	0	..	0	70	84	144	+70	0

Case No. 697, male; age at onset of diabetes forty-nine years; age at operation for gall stones, fifty-five years; anesthetic, ether. The tolerance on the day before the operation was approximately 105 grams; on the day of the operation the quantity of sugar in the urine was 35 grams, and carbohydrate in the diet 8 grams, and a minus balance continued for three days more. The patient completely recovered and remained well and active until the end of 1916, when he had a recurrence of symptoms. A gall stone was then removed from the common duct by D. F. Jones. Anesthetic, gas and oxygen and 45 cc ether administered by Freeman Allen. Acidosis was negligible and the positive carbohydrate balance maintained. This patient is now enjoying the beneficial effects of insulin.

TABLE 221.—CHART CASE NO. 697. MILD DIABETES. GALL STONES.

Date.	Diacetic acid.		Urine, total sugar, gms.	Carbo-hydrate in diet, gms.	Carbo-hydrate balance, gms.	Sodium bicar-bonate, gms.
1914						
Feb. 2 .	0	..	(0.8%)			
17–18 .	0	..	0	105	+105	8
18–19 .	+	..	35	8	− 27	12

February 18, operation for gall stones; Dr. D. F. Jones; **anesthetic ether.**

Feb. 19–20 .	+++	..	105	60	− 45	18
20–21 .	+++	..	110	34	− 75	6
21–22 .	++	..	104	85	− 20	8
22–23 .	Sl. +	..	71	110	+ 40	0
23–24 .	0	..	55	175	+120	0
24–25 .	0	..	19	110	+ 90	0
25–26 .	0	..	6	120	+115	0
26–27 .	0	..	11	120	+110	0
27–28 .	0	..	0	120	+120	0
Mar. 5–6 .	0	..	0	95	+ 95	0

Return with symptoms of obstruction of common duct.

1917						
Mar. 15–16 .	0		4	35	+ 31	0
16–17 .	Sl. +		1	50	+ 49	0

Mar. 17, operation for removal of gall stone from common duct; Dr. D. F. Jones; **anesthetic, gas and oxygen,** with 45 cc ether.

Mar. 17–18 .	+		15	20	+ 5	0
18–19 .	0		43	41	− 2	0
19–20 .	0		25	41	+ 16	0
25–26 .	0		0	74	+ 74	0

1923
July 1. Taking insulin "the last three days, I have felt more like my own self than for the last *fifteen* years." Dr. Banting and Mr. Best ,please note this quotation.

An abscess in the upper lobe of the right lung was successfully drained by C. L. Scudder. The patient, Case No. 1239, first presented symptoms of diabetes in September, 1916, at the age of forty-six years, and three months later the disease was diagnosed. During January, 1917, pulmonary symptoms developed and in

February, when he first came under my observation, after consultation with his physician and F. T. Lord, it was decided to treat the diabetes actively and the abscess of the lung expectantly for three weeks, and then operate if the pulmonary condition did not improve. From Table 222 it will be seen that the acidosis (diacetic acid and ammonia) was severe, though this was not revealed by the CO_2 tension of the alveolar air or by the blood, possibly on account

TABLE 222.—CASE 1239.[1] ABSCESS OF LUNG. OPERATION WITHOUT INSULIN IN 1917.

Date, 1917.	Diacetic acid.	Ammonia, total gms.	Total sugar in urine,	Diet in grams.				Blood CO_2, mm. Hg.	Blood sugar, per cent.	Alveolar air CO_2, mm. Hg.
				Carbohydrate.	Protein.	Fat.	Alcohol.			
Feb. 17 Spec.	+++									
Feb. 17–18	+++	..	24	..	..	..	..	..	..	37
18–19	+++	..	31	45	8	0	0	..	0.17	
19–20	++	..	19	25	5	0	0			
20–21	++++	2.4	4	10	5	0	0			
21–22	++++	2.7	0	0	0	0	0	47.7	0.14	{ 43 40
22–23	+++	2.8	2	10	5	0	0			
23–24	+++	2.6	2	0	24	0	0	..	..	37
24–25	++	..	3	0	60	0	15			
25–26	+++	2.1	8	0	92	12	30	..	..	38
26–27	++	1.9	7	0	68	24	15			
27–28	++	..	6	5	72	41	30			
28– 1	++	1.7	0	10	76	42	30			
Mar. 1– 2	++	1.4	2	15	79	61	30			
2– 3	+++	..	0	10	79	69	30			
3– 4	++	..	0	10	79	81	30	54.9	0.14	
4– 5	++	1.3	0	10	81	82	30			
5– 6	++	1.3	0	10	81	88	30			
6– 7	+++	..	1	15	84	88	30			
7– 8	++	1.2	3	20	84	82	30	..	..	36
8– 9	+	1.0	0	15	56	21	30			
9–10	+	..	0	19	51	1	30			
10–11	sl. +	..	0	24	77	46	30			
11–12	+	1.0	0	19	66	43	30			
12–13	+	..	3	24	82	61	30			
13–14	++	1.4	4	20	76	60	30	47.7	0.18	
14–15	+++	1.5	4	25	47	39	30	..	..	35
15–16	+++	1.6	8	37	46	12	30			
16–17	v. sl. +	1.1	7	49	68	13	30	..	..	33
17–18	+	0.7	20	75	33	12	0	..	..	33
	Operation: Dr.		C. L.	Scudder.	Ane	sthetic:	Gas,	and oxy	gen.	
18–19	+	1.0	23	50	58	26	30	..	..	{ 33 37
19–20	+	1.5	25	44	58	49	30			
20–21	+	1.5	9	34	56	49	21			
21–22	+	1.3	7	34	56	59	30			
22–23	+	..	6	34	63	75	30			
23–24	+	1.1	3	34	56	69	30			
24–25	+	..	2	34	63	85	30			
25–26	0	..	6	39	63	85	30			
26–27	+	1.0	2	29	63	85	30			
27–28	+	..	2	29	66	93	30			
28–29	+	0.8	2	29	66	93	30			
29–30	+	..	2	31	68	90	30			
30–31	+	..	0	37	69	88	30			
April 2– 3	0	..	0	40	74	93				
May			Sinus	healed.						

Weight at entrance, 133 pounds; weight March 16, 132 pounds; no alkalis given.

[1] This is about the last of my cases to receive alcohol. He renounced diet, despite his gain in tolerance and well-being, and died February 5, 1920. American diabetic patients do better without than with alcohol.

of the pulmonary complication. The acidosis was gradually, but not entirely, overcome. When it was seen that improvement of the condition of the lung did not take place, the patient was operated upon by Dr. C. L. Scudder under gas-oxygen anesthesia. A large abscess of the right upper lobe was evacuated after removal of portions of the fourth, fifth and sixth ribs. The cavity was large, receiving into its interior one large gauze sponge. Prior to the operation fat was decreased in the diet and the carbohydrate increased. The highest tolerance for carbohydrate reached in the three weeks prior to the operation was 19 grams, but it later rose to over 85 grams and the wound closed. Today such an operation and such a result would not appear as remarkable. The case is reported as an illustration of what could be done without insulin in 1917.

(*d*) **Spinal Anesthesia.**—In operations for amputation of gangrenous legs and for the removal of the prostate this method of anesthesia has been by far the most satisfactory at the New England Deaconess and Corey Hill Hospitals. No unfavorable incident has occurred in my experience as a result of its employment. It is true that for several years the anesthetists have been physicians who have specialized in anesthetics for many years, but recently L. S. McKittrick has given his own anesthetic, operated with the assistance of nurses only, sewed up the stump "tight" without drainage and secured excellent results. The case of Fitz[1] which developed acidosis following spinal anesthesia is probably to be explained, as he implies, by deficiency in carbohydrate, for he says that the acidosis went as quickly as it came when carbohydrate was added to the diet. I have heard of a case who developed a psychosis by being conscious throughout an amputation for gangrene, and it must be acknowledged that the mental shock of experiencing an operation cannot be disregarded. Fortunately, nothing of this sort has occurred with my patients. Paravertebral anesthesia has not been used with my patients.

(*e*) **Novocaine. Cocaine.** — Local anesthesia frequently works admirably, and often shortens the period of employment of one of the group of anesthetics previously discussed. Caution is always necessary to avoid trauma of the part.

The avoidance of trauma is a fourth element in promoting surgical success. There are various kinds of trauma, not alone the trauma due to bungling surgery, the trauma due to unnecessary tourniquets, but trauma due to the employment of strong antiseptic solutions. Indeed, antisepsis often means trauma. One shudders at the free use of 1 to 1000 corrosive sublimate and of hydrogen peroxide.

---

[1] Fitz, R.: Loc. cit., p. 611,

Undoubtedly asepsis instead of antisepsis has contributed a great deal to the success of modern diabetic surgery. How delicately wounds are treated now, compared even with the period just prior to the war.

A summary of the operations and anesthetics employed in my cases is given in Table 224.

2. **Results of Diabetic Surgery.**—It is extremely difficult to evaluate or predict results in diabetic surgery. There are so many variables. The surgeon, the physician, the anesthetic, the anesthetist, the patients with their manifold varieties of diabetes, must all be considered even before the surgical lesion. Gross conclusions alone can be reached.

TABLE 223.—SURGICAL OPERATIONS UPON DIABETIC PATIENTS **Before** 1917.

Operation.	Total cases.	Anesthetic.	Successful cases.	Fatal cases.
Gall-stones	4	Ether	697	
		Gas and oxygen, with 45 c.c. ether . . .	697[1]	
		Ether		273[2]
		Ether		639[3]
Appendicitis	3	Ether	29	
		Ether	348	
		Ether		855[4]
Cancer of uterus	1	Ether	799	
Cancer of breast	1	Gas and oxygen and ether	1088	
Cancer of bladder	1	Ether	498	
Cancer of bladder	1	Ether	576	
Cancer of bladder	1	Ether		939[5]
Prostate	5	Ether	348	
		Spinal anesthesia . .	559	
		Gas and oxygen . .	599	
		Spinal anesthesia . .	833	
		Spinal anesthesia . .	1086	
Drainage of bladder	1	Novocain	1042	
Fibroid	3	Ether	120	
		Ether	127	
		Nitrous oxide . . .		721[6]
Extensive perineal repairs	3	Ether	60	
		Nitrous oxide, oxygen and ether sequence .	173	
		Ether	368	
Exploratory laparotomy	1	Ether	333	
Abscess of lung	1	Gas and oxygen . .	1239	
Mastoid	1	Ether	503	

The data regarding my cases, excepting operations for gangrene and carbuncle, up to January 1, 1917 are grouped in Table 223. Here are 27 cases with 5 deaths, a mortality of 18 per cent. Of

[1] Two years after first operation, stone removed from common duct.
[2] Complicated with pernicious anemia.
[3] Gall stones, coma. Today an avoidable death.
[4] Seen only once, four days after operation.
[5] Died of pulmonary embolism.
[6] Complicated with severe anemia.

these deaths perhaps 2 or 3 could be avoided if a similar operation should take place today. Among the severe cases with abdominal infections, there were 3 deaths, leaving but 2 deaths for the remaining 20 operations or a mortality of 10 per cent. One of these deaths was from pulmonary embolism and the other was complicated by severe anemia. Oddly enough all the fatal cases in this series took ether, but the number of cases is too small to attach great importance to that, especially since most of the successful cases at that period were ether cases too.

In comparison with these *former 27 cases* are *61 operations* upon diabetics of my series *since April 1, 1919*. In this table, Table 224, likewise, operations for gangrene and carbuncle are omitted. The change in mortality is notable. Instead of 18 per cent it has now fallen to 9 per cent. A brief description of the larger groups of cases comprising these tables follows.

Prostatectomy.—Ten cases were operated upon and all recovered. This is all the more noteworthy because an operation for removal of a prostate is a two-stage operation; there is a tedious convalescence and the urine, besides being infected, often contains sugar. Case No. 348 caused considerable apprehension after the operation because of the development of acidosis, undoubtedly due to the use of ether as an anesthetic. (See p. 622.) Case No. 559, with onset of diabetes at seventy-three years, was operated upon at seventy-four years, January 14, 1913. Spinal anesthesia was employed. Case No. 341 was the first prostatic case to take advantage of insulin. He had been under my care for thirteen years and his tolerance had gradually fallen. Glycosuria persisted after operation with carbohydrate, 80 grams; protein, 43 grams and fat, 87 grams, despite 15 units insulin daily, explained by the slight infection which accompanies such an operation, rather than by the 80 grams of carbohydrate. Eventually he became sugar-free with 23 units daily; thirty-seven days after operation remained so with 5 units and a month later with none. Case No. 2765 counts as a successful case so far as hospital records go, but he actually died a few days later. Contrary to entreaty and against advice he left the hospital twelve days after operation. It was learned later that the catheter which he still wore in his bladder became clogged, urinary retention resulted and his death occurred from uremia. Until discharge his recovery had been uninterrupted. None of these cases have shown the remarkable increase in tolerance for carbohydrate following the operation which has sometimes been observed by others, if we exclude Case No. 341 who received insulin. In his instance the regaining of tolerance may be ascribed to the persistent and consistent treatment following operation and it may be that the noted gains in tolerance observed by others can be attributed to the same cause.

TABLE 224.—SURGICAL CASES OF DIABETES Since APRIL 1, 1919.

Case No.	Date of Onset of diabetes.	Date of Operation.	Nature of Operation.	Anesthetic.	Age at operation.	Immediate result.	Present condition.
			Abscesses:				
2798	May, 1921	Aug., 1922	Ischiorectal	G.	40	R.	A.
2463	May, 1919	Jan., 1922	Liver	G.O.	32	D.	
2084	June, 1919	1920	Axillary	CHCl₃¹	4	R.	A.
1880	April, 1916	Aug., 1921	Axillary	G.	48	R.	A.
1782	Sept., 1919	May, 1921	Scalp	None	24	R.	A.
1758	June, 1919	Feb., 1920	Axillary	G.	27	R.	D.
1623	July, 1912	Sept., 1919	Ischiorectal	G.O.	46	R.	D.
1521	Jan., 1919	Nov., 1921	Appendix	G.O.	54	R.	A.
1406	Aug., 1916	Aug., 1921	Sublingual	G.	55	R.	A.
436	May, 1909	1921	Thigh	G.	32	R.	A.
2018	Nov., 1920	Jan., 1921	Cæsarean	L.	32	R.	A.
2018	Nov., 1920	Oct., 1922	"	L.	33	R.	A.
			Cancer				
2742	Jan., 1916	July, 1922	Tr. colon	L.	60	D.	
2524	May, 1911	Feb., 1921	Rectum	S.	50	R.	A.
2116	Sept., 1915	Mar., 1921	Liver	G.O.	65	D.	
2070	Jan., 1921	Feb., 1921	Bladder	E.	59	R.	A.
2057	Jan., 1921	Nov., 1921	Bladder	S.	60	R.	D.
2034	1920	Jan., 1921	Pancreas	..	52	R.	D.
1789	Jan., 1916	April, 1920	Stomach	E.	56	R.	A.
1650²	June, 1897	1919	Penis	S.	73	R.	D.
1154	May, 1908	Jan., 1921	Stomach	E.	70	R.	D.
585	Feb., 1909	Mar., 1920 April, 1922	} Cataract	L.	61	R.	A.
1781	Feb., 1919	Mar., 1920	Cataract	L.	55	R.	A.
1631	Jan., 1916	Sept., 1919	Exploratory laparotomy	G.O.	45	R.	A.
2605	Mar., 1922	April, 1922	Gall stones	G.O.	47	R.	A.
2373	Sept., 1921	Sept., 1921	" "	E.	53	R.	A.
1785	Dec., 1919	Mar., 1920	" "	G.O.	59	R.	A.
1592	June, 1917	July, 1919	" "	G.O.E.	28	R.	A.
992	July, 1912	May, 1922	" "	G.O.	52	R.	A.
870	April, 1905	Feb., 1922	" "	G.O.	52	D.	
18	Aug., 1897	Nov., 1919	" "	G.O.	58	R.	D.
1425	Nov., 1916	April, 1920	Hemorrhoids	L.	62	R.	D.
2729	Mar., 1922	June, 1922	Hernia	S.	21	R.	A.
1983	April, 1920	Nov., 1922	" (Umbilical)	L.	47	R.	A.
2174	Mar., 1921	Oct., 1921	Fibroid	G.O.	44	R.	A.
2069	July, 1918	Jan., 1921	"	E.	45	R.	A.
1974	May, 1910	Sept., 1922	"	E.	47	R.	A.
2192	June, 1920	Aug., 1922	Mastoid	G.	29	R.	A.
3072	Feb., 1920	Mar., 1923	Prostate	S.S.	54	R.	A.
2765	1917	Aug., 1922	"	S.	69	R.	D.
2590	May, 1919	April, 1922	"	S.	63	R.	A.
2219	1918	Dec., 1922	"	E.	65	R.	A.
341	May, 1910	May, 1923	"	S.	75	R.	A.
2896	Jan., 1920	Nov., 1922	Thyroid	G.O.	55	R.	A.
2796	Mar., 1922	Oct., 1922	"	G.O.	57	R.	A.
2796	Mar., 1922	Nov., 1922	"	G.O.	57	R.	A.
2722	June, 1922	June, 1922	"	G.O.	46	R.	A.
2676	Apr., 1922	Sept., 1922	"	G.O.	36	R.	A.
2544	Sept., 1921	Feb., 1922	"	G.O.	35	R.	A.
2521	Jan., 1922	Mar., 1922	"	G.O.	26	R.	A.
2473	Sept., 1921	June, 1922	"	G.O.	54	R.	A.
2272	Nov., 1920	Sept., 1921	"	L.	42	R.	A.
2272	Nov., 1920	Oct., 1921	"	L.	42	R.	D.
2142	Aug., 1907	Oct., 1921	"	M.Sc.G.O.	44	R.	A.
2142	Aug., 1907	Dec., 1921	"	Sc.G.O.	44	R.	A.
1868	Oct., 1918	Aug., 1920	"	Sc.M.	48	D.	
1836	Jan., 1919	Sept., 1920	"	L.	42	R.	A.
2373	Sept., 1921	Sept., 1921	Ventral suspension	E.	53	R.	A.
1970	Oct., 1913	Jan., 1922	Excision of cyst in lip	L.	51	R.	A.
1866	Apr., 1914	July, 1921	Opening rt. antrum	L.	38	R.	D.

¹ 2 cc or 30 drops.
² Thirteen subpectoral injections of salt solution given by nurses at Corey Hill Hospital without an abscess.

Abbreviations.—G., gas; G.O., gas oxygen; CHCl₃, chloroform; L., local, novocaine; S., spinal anesthesia; E., ether; M, morphine; Sc., scopolamine.
R., Recovery; D., death; A, alive.

Disease of Thyroid Gland.—Of the 14 operations upon my dia-betics for disease of the thyroid gland by F. H. Lahey, there has been but 1 death. One of these patients, Case No. 2142 has gained 41 pounds, or 56 per cent of her weight prior to operation.

Removal of Uterine Fibroids.—Six cases have been operated upon with 1 death. This occurred in Case No. 721. The age of the patient at onset of the diabetes was forty-five years and at operation forty-nine years. Operation was forced because of repeated hemor-rhages. On entrance to the hospital April 21, 1914 the glycosuria was 3 per cent and diacetic acid was present. The patient became sugar-free on May 7, with a tolerance for 15 grams carbohydrate, but shortly after grew worse and acidosis reappeared. The hemor-rhage left no alternative and operation was performed (anesthetic, nitrous oxide) with a fatal issue forty-eight hours later. Today with transfusion, insulin and an appropriate diet, it is probable that even this patient might be saved.

Glycosuria disappeared for years following the operation upon Case No. 127 for fibroid of the uterus, the only instance of this type in my series. The age at onset of the diabetes was thirty-nine years and at the time of operation, forty-seven years. Following the operation, performed by M. H. Richardson in 1906, there was marked suppuration of so extensive a character that drainage was established through the abdomen, the vagina and rectum. The patient at length recovered and nine years after operation was in good health and I thought the sugar had disappeared permanently, but twelve months later a specimen of this patient's urine contained, 104 grams sugar. On February 27, 1922, the blood sugar was 0.26 per cent and the non-protein nitrogen 40.8 mg. per 100 cc blood. The urine contained a slight trace of albumin and 0.1 per cent sugar, but the patient was wretched with headaches and failing vision due to hemorrhagic retinitis. In August, 1923, she is in the hospital with coronary thrombosis, but her general health is much improved, despite a blood-pressure of 154/90 mm. Hg. She is sugar-free with carbohydrate 79 grams, protein 45 grams, fat 112 grams.

Hysterectomy for fibroids does not always affect the diabetes favorably. Case No. 2174 came through the operation most satisfactorily, but her tolerance for carbohydrate, which was 173 grams before the operation, fell to less than 61 grams of carbohydrate even with the help of 10 units of insulin. Gradually, however, insulin has saved the day and she is now, July, 1923, in good con-dition. Perhaps latent infections (teeth) may have had something to do with the loss of tolerance. At any rate the patient has shown a rheumatoid arthritis.

Cancer was the cause of operation upon 9 patients and there were 2 deaths. There were 7 patients operated upon for gall stones in the recent series with 1 death, due to an aneurysm of the heart. The thyroid was operated upon 14 times with 1 death, and that in 1915, and due more to the physician than the surgeon. Operations were also successfully preformed for cataracts (2); Cæsarean sections (2); exploratory laparotomy (1); hemorrhoids (1); hernia (2); ventral suspension (1); mastoid (1), in addition to other operations not listed, such as those upon the tonsils of which there were a good many. Of rather unusually severe abscesses there were 10 operated upon with 1 death. These data should certainly encourage physicians and surgeons to feel free to operate upon any surgical condition which arises in diabetes.

The Mortality in Diabetes Following Surgical Intervention in Other Hospitals.—At the Massachusetts General Hospital for the five years preceding 1918, Fitz[1] found that of 45 operations performed a fatal issue ensued in 13 instances, or 30 per cent. Analysis of his figures shows that for the 20 patients with infections or gangrene it was 50 per cent, but for the 25 non-infected cases it was but 12 per cent.

For a subsequent five years ending 1922, at the same institution Young[2] reports 99 surgical cases with 16 deaths, which represents a lowering of the mortality by one-half. A few of Young's cases, though surgical in nature, were not operated upon for one reason or another. Several of the deaths could not be attributed to the surgical operation. Among the 99 cases was a group of 10 surgical emergencies, acute abdominal conditions or fractures, with 2 deaths. Various surgical conditions, non-septic, made up another class of 46 cases with but 3 deaths. Gangrene was represented by 29 cases. Three refused operation and were discharged, 3 died and 4 recovered without operation. Of the remaining 19 cases who were operated upon there were 4 who died. Finally, there were 15 cases of sepsis with 4 deaths. The anesthetic employed was gas and oxygen in 28 cases, spinal anesthesia in 15 cases, local anesthesia in 10 cases and ether in 33 instances. The mortality following ether was not especially high, but it was noted that 2 of the ether cases had as high as 9 per cent of sugar in the urine following operation. Infection of clean wounds occurred in 15 instances, 11 infections taking place in 22 amputation stumps.

Ignorance of their having diabetes characterized 28 of the 99 surgical diabetics at the Massachusetts General Hospital. At one stroke this lack of knowledge of an existing diabetes shows the large number of undiscovered cases of diabetes which are in our midst, the opportunity for preventive medicine, and the contrast which prevails between the type of diabetic patient treated at a

[1] Fitz: Med. Clin. of North America, 1920, **3**, 1107.
[2] Young: Boston Med. and Surg. Jour., 1923, **188**, 767.

general hospital and one largely devoted to the care of private patients. At the latter it is extremely rare for a diabetic to enter, undiagnosed.

Strouse[1] states that of 38 operations upon diabetics in the fifteen years preceding 1916 at the Michael Reese Hospital in Chicago the deaths amounted to 31 per cent, but there were no deaths among 8 patients who were properly prepared for operation.

Karewski[2] reports that 11.8 per cent of 68 diabetic patients died of coma after operations on aseptic tissues, and 21.7 per cent of 69 cases after operations on infected tissues. Berkman[3] reports 2 deaths among 26 cases at the Mayo Clinic during 1915.

From the above reports of various clinics it can readily be seen that today the diabetic surgical mortality is less, but that, as heretofore, diabetic surgical mortality in the presence of an infection is doubly high. It is appropriate, therefore, to consider next those commonest of infections in diabetes, carbuncles and gangrene.

3. **Carbuncles.**—Today as formerly I dread a carbuncle in a diabetic more than any other surgical complication. The mortality, I suspect, is very high outside the hospital, and in the hospital I know this to have been the case, though statistics are not accurate enough to show it. *Promptly treated carbuncles in the hospital do well; the neglected carbuncles raise the mortality.* In compiling statistics it is difficult to discriminate from the records whether to classify a case as a boil or a carbuncle. Many patients with small carbuncles undoubtedly recover both in and outside hospitals, but there are many insignificantly appearing infections which develop into enormous carbuncles, and their hosts suffer for weeks, waste away and die in coma.

One of the most distressing instances of a neglected carbuncle with subsequent multiple infections is that of Case No. 513. It is very easy to see today that the medical treatment which he received in 1915 was poor, though well intentioned. As an illustration of the ravages of a carbuncle and undernutrition the case is described in some detail. It is remarkable for: (1) An average loss of weight of 1.6 kilograms (3.5 pounds) daily for eleven days; (2) the excretion of between 31.6 and 37.8 grams nitrogen daily for the six days preceding death; (3) a dextrose-nitrogen ratio of 3.67:1, when nearly fasting; (4) a variation in the daily excretion of sodium chloride between the limits of 3.3 grams and 35.8 grams.

The onset of diabetes was in October, 1911, at the age of thirty-three years, and the patient first came under observation in July, 1912. At that time, while at the hospital, he became free from

[1] Strouse: Chicago Clinics, April, 1916, p. 37.
[2] Karewski: Deutsch med. Wchnschr., 1914, **40**, 8.
[3] Berkman: Jour.-Lancet, 1916, **36**, 309.

TABLE 225.—CASE No. 513. MULTIPLE CARBUNCLES. SEVERE ACIDOSIS. RAPID LOSS OF WEIGHT. HIGH URINARY NITROGEN.

Date	Volume, c.c.	Diacetic acid	NaCl	Nitrogen, gms	Ammonia, total gms.	D:N ratio	Total gms.	Diet in grams — Carbohydrate	Protein	Fat	Alcohol	Calories	Carbohydrate balance, gms.	NaHCO₃, gms.	Naked weight of patient, pounds.	Blood sugar, per cent.	Alveolar air, CO₂, Tension in mm. Hg.
1912																	
July 14–15	2010	++++			1.7		64	120					56	12	150		29
18–19	2310	+					53	135					82	37	160		25
19–20	4080	0					98	135					37	37	160		28
27–28	1800	0					36								153		33
1914																	
July 24	2500	Sl. +					75						+++				33
1915																	
July 29	—	++++		4.4	1.4		24	Fasting save						32	138	0.37	31
29–30	1900	++++		9.4	3.0	2.55:1	31				32	224		48	138		27
30–31	3100	+++					14				48	336	−31	48	137		42
31–1	2400	+++			3.7		9				48	336	−14	48	138		33
Aug. 1–2	2200	++++			3.7		13				48	336	9	48	140		42
2–3	2200	+++			3.2		6				48	336	−13	40	142	0.24	33
3–4	1600	+++		9.3		0.65:1	10				48	336	6	32	145	0.24	37
4–5	1700	++		10.4	2.2	0.96:1	10				48	336	−10	24	147		51
5–6	1600	++		12.5	2.1	0.80:1	6		18	15	44	515	−10	16	146	0.26	53
6–7	1600	+		12.5	1.3	0.48:1	3		18	15	44	515	−6	16	145	0.24	54
7–8	1600	++		10.9	1.5	0.28:1	10		34	21	0	325	−3	16	148		54
8–9	1700	+		11.6	1.2	0.86:1	4		50	27	0	443	−10	8	146	0.30	52
9–10	2000				0.8			1	58	42	0	614	−3			0.26	53

10-11	1800	+	4.7	13.0	0.8	0.85:1	11	1	66	58	0	790	− 10	0	149		45 49
11-12	2200	:	:	13.8	:	:	:	1	66	58	0	790	−	0	146	0.23	
12-13	2200	:	3.3	14.3	:	0.63:1	9	1	60	58	0	790	−	0	147	:	49
13-14	2400	0	:	:	:	:	0	Fasting	:	:	:	:	8	0	143	:	45
14-15	2000	0	:	:	:	:	0	:	:	:	:	:	0	0	146		
15-16	1200	+	:	:	:	:	5	1	73	75	0	971	− 4	0	148		
16-17	1400	+	:	:	:	:	8	1	73	75	0	971	− 7	0	149		
17-18	1400	++	:	:	:	:	19	1	73	98	0	1178	− 18	0	149	:	44
18-19	2000	+	:	:	:	:	40	1	73	98	0	1178	− 39	0	149		
19-20	2200	++	:	:	:	:	18	Fasting	:	:	:	:	− 18	0	145		
20-21	2200	+	:	:	:	:	22	:	:	:	:	:	− 22	0	143		
21-22	2600	+	:	15.8	:	1.65:1	26	:	:	:	:	:	− 26	0	139		
22-23	2200	+	:	:	:	:	22	:	:	:	:	:	− 22	0	138		
23-24	1900	+++	8.7	17.5	2.1	2.63:1	46	0	37	49	0	589	− 46	0	136		32
24-25	2600	++++	13.9	27.0	2.9	3.07:1	83	0	45	73	23	998	− 83	0	132		24
25-26	2800	+++	12.3	24.4	3.0	3.69:1	90	0	45	67	23	953	− 90	0	131		25
26-27	4300	+++	12.0	32.7	4.2	3.67:1	120	0	31	46	11	615	−120	0	:	0.35	25
27-28	4000	+++	20.0	31.6	4.5	3.67:1	116	0	14	18	0	218	−116	80	:	:	22
28-29	5600	++++	35.8	35.3	5.0	3.17:1	112	Fasting	:	:	:	:	−112	96	:	:	22
29-30	6600	++++	35.6	36.9	4.8	3.39:1	125	0	12	10	0	138	−125	96	114	:	29 28
30-31	6000	+++++	16.8	32.4	4.4	2.96:1	96	No food retained	:	:	:	:	− 96	80	:	0.31	26
31-1	6000	+++++	9.6	37.8	4.8	1.90:1	72	No food retained	:	:	:	:	− 72	64	115	:	30 19
Sept. 1-2	:	++++	4.8	14.4	1.8	:	:	No food retained	:	:	:	:	:	40	114	0.33	19 16

acidosis, but not from sugar. During the next three years he worked hard in a market, living upon a partly restricted diet. He was not seen except during August, 1912 and July, 1913. Upon July 29, 1915 he tottered into the office with a carbuncle on the neck of *eleven* days' duration, and at once entered the New England Deaconess Hospital. During the first two weeks (July 29 to August 12) in the hospital the change in the condition of the patient was favorable, and the surgeon said the carbuncle did as well as with a non-diabetic patient. Deep-seated abscesses then began to appear in various parts of the body, and the patient began to lose weight, and in the last ten days before his death, on September 2, failed rapidly. His condition was most pitiable, complicated as it was, with the pains of multiple carbuncles, extreme weakness, and septicemia, due to an infection with staphylococcus aureus. Death occurred thirty-five days after entrance. (See Table 225.)

The weight of the patient July 30, was 62.7 kilograms (138 pounds) and on August 6, 66.7 kilograms (147 pounds), although the total calories ingested by the patient during these seven days amounted to 2531, or 362 per day. Therefore this gain in weight must have been due to a retention of water. Explanation of this is partially afforded by the 288 grams of sodium bicarbonate given during these seven days. On August 5, the quantity of sodium bicarbonate had been reduced to 24 grams, and during the following five days was reduced still more, until on August 10, it was entirely omitted. Yet during this period the weight continued to rise 0.8 kilogram (1¾ pounds). Edema was manifest, but not very marked, even when the weight was greatest. During the following nine days, August 11 to 19, no sodium bicarbonate was given, and the weight rose 0.3 kilogram more; but from this period on it steadily fell, and in eleven days, August 19 to 30, dropped from 67.8 kilograms (149 pounds) to 51.8 kilograms (114 pounds) after death, a loss of 1.6 kilograms (3.5 pounds) per day.

The striking *loss of* 1.6 *kilograms* (3.5 *pounds*) *body weight daily for eleven days,* and the coincident increase in sugar and nitrogen excreted, suggest very important changes taking place in the metabolism. That this loss was connected with disintegration of body protein as well as of fat in addition to loss of fluid is undoubted, because, as earlier noted, the *nitrogen excretion was between* 31.6 *and* 37.8 *grams daily for six days before death, while for twenty-five days before death the caloric intake had been under* 600 *calories daily.* In this patient the disease was not extremely severe when the carbuncle developed, but it was made severe by the infection and the diet.

All diabetics should be warned against becoming infected from others in the household. This may readily take place. The husband of Case No. 1245 had boils, his wife contracted carbuncles. The length of one of the crucial incisions in her back was 10 inches, yet she recovered under the care of R. C. Cochrane. No more extensive carbuncle has come under my supervision. This woman developed diabetes in 1912, at the age of forty-four years. She first came under my observation in 1917 and in 1922 caught a carbuncle. When both the surgical and medical condition appeared stationary, she was given iletin (insulin, Lilly) which appeared to help materially in her recovery, though the decrease in acidosis and gain in tolerance in this patient took place coincidently with her acquiring a disgust for food, maintaining her insulin, and reducing her diet to 10 calories per kilogram body weight. The case is also notable because when insulin was eventually omitted, the patient continued to tolerate 65 grams of carbohydrate, which she was able to increase to 79 grams soon after her discharge from the hospital.

Two other cases, 1 of my own and 1 of Christie's, deserve mention because they recovered with treatment quite different from what I suspect either he or I would employ today.

A case, apparently hopeless with carbuncle, can get well. Such was Case No. 817; age at onset of diabetes, seventy-two; first seen a year later, in January, 1915, ten days after the beginning of a carbuncle. Urine 2400 cc, 4.2 per cent of sugar. Examination showed two carbuncles on back of the neck, extensive ulceration on the right side of the neck and another area of ulceration in front. The physician described him as "drowsy by day and delirious by night." On account of his age and pitiable condition, it was debated by those in attendance as to whether it was justifiable even to attempt further medical or surgical treatment. Finally fasting was begun, with the result that he became sugar-free, and, except for a brief interval, remained so for two years.

In July, 1915, the patient was eating vegetables, a little fruit and potato twice daily, and felt well save for extensive pruritus. The insomnia which this caused made him miserable, but he was well enough to relieve it by spending his evenings at Revere Beach picture shows. Upon inquiry the patient was found to be alive and well in May, 1923, at eighty-one years of age.

Christie's[1] case was severe, frequently showing high dextrose-nitrogen ratios while taking 12 grams sodium bicarbonate daily, was fasted eleven days, and was finally discharged sugar-free upon a diet containing carbohydrate, 60 grams; protein, 55 grams; and fat, 225 grams. No operation upon the carbuncle was performed.

The success which Dr. Cochrane has had in the treatment of

---

[1] Christie: Jour. Am. Med. Assn., 1917, **68**, 170.

carbuncles of my patients can be attributed to prompt surgical intervention, the operation usually taking place upon the day of admission. All my surgical consultants agree that any infection in a diabetic is an emergency injuring a diabetic's tolerance for carbohydrate and demanding immediate operation. In fact, so intimately are tolerance and infection associated that each serves as an index of the state of the other. His procedure has been to make a wide crucial incision extending through the zone of induration. The flaps thus formed have then been undercut, parallel to the skin, to the full extent of the crucial incisions. This establishes complete drainage of the infection and in no case has it been necessary to enlarge the original openings. The wounds have then been packed with gauze, soaked in hot boracic acid solution, and a superficial dressing of the same character applied which has been changed every two hours. At the end of twenty-four hours the packs are removed and, hemorrhage having ceased, Dakin's solution or dichloramine-T dressings are begun. In his opinion the wounds clear up most rapidly under this routine. It is rarely necessary to skin graft even the large carbuncle wounds, although they have not been excised, but should it be necessary, the use of Dakin's solution has furnished a field of flat, sterile granulations most favorable for the purpose.

Vaccines have not been employed recently with my patients, though they were used in certain successful cases treated many years ago.

During the activity of the carbuncle the diet of the patient has usually been limited to about 50 grams of carbohydrate, protein, 1 gram per kilogram body weight and sufficient fat to furnish a total intake of 15 to 20 calories per kilogram body weight. It has been recognized that the urine would not become sugar-free during the presence of an infection even with insulin in liberal doses.

4. Gangrene.—Gangrene was found by Morrison[1] to be a contributary cause of death in *23 per cent* of 775 fatal cases of diabetes in Boston during the years 1895 to 1913. It has occurred in 84 cases or 3 per cent of my series. Two per cent of my living cases of diabetes have had gangrene and 6 per cent of the fatal cases. This gives an inadequate impression, however, of the frequency of gangrene in my diabetic clientèle. A much better idea of its importance is seen by a study of Table 226 in which its frequency according to the age of the patient is recorded. Here it appears that 1 in every 5 of my patients who developed diabetes above the age of seventy also developed gangrene. The frequency was but half as great in those who acquired diabetes a decade earlier, between

---

[1] Morrison: Loc. cit., p. 125.

the ages of sixty-one and seventy years, though in that decade more frequent than in all preceding decades combined.

TABLE 226.—GANGRENE IN RELATION TO AGE AT ONSET OF DIABETES.

Age at onset of diabetes.	Total cases of diabetes.	Cases of gangrene.	
		No. of cases.	Per cent.
Under 30 years	683	4	0.6
31–50 "	1080	26	2.2
51–60 "	581	23	3.6
61–70 "	226	23	10.0
71–80 "	41	8	19.5

More than twice as many males (58) as females (26) developed gangrene.

The average age at which the gangrene developed was sixty-one years. Arranged by decades, as is done in Table 227, the percentage distribution according to age at onset of gangrene is still more plainly shown. The youngest patient to develop gangrene was aged thirty-six years and the age of the oldest patient was seventy-four years.

TABLE 227.—AGE AT ONSET OF GANGRENE OF 84 DIABETIC PATIENTS.

Years.	No. of cases.	Age at onset of gangrene, average years.
31–50	8	44
51–60	28	56
61–70	40	65[1]
71–80	8	72

Gangrene does not occur as a cause of death in 49 fatal cases of diabetes reported by Muryama and Yamaguchi in Japan.

Gangrene seldom occurs in the young diabetics or in the early years of diabetes. Out of 84 cases there were but 8 who acquired gangrene in the first half century of life, and all but 1 of these cases were seen by me prior to 1917. By comparing Table 226 with Table 227, it will be found that none of the 4 patients whose diabetes began under the age of thirty years developed gangrene before thirty-one years old, that of 26 cases whose diabetes began between thirty-one and fifty years there were but 8 who developed gangrene before fifty-one years old, but that when the sixth decade is reached the interval between onset of diabetes and onset of gangrene is short. In fact, upon studying my data in detail there were discovered but 13 cases out of 84 who developed gangrene during the first year of diabetes. With 16 the duration was between one and four years. Twenty-four of the patients had the disease five to ten years, 23, eleven to twenty years, and there were 3 patients

[1] Age at onset of 3 cases estimated.

whose diabetes extended over twenty-one years, and in one of these, Case No. 1924, thirty years of diabetes elapsed between its onset at twenty-three years of age and the date he acquired gangrene. In this patient when the gangrene did develop it was of the fulminating type, of ten days' duration. He entered the hospital with a temperature of 102.4° F. He was nearly pulseless after the operation and died on the third day of uremia. The blood sugar rose from 0.27 per cent before to 0.55 per cent after the operation and the non-protein nitrogen similarly rose from 39.6 mg. to 61.8 mg. If a blood culture had been taken prior to the operation, one could speak more definitely of the hopeless condition in which the patient was received. Advancing years of duration of diabetes, as well as advancing years of life are therefore effective in the production of gangrene.

TABLE 228.—DURATION OF DIABETES PRECEDING GANGRENE.

Years of diabetes.	No. of cases.	Years of diabetes.	No. of cases.
Under 1	13	5–10	24
1–3	6	11–20	23
3–4	5	21–30	3
4–5	5	Uncertain	5

A Wassermann reaction was recorded for 28 of the cases and in 3, (11 per cent), was positive in contrast to 1.6 per cent of positive reactions for 1000 tests in my series. For 300 cases of diabetes over the age of fifty years, the reaction was also positive in 1.7 per cent. Therefore, a *positive Wassermann reaction or history of syphilis was about seven times as common among those having gangrene as among* 1000 *cases of diabetes, or among* 300 *diabetics over fifty years of age.* Of the diabetics having syphilis, 10 per cent had gangrene. Of all the diabetics, 2.8 per cent had gangrene. Each case of gangrene should be studied with especial care for the signs of syphilis.

Alcoholism, sufficient to lead to delirium tremens, was observed in but one patient, Case No. 2523.

The causes of gangrene develop slowly, and consequently gangrene itself is usually preceded by a long duration of symptoms. Charcot pointed out intermittent claudication as a precursor of gangrene, and coldness of the extremities and numbness and pains in the feet are common signs of approaching danger.

The prophylactic treatment of gangrene is seldom preached, but it is important. Root found the average weight of 22 of my cases of gangrene to be 201 pounds. Remember 1 diabetic in 5 after the age of seventy acquires gangrene and that for eighteen years in Boston 1 diabetic in 5 died with it as a contributory cause. Unfortunately, one cannot hold out this incentive to a diabetic, "if you keep sugar-free, you will avoid gangrene," but he can be told that if sugar-free, there is less chance of his developing it. All the measures which are suddenly advised when gangrene appears should have been adopted in a modified and appropriate form years before its appearance. (a) First and foremost, the emphasis in prophylaxis must be placed on treatment of the diabetes; (b) second, upon cleanliness of the feet, any diabetic fifty years of age better bathe his feet as carefully as his face if he wishes to avoid gangrene; (c) third, upon those conditions which might predispose to an infection by abrasion of the feet. New shoes should be worn but a few hours, and blisters which may have formed pricked only under aseptic precautions; flat-foot plates should be used with care; corns and toe nails are to be cut only after thorough cleansing of the part and with good instruments and in a good light; strong liniments are to be avoided; and the dangers of hot-water bags and heaters made vivid to the patient. Patients must be drilled to report any injury to the skin so soon as it occurs; (d) maintenance of a good circulation in the legs is a fourth preventive measure. Muryama and Sakaguchi did not have a single case of death from gangrene in their 49 fatal diabetics, and this despite the marked arteriosclerosis of Japanese diabetic patients. The Japanese wear thick socks and sandals which do not compress the feet. Patients predisposed to gangrene must be urged to walk for short intervals several times a day, and regularly three times a day to go through such gymnastic exercises as will bring about a free flow of blood in the feet, and should be told not to remain long in one position. The legs are not to be crossed. Bertnard Smith uses with his diabetics the groups of exercises which he found useful in the treatment of heart disease in the army.[1] When sitting, it is desirable to use a foot rest. Massage is useful. Hot foot-baths should be encouraged, and hot-air baths may be employed. In carrying out any special procedures of this nature, care should be taken to make the patient comfortable during the treatments. Whereas active hyperemia will improve the circulation, passive hyperemia is dangerous and should never be employed, save with quick alteration to active hyperemia. The surgeon should never employ a tourniquet in these cases at operation. Many of the measures advocated by Stetten[2] and Bernheim[3] for the treatment of actual gangrene are applicable here.

"Buerger[4] has suggested that certain passive exercises may be

[1] Smith, B.: Jour. Am. Med. Assn., 1919, **72**, 103.

[2] Stetten: Jour. Am. Med. Assn., 1913, **60**, 1126.

[3] Bernheim: Am. Jour. Med. Sci., 1922, **163**, 517.

[4] Buerger: Surgical Diagnosis and Treatment by American Authors, Ed. by Ochsner, A. J. Lea & Febiger, Philadelphia, 1920, **4**, 810.

of value in inducing hyperemia or rubor in the affected limb, and therefore, therapeutically beneficial in increasing the blood supply.

"This method is the logical therapeutic outcome of Buerger's method of diagnosticating impairment of circulation of the lower extremities, in that it uses the phenomenon of induced rubor, or induced hyperemia (see section on Diagnosis) in a therapeutic way. If the method is carried out daily for a sufficiently long period, it is of greater value in improving the circulatory conditions and in increasing the blood supply, than any of the other mechanical or thermal means that are at our disposal.

Buerger's Passive Exercises.—"The affected limb is elevated with the patient lying in bed, to from 60 degrees or 90 degrees above the horizontal, being allowed to rest upon a support for thirty seconds to three minutes, the period of time being the minimum amount necessary to produce blanching or ischemia. As soon as blanching is established, the patient allows the foot to hang down over the edge of the bed for from two to five minutes, until reactionary hyperemia or rubor sets in, the total period of time being about one minute longer than that necessary to establish a good red color. The limb is then placed in the horizontal position for about three to five minutes, during which time an electric heating pad or hot-water bag is applied, care being taken to prevent the occurrence of a burn. The placing of the limb in these three successive positions constitutes a cycle, the duration of which is usually from six to ten minutes. These cycles are repeated over a period of about one hour, some six to seven cycles constituting a seance.

"It is well to begin with about 3 seances daily, that is, 3 treatments daily, gradually increasing the number of seances until the patient allows the seances to occupy at least six or seven hours a day, that is every alternate hour during the daytime. During the hours of rest, heat is applied continuously in the form of an electric pad, hot-water bag, hot-air apparatus or electric lamp.

"In the opinion of the author, this method does far more to improve the circulation than either the application of superheated air (so-called baking treatment), or the diathermic treatment.

"The length of time of its application may in some cases depend upon the pain which may be induced by elevation of the foot. In some cases the symptoms may necessitate a diminution in the period of elevation." This method has been used most successfully by F. G. Brigham in an obstinate case, Case No. 1934, which had resisted many other forms of treatment.

Gangrene in an upper extremity appears in the list but once. This pathetic instance, just before the advent of insulin, occurred in one of my most faithful patients, Case No. 600, a lady of fifty-seven years, eleven years after the onset of diabetes. She developed a paronychia of the left thumb. This was incised by a surgeon of considerable experience. The wound grew worse, sugar appeared in the urine and the patient radically restricted her diet to become sugar-free, but without success, because of the infection. Several days later I learned that she was doing badly and she entered the New England Deaconess Hospital. Neither surgical nor medical treatment was of avail. The infection spread into the hand and eventually gangrene appeared. By this time the patient had a septicemia from which she died without coma.

Both lower extremities were affected with gangrene in 7 instances, and amputation of each leg was required. Case No. 343, with onset at fifty-eight years of age, lost one leg from gangrene when sixty-two years of age, and the other leg two years later, death resulting at the age of sixty-five. Case No. 355 died of angina pectoris four years and eight months after the second operation, sugar remaining absent from the urine during nearly the whole of this period. An amputation of both legs is not necessarily of bad prognosis, because but 1 of 7 such patients has succumbed within a twelve-month. One lived nearly five years after the second amputation, 2 lived over one year and 3 are now living. Case No. 1509, though legless, conducts a large manufacturing business three years after the second operation. Consider how hopeless he appeared in 1919. (See Table 229.)

The condition of the arteries and veins of extremities amputated for gangrene has been carefully investigated by Buerger.[1] He writes: "A study of the condition of the arteries and veins in limbs amputated for so-called diabetic gangrene reveals the fact that in each and every instance we are dealing not with a gangrenous process due to the diabetes *per se* but a mortifying process dependent upon extensive arterial disease. . . In short, characteristic for so-called diabetic gangrene is the presence of the typical lesions of athero- or arteriosclerosis. These differ in no way from the lesions of the arteries of the arteriosclerotic or senile gangrene, and justify the conclusion that in diabetic gangrene we are dealing with an atherosclerotic or arteriosclerotic process."

If one needs to be convinced of the *uselessness of attempting to save most gangrenous legs*, the specimens removed at operation should be studied. These show how hopeless it is to expect the arteries to regain their function. Regret is felt, not for the removal of the leg at the time, but rather that it had not been removed earlier. Extensive thrombosis of a leg precludes healing.

The value of the roentgen-ray in reaching a conclusion as to the desirability of operation is considerable. One obtains in this way both an idea of the condition of the arteries, but also of the presence of necrosed or necrosing bone.

---

[1] Buerger: Arch. Diag., April, 1915.

TABLE 229.—CASE NO. 1509. ONSET OF DIABETES AT THIRTY-FIVE YEARS. OPERATION FOR GANGRENE OF ONE LEG, AT FORTY-EIGHT YEARS, BY R. C. COCHRANE; OF REMAINING LEG, AT FORTY-NINE YEARS, BY J. C. O'CONNELL.

Date.	Diacetic acid.	Nitrogen, gms.	Ammonia, total gms.	Sugar in urine, total gms.	Diet in grams.				Carbohydrate balance, gm.	Bloor's blood fat, per cent.	Blood sugar, per cent.	Blood CO₂, vol. per cent.	Alveolar air, CO₂ mm. Hg.
					Carbohydrate.	Protein.	Fat.	Calories.					
1919 June													
19–20	++++	..	3.2	67									
20–21	++++	16.0	2.8	75	20	27	22	495	−55	..	..	..	26 / 24
21–22¹	+++	18.4	2.6	82	34	18	5	253	−48	1.588	0.197	..	28 / 27
23–24	+++	17.8	4.4	101	33	42	13	417	−68	..	..	..	24
24–25²	++	13.0	3.2	52	33	28	11	343	−19	0.890	0.182	..	24
26–27	++	20.0	3.1	77	33	57	10	450	−44		0.250	41	29
28–29	+++	22.8	4.0	87	29	45	14	..	−58				25
29–30	+++	22.0	3.1	56	29	41	13	..	−27				29
July													
30–1	+++	18.2	3.3	42	0	0	0	..	−42				25
1–2	+++	16.0	3.7	46	0	0	0	..	−46	0.600	0.210	33	29
2–3	++	16.6	2.8	26	0	0	0	..	−26				
3–4	++	15.6	3.6	30	0	0	0	..	−30				32
4–5	++	15.0	2.7	20	5	14	0	76	−15	0.780	0.194	..	31
5–6³	++	..	3.1	20	0	8	3	59	−20				
7–8	++	15.0	3.1	38	15	29	10	316	−23				31
8–9	++	..	..	45	20	45	20	545	−25				28
9–10	++	..	..	48	23	60	23	644	−25				27
11–12	++	..	2.7	49	20	60	22	623	−29				29
12–13	++	..	2.1	47	22	44	15	495	−25				27
14–15	++	..	1.5	25	23	60	18	599	− 2				28
15–16	++	..	1.5	24	18	66	25	666	− 6				26
18–19	..	..	1.5	13	23	58	32	717	+10				
19–20	0	..	1.4	12	23	59	29	694	+11				
20–21	0	..	..	17	27	64	34	670	+10				
21–22	..	..	..	7	33	56	26	590	+26				
22–23	\	..	..	2	38	59	32	704	+36				29
23–24	Slt +	..	..	0	41	73	46	888	+41				27
1920.													
June, amputation of second leg (gas-oxygen anesthesia).													

TABLE 230.—DIABETIC GANGRENE WITH AMPUTATION OF BOTH LEGS.

Case No.	Age at onset of diabetes.	Age at first amputation.	Age at second amputation.	Outcome.	
				Dead at age.	Alive at age.
2727	53	62	62	63	
2339	63	70	71	71	
1932	47	61	63	..	63
1509	35	48	49	..	52
895	55	67	71	..	72
355	58	73	74	79	
343	58	°62	64	65	

¹ First operation.
² Second operation.
³ Amputation (spinal anesthesia).

Treatment.—The dietetic treatment of cases with gangrene is simple and along the lines already described for surgical cases in general. (See p. 615.) The diabetes of these patients is essentially mild, as is almost invariably the case in those over sixty years of age. The chief factor is not to make it worse by rigid curtailment of carbohydrate and calories on the one hand or by overnutrition on the other. All dietetic changes should be gradually made. Already on p. 617 occasion was taken to show how the convalescence from an operation could be utilized to benefit the diabetes. This is still more strikingly shown in Table 231 in which my associate, H. F. Root,[1] has tabulated the changes back toward the normal of the blood sugar before operation and in successive weeks thereafter of 7 patients. Before operation the average blood-sugar percentage was 0.23 and at discharge 0.13.

TABLE 231.—BLOOD SUGAR PERCENTAGES OF 7 CASES OF DIABETIC GANGRENE. (ROOT.)

(Before Breakfast.)

		After operation.			
Case.	Before operation.	First week.	Second week.	Third week.	At discharge.
I	0.30–0.29	0.37–0.30	0.25	0.24	0.15
II	0.35	0.32	0.22	0.19	0.16
III	0.36	0.36	..	0.20	0.15
IV	0.23	....	0.20	0.17	0.11
V	0.26–0.13	0.24	0.16	0.13	0.13
VI	....	0.17	0.19	0.10	0.10
VII	0.12–0.14	0.15	0.13	0.11	0.14
Total 7 . Average:	0.27	0.26	0.19	0.19	0.13

Examples of the composition of the diets of the 7 cases of gangrene whose blood sugars have been set forth in Table 231 can be seen in Table 232. The total calories eventually were still low, but these patients were old and immediately after the operation were bedridden and so required little food. In fact, one is anxious to prevent gain in weight in order to protect the stump when the artificial leg is worn.

The *use of insulin with cases of gangrene is the same as with any elderly diabetic of long duration having an infection.* Response to insulin is definite, but not so prompt as with youthful diabetics or with those in whom the diabetes is of shorter duration. Its aid makes one still more free to operate early. These are the cases who often can give up insulin after a few weeks. Use too little rather than too much insulin, seldom over a maximum of 30 units a day and soon this dose can be reduced. To inquirers

---

[1] Root, H. F.: Boston Med. and Surg. Jour., 1922, **187**, 875.

about the employment of insulin in gangrene one can say—use it to enable you to hasten the removal of the gangrenous area.

TABLE 232.—AVERAGE DAILY DIETS OF 7 CASES OF DIABETIC GANGRENE. (ROOT.)

Case.	Time in hospital.	Diet.			First week.			Second week.			Third week.			At discharge.		
		C. Gr	P. am	F. s.	C. Gr	P. am	F. s.	C. Gr	P. am	F. s.	C. Gr	P. am	F. s.	C. Gr	P. am	F. s.
I . . .	7 days	78	52	10	58	44	24	50	58	38	59	62	47	75	71	54
II . . .	1 meal	20	23	0	77	43	20	58	40	33	63	51	44	96	67	54
III . . .	Immediate operation	..	..	..	114	51	10	69	42	34	68	47	35	114	59	65
IV . . .	1 day	32	34	45	38	23	34	33	35	48	30	33	57	45	41	70
V . . .	8 days	41	25	24	75	33	33	58	43	69	69	54	82	86	64	86
VI . . .	Immediate operation	..	..	..	71	45	43	70	65	80	..	..	..	60	68	72
VII . . .	17 days	51	42	46	32	44	33	35	44	50	41	50	73	65	55	75
Total 7 . .	Averages:	44	35	25	66	40	28	53	47	50	55	50	56	77	61	68
	Calories:	543			681			838			923			1164		

C = carbohydrate.   P = protein.   F = fat.

The treatment of actual gangrene demands the closest cooperation between a physician and a real surgeon. Undoubtedly the writer sees the bad rather more often than the favorable cases and his views may be guided somewhat by this circumstance. Nevertheless, *it is heart-rending to listen to the histories told.* A patient develops gangrene in November, is treated by her local physician and surgeons of two well-known hospitals, who advise her to wait until the affected part drops off, and enters the hospital penniless in June at 7 P.M. The leg is so foul smelling that by 9 P.M. all are glad to have it removed and the patient after a good night, smilingly meets a group of visiting doctors in the morning. Think of those months of suffering! (Incidentally this old lady showed a positive Wassermann reaction.) Another patient enters with fever and glycosuria and is immediately operated upon to give him his only chance, though the surgeon is protected by a previous blood culture which ultimately proves positive. He has been having medical treatment, though on inquiry it is learned that gangrene has been present for two months and fever present for a week during which latter period he has not seen his physician! It is only fair in such cases to protect the reputation of the surgeon, who is called so late, by taking a blood culture of the patient, although operation would not necessarily be deferred for the report, and the life of the surgeon by warning him of the danger of infecting himself with the septic organism or spirochetæ.

A gas bacillus infection of the amputated stump of the right thigh occurred in 1 patient. This woman, Case No. 1759, entered the hospital two months after the beginning of infection with the leg red and swollen and the foot a mass of purulent inflammation and gangrene. There was also a beginning gangrene of the middle toe of the left foot. The diabetes was comparatively mild and with slight acidosis, but the pulse was 120. A high thigh amputation was performed under spinal anesthesia without shock to the patient, but she died three days later with a gas bacillus infection. *The patient was fifty-seven years old, the diabetes of six months' duration and in all she had dieted two days.* What a needless death!

Gangrene deserves aggressive treatment on the part of physician and surgeon from start to finish. It is easy to understand why Stetten[1] and Bernheim[2] were successful in many of their cases and avoided operation. Bernheim's treatment as described was energetic and planned to combat the ischemia of the part, by rest in bed, exercises of the bloodvessels by promoting their contraction and dilatation with hot and cold plunges three times a day, heat for an hour at a time, the electric vibrator and the use of bromide and codein, with the expectation that eventually after weeks of treatment the circulation would improve. So long as the consulting surgeon agrees that satisfactory progress is taking place, well and good, but, if this referee is in doubt, operate immediately.

Indications for Operation in Gangrene.—The question continually arises whether the patient shall be operated upon for gangrene. Many factors must be taken into account, but the most important is the evident improvement or non-improvement of the patient. In an individual who has the dry type of gangrene which is plainly becoming localized, it is easy to decide to defer operation. It is quite as easy to decide to advise immediate operation when there is a history of rapidly progressing moist gangrene in the course of a few days. With the intermediate cases it is often a nice question as to whether prolonged local treatment will bring about recovery. If the patient has shown signs of improvement, despite the presence of considerable quantities of sugar or even acid in the urine, the chances for further improvement are probable if these are removed without causing permanent undernutrition. It is true that apparently hopeless cases may clear up, but the physician should control his own opinion every time as to the favorable progress of the

---

[1] Stetten: Loc. cit., p. 639.
[2] Bernheim: Loc. cit., p. 639.

disease by that of his surgical colleague. Do not go as far as possible to the brink without surgical interference. If, however, the urine of the patient has been sugar-free and the diet fairly liberal without improvement, it is best to operate. Procrastinating medical methods often do more damage than prompt surgical intervention. The chief task of the medical or surgical consultant is to bring to an end dangerous delays and to secure action.

Pain is an indication for operation, and I have been thankful that the operation was performed for this reason in certain diabetics whose gangrene was comparatively slight. The pain attendant on the marked arteriosclerosis in the leg was too great to witness, much less to bear, and it was a relief to see the change in the comfort of these elderly people when the leg had been removed.

The financial aspect of gangrene is a serious factor. The medical treatment of gangrene during weeks and months in home or hospital is far more expensive than early surgery. It is likewise far more wearing on the patient's nerves. So many of these late cases come to me in financial straights and so few pay my surgical colleagues anything that I am almost ashamed to look the latter in the face. The treatment of gangrene is exacting for the surgeon and it is by no means completed in a visit or two.

Each year I grow more bold in advising early operation for gangrene. One sees so many patients who are able to enjoy life after the amputation of a limb and hear of so few recoveries with enjoyment of life after months of medical treatment that I cannot help urging surgery at an early stage.

TABLE 233.—DURATION OF LIFE OF DIABETIC PATIENTS AFTER ONSET OF GANGRENE.

Cases.		Years of life after onset of gangrene.											
Condition.	No.	Under 1	1	2	3	4	5	6	7	8	9	10	12
Fatal . .	50	32	1	4	3	2	3	2	1	2			
Living . .	26	5	7	4	1	3	1	1	1	2	..	..	1
Uncertain .	8												

Results of Treatment for Gangrene.—The duration of life of diabetic patients after the onset of gangrene has varied in my 84 cases from less than one year to twelve years. The details are shown in Table 233. Among the 50 fatal cases, 32 succumbed to the disease within the first year, whereas among the 26 living cases 21 are known to have survived it. It is evident that if the patients pass the first year, they can look forward to a considerable period of life. Of the 43 cases treated surgically, 21 are still alive, while 15, or 35 per cent, died during the first year; but of the 41 cases treated medically, 17 or 42 per cent, succumbed during the same period. Forty-three cases (51 operations) of gangrene have been operated upon in my series with fifteen deaths. Restricting the number of cases to those operated upon at the Corey Hill and New England Deaconess Hospitals since April 1, 1919, there have been 25 cases and 7 deaths. At one time at the Deaconess Hospital there was a series of 7 consecutive recoveries after amputation for gangrene.

Spinal anesthesia was employed in 18 cases of gangrene with 6 deaths. Gas-oxygen anesthesia or nitrous oxide (1 case) was used, supplementing or supplemented by spinal anesthesia or ether in 10 cases with 1 death.

At the Boston City Hospital 32 cases of diabetic gangrene were operated upon between the years 1916 and 1922. The statistics relating to these cases were compiled by Dr. Horace Binney, who has kindly placed them at my disposal. Thirteen of the 32 cases recovered and 7 of the 19 fatal cases died of coma. The age of the patients ranged between forty-three and seventy-eight years, the average being sixty years. The duration of the diabetes in 16 of the cases before the development of gangrene, as recorded, varied between two months and twenty-four years, the average being four and eight-tenths years. The duration of the gangrene varied from a few days to *one year!* The average interval between admission to the hospital and operation was nine days. The site of operation was the thigh in 18 instances with 13 recoveries, the leg in 5 with 5 recoveries, and the foot in 7 with 4 recoveries. Spinal anesthesia was given in 11 cases with 8 recoveries, ether in 8 with 5 recoveries, gas and oxygen in 7 with 6 recoveries, novocaine in 3 with 2 recoveries, and chloroform in 2 with 2 recoveries. Gangrene occurred in the upper extremity, finger, in 1 instance and recovery ensued.

A writer in another city recently reports 25 cases of gangrene of the toes or foot treated at a large hospital between 1917 and 1922. Eleven cases were not operated upon and of this number 6 died. Of the 14 cases who underwent operation there were 8 deaths. Thus, of the 25 cases there were 14 deaths in the hospital and the author adds that 6 others were discharged with death imminent. Five cases were saved out of 25 admissions!

A. T. Jones[1] of Providence, R. I. reports that 8 cases coming

---

[1] Jones, A. T.: Boston Med. and Surg. Jour., 1923, **188**, 483.

for treatment of gangrene of the lower extremities were operated upon and there were but 2 deaths. Operation upon the second gangrenous extremity of 1 of these patients was refused on account of a high percentage of blood sugar.

It is inappropriate here to discuss in detail the surgical treatment of gangrene. My observation of the surgeons who operate on my cases shows that constant improvements are taking place in their methods of treatment. There has been a tendency to exact localization of treatment to the area involved, to dry dressings in preference to wet dressings, to the use of the war antiseptics, and to the least possible manipulation of the part. Increasingly often amputation is done below rather than above the knee and in many of the recent cases, so sure are these operators of their technic that the wounds are closed without drainage. It is two years since any anesthetics save spinal anesthesia or gas and oxygen have been employed. During the operation the use of a tourniquet is avoided.

The choice of the site of amputation is increasingly in favor of the leg over the thigh. With removal of the leg there is less shock and the opportunity for adjustment of an artificial leg is far better. Difficulties with the stump are by no means confined to the stump of the leg, but occur with that of the thigh as well. All the surgeons who have operated upon my patients in recent years have favored an amputation below the knee. They have not considered the absence of a palpable pulse in the popliteal space a contraindication to the low site for amputation. It is possible that my cases have been seen at an earlier period in their course and so are more favorable subjects. The thigh was amputated in 12 cases with 5 fatalities, the leg was amputated in 25 cases with 7 fatalities. There were 14 operations upon the foot with 4 deaths and the fatal operation upon the hand has been mentioned. Healing, following amputation of one of the central toes, was formerly most uncommon and still is rare and a long drawn out process.

If the diabetic kept his feet as clean as his face, gangrene would seldom occur. Gangrene is responsible for one-fifth of all diabetic deaths, and all diabetics above fifty years of age should be taught to avoid it.

If the beginning of gangrene were as noisily ushered in as an attack of biliary or renal colic the results of treatment would be far different. Death from gangrene today is usually the result of procrastination on the part of the physician and patient, and in the past was often associated with the inauguration of a fat-protein diet and ether anesthesia. Surgery often receives, but seldom deserves, the blame of a fatal issue.

L. PREGNANCY AND DIABETES.

If a pregnant woman acquires diabetes, my advice would be to allow the pregnancy to continue until contraindicated by inability to control the diabetes. This was the course followed in 1914 and 1916 with Case No. 812 and Case No. 1070, respectively. The results were favorable then and should be infinitely safer now.

If a diabetic becomes pregnant, it is more serious. In 1915, pregnancy was encouraged in *one* diabetic, but that is the only case in my series in which such sanction has been unequivocally given. Subsequent events justified the decision, as recorded below in discussion of Case No. 436. It was not advised in Case No. 2218, but when it did occur was allowed to go on to termination in the belief that earlier interruption of the pregnancy would have led to no better results.

A transient glycosuria in pregnancy may subsequently result in a permanent diabetes.

The Cheerful and the Tragic Aspects of Diabetes in Pregnancy.— The treatment of diabetes in pregnancy so much more agreeable today than a decade ago.

The introduction of blood-sugar tests conduces to peace of mind, because it allows the differentiation of those cases which resemble renal glycosuria from the true diabetics, and the demonstration that a pregnant diabetic responds to the same rules of dietetic treatment as the non-pregnant diabetic gives hope. Of course the prognosis was formerly horrible for the diabetic who became pregnant, because she broke the two cardinal rules of diabetic treatment: She overate tremendously and thus made her innocent diabetes severe, and second we doctors made it worse by curtailing carbohydrate to the limit while forcing protein and fat to the extreme in order to give her calories and—coma. No wonder these women died or that eight years ago Dr. Hubbard and I compelled Case No. 812, a doctor's wife, from New Hampshire, six months pregnant, with 6 per cent sugar, to enter the New England Deaconess Hospital and promise to remain until delivery. True, she did have a little acidosis after her Cæsarean section, because we ignorantly gave her ether, but fortunately we did know enough, even then, to protect her liver with extra carbohydrate the day before the operation and to limit the soda to a total of 13 grams in three days. These errors, acidosis due to ether and the giving of soda, were corrected in subsequent cases by operating under the influence of novocaine. This summer, 1923, while the patient was in Boston to learn the use of insulin she read a letter from *the* boy, her only child (!), to the Tri-State Medical Society: "Papa is working all day and singing all night." And to show the effect of insulin, a few weeks later after the evening New England Deaconess Hospital Diabetic Clinic held at the New York Academy of Medicine, she was discovered dancing with her friend at a neighboring café in the early morning hours.

TABLE 234.—CASE NO. 812. PREGNANCY AND DIABETES. CÆSAREAN SECTION.

Date.	Urine.				Carbo-hydrate, gms.	Carbo-hydrate balance. gms.	Blood sugar.	NaHCO₂. gms.	Weight.	
	Diacetic acid.	Nitro-gen.	Ammo-nia.	Total sugar, gms.					Mother, pounds.	Child, pounds.
Dec.29,1914	0	..	..	6.4%	..	..	..	0	6 mos. pregnant	
1915				6.4%						
Jan. 5	+	..	..	6.4%	..	..	..	0	158	
5– 6	+	..	1.3	31	120	+ 90	..	0		
6– 7	+	..	..	40	130	+ 90	..	0		
7– 8	Sl. +	..	..	20	120	+100	..	0		
8– 9	+++	..	0.5	Tr.	30	+ 30	..	0		
9–10	..	..	..	0	45	+ 45	..	8		
10–11	+++	..	..	0	45	+ 45	..	8		
11–12	+++	..	3.0	0	45	+ 45	..	8		
12–13	+++	..	..	0	40	+ 40	..	8	160	
13–14	+++	..	..	0	55	+ 55	..	12		
14–15	++++	..	2.2	0	65	+ 65	..	12		
16–17	++++	..	..	0	75	+ 75	..	12		
17–18	+++	..	..	0	85	+ 85	..	8		
20–21	+	..	1.1	0	90	+ 90	..	2		
22–23	++	..	..	0	95	+ 95	..	2		
24–25	++	..	..	0	100	+100	..	2	153	
25–27	+	..	..	0	100	+100	..	2		
27–29	++	..	..	0	100	+100	..	2		
29–30	+	..	..	0	100	+100	..	2		
30–31	+++	..	..	0	100	+100	..	2		
31– 1	++	..	..	0	100	+100	..	2		
Feb. 1– 2	++	..	..	0	100	+100	..	2		
2– 3[1]	0	..	..	0	100	+100	..	0		
5– 6	Trace	10.6	..	0	110	+110	..	0		
							After dinner			
13–14	Trace	..	..	—	110	+110	0.25%	0	157	
15–16	Trace	9.8	1.3	7	110	+105	..	0		
17–18	+	..	..	..	..	..	Fasting			
18–19	Trace	..	..	0	110	—	0.16%	0		
23–24	+	..	1.6	..	110	—	..	0		
27–28	Trace	..	..	8	144	+135	..	0		
Mar. 3– 4	Trace	..	..	4	140	—	..	0		
4– 5	Trace	..	0.6	0	..	..	..	0		
8– 9	Trace	..	1.0	—	..	..	..	0	157	
18–19	0	12.7	1.0	0	..	..	..	0		
19–20	Sl. +	12.4	..	0	..	..	..	0		
20–21	Sl. +	12.6	..	0	..	..	..	0		
21–22	Sl. +	10.9	..	0	..	..	..	0		
22–23	Sl. +	12.0	..	0	..	..	..	0		
23–24	0	11.3	0.9	0	130	+130	..	0		
24–25[2]	+++	8.8	0.8	0	5	+ 5	..	0	Delivery	8
25–26	+++	14.1	2.2	3	25	+ 22	..	0		
26–27	++++	8.7	1.8	0	0	0	..	10		
27–28	++	7.4	2.1	1	30	+ 29	..	2		
28–29	++	12.3	1.5	0	60	+ 60	..	1		
29–30	+	13.5	1.1	0	70	+ 70	..	0		
30–31	++	14.3	1.9	0	70	+ 70	..	0		
31	+	13.8	1.1	0	85	+ 85	..	0		
April 1– 2	+	..	..	0	85	+ 85	..	0		
7– 8	+++	..	1.1	0	82	+ 82	..	0		
8– 9	+	..	0.95	0	77	+ 77	Fasting	0		
11–12	0	..	..	0	82	+ 82	0.20%	0		
22	+	..	..	0	..	..	..	..	131	7¾
May 20	0	..	..	0	..	..	..	..	130	9½

[1] Observe decrease of ferric chloride reaction with elimination of sodium bicarbonate.
[2] Delivery by Cæsarean section. J C. Hubbard. Anesthetist, Freeman Allen. Anesthetic, ether. Observe appearance and persistence of acidosis after operation. In a subsequent operation upon Case No. 1070, p. 659, novocaine was employed. Albumin at no time exceeded the slightest possible trace, and casts were never present in the sediment except just after delivery.

A previous pregnant diabetic, Case No. 605, really was responsible for the success attained with the patient just described. She came to the office once, was not seen again, and was not followed from start to finish. Her outlook appeared good, and advice was given against the interruption of pregnancy. At a subsequent date, because a physician to whom she went found no sugar in a single specimen of urine and an osteopath discovered it in another, she renounced regular medicine until the sixth month. She then consulted her original physician, who was shocked when he obtained 3.8 per cent sugar with diacetic acid and albumin. She died a few hours after the pregnancy was terminated under ether (!), the baby was lost, and the husband committed suicide, as did also the next patient, Case No. 671. This young woman married having diabetes, though unaware of its presence, underwent abortion at her first pregnancy and when, contrary to advice, she became pregnant a second time, ended her life in despair. Her course was not so very different from Case No. 1722, who likewise despairing of help with diet, deliberately became pregnant in order to shorten her life and died in the seventh month of pneumonia, during which coma appeared.

Diabetes developing in pregnancy or pregnancy in a diabetic is, therefore, a serious event, though the latter the more so. The diabetes is amenable to treatment, but it tests one's skill. From beginning to end the patients must be watched, the urine examined weekly, bi-weekly, and daily near term. These pregnant creatures are unstable anyway, and severe acidosis can appear in a few hours. As delivery approaches, one must never forget the lesson of Carlson's[1] pregnant dog, who survived complete pancreatectomy until the protecting pancreases of her fetuses were lost to her at their birth.

Pregnancy in Diabetes of Many Years' Duration Occasionally Safe.—Pregnancy may occur in a diabetic even though the diabetes has been of years' duration. Case No. 1207, first showed diabetes in 1895 and became pregnant for the eleventh time twenty-three years later and had a healthy baby. The range of duration of the disease before pregnancy varied between a few weeks and four and a half years for 11 of my series. Case No. 2218, a nurse, developed diabetes in March, 1921, was married August, 1921, became pregnant February, 1922. She came under my observation May 24, 1921 with a diet of the Newburgh and Marsh type, and, perhaps because I was skeptical and changed her diet or perhaps because of the severity of her diabetes, died a year later in the sixth month, July 7, 1922, of coma.

---

[1] Carlson and Ginsberg: Am. Jour. Physiol., 1914, **36**, 217.

A young diabetic, hereditarily notable, (see p. 129) Case No. 436, was allowed to become pregnant at twenty-five years of age, three years after her marriage. She represents the happy results which can be secured in a patient of this type, and her case illustrates the rise in tolerance for carbohydrate, which is sometimes noted during the last months of pregnancy. The full description of this patient is as follows:

TABLE 235.—CASE No. 436. ILLUSTRATION OF RISE IN TOLERANCE FOR CARBOHYDRATE DURING PREGNANCY.

Date.	Vol., cc.	Diacetic acid.	Ammonia, total grams.	Urine sugar, total grams.	Carbohydrate.	Carbohydrate balance, grams.	Naked weight of patient, pounds.	Blood sugar, per cent.
1909.								
May	..	..	..	8%				
1911			Married June, 1911.					
July 31	1250	0	–	45	–	–	152½	–
1912								
Jan. 9	1020	+	–	22	–	–	151½	
June 11	960	+	–	2	–	–	–	
1913								
Mar. 22	810	+	–	2	–	–	146¼	
Dec. 23	1200	++	–	21	–	–	–	
1914								
Jan. 9	1050	++	–	11	–			
23	1140	++++	–	0	–			
Sept. 18	900	++	–	11	20	+9	–	
Dec. 5	1200	+++	2.52	0	–	–	–	
1915								
April 12	960	++	1.8	0	15	+15		
			Pregnancy began August, 1915.					
Aug. 27	630	+	–	0	–	–	–	
Sept. 20	–	++	–	0	–	–	–	
Oct. 13	1230	++	2.3	0	–	–	133½	
Nov. 4	960	+++	1.0	0	..	+10	133½	
24	960	+++	2.2	0	45	+45	–	0.13
Dec. 15	900	0	–	0	75±	+75	–	
1916								
Jan. 6	1140	Slight +	1.5	0	60	+60	–	
12	992	–	1.1	2	–	–	±	0.20
April 4	1440	+	1.9	Trace	55	+55	152½	0.30
			Successfully confined of 9½ lb. boy, April 30, 1916.					
April 25	1260	++	1.3	0	0			
May 25	1050	+	2.6	0	50	+50	–	
June 22	1530	0	..	0	50	+50		
1917								
Mar. 28	780	++	1.4	0	20±	20±		

Case No. 436 first came under my observation August 1, 1911, with onset of diabetes at the age of twenty, in May, 1909, when 8 per cent of sugar was found. The family history is remarkable in that the mother died of diabetes at the age of fifty-five, having probably had the disease ten years, and five uncles and aunts, of whom one is Case No. 759, p. 128 have had the disease. The past history was negative except that the onset of the disease took place coincidentally with the death of the patient's parents. The patient was overweight. Physical examination was negative. The course of the disease in the patient is shown by the annexed chart. (Table 235.)

Sugar was constantly present in the urine from May, 1909, until January 23, 1914, when a prolonged, energetic attempt was made to remove it. However, it quickly returned; it again disappeared, although with the presence of considerable acidosis, on December 5, 1914, this time with the help of fasting treatment. Thereafter it remained absent, and the patient acquired a tolerance for 15 grams of carbohydrate and lived strictly within this limit, even though considerable acidosis existed.

The patient became pregnant, the last catamenia being August 4, 1915, and it was observed that the tolerance for carbohydrate gradually increased. From the chart is will be seen that it finally rose to at least 60 to 75 grams. During the pregnancy the diet was halved one day each week. Confinement took place uneventfully on April 30, 1916, and the patient was delivered of a 9 pound boy. September, 1923, finds both mother and child in good condition, but she should have insulin as a safeguard against complications.

TABLE 236.—PREGNANCY AND DIABETES.

Case No.	Duration of diabetes before pregnancy, years.	Duration of diabetes to July, 1923, or death, years.
DIABETES WITH ONSET BEFORE PREGNANCY.		
436	3.0	12.0
439	0.3	1.6
604	4.2	4.0
671	1.8	2.5
729	4.5	7.6
881		
1722	1.2	1.4
2218	0.8	1.2
102	At or before pregnancy	22.0
461	" "	1.0
608	" "	0.6
DIABETES WITH ONSET DURING PREGNANCY.		
106		0.8
306		26.0
812		8.5
854		8.0
1018		13.0
1070		1.4
1207[1]		28.0
1389		6.0

[1] This patient is alive. Diabetes was discovered during her first pregnancy in 1895, and she gave birth to a daughter, her eleventh pregnancy, in July, 1918, at the age of forty-three years.

Onset of Diabetes During Pregnancy.—During pregnancy diabetes may develop, and this appears to have happened in 8 cases out of 19. The statistics, however, are not very much more reliable than those relating to trauma, because in so few instances accurate data exist about the urine before the onset of pregnancy. It would appear from Table 236, p. 653, which is inserted more as an attempt to begin a series of accurate data than as a contribution to the subject, that those women who develop diabetes during pregnancy have a more favorable outlook than those who contract pregnancy during diabetes.

A Transient Glycosuria in Pregnancy May be Followed by a Permanent Diabetes.—This is important for the doctor, first, because it again is a reminder of the necessity of seriously regarding all glycosurias, and second, because it suggests a good opportunity for preventive medicine in patients of this type. These individuals should never grow fat. Of this number there have been quite a group. I cite but one in detail, Case No. 309. This case showed sugar in 1897 during pregnancy, but following confinement, with resulting dead baby, it disappeared, but returned in nine years in the form of moderate to severe diabetes. The association of this case with gall stones and with involuntary fasting is described on p. 477. Foster[1] also observed: ". . . there had been a pronounced glycosuria during two pregnancies which had entirely subsided after the birth of each child so that there was no sugar in the urine, and no dietetic restriction was employed. During the third pregnancy there was observed not only glycosuria, but also a moderate increase of thirst and following the termination of this pregnancy the sugar excretion and the symptoms persisted."

Glycosuria, Diagnostic of Pregnancy.—Glycosuria may be diagnostic of pregnancy, recur with repeating pregnancies and disappear later.

I am indebted to Dr. Franklin S. Newell for a part of the following data. Sugar appeared in the first pregnancy of Case No. 438, aged twenty-five years, but ceased immediately after confinement. In the summer of 1910, it recurred, but a miscarriage took place. The urinary analysis of August 29, 1911, showed 0.6 per cent sugar, no diacetic acid. The nitrogen was 12.6 grams—no casts, pus or blood. In March, 1913, the patient considered herself pregnant, but the urine at that time and at subsequent examinations soon after failed to show sugar, and time showed that pregnancy did not exist. Pregnancy did occur in December, 1913, and a trace of sugar showed throughout, only to disappear after confinement in September, 1914. She died while pregnant in 1919, due to influenza and pneumonia.

[1] Foster: Diabetes Mellitus, Lippincott, 1915, p. 99.

Another similar instance is Case No. 256, who consulted me first in May, 1909. In four pregnancies, since the first, sugar has appeared, but in the intervals between pregnancies the urine remains sugar-free, and of four blood-sugar tests the highest value obtained has been 0.11 per cent.

The diet of the patient during her second pregnancy was gradually changed from one containing 160 grams of carbohydrate to one containing about 125 grams, at which it remained until after confinement. Sugar was constantly present until confinement on August 20, when the patient was successfully delivered of a boy. By September 18, the sugar had disappeared, and remained absent until a third pregnancy, one year later. The high specific gravity, 1038, in May, 1909, shows that the percentage of sugar at this time also must have been high, and it is fair to infer that if this patient had not been promptly treated the disease might have taken a serious turn. As it is, one likes to believe that it illustrates the efficacy of prompt, early treatment. At her last visit in 1923, this patient's weight was 138 pounds, and the standard weight for a woman of her years and height is 154 pounds.

Frequency of Glycosuria During Pregnancy and its Treatment.— Glycosuria occurring during pregnancy is most frequent and varies according to the zealousness with which it is sought. It may be negligible and often is, but the cases cited above show the earnestness with which it should be regarded. Modern data about its frequency during any of the months of pregnancy are lacking, but I suspect if the specimens of urine collected several times daily, before and after meals, were individually examined for a series of months, there would be comparatively few women who did not at times show a trace of sugar. A glucose tolerance test is said to be followed by glycosuria in the early months of pregnancy.

The diagnosis between diabetes and a condition resembling renal glycosuria is dependent upon tests of the blood sugar. A fasting blood sugar of 0.1 per cent or a blood sugar after a meal of 0.14 per cent or less and after a glucose tolerance test 0.16 per cent or less is reassuring. In former days the demonstration that the twenty-four-hour specimen of urine contained less than 10 grams of sugar allowed a favorable prognosis and suggested renal glycosuria, but today it is quite likely that with single specimen tests of the urine, as suggested by Gray, see p. 335, one can distinctly prove it.

The whole aspect of the treatment of the patient alters when the chemical findings indicate the absence of true diabetes. However, I am so skeptical of a renal glycosuria, save after a duration of years of observation, that advice given to the patient is to lower the carbohydrate about one-third, restrict actual sugar, substitute fruit for desserts, and above all keep a trifle underweight. Such a regimen represents only a moderate dietary restriction and should be welcomed in contrast to the rigorous restrictions which such patients formerly received.

Motzfeldt[1] also comments upon the similarity of the glycosuria of pregnancy to renal glycosuria, but he joins in the warning that such a glycosuria may change to renal diabetes. In one case with hypoglycemia, after the interval of a year he found hyperglycemia. He gives an excellent bibliography.

Diagnostic Tests of Pregnancy Based on Glycosuria.—Diagnostic tests for pregnancy are reported by Kamnitzer and Joseph,[2] based upon determinations of the glycosuria after injections of phlorhizin. The value of the test is restricted to the first three months. An alimentary test for pregnancy was described by Frank and Nothmann.[3] Küstner[4] believes this is not confined to pregnancy but is related to certain other conditions, such as the functioning of the ovaries. Bauer's[5] researches on the subject indicate likewise that such tests, 100 grams glucose on an empty stomach, are of value only in the first three months. All the women, pregnant for less than three months, showed glycosuria after the test, while this was evident in only 66 per cent of the other pregnant women and only in one of the 30 non-pregnant women. Levulose, 100 grams, as a test was used by Gottschalk and Strecker,[6] and according to them a positive levulosuria is diagnostic, but a negative result does not exclude pregnancy. They, too, considered it of especial value in the early months. Welz and Van Nest[7] in a series of cases found no error in the first three months when the test was positive. In no case was there a positive glycosuria without pregnancy, though blood-sugar estimations were as high as 0.216 per cent.

The range for blood sugar in pregnant women is the same as the blood sugar in non-pregnant women—namely, 0.09 to 0.11 per cent —and according to Rowley,[8] the average value in 53 determinations during pregnancy was 0.11 per cent. (The average value of the blood sugar in 32 observations of fetal blood taken from the umbilical cord was 0.09 per cent.) The average value for 22 observations of the blood sugar on the second day postpartum was 0.14 per cent. Muscular exertion, anesthesia, ether, are factors to be considered in the postpartum hyperglycemia.

[1] Motzfeldt: Acta Medica Scandinavica, Stockholm, 1922, **57**, 10.
[2] Kamnitzer and Joseph: Med. Klin., 1922, **18**, 396.
[3] Frank and Nothmann: Jour. Am. Med. Assn., April, 1921, p. 1141.
[4] Küstner: Klin. Wchnschr., 1922, **1**, 312.
[5] Bauer's: Zentralbl. f. Gynäkol., Leipzig, 1922, **46**, 1413.
[6] Gottschalk and Strecker: Klin. Wchnschr., 1922, **1**, 2467.
[7] Welz and Van Nest: Am. Jour. Obst. and Gynec., 1923, **5**, 33.
[8] Rowley: Am. Jour. Obst. and Gynec., 1923, **5**, 23.

Lactose is often sought in the urine, both before and after confinement, but no very satisfactory tests are available, see p. 357.

Treatment of Diabetes in Pregnancy.—The treatment of diabetes in pregnancy is along the very same lines as the treatment of diabetes apart from pregnancy, simply bearing in mind the sudden transitions which may occur in these individuals and the pains which must be taken to adapt the diet to their dietetic whims. There is no harm in keeping them undernourished until term, because thereby the mother will very likely be in better condition and perhaps delivery easier because of a smaller baby.

Insulin will doubtless save the lives of many pregnant diabetic women. As yet experience with it is awaited. These diabetic cases are often mild, and one must be cautious before giving many units. Its adaptation to the individual must be carefully considered. For the use of insulin reference should be made to p. 44.

The Metabolism of Pregnant Women.—The metabolism of 3 diabetic patients during pregnancy presented no abnormalities, either as compared with normal women in similar condition or with 2 patients compared with themselves at an earlier or later period when not pregnant and yet diabetic. If one allows for the restrictions of diet to which these patients were submitted, it is justifiable to conclude that their metabolism may be considered to conform to the conclusions of Carpenter and Murlin:[1] namely, that the metabolism of pregnant women is slightly more (about 4 per cent) than that of women in complete sexual rest.

A brief abstract of the metabolism of one of these patients, Case No. 436, is given, but the influence of undernutrition, acidosis, and nitrogen excretion entered so largely into the metabolism of the second patient, Case No. 1070, that a more detailed description of the observations upon her metabolism is entered into. The studies upon this latter patient show the extremes to which the low diet was carried a few years ago and the results which accompanied that diet. If she could only have been treated a few years later! As it was, she lived to enjoy her healthy baby for some months.

The data of the metabolism of Case No. 436 (see p. 658) for the 5 observations extending over the period from December 7, 1914, to October 26, 1922, are recorded in Table 237. The metabolism varied between −7 per cent before pregnancy to +5 and +10 per cent during pregnancy and fell to +3 per cent six months after confinement and to −12 per cent, October 26, 1922, seven years later.

---

[1] Carpenter and Murlin: Arch. Int. Med., 1911, **7**, 184. Murlin and Bailey: Jour. Am. Med. Assn., 1912, **59**, 1522; Arch. Int. Med., 1913, **12**, 288.

TABLE 237.—THE METABOLISM OF A DIABETIC BEFORE, DURING AND AFTER PREGNANCY. CASE No. 436. ONSET OF DIABETES AT TWENTY-TWO YEARS IN MAY, 1909. SUCCESSFULLY CONFINED APRIL 30, 1916. MOTHER AND CHILD IN GOOD CONDITION SEPTEMBER, 1923. HEIGHT, 161 CM.

Date.	Body weight, naked, kg.	Average pulse-rate.	Carbon dioxide per min., cc.	Oxygen per min., cc.	Respiratory quotient.	Heat output per 24 hrs.		Total heat greater (+) or less (−) than predicted (H. and B.), per cent.	NH_3, gm.	Diacetic acid.	Urinary nitrogen per 24 hrs. (preceding day), gm.	Urinary sugar per 24 hrs., gm.	
						Total cal.	Per kg. body weight, cal.						
1914. Dec. 7- 8	63 6	66	151	194	0.78	1339	21	− 7	1 6	+ + +[1]	6 3	4[1]	
1916. Jan. 13–14	61.3	..	176	214	0.82	1487	24	+ 5	1.2[1]		10.9	2[1]	Pregnancy.
Mar. 21–22[2]	65.8	86	191	228	0.84	1598	24	+10	..	0[1]	11.3	0[1]	
1918. Nov. 7- 8	58.5	..	155	210	0.74	1429	24	+ 3	1 9				
1922. Oct. 26	58.3	79	137	173	0 79	1193	20	−12	0 2	+	9 2	38	

[1] For the preceding twenty-four hours.
[2] A healthy child was born April 30. 1916.

The behavior or the respiratory quotient for the five periods is significant. In the first period before pregnancy, upon December 7, 1914, this was found to be 0.78. At the second observation, January 13, 1916, during the fifth month of pregnancy, it rose to 0.82 along with a clinical rise in tolerance for carbohydrate, as shown in Table 237. At the third observation, March 21, 1916, it rose again to 0.84, corresponding to the still greater improvement in tolerance. Six months after confinement, in November, 1916, the tolerance for carbohydrate had decreased and the condition of the patient was not so good. In line with these clinical facts is the respiratory quotient, which fell to 0.74. Seven years later the metabolism was lower, but the respiratory quotient higher, 0.79, corresponding to the excellent condition of the patient.

The diabetes of Case No. 1070 began in May, 1916, when the patient was twenty-six years and ten months old and six months pregnant. She came under observation June 19, 1916, and died October 11, 1917, in coma. The physical examination at the first visit was negative except for the pregnancy. The urine contained 5 per cent of sugar and the acidosis was severe, but with appropriate treatment the patient was made sugar-free and acid-free readily. The course of the case is shown in Table 238.

During the first period of observation (A), the diabetes was of moderate severity. On June 29, 1916, the urine was sugar-free and the acidosis moderate and the metabolism −5 per cent or 23 calories per kilogram body weight. The respiratory quotient was 0.78. For the seven days preceding the estimation of the metabolism, owing to the restrictions of diet to render the patient sugar-free and acid-free, the total calories ingested in the food amounted to but an average of 306 calories daily, the equivalent of 5 calories per kilogram body weight, which must be still more reduced on account of calories lost as sugar and acid bodies in the urine. Between June 22 and 29, Case No. 1070 gained about 2 kilograms, doubtless through retention of water.

The patient entered the hospital a second time (B) on August 31, 1916, and remained until September 26, 1916. The diabetes still remained moderately severe. Confinement was uneventful, occurring on August 31 by means of a Cæsarean section under local anesthesia, performed by Dr. J. C. Hubbard. Section B, of Table 238 shows the condition of the patient while she was in the hospital during this period; no observations were made of the metabolism.

The third entrance of the patient to the hospital (C) occurred on February 27, 1917, because of recurrence of sugar. The diabetes had now become severe in type, and this persisted. As upon the first admission, she rapidly became sugar-free and acid-free, but

TABLE 238.—THE METABOLISM OF A DIABETIC (CASE No. 1070). DURING PERIODS OF MODERATE SEVERITY: A (PREGNANCY), AND B (CONFINEMENT). DURING PERIODS OF EXTREME SEVERITY: C (ACIDOSIS WITH SUBSEQUENT UNDERNUTRITION), AND D (PRECEDING COMA).

(Age, June 19, 1916, twenty-seven years; height, 162 cm. Subject postabsorptive, except in experiments beginning October 2, 1917.)

Date and degree of severity.	Body wgt., naked, kg.	Blood sugar, per cent.	Vol. of urine, cc.	CO₂ in blood, vols., per cent.	CO₂ in alveolar air, mm. Hg.	Diacetic acid.	NH₃, gm.	Urinary nitrogen, Total gm.	Urinary nitrogen, Per kg., gm.	Urinary sugar per 24 hours, gm.	Carbohydrate, gm.	Protein, gm.	Fat, gm.	Calories.	Carb. bal., gm.	Pulse-rate.	Heat output Total.	Per kg., cal.	Per cent. H. and B. stand.	Respiratory quotient.
A (Mo.) 1916.																				
June 22–23 .	..	..	3100	..	..	++	1.9	13.3	0.240	93	100	25	0	500	+5	..				
June 23–24 .	55.1	0.28	2500	30.4	19	++	..	..	..	65	90	20	0	440	+25					
June 24–25 .	55.6	..	2900	..	21	++	1.6	..	..	41	90	20	0	440	+50					
June 25–26 .	55.6	..	1500	..	..	++	1.7	..	..	12	65	15	0	320	+55					
June 26–27 .	56.6	0.18	2000	44.9	29	++	..	..	..	4	50	10	0	240	+45					
June 27–28 .	56.6	..	2000	..	28	+	..	4.0	0.070	0	30	5	0	140	+30					
June 28–29 .	57.0	..	1800	..	26	0	..	..	..	0	10	5	0	60	+10					
June 29–30 .	57.4	0.13	2100	..	21	+	..	3.6	0.065	0	10	5	0	60	+10					
June 30–July 1	56.7	..	2400	33.3	25	0	..	..	..	0	30	15	0	180	+30					
July 1–2 .	57.0	..	1800	..	25	0	..	..	..	0	40	30	10	370	+40					
July 2–3 .	57.9	..	1800	..	25	0	..	..	..	0	60	30	10	450	+60		1310	23	− 5	0.78
July 3–4 .	57.4	..	1800	..	26	0	1.2	..	..	0	60	50	30	710	+60					
July 4–5 .	57.4	..	2100	..	26	0	..	..	..	0	60	65	40	860	+60					
July 10–11 .	55.5	0.18	2200	..	25	0	..	..	..	0	65	70	110	1530	+65					
July 14–15 .	55.6	0.13	2300	..	..	0	..	..	..	0	65	70	105	1485	+65					
B (Mo.).																				
Sept. 1–2 .	..	..	700	..	..	0	..	..	..	0	5	20	30	370	+5					
Sept. 2–3 .	..	..	900	..	28	+	..	..	..	0	50	20	30	550	+50					
Sept. 3–4 .	..	..	800	..	29	+	..	..	..	0	45	35	35	635	+45					
Sept. 4–5 .	..	..	660	..	32	+	..	..	..	0	45	35	35	635	+45					
Sept. 5–6 .	..	..	800+	..	33	0	..	..	..	0	70	45	55	955	+70					
Sept. 25–26 .	49.7	..	2570	..	..	0	..	..	..	0	85	80	180	2280	+85					

C (S.) 1917.																				
Mar. 1– 2	50.6	0.33	700	..	29	+++	..	..	..	12	0	0	0	0	−10	..	..	..	..	..
Mar. 2– 3	50.5	..	1600	..	31	+++	..	..	..	6	0	0	0	0	− 5	..	..	..	..	..
Mar. 3– 4	51.3	..	1900	..	..	+ +	..	..	..	0	0	0	0	0	0	..	..	..	..	..
Mar. 4– 5	52.2	..	2300	..	..	+	..	..	..	0	10	5	0	60	+10	..	..	..	..	..
Mar. 5– 6	50.4	0.24	2000	..	..	0	..	7.4	0.145	0	10	35	0	180	+10	59	1073	21	−18	0.78
Mar. 6– 7	51.0	0.26	1720	..	..	0	..	7.5	0.145	0	20	55	0	260	+20	..	..	..	..	..
Mar. 7– 8	50.9	..	2000	..	..	0	..	..	..	0	30	60	0	320	+30	..	..	..	..	..
Mar. 8– 9	51.3	0.32	2400	..	..	0	..	..	..	6	45	60	0	360	+40	..	..	..	..	..
Mar. 9–10	52.2	..	2100	..	..	0	..	..	..	6	0	65	0	440	0	..	..	..	..	..
Mar. 10–11	52.2	..	2200	..	..	0	..	..	..	0	15	0	0	0	+15	..	..	..	..	..
Mar. 11–12	50.4	..	2100	..	..	0	..	..	..	0	15	50	50	710	+15	..	..	..	..	..
Mar. 12–13	50.9	..	2700	..	..	0	..	..	..	0	15	50	65	845	+15	..	..	..	..	..
Mar. 13–14	51.1	..	2100	..	..	0	..	..	..	0	20	50	80	980	+20	..	..	..	..	..
Mar. 14–15	50.6	..	1900	..	..	0	..	..	..	0	25	55	90	1090	+25	..	..	..	..	..
Mar. 15–16	51.7	..	1200	..	..	0	..	..	..	0	30	50	90	1130	+30	..	..	..	..	..
Mar. 16–17	51.2	0.23	2000	..	..	0	..	..	..	0	15	45	100	1220	+15	..	1013	20	−23	0.84
Mar. 17–18	50.9	..	1675	..	..	0	..	..	..	0	20	50	70	870	+20	..	..	..	..	..
Mar. 18–19	51.2	..	2000	..	..	0	..	..	..	0	0	0	100	1180	..	..	..	..	..	..
D (S.).[1]																				
Sept. 30–Oct. 1	..	..	2480	..	17	++++	2.9	7.7	0.170	17	0	0	0	0	0	101	1181	26	− 6	0.71
Oct. 1– 2	45.4	0.34	3200	27.5	13	++++	3.2	7.0	0.155	25	65	20	0	340	+40	101	1154	25	− 8	0.68
Oct. 2– 3	45.7	0.42[2]	3980	..	13	++++	4.8	9.6	0.210	76	80	25	0	420	+ 5	..	1282	28	+ 2	0.70
Oct. 3– 4	..	0.40[2]	3900	27.5	15	++++	4.7	12.0	0.265	113	95	25	0	480	−20	99	1208	26	− 4	0.67
Oct. 4– 5	..	..	4575	26.1	14	++++	..	11.0	0.240	96	80	25	0	420	−15	89	1101	24	−13	0.71
Oct. 5– 6	..	0.42[2]	4065	..	14	+ +	3.7	9.0	0.195	70	80	25	2	420	+10	..	..	..	..	..
Oct. 6– 7	..	..	3500	27.5	12	++++	..	5.6	0.125	56	90	25	1	480	+35	..	..	..	..	..
Oct. 7– 8	45.0	0.32[2]	5500	..	13	++++	3.9	9.4	0.210	105	80	25	2	430	−25	..	..	..	..	..
Oct. 8– 9	..	..	3750	23.2	12	++++	3.2	10.5	0.235	89	70	20	2	380	−20	..	1157	27	− 4	0.71
Oct. 9–10	..	0.24	4190	..	14	++++	5.3	12.1	0.270	89	50	30	..	395	−40	..	1209	26	− 8	0.74
Oct. 10–11	..	0.67	1200	14.5	11	+ +	..	..	..	..	..	..	..	..	..	..	..	..	..	..
Oct. 11	..	..	..	18.8	..	..	..	..	..	..	..	..	..	..	..	..	..	..	..	..

[1] Specimens of urine on June 19 and June 21, 1916, contained respectively 4.6 and 5 per cent sugar.

[2] In period October 2–9, 1917, the blood sugar was not determined before breakfast as was usually done.

the blood sugar was not so easily controlled and amounted to 0.23 per cent within five days of her discharge. The metabolism, upon March 6, 1917, was −18 per cent or 21 calories per kilogram body weight, with a respiratory quotient of 0.78. The total energy in the diet for the five days preceding the observation upon the metabolism amounted to 240 calories, or no more than 1 calorie per kilogram body weight per day, and twelve days later when the calories were 17 per kilogram the metabolism was −23 per cent. The metabolism of this patient should be contrasted with that of individuals after a period of five days of fasting. The fasting subject, Miss L., following five days of fasting showed a metabolism of −5 per cent; Miss L., after four days of fasting showed a metabolism of −8 per cent.

The behavior of the respiratory quotient is also noteworthy. At the first observation in this period (March 6, 1917) it was 0.78, the same as on June 29 to 30, 1916. As previously stated, the patient continued to live upon a low diet for a prolonged period, and at the end of this time (upon March 17 to 18, 1917) with continued low diet the respiratory quotient rose to 0.84. Acidosis was absent.

The fourth admission to the hospital and final period of observation of this patient began on September 30 and extended to her death in coma on October 11, 1917. The patient was now in the severest state of diabetes and the acidosis was intense, but in the light of present knowledge I consider that these conditions were artificially induced and that even then the possibility for improvement was not abolished, although insulin was unknown. The dextrose-nitrogen ratio had by no means reached its limit. The treatment consisted of the free administration of fluids and a diet without fat but containing 50 to 95 grams of carbohydrate daily and a small quantity of protein. I hoped with this to force back her tolerance, having in mind the rising respiratory quotients which other patients had shown in extreme inanition. Of course I was groping in the dark. During nine days of this period the patient took 418 calories daily, amounting to 9 calories per kilogram body weight per day, or calories, if one subtracts the calories represented by the sugar in the urine, per kilogram body weight per twenty-four hours. The metabolism at this time, therefore, really represents the metabolism during a ten-day fast. As the patient took a little food during the day, the metabolism was not actually a fasting metabolism, but practically must be considered as nearly its equivalent. The metabolism of this patient, therefore, represents an endogenous metabolism preceding death in coma which is quite the reverse of the exogenous metabolism observed usually and described with Case No. 1412 (p. 207) who had been overeating.

The metabolism of this patient while pregnant was −5 per cent. A year later it was −18 and −23 per cent. Upon her return to the hospital (ten days before her death in coma) it rose to −6 per cent, despite the extreme undernutrition. From this point onward until death it varied unessentially from −13 to +2 per cent, the last observation being −8 per cent two days before the patient's death. What is more significant, however, is the series of low quotients, varying from 0.67 to 0.74, between October 1 and 9, inclusive, which are indicative of a high fat metabolism. *In contrast to these low quotients is the quotient 0.84 previously obtained seven months before. Conditions were essentially the same in these two periods so far as underfeeding was concerned, but in the former instance acidosis was absent and in the latter acidosis was present. In the former period the metabolism was −18 per cent and −23 per cent, in the latter −4 per cent and −8 per cent.* The patient weighed 10 per cent less in the later period, yet it is evident that the body still contained enough fat to lead to acidosis as a result of the lowering of the ability to oxidize carbohydrate. In comparison with the earlier data and taking into consideration the prolonged low diet and the great variation from standard weight amounting to −20 per cent and a nitrogen excretion of 0.22 gram per kilogram body weight, it is clear that the metabolism was relatively increased just before death, although by normal standards it was near the normal zone. *The only factor which appears responsible for the increase in the metabolism at this time is the presence of acidosis.*

The rise in the respiratory quotient to 0.74 on the last day of observation is similar to that noted with Case No. 1412 under like conditions, *i. e.*, before death in coma.

The last hours of Case No. 1070 were atypical. Notwithstanding the low values for carbon dioxide in the alveolar air just preceding death the respiration of this patient was not such as to attract attention and was not that characteristic of Kussmaul's coma. See p. 83. With the few other patients treated by undernutrition and later coming under observation with coma, the writer has also observed the absence of stormy respiration, such as was formerly seen with patients living upon large diets. It is possible that the difference in respiration may be attributed simply to the weakened condition of the patient in one instance and the sudden appearance of coma while in stronger physical condition in the other.

M. RENAL GLYCOSURIA.[1]

A diagnosis of renal glycosuria is dangerous unless the element of time is added to the four other cardinal requirements, namely,

[1] For literature see Labbé (Ann. de méd., 1922, **11**, 273) and Lewis (Arch. Int. Med., 1922, **29**, 418).

a persistent glycosuria, which is relatively independent of the diet, and the absence of hyperglycemia as well as of the symptoms of diabetes.

The more carefully these cases are studied certain resemblances to true diabetes are found. Diabetes is hereditary and familial, and so is renal glycosuria. Cammidge, Graham, Johnson,[1] and Salomon report hereditary cases and a few years ago I described the instance[2] of a mother with two children, Cases Nos. 1266 and 1612, and have recently encountered a father and son, Cases Nos. 2636 and 3158 with histories of ten years and one and a half years, respectively, who conform to all tests with blood and urine. It is noteworthy that hereditary diabetics as a rule are mild diabetics. (See p. 129.)

Different types of severity exist among renal glycosurics just as in true diabetes. My cases above cited voided small quantities of sugar in the urine, but Case No. 2165 with renal glycosuria for twenty-seven[3] (!) years voided 58 grams in twenty-four hours, yet the highest percentage of blood sugar was 0.1 per cent after a meal of about 75 grams carbohydrate. Case No. 2279, excreted even 87 grams, yet his highest blood sugar in nineteen months either before or after a meal has been 0.14 per cent. Moreover it is quite conceivable that different renal glycosurics may exist at different blood-sugar thresholds.

Pregnancy is frequently accompanied by glycosuria which is apparently benign, the glycosuria is occasionally repeated in successive pregnancies and sometimes this apparently innocent glycosuria changes over after a term of years into true diabetes. The nearer the glycosuria of pregnancy is shown to approach renal glycosuria, the more the cases of idiopathic renal glycosuria waken one's apprehensions.

The blood-pressure is not raised and the kidneys are not damaged by renal glycosuria. My case of twenty-seven years' duration, Case No. 2165, had a blood-pressure of 130/80, pulse 80, no arteriosclerosis, heart normal. There was but the slightest possible trace of albumin in the urine, no casts, blood or pus. The phenolphthalein excretion was 62 per cent in two hours and ten minutes. Despite his heavy intake of protein, as shown by an excretion of 21.3 grams urinary nitrogen in twenty-four hours, the non-protein nitrogen in the blood was 33.6 mg. per 100 cc. Case No. 3158, aged sixty years, with renal glycosuria for at least ten years, showed 34 per cent excretion of phenolphthalein, but his renal glycosuric son 70 per cent.

[1] Johnson: Rev. in Jour. Am. Med. Assn., 1922, **79**, 88; ibid., 1922, **80**, 70.
[2] Joslin: Oxford Medicine, London, 1st ed., 1921, **4**, 140.
[3] Joslin: Med. Clin. North America, 1921, **4**, 1723.

Hagedorn[1] discusses persistent and intermittent glycosurias under varying conditions of the blood sugar in a monograph in Dutch.

A so-called "renal diabetes" meaning thereby a small excretion of sugar with a remarkably high and prolonged hyperglycemia, accompanying organic disease of the kidneys, exists. It is discussed by Lewis.

The glycosuria was slightly orthostatic in Labbé's patient whom he had observed from the age of six to sixteen years. There was also an orthostatic albuminuria with slight impairment of renal function though the child was in good health.

The prognosis of a case of renal glycosuria is good, since the patient may live at least twenty-seven years, but it must be guarded because of the possibility of the change of a supposed renal glycosuria into true diabetes. There are now so many cases under observation that a few years will clarify this questionable point. Folin and Berglund[2] state the following: "Renal glycosuria is by no means uncommon; most observations on 'alimentary glycosuria' represent nothing else. From a class of 100 students one can usually find at least 1, and often 2 or more, who find sugar in their own urine when learning to make the tests for sugar." These are the important cases to watch because the diagnosis rests primarily, as was said in the opening sentence, upon time.

Insulin was given to Case No. 2279, a boy with renal glycosuria under observation for two years. Upon a constant diet without insulin the blood sugar was 0.09 per cent and 0.11 per cent both before and one hour after his noon meal. When he received 5 units of insulin before breakfast and 5 units before the noon meal the percentages were 0.08 per cent and 0.08 per cent respectively.

N. DIABETES IN CHILDREN.

Even without insulin the duration of life of diabetic children doubled in the five years, subsequent to 1914, over the preceding sixteen years. What the duration will be with insulin no one can foretell. The following statement is permissible. During the year ending August 7, 1923, there were 48 children with onset under the age of sixteen years treated under my supervision in hospitals. Of these, two, Thomas D., and Mary C., died in the hospital, see pp. 38 and 317, and of the remaining children all are alive and 40 are receiving insulin. The average duration of the disease in these living children is one and nine-tenths years, while

---

[1] Hagedorn: Blodsukkerregulationen Hos Mennesket, Gyldendalske, Copenhagen, 1921.

[2] Folin and Berglund: Loc. cit., p. 164.

for such of them as had an onset in the first decade the duration already reached is two and two-tenths years. This is in contrast to the average duration of 72 fatal cases[1] in this same decade which was two and two-tenths years.

The futures of certain children arouse extraordinary interest. George B., Case No. 2007, see p. 515, showed 4.4 per cent sugar in December, 1920, at the age of five years and eight months, but now August 1, 1923, is sugar-free, fasting blood sugar 0.11 per cent, never having taken insulin, with a diet of carbohydrate 160 grams, protein 68 grams, and fat 59 grams, and has gained 5 pounds with fluctuations. This boy has two diabetic grandparents and this circumstance may be a very important factor in his improvement.

TABLE 239.—HIGH CARBOHYDRATE AND LOW FAT DIET IN A CHILD.

Case No. 2007. Age at Onset, Five years, Nine Months. December, 1920.

Date.	Urine.			Blood sugar.	Diet.				Weight, pounds.
	Diacetic acid.	Sugar.			Carb., gms.	Prot., gms.	Fat, gms.	Cals.	
		Per cent.	Gms.						
Dec. 2, 1920	0	4.4	51						
5, 1920	0	0.5	5	..	91	55	40	944	45
6, 1920	0	0.3	3	..	102	58	0	640	
7, 1920	0	0	0	..	64	33	0	388	
11, 1920	0	0	0	..	64	40	12	524	
Jan. 18, 1921	0	0	0	..	128	55	33	1029	45
July 27, 1921	0	0	0	..	152	68	42	1258	46½
Nov. 28, 1921	0	0	0	..	155	70	44	1296	48¼
June 8, 1922	0	0	0	0.09[2]	165	70	44	1336	
Aug. 10, 1922	0	0	0	..	175	75	44	1396	
Oct. 31, 1922	0	0	0	0.13[2]					
Jan. 20, 1923	0	0	0	0.21[3]	175	75	44	1396	
Mar. 19, 1923	0	0	0	0.15[4]	178	75	44	1408	50
Aug. 1, 1923	0	0	0	0.11	160	68	59	1443	51

On August 5, 1923, this child, although sugar-free in a twenty-four-hour specimen, would show urinary sugar if the carbohydrate for breakfast exceeded 33 grams but after twice the quantity at noon and night the Benedict test remained clear. He will receive insulin for prophylactic as well as therapeutic purposes. Table 239.

Olive H., Case No. 2962, began to have diabetes at twelve years of age in December, 1922, and a month later the urine contained

[1] Joslin: Boston Med. and Surg. Jour. (The Shattuck Lecture), 1922, **186**, 833.
[2] 3° after dinner.
[3] 1° after lunch.
[4] 1½° after lunch.

9 per cent sugar.   She is now sugar-free, blood sugar 0.07 per cent, taking carbohydrate 155 grams, protein 68 grams, and fat 88 grams, without insulin which she gladly gave up February 9, 1923, because a reaction occurred, and has not yet needed to resume it, September 9, 1923.   Aravess, Case No. 3078, is a similar instance, the onset having occurred in January, 1923, with 6 per cent sugar in March. She now takes, July 19, 1923, carbohydrate 115 grams, protein 51 grams, and fat 84 grams, and her insulin was stopped in June.   Will these girls later require their insulin again?

For possible recoveries from diabetes in childhood, see p. 161.

Diabetes is more and more frequently seen in children.   In Frerich's series the children in the first decade comprised 1 per cent, in my series prior to 1917, 4.7 per cent, and among my last 1000 cases there were 6.5 per cent.   Cochmann reports a case of diabetes in an infant four months of age.   The quantity of sugar amounted to 9 per cent.   The child died when eight months old of pneumonia. Gangrene in one toe and later in a toe of the other foot is reported in a diabetic infant five months old by Ashley.   Lasalle[1] reports a case in an infant who excreted 28.5 grams sugar.   With diet this disappeared and now at four years of age the child is doing well, but must be kept upon a diabetic diet.

A *duration of life of five years or more has been attained by* 21 children out of 140 beginning in the first decade.

A *precocious development* is found frequently among those children who develop diabetes.   Twenty-two are known to have led their class or to have been distinguished in some unusual degree at school before the onset of their diabetes.

The *diabetic child is not infrequently an only child*.   It requires tact to protect such a child from too much attention.   Twenty-six of the children had no brothers or sisters.   Conversely, 15 diabetic children out of 166 children had brothers or sisters with the disease and 23 had parents or grandparents with diabetes.

Death has been due to coma in 86 per cent of 139 children under the age of sixteen years; therefore everything in the treatment of diabetic children is to be subordinated to the prevention of acidosis.

The *prognosis of a child with diabetes* is serious under any circumstances, even though insulin has been discovered, yet it is certainly unfair to base the prognosis upon the unfavorable records of the past.   There are but few cures of diabetes, but the few which are on record have most often occurred in children, and there is always the possibility that the present child is the exceptional case which may recover.   While the parents are told the usual outcome of such cases, they should be given hope.   Think of the

---

[1] Lasalle: Arch. d. Méd. d. Enfants, 1923, **26**, 423.

number of children whose lives were prolonged by routine treatment and were rewarded by the discovery of insulin. Evidence that parents appreciate this attitude and that they do not resent follow-up letters is afforded by the last sentence of a response to such a letter regarding a fatal case—"I do thank you for writing and asking about my boy," and by the Christmas cards I prize most—namely, those from the parents of my former little patients.

The prognosis is not invalidated by a high blood sugar. In Williams[1] case a blood sugar of 0.53 per cent fell to 0.11 per cent and he considered the case mild. In a patient, Case No. 2870, treated by John and myself, he found the blood sugar four and a half hours after a meal to be 0.638 per cent. This boy has done extraordinarily well with a tolerance for 180 grams carbohydrate. The children with high percentages of urinary sugar generally do well.

Growth in height and weight of diabetic children without insulin was slight, though Case No. 2007, aged five years, added 2.5 inches to his stature and 5 pounds to his weight in two and a quarter years. Rexane, Case No. 894, grew 6.5 inches and gained 14.2 pounds in the eight years of diabetes before her death at the age of ten years. Her height was then 45.5 inches without shoes and her weight 47.4 pounds without clothes. She was, therefore, about 7 inches under height and about 20 pounds under weight for the average child. From the age of two she was kept alive by faithfulness and cheerfulness, only to die in coma, December 28, 1922, just before she was to begin insulin. As a rule without insulin many of these tiny diabetics became pathetic, feeble beings, old in facial aspect and in manners, but dwarfs in size. Not so with Rexane!

The *growth with insulin* may be excessive as with Alice, Case No. 2802. The peculiar nephritic, myxedematous aspect of such children was noted by Allen and is mentioned upon p. 62. Banting and Geyelin have also observed this abnormal adipose appearance with some of their cases.

How many pounds should be gained in one year by a diabetic child? Normal boys up to the age of ten should average an increase of about 6 pounds a year and thereafter up to sixteen years about 8 pounds; the girls, a trifle less. Consequently, if a diabetic child gains a pound a month, or even three-quarters of a pound a month until he is within 10 per cent of his standard weight, that should suffice.

The food requirements of normal boys and girls are given by

---

[1] Williams: Arch. Int. Med., 1923, **23**, 546. Personal communication regarding his case, 1936.

Holt. These values appear extraordinarily high to one accustomed to the diets of diabetic children.

TABLE 240.—SUGGESTED TOTAL DAILY CALORIES (FROM DR. HOLT'S PAPER ON "THE FOOD REQUIREMENTS OF CHILDREN.")[1]

Age, years.	Boys.					Girls.				
	Average weight.		Calories per		Total daily calories.	Average weight.		Calories per		Total daily calories.
	Kilos.	Pounds.	Kilo.	Pound.		Kilos.	Pounds.	Kilo.	Pound.	
1	9.5	22	100	45	950	9.3	21	101	45	940
2	12.2	27	93	42	1135	11.8	26	94	43	1110
3	14.5	32	88	40	1275	14.1	31	87	40	1230
4	16.4	36	84	38	1380	15.9	35	82	37	1300
5	18.2	40	82	37	1490	18.2	40	78	36	1410
6	20.0	44	80	36	1600	20.0	44	76	34	1520
7	21.8	48	80	36	1745	21.8	48	76	34	1660
8	24.0	53	80	36	1920	23.9	53	76	34	1815
9	26.4	58	80	36	2110	26.2	58	76	34	1990
10	29.1	64	80	36	2330	28.5	63	77	35	2195
11	31.4	69	80	36	2510	31.5	69	80	36	2520
12	34.2	75	80	36	2735	35.8	79	80	36	2864
13	38.0	84	80	36	3040	40.6	89	79	36	3210
14	42.5	94	80	36	3400	45.0	99	74	34	3330
15	48.2	106	80	36	3855	48.3	106	67	30	3235
16	54.5	120	75	34	4090	51.0	112	62	28	3160
17	57.5	127	69	31	3945	52.6	116	58	26	3060
18	59.8	132	62	28	3730	52.8	117	56	25	2950
Adult	68.0	150	48	22	3265	60.0	132	44	20	2640

TABLE 241.—DIETS OF NORMAL AND DIABETIC CHILDREN COMPARED IN GRAMS OF FOOD PER KILOGRAM BODY WEIGHT.

Observer.	Age.	Carb.	Prot.	Fat.	Cals. per kilo.	Weight in per cent of normal for age.
Holt and Fales . .	4 yrs., 5 mos.	10.1	3.3	3.2	83	
Newburgh[2] . . .	4 " 5 "	1.1	2.1	7.8	83	+6
Horace Gray . . .	4 " 5 "	7.8	2.9	3.3	73	−6

A comparison is made in Table 241, of the diet in grams of carbohydrate, protein, and fat per kilogram body weight which a normal child should receive according to Holt with the diet of two diabetic children. This method was first used for carbohydrate in diabetics, I believe, by Root and Miles.[3] One of the patients was

[1] Holt and Fales: Am. Jour. Dis. Children, 1921, **21**, 1.
[2] Personal communication.
[3] Root and Miles: Jour. Metab. Research, 1923, **2**, 177.

under the care of Newburgh,[1] the other under one of my associates. Attention is directed to the protein which the Ann Arbor writer actually gave his child as well as to the high fat and low carbohydrate in his diet compared with the normal fat and attempt at normal carbohydrate in the diet of the other child. The future careers of these two children the profession will watch with interest.

The carbohydrate intake of healthy children has also been investigated by Holt and Fales. Among 100 healthy children from one to eighteen years of age, they found that the quantity of carbohydrate taken per kilogram body weight averaged 10 grams. "Of this 51 per cent was sugar, including lactose, saccharose and fructose, and 49 per cent was starch. The carbohydrate in the diet of the infant is almost all sugar, that of the nursing infant entirely lactose, that of the artificially fed infant usually a mixture of lactose with saccharose or maltose and dextrins."[2]

On account of the possible importance of the variety of sugars ingested, their table is inserted and to it I have added a column showing the percentage of fruit sugar to the total sugar in the diet.

TABLE 242.—AVERAGE AMOUNTS OF DIFFERENT SUGARS TAKEN.[3]
BOTH SEXES—AVERAGE GRAMS DAILY.

Age, years.	No. of cases.	Lactose.	Saccharose.	Fruit sugars.[4]	Other sugars.	Total sugars.	Fruit sugars, per cent of total.
1– 2	7	30	9	24	..	63	38
2– 3	11	33	19	40	2[5]	94	43
3– 4	10	34	12	27	..	73	37
4– 5	12	36	26	24	1[6]	87	28
5– 6	10	35	39	37	3[7]	114	32
6– 7	8	29	55	33	..	117	28
7– 8	5	24	69	38	1[5]	132	29
8– 9	9	40	64	57	..	161	35
9–10	9	39	76	43	1[5]	159	27
10–11	9	44	53	59	..	156	38
11–12	4	42	59	44	5[6]	150	29
12–13	3	48	48	35	..	131	27

Children make exceptionally good patients. This is probably due to an early discovery of the disease and to vigorous treatment.

[1] Newburgh and Marsh: Med.. Clin North America, 1923, **6**, 1125.

[2] Holt and Fales: Am. Jour. Dis. Children, 1922, **24**, 55.

[3] Holt and Fales: Am. Jour. Dis. Child., 1922, **24**, 51.

[4] This includes all sugars occurring in fruit taken; largely fructose, but includes considerable saccharose and occasionally very small amounts of starch.

[5] Honey (levulose and dextrose).

[6] Maltose.

[7] Honey and maltose.

Almost invariably children become sugar-free for a shorter or longer period. The diet is borne unusually well, and, as a rule, without complaint. In a very few favorable cases growth takes place as in healthy children, and it is this temporary growth which often deceives the physician and relatives into believing that the disease has disappeared, and has led to relaxation in treatment. In other cases growth is retarded. In such instances it is encouraging to remember that Osborne and Mendel[1] state, as a result of their experiments upon animals, that "after periods of suppression of growth even without loss of body weight, growth may proceed at an exaggerated rate for a considerable period. This is regarded as something apart from the rapid gains of weight in the repair or recuperation of tissue actually lost. Despite failure to grow for some time the average normal size may thus be regained before the usual period of growth is ended." Catamenia has returned in two of the girls who took insulin temporarily.

The methods of treatment of children with diabetes are precisely those of adults. Rigid dieting offers more comfort to the child than freedom in eating, and furthermore, I am convinced that rigid dieting is more effective in prolonging life than neglect to follow dietetic rules. Case No. 813, a little boy, remained sugar-free for a considerable length of time after returning home from the hospital. He was then given cherries to eat, which was not in accordance with his diet. From that time on it was difficult to maintain adherence to rules.

Parents occasionally renounce regulation treatment and adopt quack methods. In not a single instance has the child done as well as before the change was made. Later on the parents repent, but the harm is done and my statistics pay the penalty.

The diet of children with diabetes from the age of two upward requires surprisingly few modifications from that of an adult. Especial pains should be taken in the preparation of the vegetables, for children eat fast and occasionally diarrhea results. Strange to say, more frequently the complaint is of constipation. Children's specialists, accustomed to dealing with children of delicate digestions, sometimes err in making the diet too simple.

The *quantity of protein* required by the child is proportionately more than that of an adult. Three grams of protein per kilogram body weight is the amount which the normal child of about four years requires. As age advances this gradually decreases to 1.5 grams or 1 gram for the adult. The following table shows the nitrogenous urinary excretion of 4 healthy children selected for their

Osborne and Mendel: Am. Jour. Physiol., 1916, **40**, 16.

health and size from among the playmates of some of my diabetic children.

TABLE 243.—THE NITROGEN AND SALT IN THE URINES OF FOUR HEALTHY CHILDREN.

Date.	Name.	Age.	Height, inches.	Weight.	Volume, cc.	Specific gravity.	NaCl, gms.	Nitrogen, gms.	Calculated protein per kilogram body weight.[1]
1916.									
Oct. 18–19	C. P.	2 yrs. 10 mos.	38½	33 lb.	670	1015	3.4	6.2	2.8
19–20	..	...	..	...	960	1013	5.9	5.5	2.5
20–21	..	...	..	...	560	1015	3.2	4.3	2.0
20–21	R. B.	4 yrs. 3 wks.	41	34 lb. 14 oz.	590	1016	2.4	6.0	2.6
23–24	..	...	..	...	1135	1016	3.9	7.7	3.3
26–27	..	...	..	...	630	1017	3.8	5.2	2.2
20–21	A. C.	4 yrs. 2 mos.	42	38 lb.	540	1019	5.0	5.4	2.1
21–22	..	...	..	...	350	1030	3.3	5.6	2.2
22–23	..	...	..	...	452	1022	3.3	5.0	2.0
24–25	D. J., Jr.	3 yrs. 6 mos.	40¾	41 lb. 13 oz.	870	1014	3.5	6.9	2.5
25–26	..	...	..	...	890	1013	3.2	6.6	2.4
26–27	..	...	..	...	730	1014	3.1	6.4	2.3

The quantity of protein in broth must be considered in planning the diet of children. One specimen of broth showed 36 grams to the liter.

The *quantity of carbohydrate* is determined by the same methods as in adults. Tolerance tests are demoralizing, because the child cannot reason out why so much food of the character he enjoys should be good for him one day and not the next. It is better policy to keep the carbohydrate low rather than near the toleration limit. The Eskimo children have little carbohydrate and thrive, and so ought diabetic children with practice. New tests in treatment should be worked out upon adults; a colt needs a steady rein. In giving carbohydrate to a child, do not forget that the addition of 5 grams carbohydrate to the diet of a child weighing 15 kilograms is proportionately equal to the addition of 10 to 20 grams to that of an adult.

The restricted diet of children may possibly conceal dangers due to the absence of salts of one kind or another. To avoid such a contingency, raw vegetables are prescribed freely and a little cream for the sake of the calcium.

It is better not to give children saccharin. Strict dieting must

---

[1] (Urinary nitrogen + 10 per cent) × 6.25.

be carried out for such a long period that it is kinder to the child and easier for him to give up the taste of sweets. For this reason, various diabetic breads are not to be encouraged. Meat, eggs, cream, butter, vegetables fruit and oatmeal are the standards.

Exercise has also been beneficial even when it has been violent. Case No. 785, who took no exercise and made no exertion, improved very slowly as compared with Cases Nos. 925 and 923, who played tennis and walked miles. All the children appear to be better when taking exercise. We must never forget that one-half the glycogen in the body is stored in the muscles, and that undoubtedly, fully as much of the carbohydrate ingested is burned there. A reaction occurred when one boy receiving insulin walked 10 miles in a forenoon, an illustration of the power of exercise to reduce the blood sugar. It did not appear under similar conditions when he was less strenuous.

In addition to the following illustrative cases, other cases in children are described on pp. 56, 130, 161.

Case No. 295 is reported in detail in Publication 136 of the Carnegie Institution of Washington, D. C., 1910, p. 126; and also Publication 176, 1912, p. 21. This case and the next, Case No. 304 are inserted here because of the exceptionally long duration, which may be explained by the presence of a diabetic heredity.

Case No. 295; male; born February 2, 1886; married, chauffeur; came under observation October 25, 1909; onset of diabetes at the age of fourteen years in 1900; death in coma in May, 1912.

Family History.—Father died of diabetes, complicated by appendicitis, at age of fifty-one years, having been ill with the disease for two or three years. One brother died of diabetes at the age of eleven years. The mother has gall stones. Two brothers and one sister well. The patient was married September, 1907, and has one child in fairly good health, five months old.

Past History.—A frail boy; scarlet fever, measles, chicken-pox, whooping-cough. October, 1917, typhoid fever.

Present Illness.—The date of onset is not accurately known, but during 1899 the patient was thirsty and had polyuria. In May, 1902, sugar was found in the urine. Sugar was absent from the urine for a brief period in 1904. Since the onset of the disease the patient worked steadily, rarely losing time, save during an attack of typhoid fever, and on account of a furuncle on the heel. He began his occupation as chauffeur in April, 1909.

The greatest quantity of urine noted in twenty-four hours was 12 quarts, and upon October 23, 1909, the quantity measured amounted to 10 quarts. Up to October 1, he was in fairly good health, but was then especially upset because he could not get the diet to which he had been accustomed, being forced to live, while upon a visit, chiefly upon sugar and starch. He now "eats any time."

Physical Examination.—The greatest weight, dressed, was 60.8 kilograms; on October 25, 1909, it was 49.5 kilograms. Height, 176 cm. Typical gaunt, flushed, dry appearance. Reflexes normal; eyelids red; teeth in good condition; tip of tongue red and back of tongue slightly dry; lungs and heart normal; pulse, 128, blood-pressure, 100. "Acetone" odor to breath, and whole room filled with it.

An attack of influenza in the spring of 1910 reduced the strength of the patient materially, yet he recovered sufficiently to go into the poultry business. He did not limit his diet, and it included, among other articles, 2 quarts of milk, 6 oranges, and 10 eggs daily. In February, 1911, he returned to the hospital on account of diarrhea, which had existed for some time. Under hospital care the number of stools decreased from 12 to 5 daily, and his condition improved. During 1911, the patient's condition did not change. He agreeably passed the early winter in Florida, but in February, 1912, as the diarrhea had returned, again entered the hospital for a few days. Except for emaciation and weakness and the presence of numerous furuncles, his condition had changed but little. Death took place in coma several weeks after his return home in May, 1912.

Case No. 304; female; age at onset thirteen years in 1901; came under observation at the age of twenty-one years on November 24, 1909, and died in coma on January 4, 1910, following restricted diet and unusual exertion.

Family History.—Several of the family died of diabetes, the grandmother at thirty-five, the mother at forty-one, and a brother at twenty-five; another brother has had the disease for six years. One brother well, one brother died of pneumonia at twenty-eight, a sister of diphtheria at four.

Past History.—The only illness observed was measles. Catamenia began at the age of thirteen and continued until the end. Symptoms of diabetes also appeared when the patient was thirteen. When first seen she appeared in far better condition than one would expect. She was nervous, the eyes were prominent and her hair had been falling out, but the thyroid was normal. The pulse was 92, blood-pressure 130; there were scars of tubercular glands in the neck, but the physical examination otherwise was negative. The diet was restricted, and at first the patient did well, but during the Christmas vacation she grew very tired one night at a dance, returned to Boston for school the next day, and became exhausted with the weight of a heavy bag which she carried a long distance and in a few hours was in coma.

The data regarding four children under observation at the New

England Deaconess Hospital Clinic, February 29, 1916, are recorded in Table 244. This table is reprinted in this edition partly because someone may have been interested in the outcome of these particular cases and partly because it shows the diet at a former period.

TABLE 244.—DIETARY CHARTS OF FOUR CHILDREN PRESENT OR REPRESENTED AT THE TUESDAY MORNING CLINIC AT THE NEW ENGLAND DEACONESS HOSPITAL, FEBRUARY 29, 1916.

Case No.	Age.		Diet.				Weight, kilos.	Calories, per kilo.	Duration to death, yrs.
	At onset, yrs.	Feb., 1916, yrs.	Carbo-hydrate, gm.	Protein, gm.	Fat, gm.	Calo-ries.			
894 . .	1.3	3.6	30	30	54	762	16	50	8.0
997 . .	7.7	8.0	33	59	75	1043	20	52	3.8
995 . .	6.0	6.2	44	45	84	1112	19	59	2.2
950 . .	2.1	2.7	24	41	76	944	12	79	2.9

Insulin.—The value of insulin and the methods of its employment in diabetes in children have been discussed already. (See p. 56.) In this place, save for Case No. 1616, additional cases illustrating special features will be given. The severest case in a child in the series treated with insulin was Freddie G., Case No. 1616. He has gained 9 pounds in five months, grown 1 inch and is taking 10 units insulin having required at one time 18 units. He is still 3 pounds under weight.

How small a quantity of insulin children with diabetes of two years' more or less duration require to furnish sufficient calories for growth is astonishing. Billy B., Case No. 2560, was at the top of his class. He developed diabetes when five years and five months old in June, 1921. In the subsequent eighteen months he lost 6 pounds. He then commenced insulin and in eight months upon 2 units daily has regained what he lost, or an average of three-quarters of a pound each month. His height has not changed.

Dorothy Z., Case No. 2508 was 16 pounds overweight when she developed diabetes in July, 1921 at the age of four years and six months. From her highest weight of 48 pounds she lost 21 pounds. She has gained 12 pounds in the nine months during which she has taken insulin of which she has 6 units before breakfast and 4 units before supper. To avoid showing sugar in the forenoon, the breakfast and supper hours were separated by an additional hour. Particularly with children is the mistake made of giving meals too closely together.

Buddy H., Case No. 2084, first showed diabetic symptoms when three years and three months old in July, 1919. His weight fell from 34 pounds to 23 pounds. He began insulin in March, 1923, soon contracted scarlet fever, yet despite this infection, his weight had risen to 34 pounds by October 1, 1923. He takes 8 units of insulin daily.

TABLE 245.—TREATMENT OF A CHILD WITHOUT AND WITH INSULIN DURING TWO YEARS AND EIGHT MONTHS.

Case No. 2084.   Age at Onset, Three Years and Two Months.   June, 1919.

Date.	Diacetic acid.	Urine sugar,		Diet.				Weight, pounds.
		Per cent.	Gms.	Carb.	Prot.	Fat.	Cals.	
Dec. 1, 1920	+	3.0						
2, 1920	0	2.9	17	56	41	32	774	
9, 1920	0	2.4	55	43	39	22	575	24
16, 1920	0	2.0	23	33	36	35	591	24
Jan. 9, 1921	0	2.1	24	24	39	43	639	24
Feb. 10, 1921	0	0	0	15	39	40	576	25
20, 1921	0	0	0	16	37	35	527	24
Mar. 17, 1921	0	0	0	23	38	39	595	
April 2, 1922	0	0	0	26	40	42	642	25
June 2, 1922	0	0	0	24	38	39	599	24
Oct. 3, 1922	0	0	0	27	37	49	697	
Mar. 4, 1923	0	0	0	20	36	37	557	23
Aug. 1, 1923	0	0	0	48	42	78	1062	32
Oct. 1, 1923	0	0	0	50	42	79	1079	34

In the index under "Children" will be found references to certain phases of diabetes in childhood which for the sake of repetition are omitted here.

O. DIABETES IN OLD AGE.

Diabetes frequently occurs in old age, but proportionately it is less common than formerly in my practice because of the larger number of cases of diabetes discovered in youth and also an earlier detection of the disease after middle life. The onset in 48, or 2 per cent, of 3000 of my cases, took place above the age of seventy years. It is often claimed that such patients need no treatment, and are, in fact, better off without it. With this statement the author disagrees. These patients are very uncomfortable without medical advice and very grateful to receive it. They are furthermore satisfactory cases to treat because the disease is usually mild and it is not difficult for the patient to acquire a high tolerance. Insulin is a great comfort to them, and, though at first its benefits are not realized and its subcutaneous use disliked, in the course of time they fully appreciate it, and what is more, they may in the course of a few weeks be able to omit it and retain a good carbohydrate tolerance.

The life of the individual who acquires diabetes after the age of seventy years is shortened by it. Thirty-five fatal cases lost three and two-tenths years of life on the average, according to their expectation based on age alone, and 13 living cases whose normal expectation is seven and a half years have as yet attained but four and seven-tenths years. However, there are 10 of the group who have outlived their life's expectation and perhaps, if body weight and height were considered as well, the number would be greater. Six years ago but 4 out of 25 patients had attained this distinction.

The treatment of elderly patients must be undertaken with great caution. One should hesitate to interfere with the daily habits of any individual who has succeeded in living over three score years and ten. But if upon thorough study of the case it appears that the patient is losing ground or is hampered by diabetic symptoms or complications, there should be no hesitation in carrying out active treatment. Bearing in mind the vulnerable kidneys of elderly patients, acidosis should be avoided under all circumstances. Dietetic changes should be so slowly introduced as to disturb the equilibrium as little as possible. Do not confine the patient to bed. The Test and Maintenance Diet card may be employed though it is usually desirable to adhere to the grams of carbohydrate, protein, and fat and to adjust the composition of the individual foods to the desires of the patient. These cases should never be kept long on a low diet and one seldom allows the calories to fall below 600. Even if a few tenths of sugar persist for a few days, one can increase the diet to 15 and perhaps 20 calories per kilogram body weight and feel confident that glycosuria will disappear and then gradually work up to a full diet. With insulin one can proceed more rapidly, but 30 units may be required for months in certain refractory cases. Whether treated with or without insulin, elderly patients improve very gradually but with a little patience the improvement is far more than one is apt to expect.

A lowered caloric intake is suitable and satisfactory for most patients with advanced years, but occasionally there is one who fails to gain weight or even to keep comfortable on 30 calories per kilogram. Such cases deserve study. In one instance of this kind the basal metabolism was high, +16 per cent, but on another occasion +0.9 per cent. Nervousness and restlessness plainly were concerned with caloric needs. These patients must be fed by their clinical requirements rather than by rule of thumb.

The causes of death of these patients were not what one would expect. Cancer occurred but twice among the 30 for whom the final diagnosis was learned, whereas pulmonary tuberculosis appeared twice. There were 5 deaths from coma, confirming the mild character of the disease. Pneumonia claimed but 5 patients. To arteriosclerosis, cerebral hemorrhage and heart disease are attributed 9 deaths. Strange to say, gangrene occurs but twice in the list.

Elderly patients are often easily depressed, easily lose their appetite, easily acquire indigestion, and the danger of acidosis is by no means slight. The patient should be considered from a broad stand-point, and the diabetes viewed with a proper perspective.

Illustrative cases of the success of treatment of diabetic patients of advanced years are numerous. Case No. 629, cited in detail under Tuberculosis, p. 572, led an active life until the age of seventy-eight years, took up politics, and died at the age of eighty-four years. Case No. 559, was in good health five years after onset of diabetes at the age of seventy-two years and four years following the removal of the prostate gland, but he succumbed a year later at the age of seventy-eight years to tuberculosis. Case No. 687, from being a semi-invalid, was able to enjoy life for several years, still has a tolerance of 100 grams carbohydrate, but unfortunately is blind. When I first saw her at the age of seventy-five years, the urine contained 7 per cent of sugar. Case No. 90, who developed diabetes at the age of seventy-nine, lived ten years, during which time she made frequent trips to the tropics, and finally died in England. Case No. 899, in whom diabetes was known not to have been present at the age of eighty-two, but in whose case sugar was found at the age of eighty-three, was according to a letter from her daughter "wonderfully improved by treatment and remains sugar-free." She was one of the few patients whose tolerance came back to such an extent that she could eat rich pastry without the return of glycosuria. At the age of eighty-six years she died of hemiplegia. Other cases of old people treated recently but with insulin are recorded on p. 43. Old age is no excuse for neglect of diabetic treatment.

P. CASES OF DIABETES OF TWENTY OR MORE YEARS DURATION.[1]

The duration of the diabetes in 2.2 per cent (65) of the 3000 cases studied has been twenty or more years. In 1917, it was 1.9 per cent (23) in 1187 cases. The males predominated, comprising 71 per cent of the group in contrast to 57 per cent for the entire series. The reason for this difference is readily explained

[1] For a study of my cases of diabetes of fifteen or more years' duration, see Hornor and Joslin: Am. Jour. Med. Sci., 1918, **155**, 47.

since 17 of the cases were discovered through an examinition as a matter of routine and 25 others through examination of the urine for life insurance. Of the 25 cases discovered at life insurance 23 were males.

The importance of obesity both as a predisposing and as a favorable prognostic condition is borne out by the fact that it was present in 62 of the 65 patients.

Heredity was present in 15 of the 65 cases, a proportion similar to the incidence for the entire series.

Syphilis was unimportant in this group of diabetics as in the entire series. Wassermann reactions were done on 37 of the patients. In only 1 to whom the test was applied was a Wassermann reaction positive. This case had other clinical evidence of old syphilis.

A severe type characterized 6 of the 65 cases. Fourteen were moderately severe and 45 mild. There was but 1 of these patients who neglected treatment completely, 18 others were treated in a lax manner, 33 were treated with moderate rigidity, and 13 strictly.

All but 3 of the 40 living cases are known to have been sugar-free at some time after the discovery of glycosuria. Five of the 25 fatal cases were never known to be sugar-free from the time of the first visit until death.

Coma was the cause of death of 20 per cent (5) of the 25 fatal cases. Four died of angina pectoris, 2 of arteriosclerosis, 1 each of senility and of nephritis. Cancer was the cause of death in 3 more cases, pulmonary tuberculosis in 1, 5 died of acute infections, and 3 unknown causes. Strangely enough none died of gangrene though some had recovered from it.

The natural expectation of life was exceeded by 24 per cent (6) of the 25 fatal cases and 15 per cent (6) of the living cases. If this expectation of life be corrected for the number of pounds overweight at time of maximum weight for the 11 fatal cases for whom data exist complete, it may be stated that 64 per cent (7) lived longer than the average duration at that weight and 1 equaled the duration. Similarly sufficient data are available for 34 of the living cases to show that already 53 per cent (18) have outlived their corrected expectation of life and another has equaled such an expectation. In other words, Dr. Hornor has proved from these statistics that *if you are fat it is better to get thin, even at the expense of acquiring diabetes.*

The blood sugar was studied in 44 of the 65 cases. It ranged in 9 from 0.07 per cent to 0.12 per cent, in 13 from 0.12 per cent to 0.2 per cent, in 16 from 0.2 per cent to 0.3 per cent, in 6 over

0.3 per cent. Only 1 of the high values cannot be explained, 4 were not fasting and 1 was taken shortly before death.

The non-protein nitrogen varied between 15 and 40 mg. per 100 cc blood in 19 out of 26 cases. In the remaining 7 cases it was between 41 and 54 mg. per 100 cc blood.

The total blood lipoids were estimated by Bloor's method in 10 cases. In 9 the range was from 0.5 per cent to 1 per cent. The tenth case had a value of 1.3 per cent. This latter patient was living a year following the determination, despite the fact that at the same time the non-protein nitrogen was 45 mg. per 100 cc and he showed the presence of 0.12 per cent albumin in the urine.

Evidence that the disease was arrested, or at least not causing the symptoms usually attributable to diabetes, was present in 63 per cent (41) of the patients.

SECTION VII.

THE MANAGEMENT OF THE DIABETIC IN OFFICE AND HOSPITAL.

A. THE EDUCATION OF THE DIABETIC.

THE education of the diabetic is considered so important a part of the treatment of the diabetics committed to their care that the Trustees of the New England Deaconess Hospital have provided for them a school-room. This will accommodate the scholars and thus provide a favorable opportunity for the instruction of patients, relatives, and friends, and in a way a community service. For years we have crowded into one little bedroom for our talks, demonstrations and recitations, but the pressure of visitors has led to this departure in hospital work. The school-room should serve not alone for persons with diabetes, but for persons with other diseases. However, it is primarily for diabetics. Adjoining the school-room is a diabetic restaurant, and next to that a diabetic diet kitchen, and, it might be added, across the street is a diabetic boarding-house. With these facilities the problem of teaching patients should be in large measure solved and new ways found to simplify treatment.

The amount of information a class of diabetics will imbibe is astounding. The teacher benefits quite as much as the scholars in such a school. But the scholars want concrete facts. They want to see displayed in lump sugar the amount Aravess voided the day before she came in and to see her Benedict test now. They want to see the baby of the class perform a Benedict test, pick out the good and the bad tests from the rack, and say who shows acid poisoning. They like to look at the diet of one of their number for the day before he is discharged and vote whether he knows enough to leave. And if a dignified but, in this particular, ignorant doctor or relative is present who does not know the simple weight which represents 5 grams, the entire class rejoices in seeing its youngest member impressively teach the ignoramus by removing from his supply of change a buffalo nickel, which chances to represent that weight exactly. I sometimes think it foolish to resort to these

(681)

kindergarten methods, but apparently it is worth while. At any rate, I know it is worth while to tell the patients about coma and to get them to answer the question: What is the worst enemy of the diabetic, and what are the standard rules for its prevention? I never teach them premonitory symptoms, but say: "If you are sick, call it coma, and (1) go to bed," etc. (See p. 555.) The premonitory symptoms of coma are too indefinite. It is safer to call anything coma and get over it. The treatment will do no harm and it may save me the disgrace of having a patient die needlessly of coma years after in his own home.

Then, the patients like to talk, to tell their troubles, to display their knowledge, to help one another, and to be a happy, cheerful family. There is not half the fun in treating a patient alone, and it is so costly in time. I try to make the vigorous ones weed the diabetic garden nearby, but never succeed, and my only consolation is that Dr. Allen, with all his genius, confesses that at his beautiful sanatorium the patients make abominable shepherds. The garden and the sheep will serve as a good test to show what insulin will do.

Beware of the educated diabetic. It makes no difference whether you are professor, doctor, relative, nurse. You must acknowledge complete ignorance or prove the supposedly wise patient a fool. Otherwise there is no peace of mind for you in store. If the patient really does know more than you, extract his knowledge and save yourself.

Questions from a diabetic are as encouraging as from children. Do not stifle them. Foster the habit, but have the questions written down by the patient and then write the answers. That is the secret. When written, a large percentage are duplicates, but, when asked and *not* answered, are "the doctor was too busy to answer my question."

The patients must "see all nor be afraid." Tell them the best and the worst. Urge them to study their charts and to note the orders recorded. Have no secrets. Always make them realize that they have the diabetes, not you, and it is up to them to master it.

A diabetic patient upon entrance to a hospital should be made to understand that he is taking a course in diabetes. A simple diabetic textbook should be given him, and upon this he should be questioned in recitations and at other times as well. He should attend the diabetic classes on diet, treatment and insulin administration. He should be drilled in weighing food and easy opportunities for this should be afforded. For successful graduation in the course it is understood that he shall be able:

1. To demonstrate how to test a urine for sugar.
2. To serve himself with approximate accuracy without scales 75 grams of a 5 per cent vegetable.

3. To record a summary of his diet for the previous day.

4. To explain the quantity of carbohydrate which the diet contains.

5. To describe what he is to do if sugar returns in the urine.

6. To demonstrate how to give insulin.

7. To explain how to adjust insulin and diet.

8. To tell what to do to avoid coma.

Several years ago the hospital class system for diabetic patients was introduced by Dr. Mosenthal into the Vanderbilt Clinic in New York City; shortly afterward it was adopted by my former assistants, H. W. Goodall at the Boston Dispensary and F. G. Brigham at the Massachusetts General Hospital, where the diabetic clinic now includes 1000 patients. Mosenthal[1] has described the system he inaugurated and pointed out how it may serve to familiarize physicians with the treatment of diabetes, aid in the instruction of students and improve the treatment of patients. He calls attention to the necessity of limiting the number of patients in such a clinic in the same way hospitals limit the number of admissions to the wards.

B. HOSPITAL TREATMENT.

More than once I have cleared up the mysterious downward course of a case of diabetes by sending the patient to the hospital. It is surprising how benign severe cases of diabetes become when under the physician's eye. On the other hand, great caution is necessary in the treatment of severe cases of diabetes in the first few days following their entrance to an institution. Habits of life and of diet are broken, and the patient is under some excitement. Formerly coma was by no means an uncommon occurrence, because of the radical elimination of carbohydrate and the change to an excessive protein-fat diet. Now all this is altered. Nevertheless, watchful care over each patient should be exercised, and no matter how mild the case, the patient should be daily seen by the physician until his exact condition is understood. If acidosis is present, remember that what is done the first hour counts toward its cure more than what is attempted the next twenty-four. By this means threatening coma is often averted. The patient's routine should be disturbed as little as possible. Entrance to a hospital by no means eliminates his going outdoors. It is quite as harmful to rest too much as too little. The utmost simplicity of diet should be maintained. A complete physical examination of the patient should be made just prior to his discharge.

[1] Mosenthal: Med. Record, 1915, **138**, 589.

The first specimen of urine voided by the patient on entrance to the hospital gives little indication of his true condition. It is the rule to find that diabetic patients have made violent alterations in their diet in the few days preceding entrance. They have either broken all dietetic rules which they may have previously followed with considerable care, fearing that their diet is to be curtailed, or, in order to make a favorable impression upon the physician, may have lived upon a far more rigid diet than that to which they have been accustomed. This was well illustrated by Case No. 759. This patient had been free from acidosis for a considerable length of time, but, prior to her first visit to me, a diabetic relative had suggested restriction of diet, and this resulted in the appearance of a four plus diacetic acid reaction.

Hospital treatment is desirable for the untreated case of diabetes, because it gives him a liberal dietetic education. He really is attending school and acquiring knowledge which will be of value to him for the rest of his life. He learns from association with other patients, observes their mistakes and discloses his own. He gains confidence because he can observe the condition of patients as they leave the hospital and can compare it with his own upon entrance and with that of others who come later. He learns what the meaning of sugar in the urine is and how to test his urine. He has illustrated before him methods which will enable other patients and himself to become sugar-free, and, what is more important, becomes thoroughly familiar with what to do when sugar returns. The diet, which formerly was obscure, becomes simple, and he appreciates the reasons for its restrictions. Finally, the intricacies of insulin medication are soon solved. He learns the danger of too much insulin and the danger of too much food when insulin is omitted. He learns how to take his own insulin.

Hospital treatment is desirable because it affords the usually tired diabetic patient freedom from worry, and even if his diet were unchanged, such a respite would be helpful. During the last years, and particularly since the idea of a hospital school has been emphasized and the importance of education for a diabetic if he wishes to live long, the spirit pervading the hospital has changed. The prevailing attitude is one of coöperation and mutual helpfulness. Each patient is expected to teach someone else, and from each patient as he comes in the older patients expect to learn something which will benefit their particular case. It is advantageous to have some diabetic patients who are really very ill.

Hospital treatment is actually dangerous for the diabetic patient if the nurses are not conversant with the details and execution of the diabetic diet. This is now obviated to a considerable extent because physicians give more precise directions. Formerly it was about as hazardous to the patient to have a nurse without diabetic training supervise his diet as it would be to be etherized by a nurse without experience in the use of anesthetics. Excellent nurses make grave errors in the treatment of diabetic patients. It is surprising how often nurses who have been trained in the foremost hospitals err in saving and measuring the urine and in carrying out dietetic orders. Of course, the physician is responsible for the nurses' mistakes in large share. Nevertheless, it is notable how poorly a diabetic patient gets on with some nurses and how well with others. Coma ceases to exist as an emergency when the patient is under the charge of a trained diabetic nurse. The labor entailed in educating a diabetic nurse in a hospital where diabetes is rarely treated is far more than that required to teach the patient. The patient has the diabetes, not the nurse, and is consequently the one most interested. Furthermore, the patient is aided in the treatment by his own feelings and can communicate these to the physician. In a hospital he often neglects to do this, because he trusts to the nurse and often believes that whatever is done is all right and thus neglects to discuss questions which come up.

The trained diabetic is critical. If a nurse or doctor is not conversant with the diet and makes a plain blunder, confidence goes. These diabetics tolerate no mistakes in others.

Hospital treatment fails of its purpose unless the patient is discharged to the care of his physician at home with a report of his condition while at the hospital and with recommendations for future care. This entails much labor, which at times may not be appreciated by either patient or physician, but it is a duty which the hospital doctor should never neglect. It has been my custom on Tuesdays and Fridays at ten o'clock to give a clinic at the hospital for the benefit of the patients, their physicians, nurses, and relatives. Every effort should be made to interest the family physician in the care of the case, and the directions given the patient should be in such form that a busy practitioner can readily acquaint himself not only with what has been done, but how he should proceed.

The surgical diabetics in a hospital need supervision even more than the diabetics who enter medical wards. Hospital diabetic mortality is largely surgical and undoubtedly is as high as it is because of lack of intimate coöperation between physician and surgeon. The surgical diabetic is always the case to be seen first by the physician.

The annoyances from diabetic patients breaking the diet in open wards are now practically abolished. All patients are expected to have the urine free from sugar. It does not take long for the patient to learn that although he may "cheat the doctor, he cannot cheat the disease." Charity patients must be told that charity ceases when the diet is knowingly broken. When a child breaks the diet, he should go to bed and remain in bed until sugar-free.

The weight of the patient recorded in terms of the naked weight should be taken daily at the same morning hour.

The diabetic diet in a hospital should be very simple. Emphasis should be placed upon the point that the patient shall be taught the value of each portion of food he receives. It may be easier for the hospital dietitian to have the physician specify the grams of carbohydrate, protein and fat which the patient is to have, but in so doing the doctor fails to treat his patients unless the nurses explain the quantity of carbohydrate, protein, and fat in each different article of food. From the first day of entrance to the hospital the patient should begin to learn his diet, and unless his food is given to him in forms which he can easily duplicate upon leaving the institution, his hospital stay is a failure. Almost anybody can get a diabetic patient sugar-free, but the education of the patient to care for himself upon leaving the hospital constitutes more than 90 per cent of the treatment.

Simplification in weighing food is accomplished by the use of scales[1] of 500 grams capacity with a movable dial which can be set at zero when an empty dish is placed upon them. Food can then be placed in the dish and the weight instantly read off. Such scales reduce the labor of weighing fully 90 per cent as compared with scales where weights must be added to a pan or lever.

C. AMBULATORY TREATMENT.

Most diabetic patients in the past have been treated in physicians' offices, and most diabetic patients in the future will continue to be treated in the same manner. It is perfectly possible to carry out good treatment under these circumstances, but it involves great patience, much time in the education of the patients, and thus necessarily expense. It is advantageous in that the habits of the patients are little changed, the whole responsibility is placed upon the patient, and from the start the diabetic treatment is made to fit into the routine of life. The danger of this method is chiefly that the patient is not seen frequently enough at the very begin-

---

[1] John Chatillon & Sons, New York.

ning of treatment, and with the alteration of diet there is a possibility of acidosis. With modern treatment, especially with the limitation of fat in the diet and thus the reduction of calories for the first days, this danger is greatly lessened. How simple the dietetic part of such treatment may be made, the Test and Maintenance Diet Card shows.

The same routine as that carried out at the hospital should be taught the patient. In general, he should be made conversant with the rules embodied in A of this section. Much time will be saved if the patient is accurately taught at the start how to save the urine, to measure the food, and to record it neatly and in a systematic manner so that the physician can quickly detect mistakes in the diet. Under no condition allow the patient to tell what he has eaten, but insist on his presenting a written record of what he has eaten. The urine should be examined and reported upon while the patient is in the office, for unless this is done the patient is apt to feel, and he has a right to do so, that he is not getting satisfactory and prompt treatment. Until a patient has been free from sugar and acid for at least a week, he should report daily to the physician in person or by telephone.

Most of my cases up to 1915 were treated as ambulatory patients. This was far more difficult under the older methods of treatment than today. With a fairly intelligent patient in a single visit the history can be taken, physical examination made, the principles of treatment explained and instruction given in the use of the Benedict test. Under favorable conditions it is then possible for a patient to attend to some of his routine work, become sugar-free and present himself for a second visit after a few days. Whereas it is seldom possible to accomplish as much at a single visit, it does show the contrast in the expense of treatment for a patient under the old and new regimen. See Case No. 1796, p. 473 as an illustration of the value of a single visit to a doctor's office. In the preface the possibility of concentrating insulin treatment in a few hours and afterwards continuing treatment at home is mentioned.

D. WHAT EVERY DIABETIC PATIENT SHOULD KNOW.

1. **Faithful Treatment Accomplishes Much.**—Faithful treatment accomplishes wonderful results, but half-hearted treatment avails little. At present it must be said that treatment usually lasts for life. Prof. Naunyn wrote: "From my experience I consider it highly probable that among the early strictly treated cases, which originally were considered severe, but later ran a favorable course, there is many a one for which one must thank this early

strict treatment, while, on the other hand, there can be no doubt that the cases which ran ultimately a severe course underwent little or no care." Not infrequently those who have diabetes outlive their normal expectation of life.

2. **Success Depends upon the Patient.**—Diabetes is a disease which depends upon the honesty and intelligence of the patient for successful treatment. It develops character, for to follow the rules of diet involves constant self-control. It is painful to see how frequently disobedience and ignorance are followed by a downward course.

3. **A Sugar-free Urine Spells Improvement.**—If sugar is entirely removed from the urine, the power of the pancreas to assimilate carbohydrate improves. If the urine is not free from sugar the patient is only holding his own, or more likely growing worse. The urine will become sugar-free, by giving this function of the pancreas less work—that is, giving the patient less carbohydrate and less food to eat.

4. **Treatment Depends upon Diet and Not Drugs.** — (*a*) **Weights and Measures Employed in Computing the Diet.** — The best diet for a patient is most readily determined by testing the effects of weighed quantities of various foods. The patient should learn how to do this for himself and should find out how much carbohydrate, protein and fat he is taking, and whether he can keep sugar-free upon it. He should own scales, unless his tolerance for carbohydrate is over 100 grams, and know how to use them and to compute the carbohydrate, protein, fat and calories in the diet, just as readily as he computes the cost of the food which he buys for his meals.

(*b*) **The Quantity of Food Required.**—The amount of food necessary for a patient is determined by his weight. The weight of a diabetic patient should always be less than his former greatest weight, because thus he can be assured that he is not overeating. In this respect it is better to emulate the Indian than the Eskimo. The individual 10 per cent and even 20 per cent below weight may not be a delight to our eyes, but if over thirty-five years of age and in this condition he is much more acceptable to the insurance company. It is often desirable for a patient to lose weight, but this should be undertaken only under the doctor's direction. Frequently it is only by losing weight that a patient regains the power to tolerate carbohydrate.

(*c*) **Distribution and Exchange of Carbohydrates.**—The carbohydrate in the diet should be divided between the three meals. Even if the 10 per cent, 15 per cent and 20 per cent vegetables are allowed, vegetables from the 5 per cent group should be taken as well. Usually it is permissible to substitute for a given quantity of 5 per cent vegetables one-half as much from the 10 per cent group, one-quarter as much from the 15 per cent, or one-sixth as much from the 20 per cent. Exchange vegetables for fruit only under advice. So-called diabetic foods often contain considerable quantities of carbohydrate, and usually contain so much protein and fat that they should not be taken by the patient without due allowance for the same. They should not be taken under any circumstances unless their composition is known.

(*d*) **Special Dietetic Rules.**—Eat too little rather than too much. With a return to normal weight sugar may appear.

All food must be eaten slowly, and the coarser the food, the more thoroughly it should be masticated.

If in doubt about a food, let it alone until you have found out whether it is allowed. Do not yield to the temptation of friends to break the diet, for if this is done the plan of treatment is upset, a week's time may be lost and several pounds of weight sacrificed.

Remember it is always possible to get articles of food which are included in a strict diabetic diet for a few meals, such as eggs, meat, butter, oil and even 5 per cent vegetables, fresh, raw or canned.

5. **Care of Teeth.**—Clean the teeth after each meal and have them cleaned by a dentist every one or two months. The teeth should always be kept in good condition. If they are to be extracted, take gas and oxygen, but no ether. Novocaine injected cautiously acts admirably.

6. **Care of Skin.**—The skin must be kept unusually clean. Take a tub bath daily, but avoid prolonged cold baths. Short cold baths are often desirable. Protect the skin from injuries. Caution chiropodists and manicurists not to draw a drop of blood. If any infection occurs, see a physician at once. Next to coma (acid poisoning) gangrene is the most dangerous foe of the diabetic.

7. **Treatment of Constipation.**—The bowels should move daily. Use an enema if necessary. Never purge the bowels, but simple laxatives, such as $\frac{1}{5}$ grain aloin, fluidextract cascara sagrada 10 to 30 drops, or compound rhubarb pills, are allowable. Bran muffins made with agar agar[1] (see p. 730) and coarse vegetables or fruit for breakfast may prove sufficient. If diarrhea occurs, go to bed, keep warm, and drink hot water.

8. **Exercise.**—Exercise freely for short periods six times a day. It is desirable to walk after meals and to arrange to get exercise

---

[1] Seaweed makes a satisfactory substitute.

44

for the upper part of the body as well as the lower.   If the accustomed exercise is not taken, eat less.

9. **Rest.**—Rest is essential.   A tired child is put to bed and
wakens refreshed; one of the most noted surgeons in our country
is not ashamed to lie down for fifteen minutes after his luncheon;
the best treatment for a failing heart in heart disease is to put its
owner in bed for a week.   Diabetic patients should rest often,
should never get tired and should avoid athletic contests.   The
diet is designed to give a rest to the pancreas.

Forget you have diabetes and rest yourself and your friends.
This is one reason for not using saccharin and the other is to avoid
the perpetuation of a sweet taste.

Wear warm clothes instead of staying by the radiator or in an
overheated room.

Mental diversion is desirable, but anxiety is harmful.

10. **Sleep.**—Sleep nine hours or more and get another hour of
rest by day.   Short periods of complete relaxation yield maximal
returns.

11. **Examination of Urine.**—To collect the twenty-four-hour
quantity of urine, discard that voided at 7.00 A.M., and then save
in a cool place all urine passed thereafter up to and including that
obtained at 7.00 A.M. the next morning.

The urine should be tested daily before breakfast, using the
combined night and morning specimen for the purpose or preferably the twenty-four-hour, mixed specimen.

12. **Prevention of Diabetic Coma.**—Not one patient in a hundred
has diabetic coma at the hospital and the reasons are simple.   If
a patient "feels sick" from any cause and always if he has fever
he must:

1. Go to bed, keep warm and get rested.
2. Be cared for by a nurse.
3. Eat less food and especially take little fat and protein,
    using orange juice or oatmeal water gruel for carbohydrate.
4. Drink liquids, 1 cupful an hour, unless excused by the
    nurse.   The liquids should be hot water, coffee, tea,
    broths.
5. Take an enema.
6. If at home send for a doctor who will first make the
    diagnosis, then protect his heart, may give him insulin
    and, if he cannot take water by mouth and retain it, may
    give it or salt solution (one teaspoonful to the pint) by
    rectum or under the skin or even wash out his stomach.

13. **Directions Regarding Use of Insulin.**—See p. 564.

TABLE 246.—SPECIMEN LEAF OF A BOOK CONSTRUCTED TO FACILITATE THE RECORDING OF DIABETIC STATISTICS.[1]

No.	First visit			Name	Address	Onset				Diagnosis Date		Death Date		Duration		Sex	S. M. W.	Race	Heredity	Familial	Etiology	Pulse	Blood-pressure	Weight			Height	Type of onset		Hospital	Cause of death	Distinctive features
	Year	Month	Day			Age		Date		Year	Month	Year	Month	Years	Months									Max.	Onset	1st visit						
						Years	Months	Year	Month																							

[1] Actual size of the page 13 x 8½ inches, and the headings cover two pages.

E. FIG. 31.—DIABETIC HISTORY CHART.

NAME   No   DATE

ADDRESS   AGE Yrs. Mos.   S M   M W   F   REF. BY DR.   ADDRESS

OCCUPATION   RACE   BORN Y   Mo

FAMILY HISTORY   F.   M.   Children / Spouse / Other relatives

Bro.   Sist.   Exercise   Sleep

HABITS. C₂H₅OH   Tobac.   C't'a or ven.   Malaria.   Meas.   Mumps.   Pert.

PAST HISTORY. S. F.   Typh.   Pneu.   R. F.   Chor.   Jaun.   Tonsil.   Diph.

ONSET. Date: Acute.   Gradual   SYMPT.   CAUSE OF EXAM.

SUGAR FIRST DISCOVERED.   Insurance / Routine

LAST PRIOR EXAM.   b. Heredity   1. Hereditary   2. Familial   c. Dietary excesses   d. Strenuous life   e. Nervous

a. Obesity   g. Arteriosclerosis   h. Syphilis   i. Traumatic   j. Pancreas, abd. pain   fatty stools

f. Infections   exophth.   tremor   nervousness   palp.   diarrhea   perspiration

k. Thyroid, size   adolescence   vom.   diab. incip.

l. Hypophysis, acromegaly   gigantism

m. Liver   n. Gout   o. Kidney   p. Gall-bladder

PREVIOUS TREATMENTS. RESULTS—

SYMPT. SINCE ONSET: Weight   Height   Date

a. Maximum: b. Loss of strength   f. Pains

At onset   c. Polyuria   g. Extremities

First visit   d. Polydipsia   h. Cramps

Substandard   e. Polyphagia   i. Mouth

j. Bowels

OTHER SYMPT.   N.   V.   P.   b. Circ.   D.   P.   e. Nervous

a. Digestive   D.   N.   d. Resp.   C.   S.   f. Vision

c. Renal   Vertigo

PRESENT COMPLAINT.

PHYS. EXAM.   General appearance   Eye grounds   Color of hair   Skin and mucous memb.
   Pupils and muscles   Glands: C.   A.   I.   Thyroid
   Hearing   Tonsils
   Pulse   Arteries   Breath: Acetone   Al. air: CO$_2$ Apparatus   Teeth
   Heart   Apex, size   Bl. pr. (recumbent): Syst.   Dias.   sounds   Breasts
   Lungs
   Abdomen   Liver   Edema   Spleen   Kidneys
   Genitals   Hernia   Knee-jerks

BLOOD.   WASSERMANN   Sugar: Per cent   Fasting   Method   CO$_2$ tension   N.P.N.   Urea N   Fat
                                        After food   Hours

URINE.   Date   Vol.   Reac.   Sp. gr.   Alb.   Nitrogen   Acetone   Diacetic   Ammonia
         Sugar: Reduction   Polar   Total gms.   Sed.

DISTINCTIVE FEATURES AND COMPLICATIONS.
   Hospital
   Operation
   Anesthetic
   Surgeon

F. FIG. 32.—HOSPITAL CHART.

ONSET
NET HEIGHT IN CENTIMETERS
NET WEIGHT IN KILOGRAMS
STANDARD WEIGHT IN KILOGRAMS

HOSPITAL

NAME

No.

Date.	Volume, cc.	Specific gravity.	Reaction.	Albumin.	Acetone.	Diacetic acid.	Sodium chloride, gm.	Nitrogen, gm.	Ammonia, total gm.	Sugar in urine. Reduction, per cent.	Sugar in urine. Total gm.	Diet in grams. Carbohydrate.	Diet in grams. Protein.	Diet in grams. Fat.	Diet in grams. Calories.	Diet in grams. Total glucose.	Glucose balance, gm.	Naked weight, lbs.	Non-protein nitrogen.	Bloor's blood fat, per cent.	Blood sugar, per cent.	Blood CO_2 volume, per cent.	Alveolar air, CO_2 mm. Hg.	Insulin. Units.	Insulin. Prep No.	Insulin. Time.

G.   Fig. 33.—Patient's Chart.[1]

No.   Name

Date.	Urine.				Weight.	Diet in grams.				Insulin units.	Breakfast.	Insulin units.	Dinner.	Insulin units.	Supper.
	Vol.	Diac.	Sugar.			Carb.	Prot.	Fat.	Cal.						
			Per cent.	Total gm.											

[1] The spacing on the original chart is so arranged as to allow for recording the various quantities of food eaten at the different meals.

H. Fig. 34.—

NAME OF PATIENT   NURSE

DATE.	ORDERS.	BREAKFAST.	FORE-NOON.	DINNER.	AFTER-NOON.	SUPPER.	NIGHT.

WATER, CLEAR BROTHS, COFFEE, TEA, COCOA SHELLS AND CRACKED COCOA CAN BE TAKEN WITHOUT ALLOWANCE FOR FOOD CONTENT. (FOODS ARRANGED APPROXIMATELY ACCORDING TO CONTENT OF CARBOHYDRATES.)

VEGETABLES
(Fresh or canned.)

5%*	10%*	15% ±	20% ±
Lettuce	Tomatoes	String beans	Potatoes
Cucumbers	Brussels	Green peas	Shell beans
Spinach	sprouts	Artichokes	Baked beans
Asparagus	Water cress	Parsnips	Green corn
Rhubarb	Sea kale	Turnip	Boiled rice
Endive	Okra	Kohl-Rabi	Boiled
Marrow	Cauliflower	Squash	Canned	macaroni
Sorrel	Egg plant	Beets	lima beans
Sauerkraut	Cabbage	Carrots	
Beet greens	Radishes	Onions	
Dandelion	Leeks	Green peas	
greens	String beans	canned	
Swiss chard	canned		
Celery	Broccoli		
Mushrooms	Artichokes		
	canned		

FRUITS

Ripe olives (20 per cent) fat	Watermelon	Raspberries	Plums
Grape fruit	Strawberries	Currants	Bananas
	Lemons	Apricots	Prunes
	Cranberries	Pears	
	Peaches	Apples	
	Pineapple	Huckleberries	
	Blackberries	Blueberries	
	Gooseberries	Cherries	
	Oranges		

* Reckon available carbohydrates in vegetables of 5% group as 3%, of 10% group as 6%.

30 grams (1 ounce) contain approximately:	Carbohydrate, gm.	Protein, gm.	Fat, gm.	Calories.
Vegetables, 5 per cent	1	0.5	0	6
Vegetables, 10 per cent	2	0.5	0	10
Shredded wheat	23	3	1	104
Uneedas, two	10	1	1	53
Potato	6	1	0	28
Bread	18	3	0	84
Oatmeal, dry weight	20	5	2	118
Oysters, six	4	6	1	49
Milk	1.5	1	1	19
Meat (cooked, lean)	0	8	5	77
Fish	0	6	0	24
Chicken (cooked, lean)	0	8	3	59
Egg (one)	0	6	6	78
Cheese	0	8	11	131
Bacon	0	5	15	155
Cream, 20 per cent	1	1	6	62
Cream, 40 per cent	1	1	12	116
Butter	0	0	25	225
Oil	0	0	30	270

1 gram protein, 4 calories.
1 " carbohydrate, 4 "
1 " fat, 9 "
1 " alcohol, 7 "
6.25 grams protein contain 1 gram nitrogen.

1 kilogram = 2.2 pounds.
30 grams (gm.) or cubic centimeters (cc) = 1 ounce.
A patient at rest requires 25 calories per kilogram body weight; approximately 1 calorie per kilo per hour.

Thomas Groom & Co., 105 State St., Boston

SECTION VIII.

FOODS AND THEIR COMPOSITION.

A. DIABETIC FOODS.

THE improvement in the treatment of diabetes owes much to the recent dissemination of knowledge regarding the composition of foods. To the United States Government we are indebted for an excellent monograph by Atwater and Bryant entitled "The Chemical Composition of American Food Materials, Bulletin No. 28, Revised Edition," which was first issued in 1906. This can be purchased by sending ten cents in coin to the Superintendent of Documents, Washington, D. C.

Diabetics everywhere throughout the world owe a debt of gratitude to Dr. W. A. Orton of the U. S. Department of Agriculture for his earnest endeavor to increase the number of agreeable vegetables. For this purpose he has brought to Washington specimens from all over the world. It is to be hoped that he will shortly publish a monograph giving the results of his work. Already there has appeared an article on the subject.[1] In England, also, the subject of gardening and vegetables for diabetics has been seriously considered by Spriggs.[2]

The State of Connecticut, from its Agricultural Experiment Station in New Haven, has also published excellent special reports on diabetic foods, and from year to year adds analyses of new preparations. So far these have been distributed upon request.

Whereas the analyses of many so-called diabetic foods are recorded, no special food is recommended. Each physician must decide the merits of any particular food for himself. As a matter of fact no special diabetic food is used at the hospital. This is not meant to disparage such foods but to show that they are accessories without which the diabetic can get along very well.

The medical profession is under great obligation to the Connecticut Agricultural Experiment Station for having provided for

---

[1] Orton, W. A.: Am. Jour. Med. Sci., 1921, **162**, 498.
[2] Spriggs, E. I.: Duff House Papers, Henry Frowde, London, 1920, **1**.

work of this character, and I regret very deeply that the appreciation of physicians and diabetic patients cannot be shown in some tangible way. Prof. Street formerly and Prof. Bailey recently have been kindness itself not alone to me but to many inquisitive patients.

What is a Diabetic Food?—The definition of a "diabetic" food formulated by the Joint Committee on Definitions and Standards is as follows:

"*Diabetic Food.*—Although most foods may be suitable under certain conditions for the use of persons suffering from diabetes, the term 'diabetic' as applied to food indicates a considerable lessening of the carbohydrates found in ordinary products of the same class, and this belief is fostered by many manufacturers on their labels and in their advertising literature. A 'diabetic' food contains not more than half as much glycogenic carbohydrates as the normal food of the same class. Any statement on the label which gives the impression that any single food in unlimited quantity is suitable for the diabetic patient is false and misleading."

Prof. Street very properly lays down the following detailed requirements which a diabetic food should fulfil:

1. It should contain very much less carbohydrate than found in a normal food of the same class—certainly not over half as much.

2. The label should bear a correct statement of the percentages of protein, fat and carbohydrate present.

3. The amounts of the different carbohydrates present should be declared on the label, *i. e.*, starch, sucrose, levulose, lactose, etc.

4. The processes of manufacture should be so standardized that uniformity of composition, within reasonable limits, will be maintained from year to year.

5. No statement should be placed on the label which would give the impression that any food in unlimited quantity is suitable for a diabetic patient.

6. In the advertisements of these foods emphasis should be put on the carbohydrate content rather than on the amount of protein present.

The narrow confines of the diabetic diet have greatly stimulated the manufacture of so-called diabetic foods. These are often serviceable, but are to be employed with discretion. Their use should be discouraged at the beginning of treatment. The patient should never become dependent upon special diabetic foods, for they are often unobtainable, always make him conspicuous, and when he acquires a disgust for foods of this class it is all the harder to abide by the original diet. When the patient buys one of these foods, unfortunately he is often given a list of other diabetic foods and a new diabetic diet list, and confusion in the diet frequently results. The patients under my care who have done best either never use special diabetic foods or only a few varieties.

The high content of protein is one of the most serious drawbacks to diabetic foods. Formerly when it was not realized that from 100 grams protein 58 grams of carbohydrate could be formed, these special foods with low actual carbohydrate content were considered a great boon. Today we look at the matter differently. The makers modernized their substitutes for breads when they lowered the caloric content by the omission of fat. It is apparent, however, that it is the province of the physician, not of the patient, to determine this tolerance; and, furthermore, it is evident from the analyses that the mere calling a product a "diabetic food" by no means establishes its right to such a name or its usefulness to the diabetic. Foods containing 60 or 70 per cent of carbohydrates are no more "diabetic foods" than potatoes, rice, or oatmeal and are no more entitled to that name.

B. COMPOSITION OF NORMAL FOODS.

The following food tables were prepared for me under the supervision of Prof. E. Monroe Bailey of the Connecticut Agricultural Experiment Station situated in New Haven, Connecticut. Prof. Bailey makes the following comments upon Tables 247 and 248.

"In the table 'Composition of Normal Foods' many of the analyses are based largely on the authority of Atwater and Bryant's compilation. In substituting or adding other analyses frequent reference has been made to Prof. Sherman's 'Food Products'[1] which is also largely quoted from the authority just named. Leach, 'Food Inspection and Analysis'[2] and various reports and bulletins of the Connecticut Experiment Station have also been freely consulted. Some new analyses made by this Station, not heretofore published, and unpublished analyses made for Dr. W. A. Orton in the Bureau of Chemistry of the U. S. Department of Agriculture are included.

"The general plan of arrangement of items in the table has been to present those foods which are essentially protein, fat and carbohydrate in the order named. In choosing analyses many discrepancies are found between the various authors. These are due partly to different methods of analysis and different forms of expression but more frequently, no doubt, to variations in the composition of the subject material itself. In such cases the analysis which represents the average of the greatest number of individual

[1] The Macmillan Company, New York, 1918.
[2] Wiley & Son, New York.

analyses or the one which, for one reason or another, seems preferable, has been used.

"The significance of the term *protein* in this table is *nitrogen* × *6.25* except in the case of milk and milk products where the factor 6.38 is more correct and has been used. *Fat* means substances soluble in ether or 'ether extract.' It is probable that many of the figures for fat in baked products are too low. Where new analyses have been inserted fat has been determined by an improved method,[1] which gives results considerably higher. *The term 'carbohydrate' is to be accepted generally in the sense of 'nitrogen-free extract' which is the percentage obtained by deducting the sum of the percentages of water, ash, protein, fat and fiber from 100 per cent.* This proximate group includes the more readily assimilable carbohydrates, such as starch, dextrins, maltose, glucose, sucrose, invert sugar, raffinose, lactose and some other less common sugars, and also carbohydrates of doubtful or undetermined availability in human metabolism such as hemicellulose complexes, vegetable gums, mucilages, etc. A critical study of some of these less familiar carbohydrates has been made by Swartz.[2] Whenever the sense of 'carbohydrate' in the table is known to be other than that just stated the explanation is given in a footnote.

"In Table 248, analyses of so-called diabetic foods, etc., are given. These are taken largely from our Bulletins 220 and 236 with the addition of new analyses made recently and not yet published and with the deletion of most of the analyses made before 1913. In many cases there are no new analyses to substitute for those thus omitted but very old analyses of commerical products of this kind serve no useful purpose. There is not the same objection to old analyses of staple articles of food.

"The general significance of the terms protein, fat and carbohydrate in this table is the same as already explained for normal foods. *Protein*, however, in those products known or declared to be made from gluten, has been estimated on the basis of the factor 5.7 and under 'Protein Preparations' protein in casein products has been estimated using the factor 6.38. The *carbohydrate* group is subdivided into two parts but it should be understood that total carbohydrate is the sum of the two. The idea of the separation is to show how much of the total carbohydrate is available, the figure in the column headed 'starch' representing this available portion so far as it has been determined or can be stated. Thus Barker's gluten Food A contains 12.4 per cent of total carbohydrate; 2.6 per cent is certainly available but the availability of the 9.8 per cent has not been determined. Wherever the figure in the

---

[1] Connecticut Exp. Station Bull., 1917, **200**, 133.
[2] Swartz: Trans. Connecticut Acad. Arts and Sci., 1911, **16**, 247.

starch column includes water-soluble carbohydrate, as for example, Cheltine Diabetic Food, the figure given probably represents all of the carbohydrate that is utilized in human digestion.

"Calories have been calculated on the basis of total carbohydrate in the conventional way. In the Cellu and Cellu-Bran products of the Womans' Baking Company the 'fat' is largely or entirely mineral oil and unavailable as is also probably much of the carbohydrate and therefore calories have not been calculated.

"In the 'Reference' column are given the dates of analyses. The symbols following the dates refer to analyses taken from Connecticut Experiment Station Bulletin 220."

TABLE 247.—COMPOSITION OF NORMAL FOODS.

MEAT PRODUCTS.

Name and description of food.	Protein, per cent.	Fat, per cent.	Carbohydrate, per cent.	Calories, per 100 gms.
Beef, fresh:				
Brisket, medium fat, edible portion .	15.8	28.5	..	319
Chuck rib, edible portion, all analyses .	19.0	13.4	..	197
Flank, edible portion, all analyses . .	19.6	21.1	..	268
Loin, edible portion, all analyses . .	19.0	19.1	..	247
Ribs, edible portion, all analyses . .	17.8	24.6	..	293
Shoulder and clod, edible portion, all analyses	20.0	10.3	..	173
Miscellaneous cuts, free from visible fat	22.4	2.9	..	116
Brain, edible portion	8.8	9.3	..	119
Heart, edible portion	16.0	20.4	..	248
Kidney, as purchased	13.7	1.9	Trace	72
Liver, as purchased	20.2	3.1	2.5[1]	119
Lungs, as purchased	16.4	3.2	..	94
Marrow, as purchased	2.2	92.8	..	844
Sweetbreads, as purchased	16.8	12.1	..	176
Suet, as purchased	4.7	81.8	..	755
Tongue, edible portion	18.9	9.2	..	158
Beef, cooked:				
Roast	22.3	28.6	..	347
Steak, round	27.6	7.7	..	180
sirloin	23.9	10.2	..	187
tenderloin	23.5	20.4	..	278
Beef, canned:				
Corned[2]	26.6	11.4	..	209
Dried and smoked[3]	32.6	7.5	..	198
Kidneys, stewed	18.4	5.1	2.1	128
Luncheon beef	27.6	15.9	..	254
Roast	25.9	14.8	..	237
Tongue, ground	21.4	25.1	..	312
whole	19.5	23.2	..	287
Tripe	16.8	8.5	..	144
Beef, corned and pickled:				
Corned beef, all analyses, edible portion	15.6	26.2	..	298
Spiced beef, rolled	12.0	51.4	..	511
Tongue, edible portion	12.8	20.5	..	236
Tripe	11.7	1.2	Trace	58

[1] Largely, or in part, glycogen.
[2] Average, 3.4 per cent salt (sodium chloride).
[3] Average, 9.7 per cent salt (sodium chloride).

TABLE 247.—COMPOSITION OF NORMAL FOODS.—(Continued.)

MEAT PRODUCTS—Continued.

Name and description of food.	Protein, per cent.	Fat, per cent.	Carbo-hydrate, per cent.	Calories, per 100 gms.
Beef, dried, salted, smoked, edible portion .	30.0	6.5	..	179
Veal, fresh:				
Breast, edible portion, all analyses . .	20.3	11.0	..	180
Chuck, edible portion, all analyses .	19.7	5.8	..	131
Flank, edible portion, all analyses .	20.1	12.7	..	195
Leg, edible portion, all analyses . .	20.7	6.7	..	143
cutlets, edible portion	20.3	7.7	..	151
Loin, edible portion, all analyses . .	19.9	10.0	..	170
Heart, as purchased	16.8	9.6	..	154
Kidney, as purchased	16.9	6.4	..	125
Liver, as purchased	19.0	5.3	..	124
Lungs, as purchased	17.1	5.0	..	113
Lamb, fresh:				
Breast, edible portion	19.1	23.6	..	289
Leg, hind, medium fat, edible portion .	19.2	16.5	..	225
Loin, without kidney and tallow, edible portion	18.7	28.3	..	330
Shoulder, edible portion	18.1	29.7	..	340
Lamb, cooked:				
Chops, broiled, edible portion . . .	21.7	29.9	..	356
Leg, roast	19.7	12.7	..	193
Lamb, canned:				
Tongue, spiced, cooked, edible portion	13.9	17.8	..	216
Mutton, fresh:				
Chuck, edible portion, all analyses . .	14.6	36.8	..	390
Leg, hind, medium fat, edible portion .	18.5	18.0	..	236
Loin, without kidney and tallow, edible portion	16.0	33.1	..	362
Shoulder, medium fat, edible portion .	17.7	19.9	..	250
Heart, as purchased	16.9	12.6	..	181
Kidney, as purchased	16.5	3.2	..	95
Liver, as purchased	23.1	9.0	5.0[1]	193
Lungs, as purchased	20.2	2.8	..	106
Mutton, cooked:				
Leg roast, edible portion	25.0	22.6	..	303
Mutton, canned:				
Corned	28.8	22.8	..	320
Tongue	24.4	24.0	..	314
Pork, fresh:				
Ham, lean	25.0	14.4	..	230
Ham, medium fat, edible portion . .	15.3	28.9	..	321
Head cheese, edible portion	19.5	33.8	..	382
Loin (chops), lean, edible portion . .	20.3	19.0	..	252
Loin (chops), medium fat, edible portion	16.6	20.1	..	337
Shoulder, edible portion	13.3	34.2	..	361
Side, lard and other fat included, edible portion	9.4	61.7	..	593
Side, lard and kidneys not included, edible portion	9.1	55.3	..	534
Brains, as purchased	11.7	10.3	..	140
Heart, as purchased	17.1	6.3	..	125
Kidney, as purchased	15.5	4.8	0.7	108
Liver, as purchased	21.3	4.5	1.4[1]	131
Lungs, as purchased	11.9	4.0	..	84

[1] Largely, or in part, glycogen.

TABLE 247.—COMPOSITION OF NORMAL FOODS.—(*Continued.*)

MEAT PRODUCTS—*Continued.*

Name and description of food.	Protein, per cent.	Fat, per cent.	Carbo-hydrate, per cent.	Calories, per 100 gms.
Pork, pickled, salted or smoked:[1]				
Ham, lean, smoked, edible portion . .	19.8	20.8	..	266
Ham, medium fat, smoked, edible portion	16.3	38.8	..	414
Ham, luncheon, cooked	22.5	21.0	..	279
Shoulder, medium fat, smoked, edible portion	15.9	32.5	..	356
Pig's tongue, pickled, edible portion .	17.7	19.8	..	249
Pig's feet, pickled, edible portion . .	16.3	14.8	..	198
Salt pork, clear fat	1.9	86.2	..	783
Bacon, smoked, all analyses, edible portion	10.5	64.8	..	625
Ham, deviled	19.0	34.1	..	383
Sausage:				
Arles, edible portion	26.8	50.6	..	563
Bologna, edible portion	18.7	17.6	0.6[2]	236
Frankfort	19.6	18.6	1.1[3]	250
Pork, as purchased	13.0	44.2	1.1[4]	454
Deerfoot Farm, cooked (analysis furnished by manufacturer)	19.9	54.2	0.3	569
Pork and beef, as purchased . . .	19.4	24.1	..	295

POULTRY.

Poultry, fresh:				
Chicken, broilers, edible portion . .	21.5	2.5	..	109
liver, as purchased . . .	22.4	4.2	2.4[5]	137
Fowls, edible portion	19.3	16.3	..	224
Goose, edible portion	16.3	36.2	..	391
Goose liver, edible portion	16.6	15.9	3.7[5]	224
Turkey, edible portion	21.1	22.9	..	291

FISH PRODUCTS.

Fish, fresh:				
Alewife, whole, edible portion . . .	19.4	4.9	..	122
Bass, whole, edible portion	19.0	1.4	..	89
Bluefish, edible portion	19.4	1.2	..	88
Butterfish, edible portion	18.0	11.0	..	171
Cod, edible portion	16.7	0.3	..	70
Eels, salt water, edible portion . . .	18.6	9.1	..	156
Haddock, edible portion	17.2	0.3	..	72
Halibut, edible portion	18.6	5.2	..	121
Herring, edible portion	19.5	7.1	..	142
Mackerel, edible portion	18.7	7.1	..	139
Perch, edible portion	19.0	2.4	..	98
Porgy, edible portion	18.6	5.1	..	120
Salmon, edible portion	22.0	12.8	..	203
Shad, edible portion	18.8	9.5	..	161
Shad roe, as purchased	20.9	3.8	2.6	128
Smelt, edible portion	17.6	1.8	..	87
Trout, brook, edible portion . . .	19.2	2.1	..	96
Trout, lake, edible portion	17.8	10.3	..	164
Whitefish, edible portion	22.9	6.5	..	150

[1] The range of salt content for cured pork products may be taken as 3 to 5 per cent.
[2] Carbohydrate range, 0.2 to 3.1 per cent.
[3] Carbohydrate range, 0.0 to 6.6 per cent.
[4] Carbohydrate range, 0.0 to 8.6 per cent.   [5] Largely, or in part, glycogen.

45

TABLE 247.—COMPOSITION OF NORMAL FOODS.—(*Continued.*)

FISH PRODUCTS—*Continued.*

Name and description of food.	Protein, per cent.	Fat, per cent.	Carbo-hydrate, per cent.	Calories, per 100 gms.
Fish, preserved or canned:				
Cod, salt, "boneless," as purchased[1] .	27.7	0.3	..	114
Halibut, smoked, edible portion[2] . .	20.7	15.0	..	218
Herring, smoked, edible portion[3] . .	36.9	15.8	..	290
Mackerel, salt, edible portion[4] . . .	21.1	22.6	..	288
salt, canned, as purchased .	19.6	8.7	..	157
salt, canned in oil, edible portion	25.4	14.1	..	229
Salmon, canned, edible portion . . .	21.8	12.1	..	196
Sardines, canned, edible portion . .	23.0	19.7	..	269
Sturgeon, caviare, preserved, Russian, as purchased	30.0	19.7	7.6	328
Tunny (tuna), as purchased . . .	21.7	4.1	..	124
canned in oil, edible portion	23.8	20.0	0.6	278
Shellfish, etc., fresh:				
Clams, long, in shell, edible portion .	8.6	1.0	2.0[5]	51
round, in shell, edible portion .	6.5	0.4	4.2[5]	46
Crabs, hard shell, whole, edible portion	16.6	2.0	1.2[5]	89
Crayfish, edible portion	16.0	0.5	1.0[5]	73
Lobster, edible portion	16.4	1.8	0.4[5]	83
Mussels, in shell, edible portion . .	8.7	1.1	4.1[5]	61
Oysters, in shell, edible portion . . .	6.2	1.2	3.7[5]	50
Scallops, as purchased	14.8	0.1	3.4[5]	74
Terrapin, edible portion	21.2	3.5	..	116
Turtle, green, edible portion . . .	19.8	0.5	..	84
Shellfish, etc., canned:				
Clams, round, as purchased	8.3	0.4	2.7[5]	48
long, as purchased	8.9	0.8	0.9[5]	46
Crabs, as purchased	15.8	1.5	0.7[5]	80
Lobster, as purchased	18.1	1.1	0.5[5]	84
Oysters, as purchased	8.8	2.4	3.9[5]	72
Shrimp, as purchased	25.4	1.0	0.2	111

AMPHIBIA.

Frog's legs, edible portion	15.5	0.2	..	64

GELATIN.

Gelatin	84.2[6]	0.1	None	338

EGGS.

Eggs, fresh:[7]				
Hen, whole egg, edible portion . . .	13.4	10.5	..	148
white	12.3	0.2	..	51
yolk	15.7	33.3	..	363

[1] Contains 14.7 per cent ash, largely salt.
[2] Contains 15.0 per cent ash, largely (12.1 per cent) salt.
[3] Contains 13.2 per cent ash, largely (11.7 per cent) salt.
[4] Contains 13.2 per cent ash, largely (9.2 per cent), salt.
[5] Largely, or in part, glycogen.
[6] Nitrogen × 5.55.
[7] In shell eggs the shell comprises from 10 to 17 per cent of the weight of the whole egg; water content ranges from 60 to 67 per cent. Sea-turtle eggs contain about 76 per cent water.

TABLE 247.—COMPOSITION OF NORMAL FOODS.—(*Continued.*)

EGGS—*Continued.*

Name and description of food.	Protein, per cent.	Fat, per cent.	Carbo-hydrate, per cent.	Calories, per 100 gms.
Eggs, fresh.				
Duck, whole egg, edible portion	13.3	14.5	..	184
white	11.1	Trace	..	44
yolk	16.8	36.2	..	393
Goose, whole egg, edible portion	13.8	14.4	..	185
white	11.6	Trace	..	46
yolk	17.3	36.2	..	395
Turkey, whole egg, edible portion	13.4	11.2	..	154
white	11.5	Trace	..	46
yolk	17.4	32.9	..	366
Guinea fowl, whole egg, edible portion	13.5	12.0	..	162
white	11.6	Trace	..	46
yolk	16.7	31.8	..	353
Plover, whole egg, edible portion	10.7	11.7	..	148
Turtle, fresh water	18.1	11.1	..	172
sea	18.8	9.8	..	163
Eggs, edible portion, cooked:				
Hen, boiled	13.2	12.0	..	161
whites	12.3	0.2	..	51
yolks	15.7	33.3	..	363
Eggs, dehydrated, average	40.6	43.7	..	556

DAIRY PRODUCTS, ETC.

Milk:				
Milk, whole	3.3	4.0	4.8	68
condensed (evaporated, concentrated)	6.9	8.2	9.9	141
sweetened, condensed (sweetened evaporated, sweetened concentrated)	7.9	9.0	54.6[1]	331
skimmed	3.4	0.3	5.1	37
sweetened, condensed	9.1	1.0	59.1[2]	282
Buttermilk	3.6	0.5	4.1	35
Kephir	3.1	2.0	1.6	37
Kumiss[3]	2.8	2.0	5.4	51
Cream, "heavy" (approximately 40 per cent)	2.1	41.0	1.5	383
"light" (approximately 20 per cent)	2.8	22.0	2.7	220
Whey	1.0	0.3	5.0	27
Milk powder (dried milk):				
From whole milk	25.3	25.3	37.5	479
From partly skimmed milk (mammala type)	25.8	14.5	49.9	433
From skimmed milk, average	34.6	1.9	50.9	359
Malted milk (milk powder with malted cereal) average	13.8	6.8	71.9	404

[1] Cane sugar, 40.6 per cent; milk sugar, 14 per cent.
[2] Cane sugar, 40.9 per cent; milk sugar, 18.2 per cent.
[3] According to Van Slyke (Leach: Food Inspection and Analysis, p. 174), Kumiss, from cows' milk, contains lactose, 5 per cent; protein, 4.1 per cent; fat (calculated), 1.2 per cent.

TABLE 247.—COMPOSITION OF NORMAL FOODS.—(*Continued.*)

DAIRY PRODUCTS, ETC.—*Continued.*

Name and description of food.	Protein, per cent.	Fat, per cent.	Carbo-hydrate, per cent.	Calories per 100 gms.
Cheese:				
American, pale	28.8	35.9	0.3	440
red	29.6	38.3	..	463
Camembert	21.0	21.7	..	279
Cheddar	26.4	32.7	3.0	412
Cheshire	32.5	26.1	4.5	383
Cottage	20.9	1.0	4.3	110
Dutch	37.1	17.7	..	308
Edam	24.1	30.3	4.6	388
Full cream	25.4	30.3	2.0	382
Limburger	23.0	29.4	0.4	358
Neufchatel	18.7	27.4	1.5	327
Pineapple	29.9	38.9	2.6	480
Roquefort	22.6	29.5	1.8	363
Skimmed milk	31.5	16.4	2.2	282
Swiss	27.6	34.9	1.3	430
Ice cream, typical	3.8	12.6[1]	19.6	207

FATS AND OILS.

	Protein, per cent.	Fat, per cent.	Carbo-hydrate, per cent.	Calories per 100 gms.
Fats and Oils:[1]				
Butter,[2] average	1.5	84.6	None	767
Oleomargarine,[3] average	0.8	92.4	None	835
Nut margarine,[4] average	1.4	84.8	None	769
Salad oils and cooking fat, typical	Trace	99.7	None	897

SOUPS AND BROTHS.

	Protein, per cent.	Fat, per cent.	Carbo-hydrate, per cent.	Calories per 100 gms.
Soups, home-made:				
Bean	3.2	1.4	9.4	63
Beef	4.4	0.4	1.1	26
Chicken	10.5	0.8	2.4	59
Clam chowder	1.8	0.8	6.7	41
Meat stew	4.6	4.3	5.5	79
Soups, broths, etc., canned:				
Asparagus, cream of	2.5	3.2	5.5	61
Bouillon, beef	2.2	0.1	0.2	11
clam, typical	1.0	0.1	0.6	7
Celery, cream of	2.1	2.8	5.0	54
Chicken gumbo	3.8	0.9	4.7	42
soup	3.6	0.1	1.5	21
Consommé	1.4	0.1	0.4	8
Corn, cream of	2.5	1.9	7.8	58
Julienne	2.7	..	0.5	13
Mock turtle	3.0	1.0	5.7	44
Mulligatawny	3.7	0.1	5.7	39
Oxtail, edible portion	3.7	1.3	7.1	55
Pea soup	3.6	0.7	7.6	51
Pea, cream of green	2.6	2.7	5.7	58
Tomato soup	1.8	1.1	5.6	40
Turtle, green	6.1	1.9	3.9	57
Vegetable	2.9	..	0.5	14

[1] Standards for fat in different States vary from 7 to 14 per cent.

[2] Average salt content, 1.6 per cent; range, 0.2 to 4.1 per cent.

[3] Average ash content (largely salt), 0.9 per cent; range, 0.4 to 3.1 per cent.

[4] Average ash content (largely salt), 2.9 per cent; range, 1.1 to 6.1 per cent.

TABLE 247.—COMPOSITION OF NORMAL FOODS.—(*Continued.*)

SOUPS AND BROTHS—*Concluded.*

Name and description of food.	Protein, per cent.	Fat, per cent.	Carbo-hydrate, per cent.	Calories, per 100 gms.
Bouillon cubes:				
As purchased, average analysis[1]	11.4	1.8	5.8	85
Prepared as directed, average analysis[2]	0.2	Trace	0.1	1
Clam extract:				
As purchased	23.2	0.2	11.8	142
Prepared as directed[3]	0.5	Trace	0.3	3
Yeast extract, as purchased	31.3	0.2	12.5	177
CEREAL PRODUCTS, ETC.				
Alimentary pastes:				
Macaroni	13.4	0.9	74.1	358
cooked	3.0	1.5	15.8	91
Noodles	11.7	1.0	75.2	357
Spaghetti	12.1	0.4	75.9	356
Vermicelli	10.9	2.0	72.0	350
Bread, soft:				
Bread, alfalfa	10.6	1.3	64.0	310
corn (Johnnycake)	7.9	4.7	46.3[4]	259
Graham	8.9	1.8	51.0	256
peanut	33.6	12.8	20.0	330
rye	9.0	0.6	52.7	252
whole rye	11.9	0.6	35.0	193
rye and wheat	11.9	0.3	51.5[1]	256
wheat, average of many analyses	9.2	1.3	52.6	259
wheat, whole	9.7	0.9	48.5	241
Bread, hard, and crackers:				
Bread, white, toasted	11.5	1.6	61.2	305
Zwieback	9.8	9.9	73.5[4]	422
Crackers, Boston (split)	11.0	8.5	70.3	402
butter	9.6	10.1	71.2	414
cream	9.7	12.1	69.1	424
egg	12.6	14.0	66.2	441
flatbread	14.9	0.5	73.6[4]	359
Graham	10.0	9.4	72.3	414
oatmeal	11.8	11.1	67.1	416
oyster	11.3	10.5	70.3	421
pilot	11.1	5.0	73.9	385
pretzels	9.7	3.9	72.3	363
saltines	10.6	12.7	68.0	429
soda	9.8	9.1	72.8	412
water	11.7	5.0	75.3	393
Pastry, etc.				
Cake, coffee	7.1	7.5	62.8	347
cup	5.9	9.0	68.2	377
frosted	5.9	9.0	64.8[4]	364
fruit	5.9	10.9	64.1	378
gingerbread	5.8	9.0	62.4	354
sponge	6.3	10.7	65.9[4]	385
Cookies	7.0	9.7	73.2	408
Doughnuts	6.7	21.0	52.4	425
Fig bars	4.6	6.6	68.1	350
Ginger snaps	6.5	8.6	75.3	405
Lady fingers	8.8	5.0	70.4	362
Macaroons	6.5	15.2	64.1	419

[1] Average salt content, 70.2 per cent.

[2] Average cube weighs 3.8 gms.; 1 cup of broth is assumed to weigh 240 gms.; salt content of prepared broth, 1.1 per cent.

[3] Salt content, 0.4 per cent.

[4] Includes fiber.

TABLE 247.—COMPOSITION OF NORMAL FOODS.—(Continued.)
CEREAL PRODUCTS, ETC.—Continued.

Name and description of food.	Protein, per cent.	Fat, per cent.	Carbo-hydrate, per cent.	Calories, per 100 gms.
Pastry, etc.—Continued:				
Pie, apple	3.1	9.8	42.8[1]	272
cream	4.4	11.4	51.2[1]	325
custard	4.2	6.3	26.1[1]	178
lemon	3.6	10.1	37.4[1]	255
mince	5.8	12.3	38.1[1]	286
raisin	3.0	11.3	47.2[1]	303
squash	4.4	8.4	21.7[1]	180
Pudding, Indian meal	5.5	4.8	27.5[1]	175
rice custard	4.0	4.6	31.4[1]	183
tapioca	3.3	3.2	28.2[1]	155
Wafers, miscellaneous	8.7	8.6	74.1	409
vanilla	6.6	14.0	71.3	438
Breakfast foods:				
Barley preparations:				
barley crystals	11.5	1.3	75.2	359
cream of barley	11.1	1.6	76.2	364
pearled barley	9.5	0.9	76.2	351
Corn (maize) preparations:				
Ceraline, corn meal, hominy, average of 9 brands	8.9	1.2	76.4	352
flakes, crisps, puffs, etc., average of 8 brands	7.4	0.3	79.2	349
hominy, cooked (79 per cent water)	2.2	0.2	17.8	82
pop corn	10.7	5.0	77.3	397
Oat preparations:				
oatmeal, groats, etc., average of 5 analyses	14.6	7.7	65.1	388
rolled oats, crushed oats, oat flakes, average of 12 analyses	15.4	6.8	64.1	379
oatmeal, boiled (85 per cent water)	2.8	0.5	11.5[1]	62
oatmeal, gruel (92 per cent water)	1.2	0.4	6.3[1]	34
oatmeal water (96 per cent water)	0.7	0.1	2.9	15
Rice preparations:				
rice flakes, puffs, etc., average of 7 analyses	8.2	0.2	79.8	354
rice, boiled (73 per cent water)	2.8	0.1	24.4	110
Rye preparations:				
cream of rye	12.0	1.6	71.9	350
rye flakes	11.4	1.5	76.2	364
Wheat preparations:				
cracked and crushed	11.1	1.7	73.8	355
Farina	11.0	1.4	75.9	360
flakes	13.4	1.4	72.5	356
parched or toasted	13.6	2.4	73.7	371
Shredded	10.5	1.4	76.2	359
Flours, meals, etc.:				
Barley flour	12.3	2.4	71.3	356
Buckwheat flour	6.4	1.2	77.5	346
Corn flour	8.5	2.1	76.0	357
Corn meal	9.2	1.9	74.4	352
Oat flour	15.1	6.4	65.7	381
Potato flour	0.5	0.3	83.0	337
Rice flour	7.3	0.6	79.3	352
Rye flour	6.8	0.9	78.3	349

[1] Includes fiber.

TABLE 247.—COMPOSITION OF NORMAL FOODS.—(*Continued.*)

CEREAL PRODUCTS, ETC.—*Concluded.*

Name and description of food.	Protein, per cent.	Fat, per cent.	Carbohydrate, per cent.	Calories, per 100 gms.
Flours, meals, etc.:				
Rye meal	13.6	2.0	69.7	351
Soy-bean flour	42.5	19.9	24.3	446
Wheat flour, entire	13.8	1.9	71.0	356
Wheat flour, Graham	13.3	2.2	69.5	351
Wheat flour, patent, average	11.4	1.0	74.8	354

VEGETABLES.

	Protein, per cent.	Fat, per cent.	Carbohydrate, per cent.	Calories, per 100 gms.
Vegetables, fresh (unless otherwise stated):				
Artichokes	2.6	0.2	15.9[1]	76
Jerusalem	2.9	0.1	16.4[1]	78
Asparagus	1.8	0.2	2.4	19
Basella	2.5	0.5	1.7	21
Beans, butter	9.4	0.6	29.1[2]	159
cranberry, young pods	0.4	None	0.6	4
medium	1.3	0.6	1.7	17
fancy	1.0	0.1	2.1	13
Lima	7.1	0.7	20.3	116
refugee, young pods	0.5	None	0.8	5
medium	1.3	0.1	3.0	18
fancy	1.1	0.1	1.4	11
string (carbohydrate range, 3.9 to 10 per cent)	2.3	0.3	5.5	34
string, cooked	0.8	1.1	1.9	21
Beets (carbohydrate range, 6 to 10 per cent)	1.6	0.1	8.8	43
cooked	2.3	0.1	7.4	40
Borage (salad plant)	3.0	0.4	0.4	17
Brussels sprouts	1.5	0.1	3.4	21
Burdock	4.5	0.1	7.4	49
Cabbage (carbohydrate range, 3–6.5 per cent)	1.6	0.3	4.5	27
Chinese	1.2	0.1	2.4	15
Carrots (carbohydrate range, 5.9–11.5 per cent)	1.1	0.4	8.2	41
Cassava, root	1.6	0.2	27.1	117
Cauliflower	1.8	0.5	3.7	27
Celery	1.1	0.1	3.3[2]	19
root	2.0	0.4	6.3	37
Chard (Swiss)	3.2	0.6	5.0[2]	38
Chayote (tayote)	0.9	0.1	5.9	28
Chenopodium	8.5	1.1	2.7	55
Chicory, root	..	..	15.0	..
leaves, Italian	1.9	0.4	0.8	14
Collards	4.5	0.6	6.3	49
Corn	3.1	1.1	19.2	99
Cucumbers	0.8	0.2	2.3	14
Egg plant	1.2	0.3	4.3	25
Endive	1.0	None	2.6	14
Finochio	1.5	0.1	1.6	13
Greens, beet, cooked	2.2	3.4	3.2[2]	52
dandelion, as purchased	2.4	1.0	10.6[2]	61
turnip salad	4.2	0.6	6.3[2]	47

[1] Chiefly inulin.
[2] Includes fiber.

TABLE 247.—COMPOSITION OF NORMAL FOODS.—(*Continued.*)

VEGETABLES—*Continued.*

Name and description of food	Protein, per cent.	Fat, per cent.	Carbo-hydrate, per cent.	Calories, per 100 gms.
Vegetables, fresh (unless otherwise stated):				
Kale	3.0	0.4	2.1	24
sea	1.4	None	3.8	21
Kohl-rabi (carbohydrate range, 3.5–14 per cent)	2.0	1.0	7.0	45
Lambs' quarters	3.8	0.6	1.7	27
Leeks	1.2	0.5	5.8	33
Lettuce	1.2	0.3	2.2	16
Mushrooms[1]	3.5	0.4	6.0	42
Okra	1.6	0.2	4.0	24
Onions (carbohydrate range, 4–14 per cent)	1.6	0.3	9.0	45
cooked	1.2	1.8	4.9	41
Orach	4.6	0.4	0.2[2]	23
Oyster plant	1.2	0.1	7.0	34
Parsnips (carbohydrate range, 6–14 per cent)	1.6	0.5	11.0	55
Peas,[3] green, cooked	6.7	3.4	14.6[4]	116
marrowfat, first grade	5.1	..	12.4	..
second grade	6.7	..	11.0	..
third grade	5.9	..	14.5	..
petits pois, first grade	3.4	..	7.0	..
second grade	4.2	..	10.4	..
third grade	4.4	..	10.3	..
sifted, first grade	5.3	..	12.2	..
second grade	5.7	..	13.1	..
third grade	5.6	..	15.5	..
Peppers, Neapolitan	1.1	0.3	5.7	30
sweet, green	0.8	0.1	4.1	21
Potatoes	2.2	0.1	18.0	82
air (tropical Asia)	1.9	0.4	16.3	76
boiled	2.5	0.1	20.3	92
cooked, chips	6.8	39.8	46.7[4]	572
mashed and creamed	2.6	3.0	17.8[4]	109
sweet (carbohydrate range, 16.5–44.5 per cent)	1.8	0.7	26.1	118
cooked	3.0	2.1	42.1[4]	199
Pumpkins (carbohydrate range, 3–14 per cent)	1.0	0.1	6.0	29
Radishes (carbohydrate range, 2.7–7.5 per cent)	1.3	0.1	5.1	27
Rhubarb	0.6	0.7	2.5	19
Roquette (Rocket salad)	0.7	0.4	0.3[2]	8
Rutabagas (carbohydrate range, 3–12 per cent)	1.3	0.2	7.3	36
Sauerkraut	1.7	0.5	3.0	23
Sorrel	2.1	0.2	0.1[2]	11
Spinach	2.1	0.3	2.3	20
cooked	2.1	4.1	2.6[4]	56
Squash	1.4	0.5	8.2	43
Tomatoes	0.9	0.4	3.3	20
Truffles	9.1	0.5	7.0	69

[1] Protein and carbohydrates largely unassimilable (E. P. J.).
[2] Starch and sugar.
[3] Fat content may be taken to range from 0.5 to 1 per cent.
[4] Includes fiber.

TABLE 247.—COMPOSITION OF NORMAL FOODS.—(*Continued.*)
VEGETABLES—*Concluded.*

Name and description of food.	Protein, per cent.	Fat, per cent.	Carbohydrate, per cent.	Calories, per 100 gms.
Vegetables, fresh (unless otherwise stated):				
Turnips (carbohydrate range, 2.3–18 per cent)	1.3	0.2	6.8	34
Vegetable marrow.	0.7	0.1	1.5	10
Italian	0.7	0.1	1.4	9
Watercress	0.7	0.5	3.7	22
Yams	1.6	0.2	23.6	103
Yautia (Tanier)	4.2	0.4	53.0	232
Vegetables, dried:				
Beans	22.5	1.8	55.0	326
frijoles	21.9	1.3	65.1[1]	360
Lima	18.1	1.5	65.9[1]	350
mesquite	12.2	2.5	77.1[1]	380
soy	38.3	14.9	26.6[2]	394
Carrots, evaporated	7.7	3.6	80.3[1]	384
Lentils	25.7	1.0	59.2[1]	349
Peas	24.6	1.0	57.5	337
cow	21.4	1.4	56.7	325
Peppers, green	15.5	8.5	63.0[1]	391
red	9.4	7.7	70.0[1]	387
Potatoes, evaporated	8.5	0.4	80.9[1]	361
Tomatoes	12.9	8.1	62.3[1]	374
Vegetables, canned:				
Artichokes (carbohydrate range, 3.2–6.1 per cent)	0.8	..	4.4	21
Asparagus (carbohydrate range, 1.6–3.3 per cent)	1.5	0.1	2.3	16
Beans, baked	6.9	2.5	17.1	119
haricots verts	1.1	0.1	2.0	13
flageolets (carbohydrate range, 9.8–12.4 per cent)	4.6	0.1	11.5	65
Lima (carbohydrate range, 9.6–16.5 per cent)	4.0	3.0	13.4	97
little green	1.2	0.1	2.8	17
red kidney	7.0	0.2	17.3	99
string (carbohydrate range, 1.5–4.5 per cent)	1.1	0.1	3.3	19
wax	1.0	0.1	2.5	15
Brussels sprouts	1.5	0.1	2.9	19
Corn[3] (carbohydrate range, 11.7–25.1 per cent)	2.8	1.2	18.2	95
and tomatoes	1.6	0.4	9.1	46
Macedoine (mixed vegetables)	1.4	..	3.9	21
Okra[4]	0.7	0.1	2.9	15
Peas[5] (carbohydrate range, 4.3–17.2 per per cent)	3.6	0.2	8.6	51
Potatoes, sweet	1.9	0.4	40.6	174
Pumpkins (carbohydrate range, 3.6–7.3 per cent)	0.8	0.2	5.6	27
Squash (carbohydrate range, 3.6–12.8 per cent)	0.9	0.5	9.8	47
Succotash (carbohydrate range, 13.9–21.3 per cent)	3.6	1.0	17.7	94
Tomatoes (carbohydrate range, 1–4.5 per cent)	1.2	0.2	3.5	21

[1] Includes fiber.
[2] About one-fourth available.
[3] Average, 0.4 per cent salt (NaCl).
[4] Average, 1.1 per cent salt (NaCl).
[5] Average, 0.7 per cent salt (NaCl).

TABLE 247.—COMPOSITION OF NORMAL FOODS.—(Continued.)

PICKLES, CONDIMENTS, ETC.

Name and description of food.	Protein, per cent.	Fat, per cent.	Carbohydrate, per cent.	Calories, per 100 gms.
Pickles, condiments, etc.:				
Capers	3.2	0.5	5.0	37
Catsup, tomato (carbohydrate range, 3–26 per cent)	1.8	0.2	10.0	49
Chili sauce (carbohydrate range, 14–28 per cent)	..	..	20.0	..
Horseradish	1.4	0.2	11.0	51
Olives, green, edible portion . . .	1.1	27.6	11.6[1]	299
ripe, edible portion	1.7	25.9	4.3[1]	257
Mustard, prepared	4.7	4.1	5.0	76
cereal added (carbohydrate range, 4–15 per cent) . . .	3.5	1.9	7.0	59
Pickles, cucumber	0.5	0.3	2.7	16
mixed	1.1	0.4	4.0	24
spiced	0.4	0.1	21.0	87
Vinegar, cider (carbohydrate range, 0.3–1.5 per cent)	None	None	0.3	1
distilled	None	None	None	..
malt	..	..	0.5[2]	..
spiced salad	..	..	10.0	..
Tarragon	..	..	0.2[2]	..
wine	..	..	0.4	..

FRUITS, BERRIES, ETC.
(*Analyses are of edible portion.*)

	Protein, per cent.	Fat, per cent.	Carbohydrate, per cent.	Calories, per 100 gms.
Fruits, berries, etc., fresh:				
Apples (carbohydrate range, 9–21 per cent)	0.4	0.5	13.0	58
Apricots	1.1	..	12.0	..
Avocadós (alligator pears)	1.1	13.7	7.1	156
Bananas	1.3	0.2	20.0	88
Blackberries	1.3	1.0	8.4	48
Cherries	1.0	0.8	16.5	77
Citrang juice	1.3	..	6.9	..
Cranberries	0.4	0.6	8.4	41
Currants	1.5	..	12.8[3]	..
Egg fruit	3.4	1.9	41.0	195
Figs	1.5	..	18.8[3]	..
Gooseberries	0.4	..	12.0	..
Grapes	1.3	1.6	14.9	79
Grapejuice (carbohydrate range, 11–20 per cent)	..	..	15.0	..
Grape fruit[4]	..	..	7.2	..
Huckleberries	0.6	0.6	16.6[3]	74
Lemons	1.0	0.7	7.4	40
juice	..	..	9.8	..
Loganberries[5]	4.6	0.6	7.2[6]	53
juice[7]	0.6	..	6.8[6]	..

[1] Includes fiber.
[2] Manufacturers' analysis.
[3] Includes fiber.
[4] Florida, California and Porto Rico, carbohydrate range, 6.6–8.2 per cent (E. M. Frankel).
[5] Jour. Indust. and Engin. Chem., 1918, **10**, 30.
[6] Invert sugar.
[7] Jour. Indust. and Engin. Chem., 1917, **9**, 1043.

TABLE 247.—COMPOSITION OF NORMAL FOODS.—(*Continued.*)

FRUITS, BERRIES, ETC.—*Concluded.*

Name and description of food.	Protein, per cent.	Fat, per cent.	Carbo-hydrate, per cent.	Calories, per 100 gms.
Fruits, berries, etc., fresh:				
Loquat	0.3	..	23.0	..
Mangoes	..	..	13.0	..
Mulberries	0.3	..	12.0	..
Muskmelons	0.7	0.3	10.0	46
Nectarines	0.6	..	15.9[1]	..
Oranges[2]	0.8	0.2	11.6[1]	51
Orange-lemon juice	0.6	..	1.8	..
Papaya (papaw)	0.8	0.1	6.3	29
Peaches	0.5	0.2	9.0	40
Pears	0.6	0.5	11.4	53
Persimmons	0.8	0.7	29.7	128
Pineapple	0.4	0.3	12.0	52
Plums	1.0	..	17.0	..
Pomegranates	1.5	1.6	17.0	88
Prunes	0.8	..	19.0	..
Raspberries, black	1.7	1.0	10.0	56
red	1.0	..	9.7	..
Sapodilla	0.6	1.4	19.4	93
Sour sop	0.8	0.1	17.2	73
Strawberries	1.0	0.6	6.0	33
Tangelo juice	0.7	..	9.0	..
Watermelons	0.3	0.1	7.0	30
Whortleberries	0.7	0.3	10.0	46
Fruits, berries, etc., dried:				
Apples	1.6	2.2	66.1[1]	291
Apricots	4.7	1.0	62.5[1]	278
Citron	1.5	1.5	78.1[1]	332
Currants	2.4	1.7	74.2[1]	322
Dates	2.1	2.8	78.4[1]	347
Figs	4.3	0.3	74.2[1]	317
Prunes	2.1	..	73.3[1]	..
Raisins	2.6	3.3	76.1[1]	345
Raspberries	7.3	1.8	80.2[1]	366
Fruits, berries, etc., canned; jellies and preserves:[3]				
Apricots	0.9	..	17.3[1]	
Apricot sauce	1.9	1.3	48.8[1]	215
Blackberries	0.8	2.1	56.4[1]	248
Blueberries	0.6	0.6	12.8[1]	59
Cherries	1.1	0.1	21.1[1]	90
Cherry jelly	1.1	..	77.2[1]	..
Figs, stewed	1.2	0.3	40.9[1]	171
Grape butter	1.2	0.1	58.5[1]	240
Marmalade, orange	0.6	0.1	84.5[1]	341
Peaches	0.7	0.1	10.8[1]	47
Pears	0.3	0.3	18.0[1]	76
Pineapple	0.4	0.7	36.4[1]	154
Prune sauce	0.5	0.1	22.3[1]	92
Strawberries, stewed	0.7	..	24.0[1]	..
Tomato preserves	0.7	0.1	57.6[1]	234

[1] Includes fiber.

[2] Florida, average of seven analyses, carbohydrate, 8 per cent; California, eight analyses, carbohydrate, 8.3 per cent (E. M. Frankel).

[3] Jams, jellies, preserves and marmalade contain 47 per cent or more carbohydrate. There is a wide variation in the sugar content of canned fruits. Pie peaches are packed in water while other grades may be found in 30, 40 or even 50 per cent syrup.

TABLE 247.—COMPOSITION OF NORMAL FOODS.—(*Concluded.*)

NUTS.

(*Analyses are of edible portion.*)

Name and description of food.	Protein, per cent.	Fat, per cent.	Carbo-hydrate, per cent.	Calories, per 100 gms.
Nuts:				
Almond	21.0	54.9	15.3	639
Almond butter	22.1	61.5	7.9	674
Beechnuts	21.9	57.4	13.2[1]	657
Brazil nuts	17.0	66.8	7.0[1]	697
Butternuts	27.9	61.2	3.5[1]	676
Cashew nuts	9.7	47.2	17.0	532
Chestnuts	6.2	5.4	40.3	235
Cocoanuts	5.7	50.6	27.9[1]	590
Cocoanut milk	0.4	1.5	4.6	34
prepared	6.3	57.4	31.5[1]	668
Filberts	15.6	65.3	13.0[1]	702
Hickory nuts	15.4	67.4	11.4[1]	714
Lichi nuts	2.9	0.2	77.5[1]	323
Peanuts	25.8	38.6	21.9[1]	538
Peanut butter	29.3	46.5	17.1[1]	604
Pecans	9.6	70.5	15.3[1]	734
Pine nuts, Pignolias	33.9	49.4	6.9[1]	608
Piniones	6.5	60.7	26.2[1]	677
Pinon	14.6	61.9	17.3[1]	685
Sabine	28.1	53.7	8.4[1]	629
Pistachios	22.3	54.0	16.3[1]	640
Walnuts, California	18.4	64.4	11.6[1]	700
black	27.6	56.3	10.0	657
soft shell	16.6	63.4	13.5	691

ALCOHOLIC BEVERAGES.

	Protein	Fat	Carbohydrate	Calories
Distilled liquors[2] (whisky, gin, rum, brandy)	..	..	None or trace	..
Wines,[3] dry (carbohydrate range, trace to 3.6 per cent)	..	..	0.3	..
sweet (carbohydrate range 0.1–40.7 per cent)	..	..	8.0	..
Cordials[4] (creme de menthe, kümmel, benedictine, anisette, chartreuse	..	..	30.0	..
Beer,[5] near (average of several brands)	..	..	5.0	..
Ale[6]	..	..	5.1	..
Malt extract, commercial	..	..	10.6	..
true, concentrated	..	..	71.3	..
Cider[7] (carbohydrate range, 0–13.5 per cent)	..	..	4.5	..

OTHER BEVERAGES.

	Protein	Fat	Carbohydrate	Calories
Tea (0.5 oz. to 1 pt. water)	..	..	0.6	..
Coffee (1 oz. to 1 pt. water)	..	..	0.7	..
Cocoa (0.5 oz. to 1 pt. water)	..	..	1.1	..
(0.5 oz. to 1 pt. milk)	..	..	6.0	..
Carbonated drinks (bottled soda, sarsaparilla, birch beer, root beer, gingerale)	..	..	8.0	..

---

[1] Includes fiber.

[2] Sugar is sometimes added to brandy. One sample examined was sensibly sweet and contained 33.5 per cent of sugar (Connecticut Exp. Sta. Bull. 227, 1920, p. 232). Range of alcohol content, 35 to 50 per cent.

[3] Natural wines contain 6 to 12 per cent alcohol; "fortified" wines, 15 to 20 per cent.

[4] Range of alcohol content, 35 to 50 per cent.

[5] Range of alcohol content for beer, generally 3 to 5 per cent; for prohibition beer (near beer), not over 0.5 per cent.

[6] Range of alcohol content, same as for beer.

[7] Range of alcohol content, generally 2.5 to 6 per cent.

TABLE 248.—COMPOSITION OF SO-CALLED DIABETIC FOODS, ETC.

Reference.	Manufacturer or agent and name of product.	Protein, per cent.	Fat, per cent.	Carbohydrate.		Calories, per 100 gms.
				Starch, per cent.	Other carbohydrate, per cent.	
	FLOURS AND MEALS.					
	Herman Barker, Somerville, Mass.:					
1919	Barker's Gluten Food "A" . . .	77.0	0.4	2.6	9.8	361
1919	Barker's Gluten Food "B" . . .	74.0	0.5	5.2	10.1	362
1919	Barker's Gluten Food "C" . . .	73.0	0.4	6.4	9.8	360
	Battle Creek Sanitarium Co., Battle Creek, Mich.:					
1916–4a	Gluten Meal	26.3	1.0	55.0	8.7	369
1919–4a	Gluten Meal	39.3	0.9	41.1	10.1	370
1914–2q	Gluten Meal, 80 per cent . . .	76.6	..	5.8	..	..
	Callard, Stewart & Watt, London:					
1909–3	Casoid Flour	82.5	1.6	None	3.1[1]	357
1916–4a	Gluten Flour	73.4	..	None	..	..
	Canada Cereal & Flour Co.:					
1919–4b	Gluten Flour	18.6	4.5	43.9	16.9	358
	Cereo Co., Tappan, N. Y.					
1919	Soy Bean Gruel Flour	46.1	18.6	0.9	21.9	443
	Cheltine Food Co., Cheltenham, Eng.					
1922	Cheltine Diabetic Food . . .	57.9	10.1	16.4[2]	3.3	401
	The Dieto Food Co., New York:					
1914–2q	Pure Whole Wheat Flour . . .	13.5	2.1	62.4	12.0	371
	Empire Flour Mills:					
1919–4b	Gluten Flour	13.1	1.1	59.1	15.5	361
	Farwell & Rhines, Watertown, N. Y.:					
1913–2p	Cresco Flour	18.1	1.0	57.2	10.2	351
1919	Genuine Gluten Flour, 40 per cent	40.5	1.5	37.0	9.4	361
1913–2p	Special Diabetic Food	27.5	2.8	40.0	16.6	362
	Federal Mill & Elevator Co., Lockport, N. Y.:					
1922	Gluten Flour	38.5	1.8	42.3[2]	6.9	367
	Gericke, Potsdam:					
1910–9	Aleuronat	76.0	3.3	..	10.5[1]	376
	Golden Rod Milling Co., Portland, Ore.:					
1919	Acme Special Flour	15.1	1.8	61.5	8.6	357
1916–4a	Gluten Flour	14.1	1.3	67.0	..	..
	O. B. Gilman, Boston, Mass.:					
1913–2p	Gluten Flour	43.2	2.0	31.4	13.1	369
	The Health Food Co., New York:					
1919	Almond Meal	50.3	15.4	None	18.0	412
1919	Bran Biskue, Gluten Bran . . .	27.7	10.5	33.8	13.9	396
1919	Diabetic Casein Flour (self-raising)	72.3	0.8	None	5.7	319
1919–4b	Gluten Flour, 40 per cent . . .	39.2	1.1	37.3	13.0	368
1919	Glutosac Gluten Flour	41.5	1.7	36.2	9.1	363
1919	Pronireu (Gluten Griddle Cake Flour)	37.9	1.2	36.6	9.1	345
1914–2q	Protosac Gluten Flour	41.9	2.0	31.5	14.8	371
1919	Protosoy Soy Flour	39.4	18.6	1.9	25.1	433
1919	Pure Washed Gluten Flour . . .	74.9	2.0	3.8	10.0	373
1919	Snow Flake Diabetic Casein Flour .	79.2	1.2	None	3.2	340

[1] Includes fiber.
[2] Includes soluble carbohydrate.

TABLE 248.—COMPOSITION OF SO-CALLED DIABETIC FOODS, ETC.—*(Continued.)*

Reference.[1]	Manufacturer or agent and name of product.	Protein, per cent.	Fat, per cent.	Carbohydrate.		Calories, per 100 gms.
				Starch, per cent.	Other carbohydrate, per cent.	
	FLOURS AND MEALS—*Continued.*					
	Hudon Hebert (Furn'r.):					
1919–4*b*	Gluten Flour	14.4	2.2	52.5	16.8	355
	Jireh Diabetic Food Co., New York:					
1919–4*b*	Diabetic Flour	14.8	2.0	50.1	20.7	360
1919–4*b*	Gluten Flour	14.4	2.1	50.0	21.9	364
1913–2*p*	Patent Barley	11.4	1.6	67.8	12.4	381
1913–2*p*	Patent Cotton Seed Flour . . .	49.1	12.7	6.0	15.3	396
1913–2*p*	Patent Lentils Flour	27.3	1.2	42.6	17.2	359
1913–2*p*	Protein Flour	31.4	2.0	48.5	8.2	370
1913–2*p*	Soja Bean Flour	42.3	18.2	None	25.8	436
1906–2*e*	Wheat and Barley Flour . . .	11.8	1.9	66.2[1]	7.3	358
	Johnson Educator Food Co., Boston, Mass.:					
1911–2*k*	Educator Standard Gluten Flour .	36.6	1.4	40.9	12.8	374
	The Kellogg Food Co., Battle Creek, Mich.:					
1916–2*s*	Gluten Meal, 20 per cent . . .	24.7	0.9	51.2	14.2	369
1919	Gluten Flour, 40 per cent . . .	47.2	1.0	30.7	10.2	361
1919	Gluten Meal, thoroughly cooked, 40 per cent	43.0	1.5	33.4	12.0	367
1912–2*m*	Gluten, 80 per cent	74.2	0.9	6.2	8.8	365
1919	Pure Gluten Meal	79.1	0.7	2.6	8.7	368
	La Societe l'Aliment "Essentiel," Nanterre, France:					
1921	Heudebert, Surazotized Gluten Flour	61.3	2.3	14.0[1]	10.9	366
1921	Heudebert, Gluten Flour with Cacao	53.6	5.8	13.8[1]	14.7	381
	Lister Bros., New York:					
1919	Lister's Diabetic Flour, self-rising .	68.3	1.0	None	9.7	321
	Lyster Bros., Whitefield, N. H.:					
1915–2*r*	Casein Flour	84.5	3.6	None	0.4	372
1916–12*a*	Diabetic Flour	79.3	3.0	None	. .	. .
	Loeb's Diabetic Food Bakery, N. Y.:					
1919	Gluten Cracker Meal	36.7	10.9	30.7	11.5	414
1919	Pure Gluten Flour	38.8	1.2	38.2	10.3	360
	Maple Leaf Milling Co.:					
1919–4*b*	Gluten Flour	12.7	1.2	61.5	11.5	354
	Thos. Martindale & Co., Phila., Pa.:					
1919	Special Gluten Flour	36.8	1.5	41.4	11.2	371
	Mayflower Mills, Fort Wayne, Ind.:					
1919	Gluten Flour	48.0	1.7	28.6	10.2	363
	A. McFarlane Co.:					
1919–4*b*	Gluten Flour	12.1	1.4	60.3	14.3	359
	P. McIntosh Co.:					
1919–4*b*	Gluten Flour	15.1	1.0	63.3	9.3	360
	Theo. Metcalf Co., Boston, Mass.:					
1913–2*p*	Soja Bean Meal, 18 per cent starch	41.0	20.0	25.0		444
1913–2*p*	Vegetable Gluten, 8.1 per cent starch	73.3	1.5	5.9	11.0	374

[1] Includes soluble carbohydrate.

TABLE 248.—COMPOSITION OF SO-CALLED DIABETIC FOODS, ETC.—(*Continued*.)

Reference.[1]	Manufacturer or agent and name of product.	Protein, per cent.	Fat, per cent.	Carbohydrate.		Calories, per 100 gms.
				Starch, per cent	Other carbohydrate, per cent.	
	FLOURS AND MEALS—*Continued.*					
	Northwestern Cereal Co., London, Ont.:					
1919–4*b*	Gluten Flour	17.1	5.0	42.1	22.0	370
1919–4*b*	Gluten Flour, 40 per cent . . .	14.2	5.3	38.7	25.6	361
	Phospho Food Co., Los Angeles, Calif.:					
1914–2*q*	Phospho D & D Special	13.7	2.2	58.6	14.4	367
	Plasmon Co., London, Eng.:					
1922	Arrowroot	19.8	0.1	62.2[1]	2.5	339
	Pieser-Livingston Co., Chicago, Ill.:					
1919	Genuine Gluten Flour	41.4	1.4	36.3	9.8	363
	Potter & Wrightington, Boston, Mass.:					
1919	Diet-Ease Gluten Flour	39.6	2.3	36.2	11.8	371
	Pure Gluten Food Co., Columbus, Ohio:					
1919	Hoyt's Gluten Flour, over 40 per cent protein	41.8	1.1	33.2	12.1	359
1919	Hoyt's Gluten Self-raising Flour, over 40 per cent protein . .	41.5	0.9	33.4	9.7	346
1919	Hoyt's Gluten Special Flour, 80 per cent protein	77.2	1.2	2.8	10.6	373
	Schulenburg Oil Mill, Schulenburg, Texas:					
1919	Baumgarten Process Allison Flour .	50.0	10.0	1.1	21.6	381
1921	Allison Flour (Cotton Seed) . .	50.4	7.9	8.8[1]	15.2	369
	Soy Bean Food Products Co., San Francisco, Calif.:					
1919	Soy Bean Flour A	41.8	19.4	0.3	24.1	440
1919	Soy Bean Flour B	44.0	14.2	0.8	26.0	411
	Sprague, Warner & Co., Chicago, Ill.:					
1919	Richelieu Gluten Flour	45.3	1.2	31.6	12.5	368
	Still Rock Spa, Waukesha, Wis.:					
1919	Curdolac Flour	56.6	2.4	5.1	17.9	340
	G. Van Abbott & Sons, London:					
1913–2*p*	Almond Flour	24.6	58.6	None	7.9	657
1913–2*p*	Gluten Flour	68.5	0.9	12.4	6.8	359
1913–2*p*	Gluten Semola	46.9	2.9	28.2	8.7	361
	Waukesha Health Products Co., Waukesha, Wis.:					
1917–2*t*	Ayos, the Improved Soja Bean Flour	41.4	16.9	0.6	24.4	418
1919	Hepco Flour	44.0	19.1	0.9	21.4	438
	White Swan Spice Co., Toronto, Can.:					
1919–4*b*	Diet Flour	8.7	1.3	61.3	16.1	356
1919–4*b*	Gluten Flour	9.8	1.5	62.3	16.0	366
	Wilson Bros., Rochester, N. Y.:					
1919	Genteel Brand Flour	29.4	2.4	49.2	6.2	361
1913–2*p*	Gluten Flour, 4/7 Standard . . .	19.0	2.1	54.6	11.8	361
1913–2*p*	Gluten Flour, Self-raising, 4/7 Standard	15.8	2.0	51.8	13.3	342
1919	Gluten Flour	45.8	2.0	28.6	11.9	364

[1] Includes soluble carbohydrate.

TABLE 248.—COMPOSITION OF SO-CALLED DIABETIC FOODS, ETC.—(*Continued.*)

Reference.[1]	Manufacturer or agent and name of product.	Protein, per cent.	Fat, per cent.	Carbohydrate. Starch, per cent.	Carbohydrate. Other carbohydrate, per cent.	Calories, per 100 gms.
	PROTEIN PREPARATIONS. *Cheltine Food Co., Cheltenham, Eng.:*					
1922	Milk Protein	84.5	1.0	None	2.4[1]	357
	Norton Truax, Chicago, Ill.:					
1919	Diaprotein.	79.4	1.5	None	1.1[1]	336
1922	Diaprotein, No. 2	79.3	1.6	None	1.2[1]	336
	Plasmon Co., London:					
1922	Milk Proteid	75.9	0.7	None	3.1[1]	322
	Menley & James, New York:					
1913–2p	Glidine	83.3	0.8	None	9.1	377
	SOFT BREADS.[2] *American System of Bakeries, Hartford, Conn.:*					
1921	Gluten Bread	26.2	6.0	23.8	6.8	281
1921	Gluten Bread A	27.8	5.9	27.6	6.1	299
1921	Gluten Bread B	28.5	5.4	27.5	5.7	295
	Canada Bread Co., Toronto, Can.:					
1919–4b	Gluten Bread	9.9	1.1	34.8	16.5	255
	The Dieto Food Co., New York:					
1914–2q	Dieto Bread, Pure Whole Wheat .	8.8	0.4	36.6	11.4	231
	Ferguson Bakery, Boston, Mass.:					
1913–2p	Gluten Bread	22.1	3.1	25.2	10.5	259
	The Health Food Co., New York:					
1919–2u	Glutosac Bread	29.8	2.6	29.5	12.3	309
1919	Protosac Bread, No. 1	36.0	4.0	20.5	7.4	292
1919	Protosac Bread, No. 2	27.0	3.5	30.5	8.4	295
	J. Heinbockel & Co., Baltimore, Md.:					
1914–2q	Diabetic Bread for Diabetes . .	8.6	1.5	40.4	11.7	256
	Jireh Diabetic Food Co., New York:					
1913–2p	Whole Wheat Bread (not fresh) .	11.3	0.7	44.9	18.2	304
	Levine Bros., New Haven, Conn.:					
1922	Gluten Bread	17.5	3.8	25.7[3]	11.7	254
	Loeb's Diabetic Food Bakery, N. Y.:					
1919	Casein Bread	40.8	10.8	None	3.4	274
1919	Casein Muffins	45.7	11.4	None	7.0	313
1919	Genuine Gluten Bread	28.4	2.1	28.6	6.9	275
1922	Genuine Gluten Bread . . .	32.6	3.6	27.2[3]	4.4	289
1914–2q	P & L Genuine Glubetic Bread .	35.3	4.1	19.2	10.0	294
	Lyster Bros., Whitefield, N. H.:					
1915–2r	Casein Bread	36.6	18.4	None	2.5	322
	Slinn-Schouldis Co.:					
1919–4b	Gluten Bread	9.2	2.6	39.0	13.4	269
	Weston Bakery, Boston, Mass.:					
1915–2r	Gluten Bread	19.0	..	28.2	..	..

[1] Lactose.

[2] It should be remembered that ordinary wheat bread contains protein 9.2 fat 1.3, carbohydrate 52.6 per cent. (See Table 247, page 709.)

[3] Includes soluble carbohydrate.

TABLE 248.—COMPOSITION OF SO-CALLED DIABETIC FOODS, ETC.—(*Continued.*)

Reference.	Manufacturer or agent and name of product.	Protein, per cent.	Fat, per cent.	Carbohydrate.		Calories, per 100 gms.
				Starch, per cent.	Other carbohydrate per cent.	
	HARD BREAD AND BAKERY PRODUCTS.					
	James Aird:					
1916–4a	Gluten Bread	13.1	0.7	59.8	15.9	362
	Arnaud, Inc., N. Y.:					
1921	Cassava Cakes	1.8	0.2	69.5	11.1	331
	Brusson Jeune, Villimur, France:					
1921	Gluten Bread	33.8	3.8	45.0	0.4	351
	Callard & Co., London:					
1922	Almond Biscuits, No. 15 . . .	34.1	48.6	3.5¹	2.8	599
1922	Bran and Almond Biscuits, No. 13 .	24.4	57.5	2.8¹	3.8	642
1922	Casoid Biscuits, No. 17	58.3	24.6	0.3¹	1.7	463
1922	Casoid Rusks, No. 8	54.3	26.6	0.5¹	4.9	478
1922	Gluten and Almond Biscuits, No. 11	65.4	23.3	3.1¹	None	484
1922	Gluten Biscuits, No. 9	60.4	23.9	3.4¹	3.9	486
1922	Gluten Cracknells, No. 7 . . .	68.7	14.7	3.4¹	4.7	440
1922	Gluten Dinner Rolls, No. 6 . . .	73.8	7.1	5.2¹	5.4	402
1922	Kalari Batons, No. 5a	44.2	42.5	1.2¹	0.1	568
1922	Parmesan Cheese Straws, No. 17 .	31.2	48.9	3.5¹	6.6	606
1922	Ponos Biscuits, No. 14	60.6	19.2	1.3¹	2.6	431
1922	Prolacto Biscuits, No. 12 . . .	59.8	20.5	0.3¹	4.7	444
1922	Soup Sippets	54.1	28.7	0.5¹	7.0	505
	Canada Bread Co., Toronto, Can.:					
1916-4a	Gluten Health Bread	15.4	3.4	57.9	13.2	376
	Cheltine Food Co., Cheltenham, Eng.:					
1922	Assorted Biscuits	18.3	16.0	51.5¹	5.3	444
1922	Brown Rusks	18.2	9.7	51.0¹	10.8	407
1922	White Rusks	22.7	14.8	48.0¹	4.6	434
1922	Manhu Diabetic Biscuits . . .	12.9	12.0	61.7¹	5.6	429
	The Dieto Food Co., New York:					
1914–2q	Dieto Crackers	13.4	9.2	54.8	13.9	411
1914–2q	Dieto Rusks	15.9	9.1	52.1	14.0	410
	Fromm & Co., Dresden:					
1913–2p	Almond-form Wafers with Chocolate	4.8	29.0	14.0	48.3	529
1913–2p	Butterbrezeln	12.3	16.5	43.1	19.6	449
1914–2q	Conglutin Drops	50.8	1.1	29.2	6.9	358
1914–2q	Conglutin-Zwieback	14.3	21.3	29.7	27.9	479
1913–2p	Crackers	12.9	7.7	58.2	10.2	395
1913–2p	Eierbiscuit	18.8	11.4	37.5	23.1	420
1913–2p	Haselnuss-Stangen	13.4	16.0	None	60.8	441
1913–2p	Luft Bread	50.9	1.0	23.4	7.3	335
1913–2p	Makronen	14.1	19.4	None	56.2	456
1913–2p	Salt-Stangen	13.0	15.6	39.1	22.1	437
1913–2p	Stangenin	14.0	13.0	51.6	12.8	431
1913–2p	Uni Bread	71.7	1.7	2.9	6.5	340
	Karl Goldscheider, Karlsbad:					
1914–2q	Aleuronat-Conglutin Cakes . . .	26.6	15.6	31.7	19.6	452
1914–2q	Butter-Brezeln	10.5	14.9	43.9	23.6	446

¹ Includes soluble carbohydrate.

46

TABLE 248.—COMPOSITION OF SO-CALLED DIABETIC FOODS, ETC.—(*Continued.*)

Reference.	Manufacturer or agent and name of product.	Protein, per cent.	Fat, per cent.	Carbohydrate. Starch, per cent.	Other carbohydrate, per cent.	Calories, per 100 gms.
	HARD BREAD AND BAKERY PRODUCTS—*Continued.*					
1914–2q	Feinste Cocosnuss-Biskuits für Diabetiker "3.6 per cent carbohydrates"	34.4	45.4	None	13.9	602
1914–2q	Feinste Vanille-Biskuits für Diabetiker, "3.6 per cent carbohydrates"	46.4	30.3	None	16.8	525
1914–2q	Honigküchen für Diabetiker, "3.6 per cent carbohydrates"	40.3	38.8	None	13.9	566
1914–2q	Saccharin-Oblaten ohne Zucker	16.5	22.6	33.5	17.6	474
1914–2q	Tee-Gebäck	7.0	27.3	18.0	42.8	517
1914–2q	Zwieback	21.3	3.6	51.7	13.6	379
	Health Food Co., New York:					
1919	Alpha	68.6	8.4	1.0	6.4	380
1919	Alpha No. 1 Best Diabetic Wafer, Casein	48.4	33.5	None	4.9	515
1919	Alpha No. 2 Best Diabetic Wafer	70.5	4.0	1.1	6.3	348
1914–2q	Diabetic Biscuit	35.9	8.8	39.8	6.8	409
1919	Gluten Cracker Dust	44.5	8.8	23.2	11.8	398
1919	Gluten Nuggets	28.8	12.3	32.2	15.4	417
1919	Glutona Bread Sticks	33.4	11.1	30.6	14.1	412
1919	Glutosac Butter Wafers	31.1	8.0	40.4	7.9	390
1919	Glutosac Rusk	34.7	5.6	34.3	12.5	376
1919	Glutosac Wafers, Plain	41.0	7.5	25.1	12.1	380
1919	Glutosac Zwieback	28.8	10.5	33.3	15.2	405
1919	No. 1 Proto Puffs	69.1	4.7	3.3	10.7	375
1914–2q	No. 2 Proto Puffs	53.6	2.1	20.7	11.5	362
1919	Protosac Rusk	32.7	5.0	39.3	7.8	364
1919	Protosoy Diabetic Wafer	46.5	15.5	10.6	14.2	425
1919	Salvia Almond Sticks	32.1	26.1	21.4	9.1	485
	Heintz Food Co., Chicago, Ill.:					
1913–2p	Gluten Biscuits	11.7	18.3	21.4	37.4	447
	Huntley & Palmer, London:					
1916–2s	Akoll Biscuits	53.6	28.3	Trace	6.2	493
	Jacob & Co., Dublin, Ireland:					
1922	Plasmon Oat Biscuit	15.4	20.7	49.3[1]	6.1	470
1922	Plasmon Plain Biscuit	18.6	15.8	42.5[1]	3.9	402
1922	Plasmon Sweet Biscuit	17.8	15.2	53.6[1]	4.6	441
1922	Plasmon Wholemeal Biscuit	20.0	16.8	47.2[1]	6.6	446
	Jireh Diabetic Food Co., New York:					
1913–2p	Diabetic Biscuit	13.2	7.4	49.6	21.2	403
1913–2p	Diabetic Rusks	14.9	8.7	47.0	21.0	410
	Johnson Educator Food Co., Boston, Mass.:					
1913–2p	Educator Gluten Bread Sticks	32.7	7.2	37.5	11.5	392
1919–4b	Gluten Cookies	20.2	0.3	63.3[1]	6.7	364
	The Kellogg Food Co., Battle Creek, Mich.:					
1913–2p	Potato Gluten Biscuit	37.9	0.5	39.5	12.1	363
1919	Pure Gluten Biscuit	78.4	1.5	2.9	6.5	365
1919	40 per cent Gluten Biscuit	40.9	1.6	35.6	10.9	364

[1] Includes soluble carbohydrate.

TABLE 248.—COMPOSITION OF SO-CALLED DIABETIC FOODS, ETC.—(*Continued.*)

Reference.	Manufacturer or agent and name of product.	Protein, per cent.	Fat, per cent.	Carbohydrate.		Calories, per 100 gms.
				Starch, per cent.	Other carbohydrate, per cent.	
	HARD BREAD AND BAKERY PRODUCTS—*Continued.*					
	Laporte & Gauthier, Somerset, Manitoba, Can.:					
1921	Croustils, Dechloridized . . .	16.6	6.1	64.8[1]	3.3	394
1921	Croustils, Simple	17.1	3.4	66.0[1]	3.8	378
1921	Croustils, Glutenized	30.3	6.7	49.9[1]	3.3	394
	La Societe l'Aliment "Essentiel," Nanterre, France:					
1921	Heudebert, Bread of Gluten . .	61.8	6.2	13.2[1]	7.5	386
1921	Heudebert, Aleurone Bread . .	64.0	5.1	11.5[1]	7.5	378
1921	Heudebert, Special Diabetic Bread	55.5	5.9	19.3[1]	6.6	379
1921	Heudebert, Rolls of Gluten . . .	9.7	8.8	66.1[1]	5.2	403
1921	Heudebert, Rusks of Gluten . .	10.8	7.6	67.4[1]	5.6	404
	Loeb's Diabetic Food Bakery, N. Y.:					
1919	Aërated Gluten Bread	47.8	11.1	26.8	3.2	411
1922	Aërated Gluten Bread	49.8	12.2	23.6[1]	7.0	431
1919	Diabetic Almond Macaroons . .	30.4	46.3	0.6	10.5	583
1919	Diabetic Bread Sticks	41.8	3.8	35.4	6.9	371
1919	Diabetic Bread Sticks, Almond .	39.4	11.7	31.2	7.1	416
1919	Diabetic Butter Cookies. . . .	36.5	12.0	31.1	8.4	412
1919	Diabetic Lady Fingers . . .	47.8	34.1	1.9	3.5	519
1919	Diabetic Sponge Cookies . .	49.7	33.8	1.9	1.4	516
1919–2*u*	Gluten Bread	42.5	11.1	27.7	8.8	416
1916–2*s*	Gluten Luft Bread	40.6	9.8	29.9	11.3	415
1919	Gluten Zwieback	38.7	3.0	36.1	10.6	368
1919	Gluten Almond Zwieback . . .	41.3	7.8	32.6	7.0	394
	Pure Gluten Food Co., New York:					
1914–2*q*	No. 1 Dainty Fluffs	79.9	0.5	10.7	0.5	370
1914–2*q*	No. 2 Dainty Fluffs	66.3	0.5	21.9	3.0	369
1916–4*a*	Dainty Fluffs	80.0	0.8	7.7	3.0	370
1914–2*q*	Gum Gluten Biscuit Crisps . . .	48.1	0.5	31.2	11.5	368
	Rademann's Nährmittelfabrik, Frankfurt:					
1913–2*p*	Diabetiker-Biscuit	29.6	19.6	25.9	18.6	473
1913–2*p*	Diabetiker-Bretzel	31.4	8.5	40.7	9.4	402
1913–2*p*	Diabetiker-Cakes	29.6	13.5	39.1	8.1	429
1913–2*p*	Diabetiker-Dessert-Gebäck . . .	22.2	42.4	5.9	21.6	580
1913–2*p*	Diabetiker-Makronen	23.2	48.0	3.0	17.6	607
1913–2*p*	Diabetiker-Stangen	17.7	44.2	21.4	8.1	586
1913–2*p*	Käsestangen	9.3	33.7	38.0	8.4	526
	R. M. Scott, Ltd., Ipswich:					
1922	Gluten and Almond Biscuit . .	23.8	19.9	44.5[1]	3.2	465
	James Strachen:					
1916–4*a*	Gluten Bread	16.9	0.6	52.7	21.3	369
	Therapeutic Foods Co., Inc., N. Y.:					
1922	Energen New Natural Gluten Bread	33.1	10.1	44.0[1]	10.2	440
1922	Dr. Charasse Gluten Bread . . .	42.7	5.8	36.0[1]	5.3	388
1922	Dr. Charasse Gluto-Kola Bread .	45.9	6.0	37.3[1]	None	387
1922	Dr. Charasse Gluto-Soja Bread .	48.6	6.9	33.3[1]	0.7	393
1922	Dr. Charasse Supreme Bread . .	45.6	6.9	35.9[1]	0.6	391

[1] Includes soluble carbohydrate.

TABLE 248.—COMPOSITION OF SO-CALLED DIABETIC FOODS, ETC.—(*Continued.*)

Reference.	Manufacturer or agent and name of product.	Protein, per cent.	Fat, per cent.	Carbohydrate.		Calories, per 100 gms.
				Starch, per cent.	Other carbohydrate, per cent.	
	HARD BREAD AND BAKERY PRODUCTS—*Concluded.*					
	G. Van Abbott & Sons, London:					
1913–2*p*	Caraway Biscuits for Diabetics .	35.6	37.5	8.6	7.3	544
1913–2*p*	Diabetic Rusks for Diabetics . .	70.9	0.8	12.6	3.4	355
1913–2*p*	Euthenia Biscuit	35.8	40.7	6.9	6.3	562
1913–2*p*	Gluten Biscottes or Rolls . . .	47.1	2.3	29.8	7.7	359
1913–2*p*	Gluten Bread or Slices	49.4	2.2	27.4	8.2	361
1913–2*p*	Gluten Butter Biscuit for Diabetics	40.2	33.2	9.0	7.6	526
1913–2*p*	Ginger Biscuit for Diabetics . .	34.6	39.4	10.9	5.8	560
1913–2*p*	Midolia Biscuit	17.6	36.4	13.4	18.2	524
1922	Soya Biscuit	39.2	25.0	11.4[1]	11.8	475
1913–2*p*	Walnut Biscuits for Diabetics . .	20.9	57.2	Trace	12.3	648
	Waukesha Health Products Co., Waukesha, Wis.:					
1919	Hepco Dodgers	42.4	16.7	1.0	21.6	411
	Weston's Bakery, Boston, Mass.:					
1915–2*r*	Gluten Cookies	27.7	..	19.6	..	..
	Woman's Baking Co., Boston, Mass.:[2]					
1921	Bran Cookies, Anice	7.4	25.9	5.2[3]	..	..
1921	Bran Cookies, Caraway	8.1	24.2	5.0[3]	..	..
1921	Bran Cookies, Cocoa Nib . . .	8.2	26.9	8.7[3]	..	..
1921	Bran Cookies, Spice	6.6	22.7	9.3[3]	..	..
1921	Bran Muffins	7.3	5.9	5.6[3]	..	..
1921	Cellu Biscuits	3.2	13.2	3.9[3]	..	..
1921	Cellu Cookies, Caraway	5.6	22.5	3.8[3]	32.0	..
1921	Cellu Cookies, Lemon	4.2	24.4	3.9[3]	..	..
1921	Cellu Cookies, Vanilla	4.3	21.3	4.1[3]	..	..
1921	Cellu Kisses	23.0	0.2	2.5[3]	25.2	..
1921	Cellu Muffins	3.8	13.6	3.5[3]	..	..
1921	Cellu Nuts	5.4	28.7	3.6[3]	23.8	..
1921	Cellu Soup Wafers	3.7	25.6	4.2[3]	..	..
	BREAKFAST FOODS.					
	Arnaud Inc., New York:					
1921	Starchless Breakfast Food . . .	2.0	0.2	70.9[3]	10.3	335
	Brusson Jeune, Villimur, France:					
1913–2*p*	Farina au Gluten	30.9	0.6	48.8	8.0	356
	Dieto Food Co., New York:					
1914–2*q*	Dieto Nut Cereal	21.6	18.4	39.5	12.3	459
1914–2*q*	Wheat and Barley Cereal . . .	11.6	2.2	61.4	14.4	369
	Farwell & Rhines, Watertown, N. Y.:					
1913–2*p*	Barley Crystals	11.5	1.3	62.7	12.5	359
1913–2*q*	Cresco Grits	17.8	1.4	54.1	14.5	358
	Health Food Co., New York:					
1919	Manana Gluten Breakfast Food .	44.8	8.7	22.0	12.5	396
1919	Protosoy (Cereal)	40.1	18.2	Trace	24.9	424

[1] Includes soluble carbohydrate.
[2] The fat in these products is largely or entirely mineral oil and unassimilable.
[3] Includes soluble carbohydrate.

TABLE 248.—COMPOSITION OF SO-CALLED DIABETIC FOODS, ETC.—(*Continued.*)

Reference.	Manufacturer or agent and name of product.	Protein, per cent.	Fat, per cent.	Carbohydrate.		Calories, per 100 gms.
				Starch, per cent.	Other carbohydrate, per cent.	
	BREAKFAST FOODS—*Concluded.*					
	Jireh Diabetic Food Co., New York:					
1913–2*p*	Whole Wheat Farina	11.7	2.3	59.5	16.3	371
1913–2*p*	Frumenty	12.3	1.7	65.4	11.9	374
	Loeb's Diabetic Food Bakery, N. Y.:					
1919	Casein Breakfast Cereal . . .	36.6	42.5	0.7	11.0[1]	576
1919	Gluten Breakfast Cereal . . .	29.2	19.4	25.5	17.8	464
	Plasmon Co., London:					
1922	Oats	17.3	8.1	57.4[2]	5.9	395
	Pure Gluten Food Co., Columbus, O.:					
1919–4*b*	Gluten Breakfast Food	40.8	0.7	35.7	12.3	361
1916–4*a*	Gum Gluten Granules	39.3	0.9	40.5	11.4	373
1919	Hoyt's Gluten Breakfast Food, 40 per cent protein	46.0	1.8	31.4	10.2	366
1919	Hoyt's Gluten Granules, over 40 per cent protein	43.8	2.6	32.2	10.1	368
	Waukesha Health Products Co., Waukesha, Wis.:					
1919	Hepco Grits	40.3	16.4	0.9	23.9	408
	MACARONI, NOODLES, ETC.					
	Brusson Jeune, Villimur, France:					
1913–2*p*	Petites Pâtes au Gluten	17.0	1.0	61.2	10.8	365
	Callard & Co., London:					
1922	Casoid Flakes	78.5	3.1	1.2[2]	None	347
1922	Casoid Vermicelli	80.0	2.7	0.5[2]	None	346
	The Dieto Food Co., New York:					
1914–2*q*	Whole Wheat Brand Macaroni .	13.9	1.1	58.7	15.0	361
	Jireh Diabetic Food Co., New York:					
1913–2*p*	Macaroni	16.9	0.9	58.8	12.6	361
	Eugene Loeb, New York:					
1913–2*p*	Home Made Noodles	41.8	5.5	36.7	5.0	384
	Loeb's Diabetic Food Bakery, N. Y.:					
1919	Gluten Noodles	37.3	3.6	36.8	10.3	370
	Pure Gluten Food Co., New York:					
1914–2*q*	Hoyt's Gum Gluten Noodles . .	36.9	1.2	41.8	10.8	369
	NUTS AND NUT PREPARATIONS.					
	Dieto Food Co., New York:					
1914–2*q*	Pine Nuts	39.7	50.0	None	2.8	620
	Chas. Lawrence Co., Boston, Mass.:					
1913–2*p*	California Paper Shell Almonds, edible portion	18.4	55.3	None	16.3	637
	Christian National Food Co., Kenilworth, N. J.:					
1916–2*s*	Christian's Protoid Nuts . . .	37.6	48.2	Trace	5.7[1]	607
	Jireh Diabetic Food Co., New York:					
1913–2*p*	Diabetic Pine Nuts (Pignolias) .	39.7	49.4	None	3.4	617

[1] Includes fiber.
[2] Includes soluble carbohydrate.

TABLE 248.—COMPOSITION OF SO-CALLED DIABETIC FOODS, ETC.—(*Continued.*)

Reference.	Manufacturer or agent and name of product.	Protein, per cent.	Fat, per cent.	Carbohydrate.		Calories, per 100 gms.
				Starch, per cent.	Other carbohydrate, per cent.	
	NUTS AND NUT PREPARATIONS— *Concluded.* *The Kellogg Food Co., Battle Creek, Mich.:*					
1913–2p	Nut Bromose (Meltose and Nuts) .	17.1	26.8	3.2	36.2	467
1913–2p	Pine Nuts	38.0	49.6	4	.2	615
	Nashville Sanitarium Food Co., Nashville, Tenn.:					
1913–2p	Malted Nut Food	24.7	42.7	3.4	24.1[1]	593
1913–2p	Nut Butter	28.0	52.6	3.8	9.2	637
1913–2p	Nutcysa	12.9	21.0	Trace	6.3	266
1913–2p	Nutfoda	20.8	8.0	Trace	6.8	182
	CHOCOLATE AND CHOCOLATE PREPARATIONS. *Brusson, Jeune, Villimur, France:*					
1913–2p	Chocolate with added Gluten a la Vanille	15.9	49.7	9.2	17.2	617
	Callard & Co., London:					
1922	"Casoid" Chocolates	22.9	38.8	5.0	23.0	553
1922	"Casoid" Dessert Chocolate . .	24.9	46.1	7.9	11.3	591
1922	"Casoid" Nut Chocolate . . .	23.9	46.4	8.6	11.3	593
1922	Chocolate Biscuits	26.1	49.8	5.6	9.2	612
1922	Sugarless Chocolate	14.0	44.3	14.0	17.3	580
	Fromm & Co., Dresden:					
1913–2p	Conglutin-Diabetiker-Schokolade .	17.6	39.1	4.3	28.4	553
	Karl Goldscheider, Karlsbad:					
1914–2q	Feinste Dessert-Schokolade für Diabetiker, "9.98 per cent carbohydrates"	11.4	57.6	5.0	20.4	665
1914–2q	Feinste Mocca-Schokolade für Diabetiker, "10.26 per cent carbohydrates"	10.2	60.2	4.1	19.4	677
1914–2q	Feinste Nuss-Schokolade für Diabetiker, "11.32 per cent carbohydrates"	14.6	54.4	6.9	16.4	641
1914–2q	Feinste Orange-Schokolade für Diabetiker, "9.98 per cent carbohydrates"	11.4	57.6	5.0	19.9	664
	Loeb's Diabetic Food Bakery, N. Y.:					
1919	Almond Chocolate Bars	14.9	53.2	5.3	15.6	622
1919	Diabetic Chocolate	14.7	51.7	7.3	15.5	615
	Plasmon Co., London:					
1922	Plasmon Chocolate	13.8	29.4	38.5[2]	14.4	531
	Rademan's Nährmittelfabrik, Frankfurt:					
1913–2p	Diabetiker-Chokolade	17.5	57.6	3.8	13.1	656

[1] Includes fiber.
[2] Includes soluble carbohydrate.

TABLE 248.—COMPOSITION OF SO-CALLED DIABETIC FOODS, ETC.—(Continued.)

Reference.	Manufacturer or agent and name of product.	Protein, per cent.	Fat, per cent.	Carbohydrate.		Calories, per 100 gms.
				Starch, per cent.	Other carbohydrate, per cent.	
	COCOA.					
	Callard & Co., London:					
1922	Biogene Cocoa	33.1	17.9	11.1[1]	19.8	417
	Cheltine Food Co., Cheltenham, Eng.:					
1922	Cheltine Milk-Cocoa	47.1	15.9	8.9[1]	13.1	420
	The Dieto Food Co., New York:					
1914-2q	Dieto Cocoa	23.6	22.9	12.4	26.6	456
	Loeb's Diabetic Food Bakery, N. Y.:					
1922	Diabetic Cocoa	25.4	20.9	16.0[1]	23.1	446
	Gustav Müller, New York:					
1913-2q	Charrasse Gluto-Cacao	21.5	22.2	16.3	23.8	466
	Plasmon Co., London:					
1922	Cocoa	50.4	11.6	6.0[1]	13.1	382
	Rademan's Nährmittelfabrik, Frankfurt:					
1913	Diabetiker-Cacao	17.6	23.6	10.7	34.0	462
	SUGAR-FREE MILK.					
	Gustav Müller & Co., New York:					
1913-2p	Dr. Bouma Sugar-free Milk . .	2.4	5.3	..	..	57
	D. Whiting & Sons, Boston, Mass.:					
1919	Sugar-free Milk	6.4	9.3	..	0.2[2]	110
	FRUITS AND VEGETABLES.					
	The Diaprotein Co., Columbus, Ohio:					
	"Dieta" Brand Products:					
1921	Apple Sauce	0.2	0.6	5.8[1]	3.7	44
1921	Blackberries	0.7	0.5	2.6[1]	2.4	27
1921	Cherries, Red, Pitted	0.5	0.1	5.1[1]	3.4	37
1921	White	0.7	0.1	3.8[1]	3.5	33
1921	Peaches, Yellow	0.5	0.1	2.9[1]	2.5	25
1921	Pears, Bartlett	0.3	0.1	2.5[1]	2.7	23
1921	Raspberries, Red	0.9	0.7	3.0[1]	4.0	38
1921	Strawberries	0.6	0.4	2.0[1]	2.4	24
1921	Beans, Cut, Wax	0.8	0.1	1.2[1]	0.5	11
1921	Refugee, Green . . .	1.0	0.1	1.4[1]	0.8	14
1921	Peas, Green	3.2	0.4	3.9[1]	2.2	41
1921	Rhubarb	0.4	0.1	0.3[1]	1.9	11
1921	Spinach	3.1	0.6	0.6[1]	1.0	24
1921	Tomatoes	1.0	0.2	1.5[1]	1.3	-17
	MISCELLANEOUS PRODUCTS.					
	The Dieto Food Co., New York:					
1914-2q	Dieto Baking Powder	..	..	12.9	..	..
1914-2q	Dieto Barley Coffee	13.2	7.3	17.7	46.2	374
	Manual Freres:					
1917-2t	Longuets de Lausanne . . .	14.2	5.5	49.2	16.9	371
	Health Food Co., New York:					
1913-2p	Kaffeebrod	12.9	1.5	10.1	62.4	355
	Genevieve Jackson, Los Angeles, Calif.:					
1919	Dia-Biskit	17.6	4.8	6.1[3]	47.2	328

[1] Includes soluble carbohydrate.
[2] Lactose.
[3] Includes reducing material derived from agar-agar.

TABLE 248.—COMPOSITION OF SO-CALLED DIABETIC FOODS, ETC.—(Concluded.)

Manufacturer or agent and name of product.	Protein, per cent.	Fat, per cent.	Carbohydrate.		Calories, per 100 gms.
			Starch, per cent.	Other carbohydrate, per cent.	
BRAN PRODUCTS.					
Bran Products and Other Laxative Preparations:					
Bran, washed (Woman's Baking Co.) . .	11.2	7.4	4.6[1]	....	....
Bran (so-called "health bran" for dietetic use), average of six commercial brands . . .	15.6	4.8	55.8		329
Bran Biskue	12.1	13.1	61.0		410
Bran Zos	13.2	2.5	65.6		338
Bran-eata Biscuit	9.1	0.9	72.2		333
Brose Good Health Breakfast Food . . .	14.4	4.3	65.5		358
Cerag	11.3	0.9	73.0		345
Christian's Laxative Bread	10.0	1.4	74.6		351
Colax	1.1	0.8	82.8		343
Dietetic Bran Biscuit	9.9	5.0	69.1		361
Educator Bran Cookies	8.9	14.5	64.7		425
Educator Bran Meal	12.3	2.8	66.4		340
F.B.A. Health Biscuit	6.1	1.7	77.3		349
Fruit Nut Cereal	13.5	1.2	72.4		354
Good Health Biscuit (Kellogg)	7.7	1.2	74.5		340
Health Food Wafers	10.0	7.9	65.7		374
India (Digestive) Biscuit	12.8	2.2	66.1		335
Laxa	12.4	2.8	66.6		341
Laxative Biscuits (Kellogg)	16.7	10.8	57.7		395
Mansfield's Agar-Agar Wafers	7.1	12.0	69.9[2]		416
Oval Digestive Biscuit (H and P)	7.8	16.3	64.5		436
Uncle Sam Health Food	21.3	24.4	40.9		468
Zim	7.4	1.7	74.2		342

C. DIETETIC SUGGESTIONS, RECIPES AND MENUS.

Many books have been written containing recipes for diabetic patients. Modern methods of treatment make most of these needless. For severe diabetic patients such rules are often dangerous because of the high content in fat in the foods produced. In general patients prefer and should be encouraged to take simple natural foods rather than artificial ones. The mild cases of diabetes need no special recipes.

1. **Substitutes for Bread.**—Many of the preparations upon the market as shown by Table 248, contain as great, or even a greater, quantity of carbohydrates than ordinary bread; a few contain less; but the percentage of carbohydrate may vary from time to

---

[1] Includes soluble carbohydrate.
[2] Carbohydrate of agar-agar largely unavailable.

time. Patients, and sometimes physicians, forget that substitutes for bread must be prescribed only in definite amounts. A diabetic bread should never be prescribed without a knowledge of its content of carbohydrate, protein and fat.

The bread of one of the largest bakeries in Boston, upon analysis, showed 55 per cent carbohydrate. Bread made without milk or sugar, but with water and butter, contains 45 to 50 per cent carbohydrates. Such a bread is undoubtedly superior to many different bread substitutes upon the market. The percentage of carbohydrate in toast is greater than in plain bread, such as rye bread, Graham bread, black bread and pumpernickel, contain somewhat less carbohydrate. Never give bread substitutes early in treatment. Teach patients to live without them. Potatoes are safer than bread and a banana safer than a potato, though both contain equal percentages of carbohydrate, because the former is limited in size, usually containing about 20 grams carbohydrate, and the latter almost unlimited.

There are four types of bread substitutes.

(*a*) **Bran Bread.**—Bran is being more and more employed in the diet of diabetic patients, but it is usually bran, washed nearly free of carbohydrate. (See below.) This is neither more nor less than the use of cellulose, and this is supposed to have no effect upon the metabolism. Unfortunately, the availability of the protein, fat and carbohydrate of unwashed bran to the diabetic patient has not been determined, although there are plenty of data upon its digestibility by ruminant animals. Bread made of bran alone is not very palatable, though with the fat of bacon or butter it is liked better. It furnishes bulk and acts favorably upon constipation. It should be remembered that untreated bran contains about 56 per cent of carbohydrate of which approximately one-half is assimilable. For this reason bran biscuits bought at a restaurant often prove to be a delusion and a snare. In purchasing bran to use for washed bran go to a feed store and ask for coarse bran for cattle and not for bran for the table. The various preparations of bran, bran breads, and cookies sold under trade names often contain carbohydrate other than bran, hence the reason for their palatable taste; beware of them. They may contain over 60 per cent carbohydrate, of which less than 10 per cent is real bran. Mild diabetics get into little trouble with bran, but the serious ones often suffer.

To free bran from starch first sift in an ordinary flour-sifter. This eliminates a great deal of the finer starch, then tie the bran in cheesecloth and fasten the same on a faucet. It should be thoroughly mixed and kneaded from time to time to be sure the water reaches all portions and should be washed until the water comes away *clear.* This may require an hour.[1]

BRAN WAFERS.

Washed bran . .	2 cups	Salt and saccharine to taste.
India gum . . .	1 tablespoonful	Ginger, cloves, anise or caraway seed,
Mineral oil . . .	1 tablespoonful	½ teaspoonful, if desired.

Mix dry ingredients and then add bran and mineral oil with enough water to make a stiff dough. Knead with finger tips. Pat out and cut into thin cookies. Bake about forty-five minutes in a moderate oven until crisp.

Bran Biscuits for Constipation.—The following rule was given me by Dr. F. M. Allen:

Bran	60 gm.
Salt	¼ teaspoonful
Agar-agar, powdered	6 gm.
Cold water	100 cc (½ glass)

Tie bran (for character of bran to purchase see p. 729) in cheese-cloth and wash under cold water tap until water is clear. Bring agar-agar and water (100 cc) to the boiling-point. Add to washed bran the salt and agar-agar solution (hot). Mold into two cakes. Place in pan on oiled paper, and let stand for half an hour; then, when firm and cool, bake in moderate oven thirty to forty minutes.

The bran muffins naturally will be far more palatable if butter and eggs are added. This may be done providing the patient allows for this in the diet.

BRAN CAKES FOR DIABETICS.

Food.	Amount.	Protein, gm.	Fat, gm.	Carbo-hydrate, gm.	Calories.
Bran	2 cups				
Melted butter .	30 gm.	..	25	...	225
Eggs (whole) .	2	12	12	...	156
Egg-white (1) .	25 gm.	3	..	...	12
Salt	1 teaspoonful				
Water,					
		15	37	0	393

Mix the thoroughly washed and dry bran, well beaten whole eggs, butter and salt. Beat the egg white very stiff and fold in at the last. Shape with knife and tablespoon into three dozen small cakes. If desired, ½ gram of cinnamon or other flavoring

---

[1] Four preliminary analyses of washed bran showed the following percentages of starch: 0.6, 1.8, 2.7, 5.2 per cent. Two preliminary analyses made under the direction of Dr. K. L. Mark, of Simmons College, showed pentosan 29.8 and 33.5. The wide variations in the percentages of starch will account for the occasional occurrence of sugar in the urine following the use of bran cakes.

may be added. Each cake contains: protein, 0.5 gram; fat, 1 gram calories 11.

(*b*) **Gluten Breads.**—These breads are made by removing the sugar-forming material from the flour. It is surprising how thoroughly this can be done. I have often found the percentage of carbohydrate in one such flour to be negligible. The large quantity of protein which they contain in small bulk is objectionable.

(*c*) **Light Breads.**—French bread cut in thin slices is a possible substitute for bread, because it is bulky, gives the appearance of a large quantity, and carries much butter. Manufacturers have taken advantage of this idea, and many light breads are on the market. These breads often contain about the same quantity of carbohydrate as ordinary bread, though a few contain considerably less. Their virtue consists solely in their bulk, which allows a surface on which to spread butter. It is better for the patient to forget the taste, and to follow the advice of Case No. 2962, who replied at a clinic before the Tri-State Medical Society at the Harvard Medical School when I asked what diabetics were to do with apples—"throw them away."

(*d*) **Various Other Substances** have been used for flour in the manufacture of bread. Thus, aleuronat meal, corn cob meal, casein under various trade names, and soy bean have been employed, and the manufacturers have been most ingenious in their preparation.

Soy bean is extensively used, and probably deserves a still wider introduction into the diabetic diet. The carbohydrate in it is unassimilable. Agar-agar may be used to dilute the flour or to add to bran and also to relieve the constipation of the diabetic, which is frequently troublesome. For the last few years India gum, suggested to me by Dr. Allen, has been substituted. It is much cheaper, and is as satisfactory. India gum will thicken broth or any fluid. In the right proportions it is the fundamental for a good many palatable recipes.

2. **Substitutes for Milk.**—A few tablespoonfuls of cream are a great comfort to a diabetic patient. The average patient usually receives 120 cc to 240 cc of 20 per cent cream daily. If it is desirable to give more fat without increasing carbohydrate and protein, 40 per cent cream may be substituted.

It is economical and convenient to give either $\frac{1}{4}$ of a pint or $\frac{1}{2}$ of a pint of cream a day. This makes the quantity definite, corresponds to the customary quantity which is sold and will last either one day or two days. Twenty per cent cream is also the upper 4 ounces on a quart of milk which has stood twenty-four hours.

The fat having been removed the chief value of milk to the diabetic patient is lost. The percentage of sugar in sour milk is not much less than in fresh milk. Sugar-free milks[1] have been put upon the market on a large scale, and many of my patients, particularly children, have found them of distinct advantage. These preparations of diabetic milk will keep from one to three weeks, and are consequently of great value to patients when traveling. As a rule they are concentrated one-half. Consequently they should be diluted before being used. This is advantageously accomplished with an equal part Celestins Vichy.

Williamson suggested the following rule for the manufacture of artificial milk: "To about a pint of water, placed in a large drinking pot or tall vessel, 3 or 4 tablespoonfuls of fresh cream are added and well mixed. The mixture is allowed to stand from twelve to twenty-four hours, when most of the fatty matter of the cream floats to the top; it can be skimmed off with a teaspoon easily, and upon examination it will be found practically free from sugar. This fatty matter thus separated is placed in a glass. The white of an egg is added to it and the mixture well stirred. Then dilute with water until a liquid is obtained which has the exact color and consistency of ordinary milk. If a little salt and a trace of saccharin be added, a palatable drink, practically free from milk sugar, is produced."[2]

Rennet may be made from milk, but unless the curd is carefully washed it will contain 2 to 2.5 per cent lactose. When the rennet is made from cream, the lactose is materially diminished. Kefir contains approximately 2.4 per cent milk sugar. Von Noorden says this milk has been of great help in the treatment of diabetes in children.

Lawrence Litchfield, of Pittsburgh, gives whipped cream to his patients made according to the following rule: Add 2 ounces of 40 per cent cream to a pint of cold water in a Mason jar and have it shaken vigorously until the cream is thoroughly "whipped." Sometimes a trace of saccharin is added, usually not. "My patients like to eat this with a spoon, but, of course, it can be used in any way that is desired." It contains carbohydrate 2 grams, protein 2 grams, fat 24 grams.

BAVARIAN CREAM (DIABETIC).

Food.	Amount.	Protein, grams.	Fat, grams.	Carbo-hydrate, grams.	Calories
Cream, 40 per cent	90 cc	3	36	3	348
Water	10 cc				
Egg (1)	50 gm.	6	6	..	78
Gelatin	2 gm.	2	..	..	8
Saccharin (to sweeten), Flavoring(to taste)					
		11	42	3	434

[1] See page 727.   D. Whiting & Sons, Boston.

Soften the gelatin in cold water, then add to the cream, which has been heated. Stir until dissolved, pour on the beaten egg, cook like soft custard, turn into mold and chill.

ICE CREAM (DIABETIC).

Food.	Amount.	Protein, grams.	Fat, grams.	Carbo-hydrate, grams.	Calories.
Cream, 40 per cent .	90 cc	3	36	3	348
Water	10 cc				
Egg (1)	50 gm.	6	6	..	78
Saccharin (to sweeten)					
Flavoring (to taste)					
		9	42	3	426

Make a soft custard of the egg, 50 cc of the cream, and the water. Whip the remaining 40 cc of cream and fold into custard. The saccharin may be added to the egg. The flavoring should be added last.

Cracked Cocoa.—Cracked cocoa (cocoa nibs) makes a most useful drink for diabetic patients. This is not generally appreciated by the profession

The sample of cracked cocoa (cocoa nibs) used has been purchased of the S. S. Pierce Co., Boston. It was analyzed by Prof. Street, with the following result:

Moisture 2.83
Protein 14.69
Fat 51.42
Fiber 4.32
Ash 3.88
Starch 7.48
Reducing sugar, as dextrose direct . . . . None
Reducing sugar, as dextrose after inversion 0.94

The cocoa is prepared for the table by adding a cupful of the cracked cocoa to a quart of water and letting it simmer on the back of the stove all day, adding water from time to time. The strained infusion alone should be taken and not the nutritious grounds or nibs. Prof. Street was good enough to analyze the infusion, and wrote me: "The cocoa prepared according to directions contained 0.032 per cent of reducing sugar as dextrose direct and 0.138 per cent of total reducing sugars."

Cocoa shells are extensively used as a beverage. One cup of cocoa shells to a quart of water should be used, allow to simmer at least one-half hour. Drink the strained infusion. Cocoa shells are far cheaper than cocoa nibs.

Desserts can often be made with gelatin and this may be flavored with coffee, lemon, rhubarb, or cracked cocoa. In preparing such desserts if saccharin is used it should be added as late as possible during the cooking for it is apt to become bitter with heat. It is always a safe rule to add too little rather than too much saccharin.

Extracts.—In making agar jelly, gelatin and other desserts flavoring extracts can be used. The general rule is one teaspoonful of extract to a pint of liquid. The standard extracts and vegetable colorings can be employed. We frequently use sugar-free extracts which are made by Emma Hall[1] and known to be sugar-free. Some patients overindulge in the use of extracts by putting a teaspoonful in every cup of cocoa shells or coffee that they drink as well as by increasing the amount allowed in recipes. This should be avoided.

Sea moss farina and Irish moss are usually allowable for diabetic patients. Most of the carbohydrate in these materials is in the form of pentosans and galactans, which Swartz[2] has shown to be quite inert in the body. Unfortunately these products are sometimes adulterated with other carbohydrates. This emphasizes the fact that no matter how useful a food may be in itself, one must always be on the lookout for adulteration.

Agar-agar Jelly.

Agar-agar (powdered) 1 teaspoonful.

Water, strained cocoa shells, or coffee, $1\frac{1}{2}$ pints.

Flavoring extract 1 teaspoonful.

Mix agar with a little of the water until it forms a smooth paste. Add rest of water and boil ten minutes. Strain, flavor, color, and sweeten with saccharin as desired. Pour into molds and cool at room temperature.

LEMON JELLY (DIABETIC).

Food.	Amount.	Protein, grams.	Fat, grams.	Carbohydrate, grams.	Calories.
Lemon juice	30 cc	..	..	3	12
Water	50 cc				
Gelatin	4 gm.	4	..	..	16
Saccharin (to sweeten)					
Cream	30 cc	1	12	1	116
		5	12	4	144

Soften gelatin in a part of the cold water. Heat the remaining water and lemon juice and pour over the gelatin. Stir until dissolved. Add saccharin, strain into cups. Serve with cream.

Lime juice is used in flavoring. One teaspoonful in a glass of water makes a good beverage in hot weather. One must be very sure that the lime juice is free from sugar or contains but a trace. The proper seasoning of the food is a great help to the diabetic

[1] Woman's Baking Company, 172 Harvard Avenue, Allston, Mass.
[2] Swartz; Trans. Conn. Acad. Arts and Sci., 1911, 16, 247.

patient. So many articles are excluded from the diet that the great variety which is possible in the preparation of the food by the help of seasoning is overlooked. Horseradish, to be sure, contains 10 per cent of carbohydrate, but it would take at least 2 teaspoonfuls to contain a gram, and probably far more. Sour pickles are allowable, and other pickles made from the group of 5 per cent vegetables, provided one is assured that they have been prepared without sweetening. Mint, capers, curry, tarragon vinegar, distilled vinegar, bay leaf, cloves, ginger, mustard, paprika, anise seed, caraway seed, celery salt and onion extract may all be used as seasoning.

Five per cent vegetables furnish the bulk of a diabetic patient's diet and their variety leaves little chance for monotony. Lettuce, endive, chickory and water cress combined with other fresh vegetables furnish salad all the year round. Cabbage is inexpensive and very good. White, green, red, or Chinese cabbage chopped finely, served cooked or raw as cold slaw, may be used. Greens, chopped, can be blended in cooking as, for example, Abyssinian, senel and chard, Chinese mustard and spinach. For the last few years we have used lettuce instead of washed vegetables. It has but 2 per cent carbohydrate and is more palatable in the end. One patient for over a year before insulin days took 600 grams daily.

Miss McCullough suggests that large outer stalks of cauliflower, slightly green covering, be carefully cleaned, cut in half-inch pieces and boiled until tender. Similarly, green leaves and any small pieces of lettuce may be shredded and served as spinach. The flat, large, celery stalks with any or all leaves chopped finely answer well. Rhubarb retains its acid flavor and has proven so acceptable on addition to the diet that canning it by cold water method for future use should be encouraged.

Diabetic patients should be urged whenever possible to have a garden. This, too, enables a patient to can his own winter's supply of vegetables and the chance to enjoy a variety of vegetables during the winter which otherwise could not be obtained.

At the New England Deaconess Hospital we have seldom found trouble with canned vegetables but it is quite advantageous to use those put up especially for diabetics without the addition of sugar or salt. (See p. 727.) The small stringless beans with practically no bean in them at all are perfectly safe for general use as a 5 per cent vegetable. One must always be careful in using canned vegetables because of sugar which may have been added.

3. **Seven Menus for a Severe Diabetic.**—For menus and recipes which make them possible I am greatly indebted to Miss Alice Dike, Instructor in Household Economics at Simmons College,

to Case No. 765, and to Miss Sigrid Kenseth who has revised the original recipes to make them applicable to present day needs. The carbohydrate is designedly kept low because it is an easy matter to add to it. Similarly with more carbohydrate, more calories can be given in the form of fat. The ketogenic-antiketogenic balance is 1.2 and thus safe for an individual weighing 50 kilograms who while living upon it so regulates his activity that weight is neither gained nor lost.

The calories furnished amount to about 1400—a maintenance diet for a patient weighing about 50 kilograms and a sufficient diet for a patient who leads a quiet life.

THREE STANDARD HOSPITAL DIETS.

		Carbohydrate.	Protein.	Fat.	Calories.
Oatmeal	15 gm.	10	3	1	
Orange	200 "	20	0	0	
5 per cent					
vegetables	600 "	20	10	0	
Meat	60 "	0	16	10	
Eggs	2	0	12	12	
Bacon	30 gm.	0	5	15	
Butter	30 "	0	0	25	
20 per cent cream	240 "	8	8	48	
		58	54	111	1441[1]

DIET I.

Breakfast.	Dinner.	Supper.
Egg omelet . 1	Steak . . . 60 gm.	Egg poached . 1
Bacon . . . 15 gm.	Lettuce and toma-	Bacon . . . 15 gm.
Oatmeal . . 15 "	to salad with	Stewed tomatoes 150 "
20% cream . 80 cc	mayonnaise 100 gm.	Asparagus . . 150 "
Butter . . . 10 gm.	String beans . 100 "	20% cream . . 80 cc
Grapefruit . . 100 "	Cabbage . . 100 "	Butter . . . 10 gm.
Coffee, bran	20% cream . . 80 cc	Grapefruit . . 150 gm.
	Orange . . . 75 gm.	Bran
	Cellu bran, coffee agar	Lemon agar jelly, cocoa
	jelly, tea, bran	shells

DIET II.

Breakfast.	Dinner.	Supper.
Scrambled egg 1	Chicken . . . 60 gm.	Soft boiled egg
Bacon . . . 15 gm.	Cauliflower . . 150 "	with mayonnaise 1
Shredded wheat ½ "	Brussel sprouts . 180 "	Bacon . . . 15 gm.
20% cream . 80 cc	Lettuce . . . 30 "	Swiss chard . . 180 "
Butter . . . 10 gm.	with Cucumber 60 "	Celery . . . 30 "
Orange . . . 50 "	Butter . . . 15 "	Lettuce . . . 30 "
Coffee	20% cream . . 80 cc	20% cream . . 80 cc
Bran	Grapefruit . . 100 gm.	Strawberries . 150 gm.
	Bran, cocoa shells, maple	Tea, bran
	agar jelly	

[1] The patient is an adult. Weight, 50 kilograms. If fat in the cream is 40 per cent, the calories would amount to 1657.

DIET III.

Breakfast.	Dinner.	Supper.
Bacon . . . 30 gm.	Cod fish . . . 60 gm.	Eggs 2
Oatmeal . . 30 gm.	Bacon . . . 20 "	Chopped raw cab-
20% cream . 100 cc	Stewed tomato . 150 "	bage with diabe-
Butter . . . 15 gm.	Boiled onion . 90 "	tic mayonnaise 60 gm.
Bran, coffee	Radish . . . 20 "	Spinach . . . 150 "
	Lettuce . . . 40 "	Butter . . . 10 "
	with Grapefruit,	Orange, sliced . 100 "
	salad . . . 100 "	Cocoa shells
	20% cream . . 60 cc	Bran
	Butter . . . 15 gm.	
	Lemon and lime agar jelly	
	Bran, coffee	

Squab.—A squab when carefully boned yields 50 grams of meat. This is broiled in an oiled paper case to prevent evaporation, and when served with the escaped juices proves a favorite dish for patients. It contains about 12 grams protein and 5 grams fat. The lean part of a lamb chop yields about 30 grams of meat.

Boiled Dinner.—Corned beef, with cabbage and one other vegetable, served together as a boiled dinner, is most acceptable to male patients. A portion containing 50 to 75 grams of meat and 100 grams of each vegetable makes an excellent meal. Corned beef hash made of meat and vegetables in the same proportion could also be served for variety.

4. Diabetic Menus for a Week.

(Prepared by Miss Sigrid Kenseth, R. N., of the New England Deaconess Hospital.)

MONDAY.

Total Diet for the Day.

	Grams.	Carbohydrate.	Protein.	Fat.
Bacon	30 0		5	15
Egg (1)	 0		6	6
Chicken	45 0		12	5
Meat	45 0		12	8
40 per cent cream	150 5		5	60
Grapefruit	200 10		0	0
Lettuce	50 1		1	0
5 per cent vegetables	420 14		7	0
Butter	30 0		0	25
		30	48	119

Breakfast.

1 egg with tomato, scrambled 60 gm.   40 per cent cream with coffee 40 cc.
Bacon . . . . 30 "   Butter . . . . 5 gm.
Grapefruit . . . . . 140 "

Total: Carbohydrate, 10; protein, 13; fat, 41.

47

Lunch.

Salad with mayonnaise: Baked stuffed tomato:
Chicken . . . . . . 45 gm. Butter . . . . . . 5 gm.
Celery . . . . . . 60 " Tomato . . . . . . 90 "
Lettuce . . . . . . 60 " Celery . . . . . . 30 "
         Onion . . . . . . 15 "
Raspberry jelly with 40 per cent cream, whipped . . . . . 55 cc.
Butter . . . . 5 gm.
Tea and 40 per cent cream . . . . 10 cc.
Total: Carbohydrate, 10; protein, 19; fat, 39.

Dinner.

Meat pie: Butter . . . . 15 gm.
Meat . . . . . . 45 gm. Coffee ice cream (40 per cent
Tomato . . . . . . 60 "   cream) . . . . . . 45 cc.
Cauliflower . . . . . 90 " Grapefruit . . . . . 60 gm.
Total: Carbohydrate, 10; protein, 18; fat, 39.

TUESDAY.

Total Diet for the Day.

	Grams.	Carbohydrate.	Protein.	Fat.
Eggs (2)		0	12	12
Grapefruit	100	5	0	0
Triscuit	1	7	1	0
Bacon	30	0	5	15
Cheese	15	0	4	6
40 per cent cream	120	4	4	48
Meat	60	0	16	10
5 per cent vegetables	360	12	6	0
Butter	35	0	0	29
Lettuce	100	2	1	0
		30	49	120

Breakfast.

Dropped egg on toasted Triscuit with 40 per cent cream with coffee 30 cc.
Butter . . . . . 5 gm. Bran
Bacon . . . . . 30 " Butter . . . . 5 gm.
Total: Carbohydrate, 8; protein, 13; fat, 41.

Lunch.

Cheese omelet: Salad with mayonnaise:
Cheese . . . . . . 15 gm. Lettuce . . . . . . 50 gm.
Egg (1) . . . . . .   Cucumber . . . . . 30 "
Fried egg plant . . . . 180 " Tomato . . . . . . 30 "
Butter . . . . 5 "

Lemon Bavarian Cream (40 per cent cream) . . . . . . 50 cc.
Bran with butter . . . . 5 gm.
Tea
Total: Carbohydrate, 11; protein, 16; fat, 40.

Dinner.

Meat (croquettes) . . . 60 gm. Lettuce with French dressing 50 gm.
Tomato sauce: Cauliflower . . . . . 90 "
Butter . . . . . . 5 " Butter . . . . 10 "
Tomato . . . . . . 30 " Strawberries . . . . . 75 "
         with cream . . . . . 40 cc.

Total: Carbohydrate, 11; protein, 20; fat, 39.

WEDNESDAY.

Total Diet for the Day.

	Grams.	Carbohydrate.	Protein.	Fat.
Bacon	30	0	5	15
Lettuce	100	2	1	0
Egg and white (1)		0	9	6
Oatmeal	10	7	2	1
Olive oil	10	0	0	10
Butter	30	0	0	25
40 per cent cream	120	4	4	48
Chicken	45	0	12	5
Meat	45	0	12	8
5 per cent vegetables	300	10	5	0
Grapefruit	140	7	0	0
		30	50	118

Breakfast.

Oatmeal	10 gm.	Butter	10 gm.
1 egg, egg white(egg in nest)	1 "	Grapefruit	40 "
Bacon	20 "	Brans	2
40 per cent cream	40 cc.	Coffee	

Total: Carbohydrate, 10; protein, 15; fat, 41.

Lunch.

40 per cent cream with clam broth	20 cc.	Bran with mayonnaise, 40 per per cent cream	20 cc.
Club sandwich:		Cocoa shells	
Chicken	45 gm.	Brans	2
Lettuce	50 "	Grapefruit	100 gm.
Tomato	90 "		
Bacon	10 "		
Butter	15 "		

Total: Carbohydrate, 10; protein, 17; fat, 39.

Dinner.

Cream asparagus soup:		Veal	45 gm.
Butter	5 gm.	Brussel sprouts	120 "
40 per cent cream	30 "	Lettuce	50 "
Asparagus	90 "	French dressing:	
Mocha whip		Olive oil	10 cc.
Coffee with 40 per cent cream	10 cc.	Vinegar	10 "
Cellu-bran wafers	2		

Total: Carbohydrate, 10; protein, 18; fat, 38.

THURSDAY.

Total Diet for the Day.

	Grams.	Carbohydrate.	Protein.	Fat.
Chicken	45	0	12	5
Corned beef	60	0	16	10
Liver	30 }	0	11	17
Bacon	30 }			
5 per cent vegetables	300	14	7	0
40 per cent cream	150	5	5	60
Butter	45	0	0	38
Grapefruit	200	10	0	0
Orange	30	3	0	0
		29	50	121

Breakfast.

Grapefruit	140 gm.	Butter	10 gm.
Liver	30 "	40 per cent cream . . .	30 cc.
Bacon	30 "	Bran	
		Coffee	

Total: Carbohydrate, 8; protein, 12; fat, 42.

Lunch.

Chicken à la King:

Chicken	45 gm.	Cold slaw	60 gm.
40 per cent cream . . .	50 cc.	Sliced	
Butter	10 gm.	Orange	25 "
Green pepper	15 "	Grapefruit	60 "
Pimento	15 "	40 per cent cream with cocoa	
Mushrooms	60 "	shells	10 cc.
		Butter	5 gm.
		Bran	

Total: Carbohydrate, 11; protein, 17; fat, 42.

Dinner.

Broth		Butter	10 gm
Boiled dinner:		Cocoa Blanc Mange	
Corned beef	60 gm.	Cream	60 cc.
Cabbage	120 "		
Turnip	60 "		

Total: Carbohydrate, 10; protein, 21; fat, 42.

FRIDAY.

Total Diet for the Day.

	Grams.	Carbohydrate.	Protein.	Fat.
Bacon	40	0	7	20
Orange	90	9	0	0
5 per cent vegetables	450	15	8	0
Lettuce	100	2	1	0
Olive oil	10	0	0	10
Butter	45	0	0	38
40 per cent cream	120	4	4	48
Fat fish	60	0	12	6
Fish (haddock)	90	0	18	0
		30	50	122

Breakfast.

Orange	90 gm.	Butter	10 gm.
Bacon	40 "	Bran	
40 per cent cream . . .	30 cc.	Coffee	

Total: Carbohydrate, 10; protein, 8; fat, 40.

Lunch.

Fish chowder:		Maple whip with 40 per cent	
Haddock	90 gm.	cream	15 cc.
40 per cent cream . . .	45 "	Butter	10 gm.
Onion	30 "	Bran	
Butter	10 "	Tea or cocoa shells.	
Stuffed tomato salad:			
Tomato	90 gm.		
Lettuce	50 "		
Cucumber and celery . .	60 "		

Total: Carbohydrate, 10; protein, 24; fat, 41.

Dinner.

Tomato bouillon:
Tomato	60 gm.
Butter	5 "
Mackerel (broiled) with melt-	45 "
ed butter	10 "
Endive	50 "
Greens	150 "
Celery	30 "

Total: Carbohydrate, 10; protein, 18; fat, 41.

French dressing:
Olive oil	10 gm.
Vinegar	10 "
Pineapple jelly with 40 per cent cream, whipped . .	30 cc.

SATURDAY.

Total Diet for the Day.

	Grams.	Carbohydrate.	Protein.	Fat.
Eggs (2)	. . . . .	0	12	12
Meat	60	0	16	10
Bacon	30	0	5	15
Sardines	30	0	7	6
40 per cent cream	120	4	4	48
Butter	35	0	0	29
5 per cent vegetables	390	13	7	0
Strawberries	75	5	0	0
Grapefruit	160	8	0	0
		30	51	120

Breakfast.

Griddle cakes (1 egg) with substitute maple syrup	
Grapefruit	160 gm.
Butter	15 "

Bacon	20 gm.
Cream (40 per cent) . . .	30 cc.
Coffee	

Total: Carbohydrate, 9; protein, 10; fat, 41.

Lunch.

Tomato bisque:
40 per cent cream . . .	40 cc.
Tomato	120 gm.
Butter	5 "
Sardines	30 "
Swiss chard	120 "

Butter	5 gm.
Bran	
Sponge cake (½ egg)	
40 per cent cream . . .	10 cc.
Cocoa shells	

Total: Carbohydrate, 10; protein, 16; fat, 39.

Dinner.

Broth	
Steak	60 gm.
Bacon	10 "
Cauliflower	60 "
Mushrooms	90 "
Strawberry shortcake:	
Sponge cake (½ egg)	
Strawberries	75 gm.
40 per cent cream, whipped	40 cc.

String beans	90 gm.
Lettuce salad with mayonnaise	
Butter	10 "
Bran:	

Total: Carbohydrate, 11; protein, 25; fat, 42.

SUNDAY.

Total Diet for the Day.

	Grams.	Carbohydrate.	Protein.	Fat.
Egg (1)		0	6	6
Oysters (6)		4	6	1
Meat	90	0	24	15
Oil	15	0	0	15
5 per cent vegetables	450	11	6	0
10 per cent vegetables	45	3	3	0
Grapefruit	80	4	0	0
40 per cent cream	120	4	4	48
Butter	30	0	0	25
Bacon	20	0	3	10
		30	52	120

Breakfast.

Grapefruit	80 gm.	40 per cent cream	30 cc.
Corned beef and vegetable hash:		Butter	10 gm.
Bacon	20 "	Coffee	
Corned beef	45 "	Bran	
Cabbage	60 "		
Beets	45 "		

Total: Carbohydrate, 10; protein, 18; fat, 38.

Lunch.

Oyster stew:		Asparagus	90 gm.
Oysters	6	40 per cent cream	10 cc.
40 per cent cream	60 cc.	Lemon and lime jelly	
Butter	10 gm.		
Egg salad:			
Egg	1		
Lettuce	30 gm.		
Mayonnaise			

Total: Carbohydrate, 10; protein, 16; fat, 43.

Dinner.

Roast lamb with mint sauce	45 gm.	French dressing:	
String beans (canned)	150 "	Olive oil	15 cc.
Butter	10 "	Vinegar	10 "
Sliced cucumber	30 "	Rhubarb (pie)	90 gm.
		40 per cent cream	20 cc.
		Coffee	

Total: Carbohydrate, 10; protein, 18; fat, 39.

Recipes for Daily Menus.

Broths.—Each pound of beef, veal, chicken or lamb, or 1 pint of clams, should make 1 quart of broth. Let cool, and skim off all fat before serving.

Bouillon.—Bouillon cubes are not advisable because of their high salt content.
Salt:

Armour's	21 per cent
Steero	39 "
Oxo	62 "

Tomato Bouillon.

Tomato	60 gm.	Bay leaf	½
Broth	1 cup	Clove	1
Onion extract	½ teaspoonful	Celery salt or celery	
		tops	¼ teaspoonful

Mix all ingredients, boil twenty minutes, strain and serve.

Bran Cookies.

Washed bran	2 cups
India gum	1 tablespoonful
Mineral oil	1 "

Salt and saccharin to taste.

Ginger, cloves, anise, or caraway seed, ½ teaspoonful, if desired.

Mix dry ingredients and then add bran and mineral oil with enough water to make a stiff dough. Knead with finger tips. Pat out and cut into thin cookies. Bake about forty-five minutes in a moderate oven until crisp.

Cellu-bran Cookies.

Washed bran	2 cups
Cellu-flour	½ cup
India gum	1 tablespoonful
Spice	1 teaspoonful
Mineral oil	1 tablespoonful

Salt and saccharin to taste.

Mix as bran cakes and bake in moderate oven, being careful not to brown cookies.

Cellu-flour Cookies.

Cellu-flour	2 cups
India gum	1 tablespoonful
Flavoring extract or spice	1 teaspoonful

Salt and saccharine to taste.

Mix and bake as above.

Cellu-flour Pie Crust.

Cellu-flour	2 tablespoonfuls
India gum	1 teaspoonful

Salt and enough water to make a stiff dough.

Mix with finger tips and shape pie crust as desired before baking, bake in a moderate oven, being careful not to brown.

Cellu-flour Sponge Cakes.

Egg	1
Water	1 tablespoonful
Extract	½ teaspoonful
Cellu-flour	1–1½ tablespoonfuls

Beat white and yolk of egg separately. To the yolk add water, extract, salt and saccharin. Then add cellu-flour from 1 to 1½ tablespoonfuls, according to the consistency of the yolk. When the mixture is almost brittle add the egg white, being careful not to beat in too thoroughly. A pinch of baking powder may be used if desired. Bake in a quick oven about fifteen minutes.

Variations.—With strawberries and whipped cream, as allowed in diet, a short-cake can be made; 15 gm. of nuts chopped may be added if allowed in diet, or 30 gm. of blueberries if desired.

Cellu-flour Griddle Cakes.

Egg	1
Water	1 tablespoonful
Cellu-flour	1–2 tablespoonfuls

Salt and saccharin to taste.

Beat white and yolk of egg separately and together add water and cellu-flour, enough to make a fairly firm mixture, salt and saccharin. Fry on a hot griddle and serve with butter allowed in diet or a substitute maple syrup.

Food value: Carbohydrate, 0; protein, 6; fat, 6.

Substitute Maple Syrup.

Water	1 cup
India gum	½ teaspoonful
Maple extract	1 "
Saccharin	

Mix gum with a little water and then gradually add the remainder of cup, beating with an egg-beater until all lumps are removed. Add flavoring, saccharin and extract; serve hot.

Candy.

Agar-agar . . . .   4 teaspoonfuls
Water . . . .   1000 cc.
Flavoring (wintergreen, peppermint, spearmint or vanilla).
Dissolve agar in water. Bring to a boil and boil twenty minutes. Cool after adding flavoring and saccharin and cut in squares.

Cheese Custard.

Egg   1
Milk   . . . .   120 cc.
Grated cheese . . . .   10 gm.
Beat egg, add pinch of salt, milk and cheese. Beat and bake as two custards in a pan of water in oven.

Cream . . . .   60 cc.
Water (may be used if milk is not allowed in diet) . . . . . .   30 "

Food value with milk: Carbohydrate, 6; protein, 13; fat, 14.
Food value with cream: Carbohydrate, 2; protein, 8; fat, 18.

Cheese Salad.

Cream cheese . . . .   15 gm.
Pimento . . . .   10–15 "
Dice pimento and mix with cheese allowed. Shape into small balls and serve on lettuce, 25 gm.
Food value: Carbohydrate, 1; protein, 5; fat, 5.

Irish Moss Blanc Mange.—Soak small amount of moss in cold water ten minutes. Pour off water and add to moss 60 cc of 40 per cent cream and 120 cc of cocoa shell liquid. Bring to boil and boil until a drop jellies on a coldplate. Then flavor with vanilla, ½ teaspoonful, and saccharin. Strain and mold.

Custard.

Egg   1
Cream . . . .   60 cc.
Milk   . . . .   120 "
    or
Cream . . . .   60 "
Water . . . .   120 "
Flavoring, saccharin, nutmeg if desired.
Beat egg thoroughly, add cream, milk, etc. Bake as two custards in a pan of water. Any combination of milk and cream if figured correctly may be used.
Food value of each custard with milk: Carbohydrate, 4; protein, 6; fat, 11.
Food value of each custard with water: Carbohydrate, 1; protein, 4; fat, 9.

Agar-agar Jelly.

Agar-agar (powdered) . . . .   1 teaspoonful
Water, strained cocoa shells, or coffee . . . .   1½ pints
Flavoring extract . . . .   1 teaspoonful
Mix agar with a little of the water until a smooth paste. Add rest of water and boil ten minutes. Strain, flavor, color and sweeten with saccharin as desired. Pour into molds and cool at room temperature.

Suggestions:

Vanilla .	. . . .	1 teaspoonful	Coffee	1 cup
Lemon .	. . . .	1 "	Cocoa shells . . .	1 "
Orange .	. . . .	1 "	Peppermint . . .	½ teaspoonful
Lime .	. . . .	1 "	Wintergreen . . .	½ "
Raspberry .	. . .	1 "	Spearmint . . .	½ "
Strawberry	. . .	1 "	Mint and little bit of	
Pineapple .	. . .	1 "	lemon juice.	
Mapleine .	. . . .	1 "	Lemon and lime, each	1 teaspoonful

Gelatin.—One teaspoonful gelatin to 2 cups of hot water dissolved may be added to 1 teaspoonful of any of the above extracts and saccharin to taste. Gelatin is used very little because of high protein content. Gelatin may be used when agar-agar is too laxative.

Bavarian Cream.—To any of the extracts suggested, when just beginning to jell, beat in whipped cream allowed in diet.

Whips.—To any jellies, when partially jelled, beat in beaten white of egg. Cocoa and coffee together make a mocha whip.

Coffee Spanish Cream.—Dissolve ½ teaspoonful of gelatin in 5 tablespoonfuls of coffee. Pour this on beaten yolk of egg. Add 60 cc of cream and 60 cc of milk, saccharin. Cook as soft custard and when thick add to beaten white of egg. This makes two creams. Chill and mold on ice.
Food value of one cream: Carbohydrate, 2.5; protein, 5; fat, 10.

Spanish Cream.—Use maple, vanilla or other extract and dissolve gelatin in hot water instead of coffee, or use hot cocoa shells instead of hot coffee.

Snow Pudding.
Lemon juice	1 teaspoonful
Gelatin	1 "
Saccharin	2 grains
Boiling water	½ cup
1 egg white beaten stiff	

Dissolve gelatin in ½ cup of boiling water, add lemon juice, saccharin. When partly jelled add beaten egg white. Beat thoroughly and cool.
Food value: Carbohydrate, 1; protein, 3; fat, 0.

Peach Snow Pudding.
Peaches cooked (less if figured)	75 gm.

Remove peaches from juice. Dissolve in the juice 1 teaspoonful of gelatin. Add enough boiling water to make 1 cup. Add small amount of pink coloring. When partially jelled beat with an egg-beater until light and frothy. Then stir in peaches.
Food value: Carbohydrate, 10; protein, 0; fat, 0.

Custard Sauce (for any desserts).
Cream or milk	30 cc,
Egg yolk	½ (saccharin)
Water	2 tablespoonfuls

Cook as a soft custard, cool and serve.
Food value with milk: Carbohydrate, 1; protein, 4; fat, 4.
Food value with cream: Carbohydrate, 1; protein, 4; fat, 9.

Ice Cream.
Cream	60 cc.
Milk	60 "
Egg	1 "
Saccharin and flavoring	

Beat as an egg-nog and freeze. More milk and cream may be added to make enough for two meals, or cream may be used entirely if milk is not allowed in diet.
Food value: Carbohydrate, 5; protein, 10; fat, 20.

Coffee Ice Cream.
Coffee	1 cup
20 per cent or 40 per cent cream	45-60 cc.
India gum	1 teaspoonful
Saccharin to taste	

Dissolve India gum in a little water, add coffee, beat and boil until a smooth consistency. Add cream and saccharin. Put mixture in small saucepan. Place in larger pan of salt and ice. Stir from time to time until mixture freezes and is smooth. Cocoa shells may be used in the same way instead of coffee if desired.

Rhubarb Pie.—Stew rhubarb, 90 gm., in ¼ cup of water. Thicken with ¼ teaspoonful of India gum. Cool, sweeten with saccharin and put in crust which has been previously baked.

Other fillings may be made the same way, using more India gum if necessary

		C.
Cranberry	30 gm.	3
Blueberries	65 "	10
Peach	75 "	10

Suggestions.

Eggs.

Fried	Scrambled with tomato
Broiled	Baked in tomato with cheese on top.
Scrambled—onion, chives, parsley	Stuffed eggs
Omelet—plain or with asparagus, 60 gm.	Dropped eggs
Baked	Ham omelet
Hard boiled served with spinach	Egg with dried beef
Hard boiled in salad	Spanish omelet

Cheese Omelet.—Beat white and yolk of 1 egg separately. Add to yolk 15 grams of grated cheese, pinch of salt and 1 teaspoonful of water. Fold in white of egg. Beat stiff. Bake in oven until a golden brown.
Food value: Carbohydrate, 0; protein, 10; fat, 12.

Egg in Nest.—Beat white of 1 egg until very stiff with a little salt. Drop on a tin greased with mineral oil and sink whole yolk into the center of the white. Bake in a quick oven about five minutes until brown.

Scrambled Egg and Tomato.

Egg	1
Tomato	60 gm.

Beat white and yolk separately with a little salt and fold in together. Put into frying pan greased with mineral oil. Cook one minute then add 60 gm. cooked tomato pulp, stirring with a fork until done.
Food value: Carbohydrate, 2; protein, 7; fat, 6.

Fat-free Fish.	**Fat Fish.**	**Canned Fish.**
Cod	Mackerel	Salmon
Haddock	Sword fish	Tuna
Finnan haddie	Smelts	
Flounder	Fresh salmon	
Salt cod	Trout	
Lobster	Halibut, etc.	
Shrimp		

Meat, 30 gm., equals { Fat-free fish, 30 gm.   or   Fish,   40 gm.
{ Bacon,   10 "   Butter, 6 "

Meat, 30 gm., equals   Fat fish, 30 gm.

Meat, 30 gm., equals { Canned salmon, 30 gm.
{ Canned tuna,   30 "

Fish Chowder.

40 per cent cream	45 cc
Fish	90 gm.
Onion	40 gm.
India gum	1 teaspoonful
Salt	
Parsley	

Cut fish in small pieces and cook with finely chopped onion. Strain and thicken with ½ teaspoonful of India gum, add to onion and fish. Add parsley and salt. Lastly, add cream and heat in a double boiler. Butter may be added if desired.

Food value with milk (60 cc): Carbohydrate, 5; protein, 21; fat, 2.
Food value with 20 per cent cream (60 cc): Carbohydrate, 4; protein, 22; fat, 12.
Food value with 40 per cent cream (45 cc): Carbohydrate, 3.5; protein, 21.5; fat, 18.

Fish Cakes.

Fish—salt cod—(more according to fish in diet) . . . . 30 gm.
Bran . . . . 2 teaspoonfuls
India gum . . . . ½ teaspoonful
Onion extract, few drops, seasoning.

Mix all together with enough hot water or broth to shape into a cake. Fry until brown in mineral oil.

Food value: Carbohydrate, 0; protein, 6; fat, 0.

Salt cod soaked overnight and cooked can be used, taking cooked weight.

Meat.—Any lean meat can be used in a diabetic diet, pork being the only meat in which it is hard to differentiate the fat.

Meat Pie.

Meat . . . . 45 gm.
Tomato . . . . 90 "
Celery . . . . 60 "
Food value: Carbohydrate, 5; protein, 15; fat, 8.

Stew all together in one cup of broth. Pour off the broth and thicken in casserole with cellu-flour crust on it. Bay leaf, parsley and mace may be used as flavoring if desired; if diet is so small that it does not permit the use of onion, onion extract may be used, also celery salt.

Thin Stew.—This may be as above, but use a smaller amount of India gum in thickening. Any combination of vegetable may be used in making either of the above, but the value must be figured out and deducted from diet.

Meat or Chicken Croquettes.

Meat . . . . 60 gm.
Washed bran . . . . 1 teaspoonful
India gum . . . . ½ "
Broth . . . . 1 tablespoonful
Onion extract, a few drops.

Mix gum and bran together. Add to meat which has been ground up. Add broth, salt and pepper and onion extract. Shape into two croquettes. Fry in deep mineral oil until golden brown.

Food value: Carbohydrate, 0; protein, 16; fat, 10.

Chicken à la King.

Mushrooms . . . . . 60 gm.   Green pepper . . . 15 gm.
Chicken . . . . . . 45 "   40 per cent cream . . 50 cc.
Pimento . . . . . . 15 "   Broth . . . . . . 1 cup

Cook chicken, vegetables, broth and cream together one-half hour. Pour off liquid and thicken with ½ teaspoonful of India gum. Add to chicken and vegetables and serve.

Food value: Carbohydrate, 3; protein, 15; food, 36.

Club Sandwich.—Butter 4 bran wafers with 15 gm. of butter, then, using chicken, bacon, etc., as above, make 2 sandwiches.

Mayonnaise Dressing.

Yolk of egg 1
Mineral oil . . . . 3 cups
Juice of lemon . . . . ½
Salt, paprika, mustard to taste
Distilled vinegar . . . . 1–2 tablespoonfuls

Beat yolk, add lemon juice, mustard, salt, paprika, then oil drop by drop until it is thoroughly worked in, not increasing amount until you are sure it will not separate. Add vinegar to proper consistency. Allow 2 dessertspoonfuls daily.

Oil Dressing.—Equal parts of oil and vinegar. Beat with a little ice. Add salt, pepper. Remove ice and serve at once.

Any 5 per cent vegetables or 10 per cent vegetables may be served cold on lettuce with mayonnaise or French dressing.

Suggestions.

Asparagus	60 gm.		Lobster salad
String beans	60 "		Shrimp salad
String beans ⎫ Beets ⎭	30 "		Chicken and celery salad.
Tomato plain	60 "		
Tomato stuffed with cucumber			
Chopped cabbage	60 "		
Cabbage, 60 gm., with green pepper	15 "		
Cabbage, 60 gm., with pimento. .	15 "		
Radishes	30 "		
Cucumber	30 "		
Beets and carrots chopped . . .	60 "		

Stuffed Tomato Salad.—Weigh tomato after scooping inside. Chop up cucumber and celery about 50 gm. Mix together with mayonnaise. Season, refill shell and serve on lettuce leaf. Other vegetables should be used chopped up in place of cucumber and celery.

Chicken Salad.

Chicken (chopped)	45 gm.
Celery (chopped)	60 "

Mix with diabetic mayonnaise and serve on crisp lettuce, 50 gms.

Oyster Stew.

40 per cent cream	60 cc.
Oysters	6
Water	1 cup
Butter	10 gm.
Salt, etc.	

Stew oysters in 1 cup of water. Add cream and butter when oysters are cooked. Heat, add seasoning and serve.

Food value: Carbohydrate, 6; protein, 8; fat, 33.

Cream of Asparagus Soup.

Asparagus	90 gm.
40 per cent cream	30 cc.
Cold water	1 cup
India gum	½ teaspoonful
Butter	5 gm.

Cook asparagus in water, strain, add water to cream and thicken with India gum, ½ teaspoonful. Put asparagus through sieve, add to the above and serve.

Food value: Carbohydrate, 4; protein, 3; fat, 16.

Cream of Tomato Soup.

Tomato	120 gm.
40 per cent cream	40 cc.
India gum	2 teaspoonfuls
Water	½ cup
Butter	5 gm.

Heat tomato, strain and weigh. Mix India gum with cold water. Add cream and beat with turbin beater. Heat in double boiler (salt, cayenne, paprika). Add two mixtures at last.

Food value: Carbohydrate, 5; protein, 3; fat, 20.

Most any combination can be worked out of 20 per cent cream or milk to use in these recipes, when 40 per cent cream is not allowed in diet. Cream of celery and spinach soup are very good.

Gravy.—Thicken 1 cup of broth with ½ teaspoonful of India gum. Beat with a turbine egg-beater until all lumps are removed. Season as desired and serve hot.

Tomato Sauce.

Bay leaf ⎱
Tomato ⎰ 30 gm. stewed with ¼ cup of hot water.

Strain and thicken with India gum. Season with salt, pepper and a few crops of onion extract. Serve hot.

Vegetables.—Fried Egg Plant.—Cut egg plant in fairly thin slices. Parboil in salted water. Drain off water, dry thoroughly, and fry in deep hot mineral oil. Serve with butter.

Baked Stuffed Tomato.—Weigh tomato, 90 gm., scoop out inside and stew together with celery, 30 gm., onion, 15 gm., butter, 5 gm., bay leaf, salt and pepper. Refill shell and bake in oven fifteen to twenty minutes.

Coleslaw.—Chop up cabbage finely and mix with diabetic mayonnaise dressing, 1 dessertspoonful. Serve cold.

New England Deaconess Hospital Recipe for Cooking Oatmeal.

Oatmeal . . . . 1 cup
Water . . . . 4 cups

Bring to boiling-point and steam in double boiler for three hours. Multiply number of grams dry weight by 8 to find cooked weight.

D. TABLES OF EQUIVALENTS.

TABLE 249.—COMPARATIVE SCALES OF KILOGRAMS AND POUNDS, CENTIMETERS AND INCHES.

(I am indebted to Mr. Edward Clark, of the Massachusetts Institute of Technology, for the preparation of these scales.)

Kilograms to pounds.　　　　　Centimeters to feet and inches.

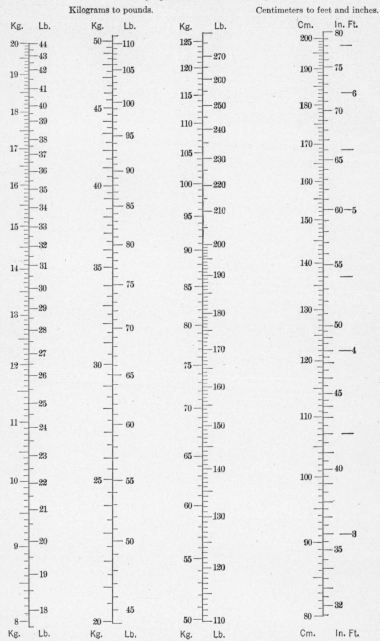

E. EQUIVALENTS USEFUL IN DIABETIC WORK.[1]

TABLE 250.

1 gram O_2 (T. = 0° C.   Tension, 760 mm. mercury) = 0.7   liters.
1 gram CO_2 (T. = 0° C.   Tension, 760 mm. mercury) = 0.5091 liters.

1 liter O_2 (T. = 0° C.   Tension, 760 mm. mercury) = 1.4285 gm.
1 liter CO_2 (T. = 0° C.   Tension, 760 mm. mercury) = 1.9642 gm.

According to Zuntz[2] the quantity of oxygen which has been used and the quantity of carbon dioxide which has been produced in the combustion of protein represented by the excretion of 1 gram of urinary nitrogen is, at 0° C. and a pressure of 760 mm. Hg., as follows:

1 gram urinary nitrogen equivalent to 8.44 grams O_2, or 5.91 liters.
1 gram urinary nitrogen equivalent to 9.33 grams CO_2, or 4.75 liters.

1.0 ounce . . . .   28.4   grams
1.0 pound . . . .   454.0   "
2.2 pounds . . . .   1.0   kilogram

1 fluidounce . . . .   29.6   cubic centimeters
1 quart . . . .   946.0   "   "

1000 grams . . . .   1.0   kilogram
1000 cubic centimeters . . . . .   1.0   liter

1.0 meter . . . .   39.37 inches
1000.0 meters . . . . 3281.00 feet
1609.3 meters . . . . 5280.00 feet or 1 mile.

---

1 horizontal kilogram-meter requires expenditure of 0.0005 calorie.
426.5 vertical kilogram-meters represent the heat equivalent of 1 calorie.

[1] See Table 150, p. 399 and Table 152, p. 401.
[2] Zuntz u. Schumburg: Physiologie des Marsches, Berlin, Hirschwald, 1901, p. 361.

SECTION IX.

HARRIS AND BENEDICT PREDICTION TABLES.

The Harris and Benedict formula employed for men is:

$$h = 66.473 - 13.752w - 5.003s - 6.755a$$

in which h represents the heat-production per twenty-four hours, w the nude body weight in kilograms, s the height without shoes in centimeters, and a the age in years. For a male, aged twenty-four years, height 170 cm., and weight 63 kilograms, and assuming the metabolism obtained by observation to be 1783 calories, the calculation would therefore be as follows:

$$h = 66.473 - (13.752 \times 63) - (5.003 \times 170) - (6.755 \times 24) = 1621 \text{ calories;}$$

$$\frac{\text{observed metabolism (1783)} - \text{predicted metabolism (1621)}}{1621} = 10 \text{ per cent H. and B.}$$

For women the formula is:

$$h = 655.096 - 9.563w - 1.85s - 4.676a$$

Making use of the Harris and Benedict Prediction Tables the calculation of basal metabolism is as follows:

Sex . . . . Male	Factor for height and age in cm.[1]		688
Age in years 24	Factor for weight in kg.[2] . .		933
Height in centimeters 170			——
Weight in kilograms 63	Basal metabolism		1621

The DuBois method is based upon his formula for calculating the body-surface. Having obtained this, it is multiplied by the calories computed by him to be standard for square meter body-surface for age and sex.

---

[1] See page 755.

[2] See page 760.

48

(753)

The DuBois formula for ascertaining body-surface of men and women is as follows:

$$\text{Area (sq. cm.)} = \text{Weight}^{0.425} \times \text{Height}^{0.725} \times 71.84$$

in which the product of the weight in kilograms raised to the power 0.425 and the height in centimeters raised to the power 0.725 is multiplied by the factor 71.84.

The DuBois table for estimation of calories per square meter body-surface is reproduced in Table 251.

TABLE 251.—CALORIES PER SQUARE METER OF BODY-SURFACE (HEIGHT-WEIGHT FORMULA) PER HOUR FOR AGE AND SEX.

Age in years.	Males.	Females.	Age in years.	Males.	Females.
14–16 . . .	46.0	43.0	40–50 . . .	38.5	36.0
16–18 . . .	43.0	40.0	50–60 . . .	37.5	35.0
18–20 . . .	41.0	38.0	60–70 . . .	36.5	34.0
20–30 . . .	39.5	37.0	70–80 . . .	35.5	33.0
30–40 . . .	39.5	36.5			

The calculation is as follows:

Sex, male; age in years, twenty-four; height in centimeters, 170; weight in kilograms, 63.

$$\text{Area (sq. cm.)} = (\text{Weight}) \ 63^{0.425} \times (\text{Height}) \ 170^{0.725} \times 71.84 = 17,305 \text{ sq. cm.}$$
$$= 1.73 \text{ square meters}$$
$$1.73 \times 39.5 = 68.3 \text{ calories per hour}$$
$$68.3 \times 24.0 = 1639 \text{ calories per twenty-four hours}$$

Thus, by the Harris and Benedict Standards the basal metabolism of a male, twenty-four years of age, 63 kilograms in weight, and 170 cm. in height would be 1621 calories and by the DuBois Standard, 1639 calories.

In the original publication of Harris and Benedict the figures are given for the nearest tenth of a kilogram, and the nearest centimeter. It is felt that for practical purposes in the clinic data with sufficient accuracy are obtained if calculated to the nearest kilogram and the nearest 2 cm. For example, the weight of a patient may easily vary half a kilogram, according to whether water has been drunk or the rectum and bladder evacuated. As records are not kept of such data, it appears to be a false refinement of accuracy to attempt to calculate the metabolism more closely than to $\frac{1}{2}$ kilogram. Similarly, it is extremely difficult to measure an individual to within less than a centimeter. However, should more intimate data be desired, it is a simple matter to interpolate the intervening figures in the tables, as has in fact been done in the following example.

Harris and Benedict Prediction Tables. The use of these tables is better shown by example than by description.

Man, aged twenty-seven years; height, 172 cm.; weight, 77.2 kg.		Woman, aged twenty-two years; height, 166 cm.; weight, 77.2 kg.		Woman, aged sixty-six years; height, 162 cm.; weight, 62.3 kg.	
From Table 251 .	678	From Table 252 .	204	From Table 252 .	−9
From Table 253 .	1128	From Table 253 .	1393	From Table 253 .	1251
Predicted cals. .	1806	Predicted cals. .	1597	Predicted cals. .	1242

TABLE 252.—FACTORS FOR STATURE AND AGE IN MEN.

Cm.	21	22	23	24	25	26	27	28	29	30
151	614	607	600	593	587	580	573	566	560	553
153	624	617	610	603	597	590	583	576	570	563
155	634	627	620	613	607	600	593	586	580	573
157	644	637	630	623	617	610	603	596	590	583
159	654	647	640	633	627	620	613	606	600	593
161	664	657	650	643	637	630	623	616	610	603
163	674	667	660	653	647	640	633	626	620	613
165	684	677	670	663	657	650	643	636	630	623
167	694	687	680	673	667	660	653	646	640	633
169	704	697	690	683	677	670	663	656	650	643
171	714	707	700	693	687	680	673	666	660	653
173	724	717	710	703	697	690	683	676	670	663
175	734	727	720	713	707	700	693	686	680	673
177	744	737	730	723	717	710	703	696	690	683
179	754	747	740	733	727	720	713	706	700	693
181	764	757	750	743	737	730	723	716	710	703
183	774	767	760	753	747	740	733	726	720	713
185	784	777	770	763	757	750	743	736	730	723
187	794	787	780	773	767	760	753	746	740	733
189	804	797	790	784	777	770	763	756	750	743
191	814	807	800	794	787	780	773	766	760	753
193	824	817	810	804	797	790	783	776	770	763
195	834	827	820	814	807	800	793	787	780	773
197	844	837	830	824	817	810	803	797	790	783
199	854	847	840	834	827	820	813	807	800	793

	31	32	33	34	35	36	37	38	39	40
151	546	539	533	526	519	512	506	499	492	485
153	556	549	543	536	529	522	516	509	502	495
155	566	559	553	546	539	532	526	519	512	505
157	576	569	563	556	549	542	536	529	522	515
159	586	579	573	566	559	552	546	539	532	525
161	596	589	583	576	569	562	556	549	542	535
163	606	599	593	586	579	572	566	559	552	545
165	616	609	603	596	589	582	576	569	562	555
167	626	619	613	606	599	592	586	579	572	565
169	636	629	623	616	609	602	596	589	582	575
171	646	639	633	626	619	612	606	599	592	585
173	656	649	643	636	629	622	616	609	602	595
175	666	659	653	646	639	632	626	619	612	605
177	676	669	663	656	649	642	636	629	622	615
179	686	679	673	666	659	652	646	639	632	625
181	696	689	683	676	669	662	656	649	642	635
183	706	699	693	686	679	672	666	659	652	645
185	716	709	703	696	689	682	676	669	662	655
187	726	719	713	706	699	692	686	679	672	665
189	736	729	723	716	709	702	696	689	682	675
191	746	739	733	726	719	712	706	699	692	685
193	756	749	743	736	729	722	716	709	702	695
195	766	759	753	746	739	732	726	719	712	705
197	776	769	763	756	749	742	736	729	722	715
199	786	779	773	766	759	752	746	739	732	725

TABLE 252.—FACTORS FOR STATURE AND AGE IN MEN.—*Continued.*

Cm.	41	42	43	44	45	46	47	48	49	50
151	479	472	465	458	452	445	438	431	425	418
153	489	482	475	468	462	455	448	441	435	428
155	499	492	485	478	472	465	458	451	445	438
157	509	502	495	488	482	475	468	461	455	448
159	519	512	505	498	492	485	478	471	465	458
161	529	522	515	508	502	495	488	481	475	468
163	539	532	525	518	512	505	498	491	485	478
165	549	542	535	528	522	515	508	501	495	488
167	559	552	545	538	532	525	518	511	505	498
169	569	562	555	548	542	535	528	521	515	508
171	579	572	565	558	552	545	538	531	525	518
173	589	582	575	568	562	555	548	541	535	528
175	599	592	585	578	572	565	558	551	545	538
177	609	602	595	588	582	575	568	561	555	548
179	619	612	605	598	592	585	578	571	565	558
181	629	622	615	608	602	595	588	581	575	568
183	639	632	625	618	612	605	598	591	585	578
185	649	642	635	628	622	615	608	601	595	588
187	659	652	645	638	632	625	618	611	605	598
189	669	662	655	648	642	635	628	621	615	608
191	679	672	665	658	652	645	638	631	625	618
193	689	682	675	668	662	655	648	641	635	628
195	699	692	685	678	672	665	658	651	645	638
197	709	702	695	688	682	675	668	661	655	648
199	719	712	705	698	692	685	678	671	665	658

	51	52	53	54	55	56	57	58	59	60
151	411	404	397	391	384	377	370	364	357	350
153	421	414	407	401	394	387	380	374	367	360
155	431	424	417	411	404	397	390	384	377	370
157	441	434	428	421	414	407	400	394	387	380
159	451	444	438	431	424	417	410	404	397	390
161	461	454	448	441	434	427	420	414	407	400
163	471	464	458	451	444	437	431	424	417	410
165	481	474	468	461	454	447	441	434	427	420
167	491	484	478	471	464	457	451	444	437	430
169	501	494	488	481	474	467	461	454	447	440
171	511	504	498	491	484	477	471	464	457	450
173	521	514	508	501	494	487	481	474	467	460
175	531	524	518	511	504	497	491	484	477	470
177	541	534	528	521	514	507	501	494	487	480
179	551	544	538	531	524	517	511	504	497	490
181	561	554	548	541	534	527	521	514	507	500
183	571	564	558	551	544	537	531	524	517	510
185	581	574	568	561	554	547	541	534	527	520
187	591	584	578	571	564	557	551	544	537	530
189	601	594	588	581	574	567	561	554	547	540
191	611	604	598	591	584	577	571	564	557	550
193	621	614	608	601	594	587	581	574	567	560
195	631	624	618	611	604	597	591	584	577	570
197	641	634	628	621	614	607	601	594	587	580
199 . , . ,	651	644	638	631	624	617	611	604	597	590

TABLE 252.—FACTORS FOR STATURE AND AGE IN MEN.—*Continued.*

Cm.	61	62	63	64	65	66	67	68	69	70
151	343	337	330	323	316	310	303	296	289	283
153	353	347	340	333	326	320	313	306	299	293
155	363	357	350	343	336	330	323	316	309	303
157	373	367	360	353	346	340	333	326	319	313
159	383	377	370	363	356	350	343	336	329	323
161	393	387	380	373	366	360	353	346	339	333
163	403	397	390	383	376	370	363	356	349	343
165	413	407	400	393	386	380	373	366	359	353
167	423	417	410	403	396	390	383	376	369	363
169	434	427	420	413	406	400	393	386	379	373
171	444	437	430	423	416	410	403	396	389	383
173	454	447	440	433	426	420	413	406	399	393
175	464	457	450	443	437	430	423	416	409	403
177	474	467	460	453	447	440	433	426	419	413
179	484	477	470	463	457	450	443	436	429	423
181	494	487	480	473	467	460	453	446	440	433
183	504	497	490	483	477	470	463	456	450	443
185	514	507	500	493	487	480	473	466	460	453
187	524	517	510	503	497	490	483	476	470	463
189	534	527	520	513	507	500	493	486	480	473
191	544	537	530	523	517	510	503	496	490	483
193	554	547	540	533	527	520	513	506	500	493
195	564	557	550	543	537	530	523	516	510	503
197	574	567	560	553	547	540	533	526	520	513
199	584	577	570	563	557	550	543	536	530	523

TABLE 253.—FACTOR FOR STATURE AND AGE IN WOMEN.

	21	22	23	24	25	26	27	28	29	30
151	181	176	172	167	162	158	153	148	144	139
153	185	180	175	171	166	161	157	152	147	143
155	189	184	179	174	170	165	160	156	151	146
157	192	188	183	178	173	169	164	159	155	150
159	196	191	187	182	177	173	168	163	158	154
161	199	195	190	186	181	176	172	167	162	158
163	203	199	194	189	185	180	175	171	166	161
165	207	202	198	193	188	184	179	174	170	165
167	211	206	201	197	192	187	183	178	173	169
169	214	210	205	200	196	191	186	182	177	172
171	218	213	209	204	199	195	190	185	181	176
173	222	217	212	208	203	198	194	189	184	180
175	225	221	216	211	207	202	197	193	188	183
177	229	225	220	215	210	206	201	196	192	187
179	233	228	224	219	214	210	205	200	195	191
181	237	232	227	223	218	213	209	204	199	195
183	240	236	231	226	222	217	212	208	203	198
185	244	239	235	230	225	221	216	211	207	202
187	248	243	238	234	229	224	220	215	210	206
189	251	247	242	237	233	228	223	219	214	209
191	255	250	246	240	236	232	227	222	218	213
193	259	254	249	245	240	235	231	226	221	217
195	262	258	253	248	244	239	234	230	225	220
197	266	262	257	252	247	243	238	233	226	224
199	270	265	261	256	251	247	242	237	232	228

TABLE 253—FACTORS FOR STATURE AND AGE IN WOMEN.—*Continued.*

Cm.	31	32	33	34	35	36	37	38	39	40
151	134	130	125	120	116	111	106	102	97	92
153	138	133	129	124	119	115	110	105	101	96
155	142	137	132	128	123	118	114	109	105	100
157	145	141	136	131	127	122	117	113	108	103
159	149	144	140	135	130	126	121	116	112	107
161	153	148	143	139	134	129	125	120	115	111
163	157	152	147	143	138	133	128	124	119	114
165	160	156	151	146	142	137	132	128	123	118
167	164	159	155	150	145	141	136	131	127	122
169	168	163	158	154	149	144	140	135	130	126
171	171	167	162	157	153	148	143	139	134	129
173	175	170	166	161	156	152	147	142	138	133
175	179	174	169	165	160	155	151	146	141	137
177	182	178	173	168	164	159	154	150	145	140
179	186	181	177	172	167	163	158	153	149	144
181	190	185	180	176	171	166	162	157	152	148
183	194	189	184	180	175	170	165	161	156	151
185	197	193	188	183	179	174	169	165	160	155
187	201	196	192	187	182	178	172	168	164	159
189	205	200	195	191	186	181	177	172	167	163
191	208	204	199	194	190	185	180	176	171	166
193	212	207	203	198	193	189	184	179	175	170
195	216	211	206	202	197	192	188	183	178	174
197	219	215	210	205	201	196	191	187	182	177
199	223	218	214	209	204	200	195	190	186	181

Cm.	41	42	43	44	45	46	47	48	49	50
151	88	83	78	74	69	64	60	55	50	46
153	91	87	82	77	73	68	63	59	54	49
155	95	90	86	81	76	72	67	62	58	53
157	99	94	89	85	80	75	71	66	61	57
159	102	98	93	88	84	79	74	70	65	60
161	106	101	97	92	87	83	78	73	69	64
163	110	105	100	96	91	86	82	77	72	68
165	113	109	104	99	95	90	85	81	76	71
167	117	113	108	103	98	94	89	84	80	75
169	121	116	112	107	102	98	93	88	83	79
171	125	120	115	111	106	101	97	92	87	83
173	128	124	119	114	110	105	100	96	91	86
175	132	127	123	118	113	109	104	99	95	90
177	136	131	126	122	117	112	108	103	98	94
179	139	135	130	125	121	116	111	107	102	97
181	143	138	134	129	124	120	115	110	106	101
183	147	142	137	133	128	123	119	114	109	105
185	150	146	141	136	132	127	122	118	113	108
187	154	150	145	140	135	131	126	121	117	112
189	158	153	149	144	139	134	130	125	120	116
191	162	157	152	148	143	138	134	129	124	119
193	165	161	156	151	147	142	137	133	128	123
195	169	164	160	155	150	146	141	136	132	127
197	173	168	163	159	154	149	145	140	135	131
199	176	172	167	162	158	153	148	144	139	134

TABLE 253—FACTORS FOR STATURE AND AGE IN WOMEN.—*Continued.*

Cm.	51	52	53	54	55	56	57	58	59	60
151	41	36	31	27	22	17	13	8	3	−1.2
153	45	40	35	31	26	21	16	12	7	2
155	48	44	39	34	30	25	20	16	11	6
157	52	47	43	38	33	29	24	19	15	10
159	56	51	46	42	37	32	28	23	18	14
161	59	55	50	45	41	36	31	27	22	17
163	63	58	54	49	44	40	35	30	26	21
165	67	62	57	53	48	43	39	34	29	25
167	70	66	61	56	52	47	42	38	33	28
169	74	69	65	60	55	51	46	41	37	32
171	78	73	68	64	59	54	50	45	40	36
173	82	77	72	67	63	58	53	49	44	39
175	85	81	76	71	67	62	57	52	48	43
177	89	84	80	75	70	66	61	56	52	47
179	93	88	83	79	74	69	65	60	55	51
181	96	92	87	82	78	73	68	64	59	54
183	100	95	91	86	81	77	72	67	63	58
185	104	99	94	90	85	80	76	71	66	62
187	107	103	98	93	89	84	79	75	70	65
189	111	106	102	97	92	88	83	78	74	69
191	115	110	105	101	96	91	87	82	77	73
193	119	114	109	104	100	95	90	86	81	76
195	122	118	113	108	104	99	94	89	85	80
197	126	121	117	112	107	103	98	93	89	84
199	130	125	120	116	111	106	102	97	92	88

Cm.	61	62	63	64	65	66	67	68	69	70
151	−6	−11	−15	−20	−25	−29	−34	−39	−43	−48
153	−2	−7	−12	−16	−21	−26	−30	−35	−40	−44
155	1	−3	−8	−13	−17	−22	−27	−31	−36	−41
157	5	1	−4	−9	−14	−18	−23	−28	−32	−37
159	9	4	−0	−5	−10	−15	−19	−24	−29	−33
161	13	8	3	−1	−6	−11	−15	−20	−25	−30
163	16	12	7	2	−2	−7	−12	−16	−21	−26
165	20	15	11	6	1	−3	−8	−13	−17	−22
167	24	19	14	10	5	0	−4	−9	−14	−18
169	27	23	18	13	9	4	−1	−5	−10	−15
171	31	26	22	17	12	8	3	−2	−6	−11
173	35	30	25	21	16	11	7	2	−3	−7
175	38	34	29	24	20	15	10	6	1	−4
177	42	37	33	28	23	19	14	9	5	0
179	46	41	37	32	27	22	18	13	8	4
181	50	45	40	36	31	26	22	17	12	8
183	53	49	44	39	35	30	25	21	16	11
185	57	52	48	43	38	34	29	24	20	15
187	61	56	51	47	42	37	33	28	23	19
189	64	60	55	50	46	41	36	32	27	22
191	68	63	59	54	49	45	40	35	31	26
193	72	67	62	58	53	48	44	39	34	30
195	75	71	66	61	57	52	47	43	38	33
197	79	74	70	65	60	56	51	46	42	37
199	83	78	74	69	64	59	55	50	45	41

TABLE 254.—FACTOR FOR BODY WEIGHT.

	Men.		Women.			Men.		Women.	
	0.0	0.5	0.0	0.5		0.0	0.5	0.0	0.5
Kg.					Kg.				
25 . . .	410	417	894	899	75 . . .	1098	1105	1372	1377
26 . . .	424	431	904	909	76 . . .	1112	1118	1382	1387
27 . . .	438	445	913	918	77 . . .	1125	1132	1391	1396
28 . . .	452	458	923	928	78 . . .	1139	1146	1401	1406
29 . . .	465	472	932	937	79 . . .	1153	1160	1411	1415
30 . . .	479	486	942	947	80 . . .	1167	1173	1420	1425
31 . . .	493	500	952	956	81 . . .	1180	1187	1430	1435
32 . . .	507	513	961	966	82 . . .	1194	1201	1439	1444
33 . . .	520	527	971	975	83 . . .	1208	1215	1449	1454
34 . . .	534	541	980	985	84 . . .	1222	1228	1458	1463
35 . . .	548	555	990	995	85 . . .	1235	1242	1468	1473
36 . . .	562	568	999	1004	86 . . .	1249	1256	1478	1482
37 . . .	575	582	1009	1014	87 . . .	1263	1270	1487	1492
38 . . .	589	596	1019	1023	88 . . .	1277	1283	1497	1501
39 . . .	603	610	1028	1033	89 . . .	1290	1297	1506	1511
40 . . .	617	623	1038	1042	90 . . .	1304	1311	1516	1521
41 . . .	630	637	1047	1052	91 . . .	1318	1325	1525	1530
42 . . .	644	651	1057	1062	92 . . .	1332	1338	1535	1540
43 . . .	658	665	1066	1071	93 . . .	1345	1352	1544	1549
44 . . .	672	678	1076	1081	94 . . .	1359	1366	1554	1559
45 . . .	685	692	1085	1090	95 . . .	1373	1380	1564	1568
46 . . .	699	706	1095	1100	96 . . .	1387	1394	1573	1578
47 . . .	713	720	1105	1109	97 . . .	1400	1407	1583	1588
48 . . .	727	733	1114	1119	98 . . .	1414	1421	1592	1597
49 . . .	740	747	1124	1128	99 . . .	1428	1435	1602	1607
50 . . .	754	761	1133	1138	100 . . .	1442	1449	1611	1616
51 . . .	768	775	1143	1148	101 . . .	1455	1462	1621	1626
52 . . .	782	788	1152	1157	102 . . .	1469	1476	1631	1635
53 . . .	795	802	1162	1167	103 . . .	1483	1490	1640	1645
54 . . .	809	816	1172	1176	104 . . .	1497	1504	1650	1654
55 . . .	823	830	1181	1186	105 . . .	1510	1517	1659	1664
56 . . .	837	843	1191	1195	106 . . .	1524	1531	1669	1674
57 . . .	850	857	1200	1205	107 . . .	1538	1545	1678	1683
58 . . .	864	871	1210	1215	108 . . .	1552	1559	1688	1693
59 . . .	878	885	1219	1224	109 . . .	1565	1572	1698	1702
60 . . .	892	898	1229	1234	110 . . .	1579	1586	1707	1712
61 . . .	905	912	1238	1243	111 . . .	1593	1600	1717	1721
62 . . .	919	926	1248	1253	112 . . .	1607	1614	1726	1731
63 . . .	933	940	1258	1262	113 . . .	1620	1627	1736	1741
64 . . .	947	953	1267	1272	114 . . .	1634	1641	1745	1750
65 . . .	960	967	1277	1281	115 . . .	1648	1655	1755	1760
66 . . .	974	981	1286	1291	116 . . .	1662	1669	1764	1769
67 . . .	988	995	1296	1301	117 . . .	1675	1682	1774	1779
68 . . .	1002	1008	1305	1310	118 . . .	1689	1696	1784	1788
69 . . .	1015	1022	1315	1320	119 . . .	1703	1710	1793	1798
70 . . .	1029	1036	1325	1329	120 . . .	1717	1724	1803	1807
71 . . .	1043	1050	1334	1339	121 . . .	1730	1737	1812	1817
72 . . .	1057	1063	1344	1348	122 . . .	1744	1751	1822	1827
73 . . .	1070	1077	1353	1358	123 . . .	1758	1765	1831	1836
74 . . .	1084	1091	1363	1368	124 . . .	1772	1779	1841	1846

Table 255.—Heights and Weights of Men and Women of Fifteen or More Years of Age (With Clothes).[1]

MEN.

Age.	Feet and inches with shoes.																	
	5-0	5-1	5-2	5-3	5-4	5-5	5-6	5-7	5-8	5-9	5-10	5-11	6-0	6-1	6-2	6-3	6-4	6-5
16	109	111	114	117	120	124	128	132	136	140	144	149	154	159	164	169	174	179
18	113	115	118	121	124	128	132	136	140	144	148	153	158	163	168	173	178	183
20	117	119	122	125	128	132	136	140	144	148	152	156	161	166	171	176	181	186
22	119	121	124	127	131	135	139	142	146	150	154	158	163	168	173	178	183	188
24	121	123	126	129	133	137	141	144	148	152	156	160	165	171	177	182	187	192
26	123	125	127	130	134	138	142	146	150	154	158	163	168	174	180	186	191	196
28	125	127	129	132	135	139	143	147	151	155	159	164	170	176	182	188	193	198
30	126	128	130	133	136	140	144	148	152	156	161	166	172	178	184	190	196	201
32	127	129	131	134	137	141	145	149	154	158	163	168	174	180	186	192	198	203
34	128	130	132	135	138	142	146	150	155	160	165	170	176	182	188	194	200	206
36	129	131	133	136	139	143	147	151	156	161	166	171	177	183	190	196	202	208
38	130	132	134	137	140	144	148	152	157	162	167	173	179	185	192	198	204	210
40	131	133	135	138	141	145	149	153	158	163	168	174	180	186	193	200	206	212
42	132	134	136	139	142	146	150	154	159	164	169	175	181	187	194	201	208	214
44	133	135	137	140	143	147	151	155	160	165	170	176	182	188	195	202	209	215
46	134	136	138	141	144	148	152	156	161	166	171	177	183	189	196	203	210	216
48	134	136	138	141	144	148	152	156	161	166	171	177	183	190	197	204	211	217
50	134	136	138	141	144	148	152	156	161	166	171	177	183	190	197	204	211	217
52	135	137	139	142	145	149	153	157	162	167	172	178	184	191	198	205	212	218
54	135	137	139	142	145	149	153	158	163	168	173	178	184	191	198	205	212	219

Allow 1 inch for shoes and 10 pounds for clothes.

WOMEN.

Age.	Feet and inches with shoes.																
	4-8	4-9	4-10	4-11	5-0	5-1	5-2	5-3	5-4	5-5	5-6	5-7	5-8	5-9	5-10	5-11	6-0
16	102	104	106	108	109	111	114	117	120	124	128	132	136	139	143	148	153
18	104	106	108	110	112	114	117	120	123	126	130	134	138	141	145	150	155
20	106	108	110	112	114	116	119	122	125	128	132	136	140	143	147	151	156
22	107	109	111	113	115	117	120	123	126	129	133	137	141	145	149	153	157
24	109	111	113	115	117	119	121	124	127	130	134	138	142	146	150	154	158
26	110	112	114	116	118	120	122	125	128	131	135	139	143	147	151	155	159
28	111	113	115	117	119	121	123	126	130	133	137	141	145	149	153	156	160
30	112	114	116	118	120	122	124	127	131	134	138	142	146	150	154	157	161
32	113	115	117	119	121	123	125	128	132	136	140	144	148	152	155	158	162
34	115	117	119	121	123	125	127	130	134	138	142	146	150	154	157	160	163
36	116	118	120	122	124	126	128	131	135	139	143	147	151	155	158	161	164
38	117	119	121	123	125	127	130	133	137	141	145	149	153	157	160	163	166
40	119	121	123	125	127	129	132	135	138	142	146	150	154	158	161	164	167
42	120	122	124	126	128	130	133	136	139	143	147	151	155	159	162	166	169
44	122	124	126	128	130	132	135	138	141	145	149	153	157	161	164	168	171
46	123	125	127	129	131	133	136	139	142	146	150	154	158	162	165	169	172
48	124	126	128	130	132	134	137	140	143	147	152	156	160	164	167	171	174
50	125	127	129	131	133	135	138	141	144	148	152	156	161	165	169	173	176
52	125	127	129	131	133	135	138	141	144	148	152	157	162	166	170	174	177
54	125	127	129	131	133	135	138	141	144	148	153	158	163	167	171	174	177

Allow 1½ inches for shoes and 6 pounds for clothes.

[1] Association of Life Insurance Directors and Actuarial Society of America, New York, 1912, pp. 38 and 67.

CASE INDEX.

(763)

GENERAL INDEX.

A

49

$HgCl_2$.   9 x
KI -   3 ĩĩ
siĩ 20 gtt. water

110 - 50

p -   c   -   125   7 O₂ -
50   50   140 - 165

              p -   7   c -
              70   165 70